GENITOURINARY RADIOLOGY

SIXTH EDITION

N. REED DUNNICK, MD
Fred Jenner Hodges Professor and Chair
Department of Radiology
University of Michigan
Ann Arbor, Michigan

JEFFREY H. NEWHOUSE, MD
Professor of Radiology and Urology
Columbia College of Physicians and Surgeons
New York-Presbyterian Hospital
New York, New York

RICHARD H. COHAN, MD
Professor of Radiology
Associate Chair for Education
University of Michigan
Ann Arbor, Michigan

KATHERINE E. MATUREN, MD, MS
Associate Professor of Radiology and Obstetrics and Gynecology
University of Michigan
Ann Arbor, Michigan

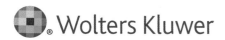

Philadelphia • Baltimore • New York • London
Buenos Aires • Hong Kong • Sydney • Tokyo

Acquisitions Editor: Sharon Zinner
Editorial Coordinator: Lauren Pecarich
Marketing Manager: Dan Dressler
Production Project Manager: David Saltzberg
Design Coordinator: Teresa Mallon
Manufacturing Coordinator: Beth Welsh
Prepress Vendor: SPi Global

9 8 7 6 5 4 3 2 1

Printed in China

Library of Congress Cataloging-in-Publication Data
Names: Dunnick, N. Reed, author. | Newhouse, Jeffrey H., author. | Cohan, Richard H., author. |
    Maturen, Katherine E., author.
Title: Genitourinary radiology / N. Reed Dunnick, Jeffrey H. Newhouse, Richard H. Cohan,
    Katherine E. Maturen.
Other titles: Textbook of uroradiology
Description: 6th edition. | Philadelphia : Wolters Kluwer, [2017] | Preceded by Textbook of
    uroradiology / N. Reed Dunnick, Carl M. Sandler, Jeffrey H. Newhouse. 5th edition. 2013. |
    Includes bibliographical references and index.
Identifiers: LCCN 2017019361 | ISBN 9781496356192
Subjects: | MESH: Radiography | Urologic Diseases—diagnostic imaging | Genital Diseases,
    Male—diagnostic imaging | Genital Diseases, Female—diagnostic imaging | Urography
Classification: LCC RC874 | NLM WJ 141 | DDC 616.6/07572—dc23 LC record available at
    https://lccn.loc.gov/2017019361

The sixth edition of this textbook is dedicated first and foremost to our uroradiology colleagues, many of whom have served as mentors and sources of inspiration to each of us. Their scientific contributions are the basis of modern uroradiology upon which this book is based.

Among our colleagues in uroradiology, we especially miss Carl Sandler, who coauthored all previous editions. He was a good friend whom we all miss dearly.

We also dedicate this book to our families, who have lovingly tolerated our devotion to this endeavor.

To Marilyn, Cory, Amanda, Sasha, Andrea, Marie, Alexa, Eleanor, Charlotte, Ian, Nathan, Jonathan, Tyler, Blake, and Spencer

To Nancy, Amy, and Ted

To Nina, Adam, Brooke, Alex, Katie, Charlie, Holly, Rebeka, and the Gabit

To Geoff, Iris, and Julian

Preface

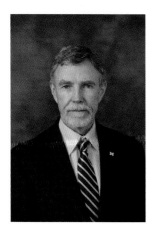

N. Reed Dunnick, MD

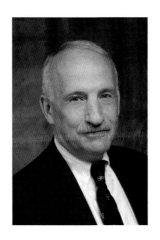

Jeffrey H. Newhouse, MD

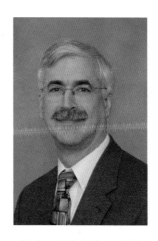

Richard H. Cohan, MD

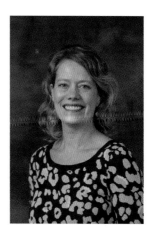

Katherine E. Maturen, MD, MS

The first edition of the *Textbook of Uroradiology* grew out of a discussion among Drs. Ronald McCallum, Carl Sandler, and Reed Dunnick at the annual meeting of the Society of Uroradiology in Scheveningen, The Netherlands, in May 1986. It was published by Williams & Wilkins in 1990. When Dr. McCallum retired, Drs. Dunnick and Sandler were joined by Drs. E. Stephen Amis and Jeffrey H. Newhouse, who had written their own textbook, *Essentials of Uroradiology*, published by Little, Brown and Company. These four authors completed the second, third, and fourth editions. Dr. Amis declined participation in the fifth edition due to his own busy schedule, and Drs. Richard Cohan and Stuart Silverman were recruited to each contribute a chapter in an area of their special expertise. After publication of the fifth edition, Dr. Sandler, a Professor of Radiology at the University of Texas, at Houston, passed away. Drs. Cohan and Katherine Maturen were recruited to participate in the creation of this, the sixth edition. The goal of the textbook remains to include material the reader *ought* to know, not everything there *is* to know.

With each revision, much new information is added. In order to keep the book a manageable size, older or outdated material is deleted. The excretory urogram, for decades the primary imaging modality of the urinary tract, is rarely, if ever performed and has been deleted. The chapter on anatomy has been removed, and pertinent information has been included in the chapter on congenital anomalies and other organ-specific chapters. The chapter on examination techniques has also been eliminated, reflecting the demise of many traditional uroradiologic examinations. The chapter on contrast material has been streamlined to focus on current usage.

Chapter authorship has often been rotated to help freshen the material. In keeping with the tradition started with the first edition, individual authorship of separate chapters has not been designated, reflecting our view that the textbook is a collaborative effort. As in prior editions, "suggested readings" are included at the end of each chapter to provide a guide for the reader who desires more detailed information on a particular topic, but no individual references were deemed necessary.

We continue to expect that the reader will find *Genitourinary Radiology, Sixth Edition*, a useful addition to his or her library and hope that this new version will be met with the same level of acceptance enjoyed by its predecessors.

N.R.D.
J.H.N.
R.H.C.
K.E.M.

Acknowledgments

We gratefully acknowledge the many contributions of individuals at our institutions as well as the highly skilled professionals at Wolters Kluwer who made this book possible.

At the University of Michigan, Carly Brandreth was essential to the process of editing and reformatting, as well as finding and cropping appropriate images.

Many thanks to Danielle Dobbs of the University of Michigan Media Division for medical illustrations; current and former University of Michigan abdominal imaging faculty and fellows Anca Avram, MD, Elaine Caoili, MD, Nicole Curci, MD, Roshni Parikh, MD, Michelle Sakala, MD, Erica Stein, MD, Peter Strouse, MD, Kara Udager, MD, and Ashish Wasnik, MD, for image examples; pathologists Amir Lagstein, MD, Bronwyn Bryant, MD, and Andrew Sciallis, MD for histologic images; and Karen McLean, MD, PhD, for intraoperative photography.

Contents

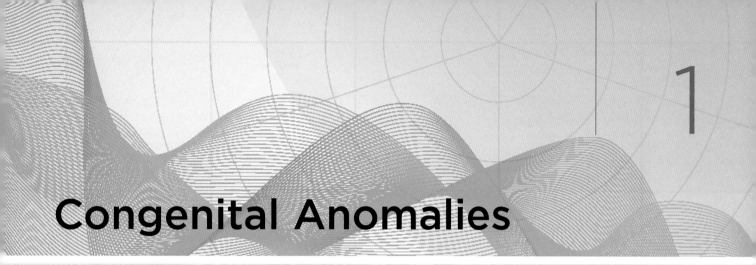

Congenital Anomalies

UPPER URINARY TRACT ANOMALIES

Kidney

Anatomy

The kidneys are paired retroperitoneal structures that parallel the psoas muscle on either side of the lumbar spine. They are composed of a variable number of renal pyramids, each of which consists of a minor calyx and its associated ducts. The base of the pyramid is formed by its overlying renal cortex and the apex is the renal papilla, which projects into a minor calyx. The papillae contain the openings of the distal collecting ducts (of Bellini), which empty into the calyces. The calyx is the cup-shaped portion of the intrarenal collecting system and the rim of the cup is the fornix. Urine drains from each calyx into an infundibulum and then into the renal pelvis.

The kidney is divided into an outer cortex and an inner medulla by the arcuate artery at the base of each pyramid. Columns of cortical tissue sometimes descend between the medullary pyramids and are often referred to as a column of Bertin. The calyces, infundibula, and renal pelvis are referred to as the "intrarenal collecting system." The renal sinus is the space around the collecting system and contains a variable amount of fat, along with branches of the renal artery, vein, and lymphatics.

The retroperitoneum is defined by fascial layers and divided into three compartments: the anterior pararenal space, the perirenal space, and the posterior pararenal space (Fig. 1.1). The anterior pararenal space contains the pancreas, the second through fourth portions of the duodenum, the ascending and descending colon, and the hepatic and splenic arteries. The perirenal space is defined by the anterior and posterior layers of Gerota fascia. These two layers may fuse in the midline or may extend across the midline without fusing, allowing communication between the two perirenal spaces. The kidney, adrenal gland, and proximal ureter are contained within Gerota fascia in the perirenal space. The posterior pararenal space contains only fat.

Anomalies of Position

Malrotation

Malrotation of a normally positioned kidney most commonly occurs as a result of failure of rotation of the kidney about its vertical axis. This results in an anterior position of the renal pelvis. It may be bilateral or unilateral, and in rare circumstances, overrotation of the kidney may result in a laterally facing renal pelvis. On computed tomography (CT), the renal pelvis will be seen projecting anteriorly (Fig. 1.2).

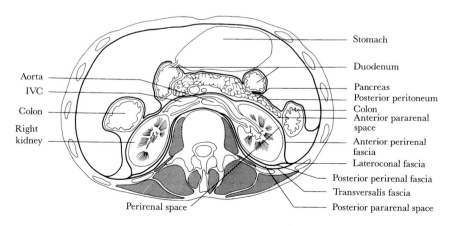

FIGURE 1.1. Retroperitoneal anatomy. (From Amis ES Jr, Newhouse JH. *Essentials of Uroradiology*. Boston, MA: Little, Brown & Co.; 1991:5, with permission.)

1

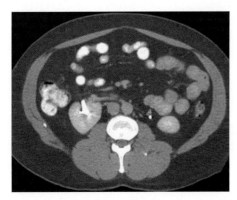

FIGURE 1.2. Malrotated kidney. On CT, the renal pelvis projects anteriorly.

Renal Ectopy

As the fetal kidneys ascend from the pelvis, each kidney acquires blood supply from the neighboring vessels. The initial supply from the external and internal iliac vessels is lost during this process, and blood supply directly from the aorta is acquired around the 8th week of development. An abnormality in acquiring such blood supply may prevent cephalic migration from occurring and result in renal ectopy or an abnormal position of the kidney. The most common form of renal ectopy is a pelvic kidney in which the kidney is located in the true pelvis or anterior to the sacrum (sacral kidney). The reported incidence of renal ectopy varies between 1:500 and 1:1,200. The exact incidence is difficult to determine, because renal ectopy is often clinically silent. With any congenital anomaly, the likelihood of finding other anomalies in the same or other organ systems is increased. Therefore, it is not unusual to find pelvic kidneys associated with a pathologic process, such as hydronephrosis or vesicoureteral reflux. Clinical symptoms related to the presence of a pelvic kidney are usually due to one of its associated conditions, such as pain from obstruction or infection related to reflux.

The findings depend on the degree of renal function in the pelvic kidney and the presence of associated abnormalities. On ultrasound, the reniform mass will be found in the pelvis with a characteristic pattern of renal sinus echoes. On CT, a functioning mass of renal parenchyma can usually be identified (Fig. 1.3). Angiography is often employed before any contemplated surgical procedure on a pelvic kidney because of the highly variable nature of its blood supply.

Intrathoracic Kidney

This rare anomaly occurs when the kidney ascends to a position higher than the second lumbar vertebra. The kidney may reach an intrathoracic location through a posterior diaphragmatic aperture that may be congenital or acquired. The anomaly is more common in males and is more commonly found on the left side. The blood supply to an intrathoracic kidney generally arises from the abdominal aorta in its normal location. Congenital intrathoracic kidney occurs in 1:15,000 births and often is diagnosed by finding a posterior thoracic mass, which appears to arise from the diaphragm on a chest radiograph.

Anomalies of Number

Renal Agenesis

True renal agenesis is the complete congenital absence of renal tissue (Fig. 1.4). This condition is to be distinguished from acquired forms of agenesis, in which renal tissue develops but atrophies during development or during childhood because of an associated malfunction. Renal agenesis occurs in approximately 1 in 1,000 births. It is thought to occur as the result of failure of formation of the ureteral bud or because of an inherent deficiency of the metanephric blastema. In the latter case, partial development of the ureter may be present. In true agenesis, ipsilateral absence of the trigone and ureteral orifice will be found in the bladder on cystoscopy. No renal artery is present, and the colon occupies the renal fossa on the affected side. The ipsilateral adrenal gland is absent in 8% to 10% of cases. Compensatory hypertrophy of the contralateral kidney almost always accompanies renal agenesis and can also be found when the other kidney is compromised by any other process, is removed, or is functionally compromised. However, the older the patient at the time of renal damage, the less compensatory hypertrophy will occur.

Genital abnormalities may also be associated with unilateral renal agenesis and, when present, suggest an etiology that also affects the mesonephric duct. In males, such abnormalities include cysts or absence of the ipsilateral seminal vesicle, absence of the ipsilateral vas deferens, hypoplasia or agenesis of the testicle, and hypospadias.

In females, renal agenesis may be associated with a unicornuate or bicornuate uterus, absence or hypoplasia of the uterus, and

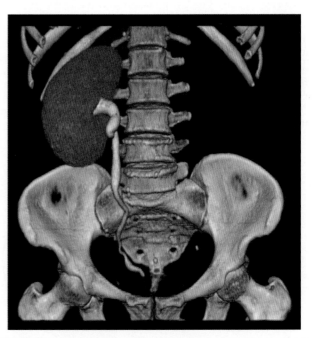

FIGURE 1.4. Renal agenesis. A volume-rendered image from a CT urogram shows a single right kidney to be present. (Courtesy of Seog Wan Ko, MD, Department of Radiology, Gwangju Christian Hospital, Gwangju, South Korea.)

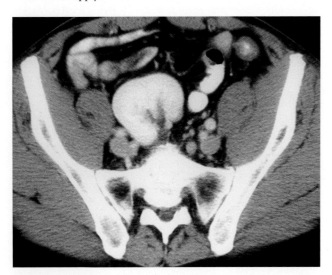

FIGURE 1.3. Pelvic kidney. A contrast-enhanced CT examination demonstrates the right kidney in the pelvis.

absence or aplasia of the vagina, the Mayer–Rokitansky–Kuster–Hauser syndrome (MRKH syndrome). Often considered the male counterpart of the MRKH syndrome, Zinner syndrome includes unilateral renal agenesis, a cyst in the ipsilateral seminal vesicle, and obstruction of the ejaculatory duct. Men with Zinner syndrome are often diagnosed during adulthood because of infertility.

Bilateral renal agenesis is extremely rare and incompatible with life. Males are affected in three-fourths of the cases. Infants with this abnormality exhibit the characteristic features of Potter facies, which include low-set ears and a prominent palpebral fold.

Renal Hypoplasia and Dysplasia

Renal hypoplasia is an unusual renal anomaly in which the kidney is at least 50% smaller than normal and contains fewer than the normal number of calyces. The condition is usually unilateral, and the kidney functions normally for its size. Most unilaterally small kidneys are acquired because of chronic ischemia, reflux (chronic atrophic pyelonephritis), or long standing obstruction (hydronephrotic atrophy). However, these conditions can be differentiated from hypoplasia by the fact that in reflux or obstruction, the calyces are abnormally cupped.

The Ask-Upmark kidney (see Chapter 10) was thought by some to be a variant of renal hypoplasia. The kidney is small, predominantly because of cortical loss in the upper pole associated with cortical indentations. However, most patients also have associated reflux and infection. The Ask-Upmark kidney is currently thought to be caused by scarring due to chronic pyelonephritis rather than a true congenital lesion.

Supernumerary Kidney

A supernumerary kidney is extremely rare. Cleavage of the metanephric blastema has been suggested as the cause for this abnormality. Most supernumerary kidneys are caudally placed and are hypoplastic. They may be connected to the ipsilateral dominant kidney either completely or by loose areolar connective tissue. A separate collecting system in the supernumerary kidney is generally present.

Anomalies of Form

Crossed Ectopy

Crossed ectopy is defined as a kidney located on the opposite side of the midline from its ureter. The crossed kidney usually lies below the normally situated kidney. In 90% of the cases, at least partial fusion between the kidneys is present (crossed-fused ectopy). In the remainder, two discrete kidneys on the same side are present (crossed-unfused ectopy). Other variations of crossed ectopy, including solitary crossed ectopy and bilateral crossed ectopy, have been described (Fig. 1.5). The anomaly is more common in males (2:1), and left-to-right ectopy is three times more common than

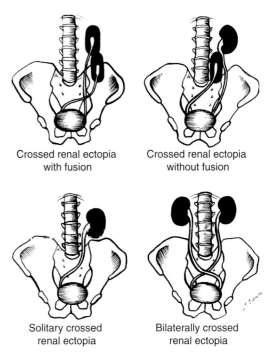

Crossed renal ectopia with fusion

Crossed renal ectopia without fusion

Solitary crossed renal ectopia

Bilaterally crossed renal ectopia

FIGURE 1.5. Schematic drawing showing the variations of crossed renal ectopy.

right-to-left ectopy. Crossed-fused ectopy has been estimated to occur in approximately 1:1,000 births.

The anomaly is thought to result because of an abnormally situated umbilical artery that prevents normal cephalic migration from occurring; in such cases, the developing kidney takes the path of least resistance and crosses to the opposite side, where cephalic migration resumes. Others have postulated that the abnormality occurs when the ureteral bud crosses to the opposite side, where it induces nephron formation in the contralateral metanephric blastema.

In most cases of crossed renal ectopy, the ureters are not ectopic and cystoscopy reveals a normal trigone. The incidence of associated congenital anomalies is low. Symptoms of crossed renal ectopy are rare; however, these patients may present in adulthood with abdominal pain, pyuria, or urinary tract infection. A slightly higher incidence of urinary tract calculi associated with crossed renal ectopy is thought to be related to stasis.

The abnormality is readily detected on cross-sectional imaging studies (Fig. 1.6). On ultrasound, crossed-fused ectopy can be

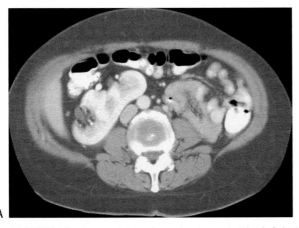
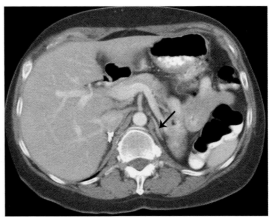

A

B

FIGURE 1.6. **Crossed-fused renal ectopy. A:** The left kidney lies in the right abdomen and is fused to the right kidney. **B:** The left adrenal gland (*arrow*) has a single limb.

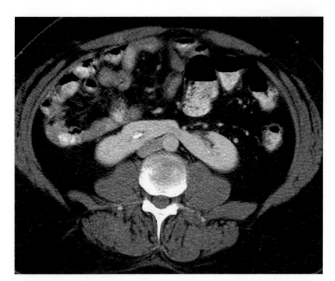

FIGURE 1.7. Horseshoe kidney. An enhanced CT demonstrates fusion of the two renal units.

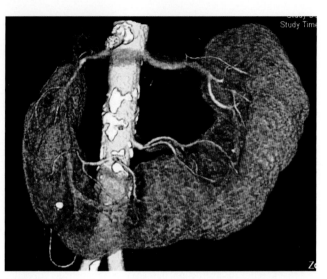

FIGURE 1.9. Horseshoe kidney. Reconstructed images from a CT urogram demonstrate multiple arteries supplying a horseshoe kidney.

identified by a characteristic anterior or posterior "notch" between the two kidneys. The blood supply to the crossed renal unit is generally anomalous; as with pelvic kidney, angiography is usually recommended before surgical procedures.

Horseshoe Kidney

Horseshoe kidney is the most common renal anomaly, occurring in approximately 1:400 births. There is a 2:1 male predominance. The abnormality occurs when the kidneys are connected by an isthmus. The anomaly is thought to occur because an abnormal position of the umbilical artery results in disturbance of the normal pattern of cephalic migration. As a result, there is contact between the developing metanephric blastema on each side that leads to partial fusion.

The isthmus of a horseshoe kidney usually consists of a band of parenchymal tissue (Fig. 1.7) that has its own blood supply. In some cases, the band consists of only fibrous tissue. Usually, the band joins the lower poles of the kidney and prevents normal rotation from occurring, so that on each side, the renal pelvis is in an anterior position. Rarely, the band connects the upper

poles rather than the lower poles. The band is usually located anterior to the aorta and inferior vena cava (IVC), but posterior to the inferior mesenteric artery, which is thought to prevent further cephalad migration from occurring. However, variations are common so that the position of the kidneys, their blood supply, their relation to the major vessels, and even the size of the kidney on either side are variable. Horseshoe kidney is commonly associated with ureteropelvic junction (UPJ) obstruction (Fig. 1.8). Many patients with horseshoe kidney remain asymptomatic throughout their lifetimes; in the remainder of patients, symptoms of obstruction, infection, or a renal calculus bring the abnormality to medical attention. A horseshoe kidney is more prone to injury with blunt abdominal trauma, presumably because it is relatively less protected in its more anterior position.

The blood supply to a horseshoe kidney is quite variable, most patients having multiple bilateral renal arteries (Fig. 1.9). The isthmus may be supplied by branches of the renal arteries or directly from the abdominal aorta, the inferior mesenteric artery, or the iliac arteries.

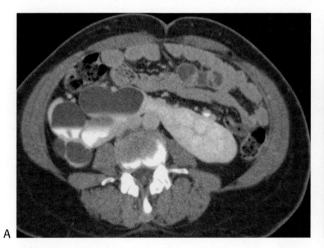
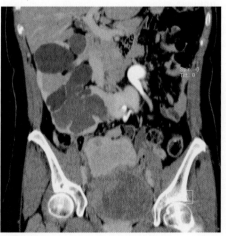

A

B

FIGURE 1.8. Horseshoe kidney with UPJ obstruction. **A:** Axial CT image reveals severe hydronephrosis of the right portion of the horseshoe kidney with only a thin rim of functioning parenchyma remaining. **B:** Coronal reformatted image. (Courtesy of Seog Wan Ko, MD, Department of Radiology, Gwangju Christian Hospital, Gwangju, South Korea.)

Imaging findings in patients with a horseshoe kidney include (1) an abnormal axis for each kidney with the lower poles more medially located than the upper poles, (2) the kidneys lie in a more caudad position, and (3) a bilateral malrotation with the renal pelves in an anterior position so that the lower calyces lie in a more medial position than the proximal ureter. On CT or MR, the isthmus of a horseshoe kidney is usually easily identified and may also be helpful in defining the relationship of the kidney to the major vessels.

Other Fusion Anomalies

Various other fusion abnormalities occur much less commonly than a horseshoe kidney or crossed renal ectopy. A doughnut kidney refers to two kidneys joined medially at their poles to form a ringlike renal mass. The lump, or pancake, kidney is a rare abnormality marked by extensive fusion between the two renal masses. The kidney is found in the midline or slightly to one side, generally no higher than the sacral promontory. The renal pelves are anterior and drain separate portions of the kidney. The ureters generally do not cross.

Renal Pelvis and Ureter

Unipapillary Kidney and Polycalycosis

The normal human intrarenal collecting system typically has 10 to 14 calyces. On rare occasions, a unipapillary kidney can be found in humans. It is more commonly found involving the left kidney and is usually associated with other significant anomalies, such as ipsilateral hypoplasia and frequent abnormalities of the contralateral kidney. Conversely, polycalycosis signifies an increased number of calyces; this is usually an isolated finding in an otherwise normal kidney.

Congenital Megacalyces

Many investigators believe that congenital megacalyces, also known as megacalycosis, is an acquired condition. The calyces are all symmetrically enlarged, although the renal pelvis and ureter are of normal size (Fig. 1.10). Furthermore, there is no history to suggest previous obstruction or reflux. Involvement is almost always unilateral, and the kidney is typically normal in size and function. Although megacalyces may be congenital, clinically silent obstruction or reflux in the distant past, perhaps even during fetal life, may be the cause. Another factor that favors an acquired etiology is that megacalycosis is typically seen in adults.

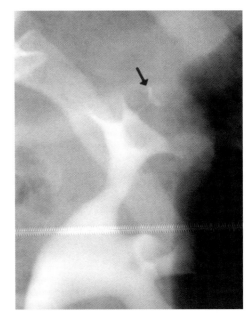

FIGURE 1.11. Microcalyx. A small, but otherwise normal-appearing calyx (*arrow*) is seen in the upper pole.

Microcalyx

A microcalyx resembles a normal calyx in every way but size (Fig. 1.11). It may arise from the renal pelvis or an infundibulum and ends at a papillary tip. The microcalyx is formed normally with a fornix and tubules draining into it.

Aberrant (Ectopic) Papilla

Most renal papilla empty into a minor calyx. In the renal polar regions, where compound calyces are common, several papillae may empty side by side into a major calyx. Rarely, a papilla may have an aberrant insertion into the collecting system and may present as a filling defect that must be differentiated from stones, tumors, or other pathologic processes. The aberrant papilla can protrude into virtually any part of the collecting system surrounded by renal parenchyma, including an infundibulum or the intrarenal portion of the renal pelvis. The resultant finding on excretory urography or retrograde pyelography is a smooth round or ovoid lucent defect in the contrast-filled collecting

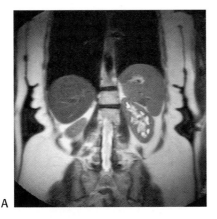
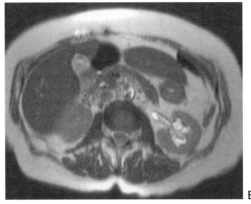

FIGURE 1.10. Congenital megacalyces. **A:** Coronal. **B:** Axial MR shows diffuse enlargement of calyces in the left kidney. The left renal pelvis is not dilated.

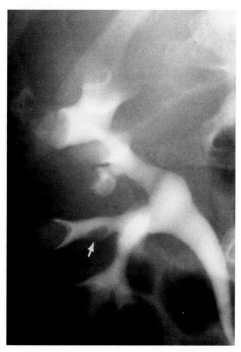

FIGURE 1.12. Ectopic papilla. A smooth ovoid filling defect (*arrow*) in an infundibulum is seen on an excretory urogram.

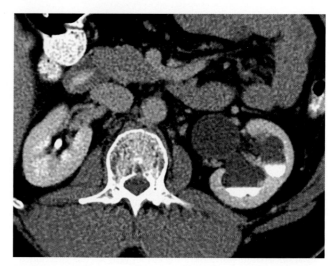

FIGURE 1.13. UPJ obstruction. Enhanced CT in excretory phase demonstrates a dilated left renal pelvis and caliectasis with layering of contrast in the dependent portions of the collecting system.

system (Fig. 1.12). The smooth border and fixed location on a margin of the collecting system tend to differentiate the finding from a tumor or stone. Oblique views may show the extrinsic origin of the papilla.

Ureteropelvic Junction Obstruction and Congenital Megaureter

Although occurring at either end of the ureter, UPJ obstruction and congenital megaureter are discussed together because of their histologic and physiologic similarities. Both conditions are caused by a deficiency and derangement of the ureteric smooth muscle fibers with associated fibrosis, resulting in a failure of normal peristalsis in the affected segment and subsequent functional obstruction. Congenital obstruction of the UPJ is a common anomaly of the urinary tract. The disorder produces caliectasis and marked pelviectasis as a result of a functional narrowing of the UPJ.

In approximately 5% of cases, extrinsic compression of the UPJ by an aberrant renal artery results in a similar radiographic pattern. Congenital UPJ obstruction is the most common cause of an abdominal mass in a neonate. The disorder is being discovered increasingly in the antenatal period because of the almost routine use of obstetric ultrasound. The abnormality may be clinically silent until adulthood, when hematuria, flank pain, fever, or, rarely, hypertension causes the patient to seek medical attention. Cases in which presentation has been delayed into the sixth or seventh decade have been reported. In some patients, it is an incidental finding on studies performed for another indication. Males are affected more often than females by a 2:1 ratio, and the left side is more commonly affected than the right for unknown reasons. A familial tendency toward the disorder has also been reported.

In some patients, symptoms may be present only during sustained diuresis, a condition known as "beer-drinker's hydronephrosis" or Dietl crisis. Such cases are attributed to a very mild UPJ obstruction, such that under conditions of normal urine flow rates, the UPJ is compensated. Examinations while the patient is asymptomatic may be normal or show only an extrarenal pelvis; the use of a diuretic renogram or a urographic study during acute symptoms has been advocated to demonstrate the underlying abnormality.

The renal pelvis and calyces are dilated, and with long-standing or very high-grade obstruction, a virtually nonfunctioning kidney may be present. The UPJ itself, which may be difficult to visualize, appears to join the renal pelvis in a higher or more medial position (Figs. 1.13 and 1.14). Care must be taken to differentiate a true UPJ obstruction (Fig. 1.15) from a large extrarenal pelvis. In the

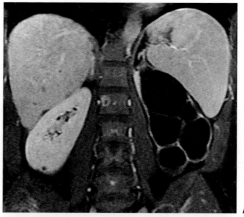

A

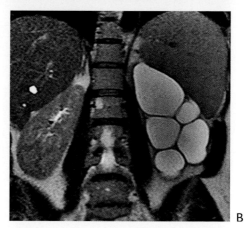

B

FIGURE 1.14. UPJ obstruction. MR images in T1 **(A)** and T2 weighting **(B)** demonstrate markedly dilated calyces.

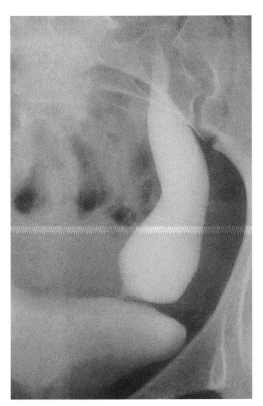

FIGURE 1.15. Primary megaureter. Excretory urogram demonstrates a markedly dilated distal left ureter.

been reported with endopyelotomy, pyeloplasty consistently corrects the defect in 85% to 90% of patients. Endopyelotomy probably should not be used in infants and has a higher failure rate in patients with extremely redundant renal pelves or long UPJ strictures.

Congenital megaureter, or *primary megaureter*, is a functional obstruction of the distal ureter. Typically, approximately 2 cm of the ureter just above the ureteral orifice is involved, and this abnormal segment is usually of normal caliber. However, the ureter proximal to this improperly functioning segment is variably dilated. It is not unusual to see this dilation involving only the distal one-third of the ureter, although if the obstruction is severe enough, significant hydronephrosis may occur (Fig. 1.16). As with UPJ obstruction, a normal-size ureteral catheter can be easily passed through the abnormal ureteral segment. Thus, this narrowing is not an anatomic stricture; rather, it is a failure of the abnormal ureteral segment to undergo normal peristalsis. It is also possible that the abnormality is a very mild narrowing or an inability to distend to the maximal normal diameter of the most distal part of the ureter. Under these conditions, every bolus, which is pushed down the ureter by a following contraction wave, has its hydrostatic pressure rise above normal as it is pushed through the limited-distensibility terminal segment. Over time, the ureter just above this segment dilates and, as any other significantly dilated ureter, is no longer capable of transmitting a normal contraction wave. Treatment for severe cases includes excision of the abnormal distal segment, surgical tapering of the dilated "normal" ureter, and reimplantation of the tapered ureter into the bladder using antirefluxing techniques.

Circumcaval Ureter

The embryology of the IVC is complex. Normally, the suprarenal IVC derives from the right subcardinal vein and the infrarenal IVC derives from the right supracardinal vein. Circumcaval ureter results when the subcardinal vein, which lies ventral to the ureter, persists and forms the major portion of the vena cava (Fig. 1.17). The right ureter is carried medially by the migration of the subcardinal vein toward the developing IVC. Symptoms of circumcaval ureter, if any, relate to the degree of ureteral obstruction.

The typical pattern is a tortuous, dilated proximal right ureter and associated hydronephrosis. The course of the proximal ureter is described as having a "reverse J" configuration before it crosses behind and around the IVC and then descends medial to the ipsilateral lumbar pedicle This severe medial deviation is the hallmark of a circumcaval ureter.

latter case, the renal pelvis may appear quite dilated; however, in the absence of caliectasis, the diagnosis of UPJ obstruction should not be entertained. Variable filling of the ureter may occur distal to the UPJ. When there is significant kinking of the UPJ, an aberrant vessel may be the cause of the obstruction.

Pyeloplasty has been considered the treatment of choice for UPJ obstruction. Percutaneous nephrostomy followed by balloon pyeloplasty or by endoscopic endopyelotomy has been reported as a primary procedure and as a secondary procedure in patients in whom surgical therapy has failed. Although success rates of up to 85% have

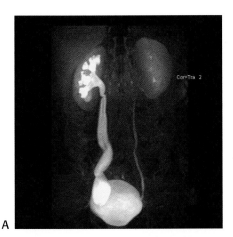
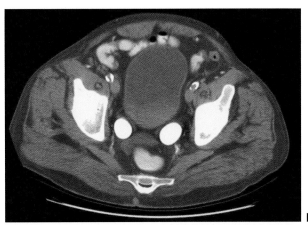

A   B

FIGURE 1.16. Primary megaureter. **A:** MR urogram demonstrates dilated right collecting system and ureter with a "beak" in the distal ureter characteristic of a primary megaureter. (Courtesy of Seog Wan Ko, MD, Department of Radiology, Gwangju Christian Hospital, Gwangju, South Korea.) **B:** Axial CT image from a different patient showing bilaterally dilated distal ureters. The more proximal ureters were normal indicating primary megaureter as the cause.

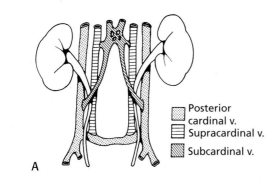

Posterior
cardinal v.
Supracardinal v.
Subcardinal v.

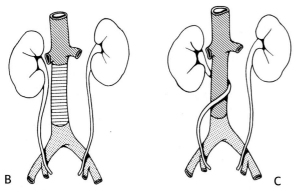

FIGURE 1.17. Embryology of circumcaval ureter. **A:** Embryologic condition, with ureter winding among three cardinal veins. **B:** Normal development of vena cava, with infrarenal portion arising from the supracardinal vein that lies under ureter. **C:** Circumcaval ureter develops when the infrarenal portion of the vena cava develops from the sub-cardinal vein, which in embryonic life is ventral to the ureter. (Modified from Fig. 9.195 in Witten DM, Myers GH, Utz DC, eds. *Emmett's Clinical Urography*. 4th ed. Philadelphia, PA: WB Saunders Co.; 1977:678, with permission.)

Duplex Collecting Systems

Duplication of the collecting system may be partial or complete. Partial duplication is the most frequently occurring congenital anomaly in the urinary tract. The duplex collecting system and its related abnormalities can result in some of the most complicated patterns detected on imaging studies in both children and adults.

The autopsy incidence of partial duplication is approximately 1 in 150 cases, whereas complete duplication is found approximately once in every 500 cases. However, the incidence in clinical series for this anomaly is up to six times higher, probably reflecting the likelihood for this anomaly to produce symptoms. Complete duplications are bilateral in up to 20% of cases.

Ureteral Anatomy

The UPJ is usually a gentle tapering of the renal pelvis as it joins the proximal ureter. The ureter remains retroperitoneal throughout its course as it crosses anterior to the common or external iliac vessels. It curves laterally and then medially before coursing submucosally in the bladder wall for about 2 cm before entering the bladder lumen at the lateral margin of the trigone. The ureterovesical junction is the narrowest portion of the ureter.

Embryology

The ureter forms as a bud from the mesonephric duct (Fig. 1.18). The normal kidney is formed when this bud invaginates the metanephric blastema and, through multiple branchings, forms

the collecting system and distal collecting ducts. Partial duplication results from the branching of the ureteral bud before it connects with the metanephric blastema. The point at which the ureteral bud branches will determine the level at which the two ureters join; this bifurcation may occur anywhere from the bladder wall to the renal pelvis. The latter will result in a bifid renal pelvis. On rare occasions, the single ureteral bud may trifurcate or may even branch into four or five segments before meeting the metanephric blastema, resulting in multiplication of the renal pelvis. Another variation occurs when one branch of a partially duplicated system fails to reach the kidney and becomes a blind-ending stump connected to the functional ureter (Fig. 1.19). This branch is sometimes short and is referred to as a ureteral diverticulum. However, because all layers of the ureteral wall are present, this branch is not a true diverticulum and is more properly termed a blind-ending ureteral bud.

Complete duplication of the ureter occurs when two separate buds arise from the mesonephric duct. These buds invaginate the metanephric blastema separately, resulting in the formation of separate upper and lower intrarenal collecting systems. Each of these systems is known as a *moiety*, and each is drained by a separate ureter. As the mesonephric duct migrates caudally during embryonic life, the ureter from the lower moiety is deposited near its expected normal location in the bladder, and its ureterovesical junction is therefore usually close to its normal position on the trigone. The ureter from the upper moiety remains attached to the mesonephric duct longer during its caudal migration and eventually connects with the bladder inferiorly and medially. The Meyer–Weigert law states that the ureter from the upper moiety will enter the bladder inferiorly and medially (the ectopic ureter) in relation to the ureter draining the lower moiety (the orthotopic ureter). The corollary to the Meyer–Weigert law is that the upper moiety often obstructs while the lower moiety may reflux.

The majority of complete and incomplete duplications are associated with normal function and are incidental findings on imaging studies. Typically, the upper moiety is the smaller of the two, containing only two or three calyces and draining approximately 25% of the kidney. In cases of incomplete duplication, the point at which the two proximal ureters join can occur anywhere, including in the bladder wall, where it may be impossible to differentiate partial from complete duplication. Cystoscopy is needed to determine whether there are one or two orifices on the side in question. In uncomplicated complete duplications, the two orifices usually enter the bladder adjacent to each other in a relatively normal position on the trigone. On ultrasound, ureteral duplication may be demonstrated on longitudinal scans as two distinct groups of renal sinus echoes. On CT, the duplication is often best demonstrated on coronal reconstructed images (Fig. 1.20). Axial scans obtained through the junction of the upper and lower pole moieties will demonstrate an absence of collecting system elements or renal sinus fat, a feature that has been termed the "faceless kidney" and may help identify duplication even in the absence of contrast enhancement (Fig. 1.21).

Three distinct abnormalities of the termination of the ureters in complete duplications can result in significant pathologic changes in the duplicated kidney:

■ Maldevelopment of the valve mechanism at the ureterovesical junction of the lower-pole ureter (resulting in reflux)
■ Ectopic insertion of the upper-pole ureter outside the bladder
■ Ectopic ureterocele also involving the ureter draining the upper moiety

Maldevelopment of the Valve Mechanism of the Lower-Pole Ureter

Improper development of the valve mechanism at the ureterovesical junction involves the orifice of the ureter draining the lower-pole moiety. This orifice may be slightly above and lateral to its

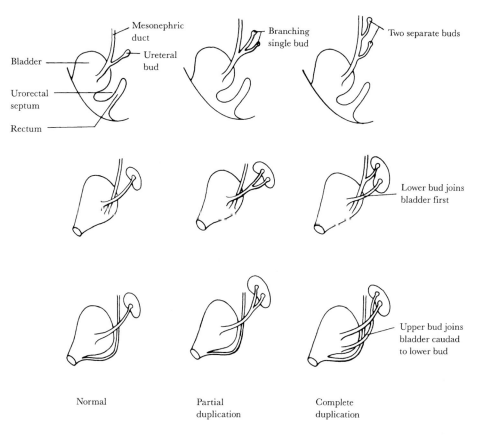

FIGURE 1.18. Embryology of duplex collecting systems. (From Amis ES Jr, Newhouse JH. *Essentials of Uroradiology*. Boston, MA: Little, Brown & Co.; 1991:258, with permission.)

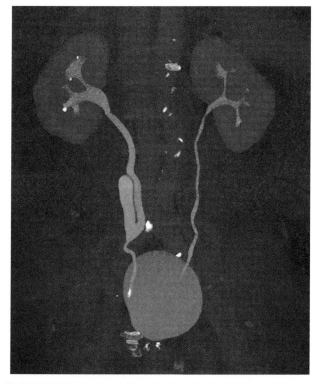

FIGURE 1.19. Ureteral diverticulum. CT urogram demonstrates a blind-ending ureteral bud in the midportion of the right ureter.

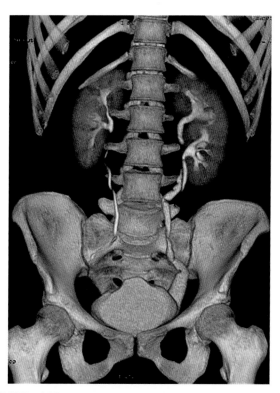

FIGURE 1.20. Duplicated collecting system. Volume-rendered CT urogram shows a left duplicated collecting system.

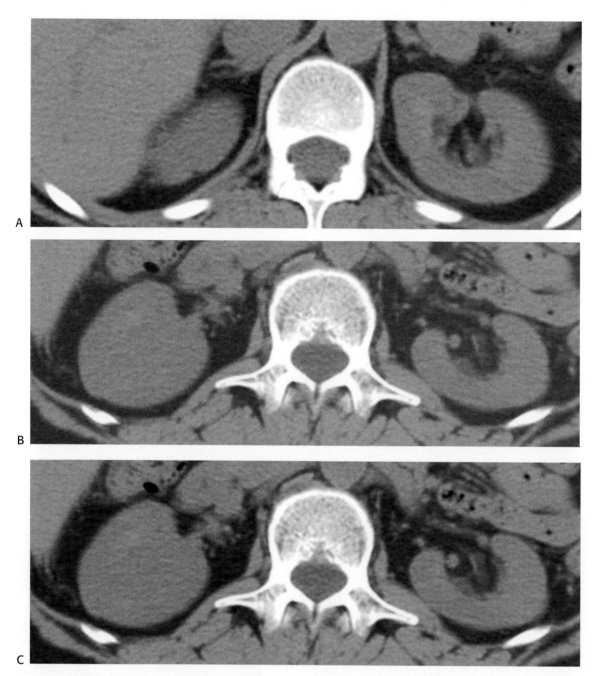

FIGURE 1.21. Faceless kidney. Unenhanced CT demonstrates no renal pelvis in the midportion of the right kidney.

normal position on the trigone. Because of this abnormal location, there is shortening of the submucosal tunnel for the distal ureter and a more direct course through the bladder wall, a condition that facilitates reflux. The incidence of reflux into the lower moiety in complete duplication is significantly higher than that for a single collecting system. Reflux into the lower moiety is the most common abnormality associated with complete duplications.

Radiographically, reflux can be demonstrated by voiding cystourethrography, which is often done as a radionuclide voiding cystogram. The spectrum of radiographic appearances ranges from reflux into a nondilated, normal-appearing lower-pole collecting system to massive dilation of the lower moiety with complete loss of function. In addition, one usually finds reflux nephropathy, including focal or diffuse lower-pole renal scarring with clubbing of the underlying calyces.

Ectopic Insertion of the Ureter

Another major abnormality associated with complete duplication is ectopic insertion of the ureter draining the upper pole. The insertion is either caudal to the orthotopic ureter or extravesical in location, resulting in obstruction and possible dysplasia of the upper moiety. More than two-thirds of all extravesical ectopic ureteral insertions are associated with complete duplication (Fig. 1.22). Remnants of the embryonic mesonephric duct can be found in the walls of the vagina, uterus, and broad ligaments in approximately one-fourth of all adult females. These vestigial structures explain

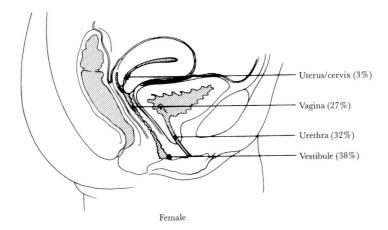

Female

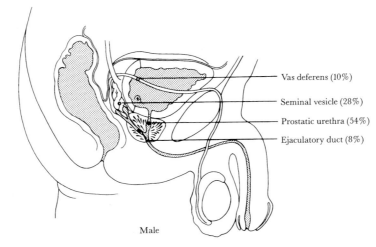

Male

FIGURE 1.22. Sites of extravesical insertions of the upper moiety ureter in completely duplicated collecting systems. (From Amis ES Jr, Newhouse JH. *Essentials of Uroradiology*. Boston, MA: Little, Brown & Co.; 1991:261, with permission.)

the ectopic insertion of the ureter into these female reproductive organs. In the male, ectopic insertion of the ureter into the vas deferens and seminal vesicles is easily explained by the fact that these organs are derived from the mesonephric duct, which also gives rise to the ureter. Ectopic ureters terminating outside the urinary tract tend to obstruct the upper moiety. Generally speaking, the more distal the ectopic orifice, the more dysplastic the upper moiety it drains.

Clinically, extravesical ectopic ureters in females are commonly beyond sphincter control, resulting in continual dribbling of urine. In males, ectopic orifices occur above the level of the external urethral sphincter. In males, a typical clinical presentation is chronic or recurrent epididymitis due to ectopic insertion of the ureter into the ipsilateral vas deferens or seminal vesicle.

Imaging findings include a dilated upper-pole collecting system and a lower-pole collecting system with reversal of its normal axis, fewer than the normal number of calyces expected, and lateral deviation of the proximal ureter due to the medial location of the dilated ureter from the nonfunctioning upper pole. Ultrasound typically shows an echo-free cystic area in the medial upper pole of the kidney (Fig. 1.23A). This represents the dilated upper collecting system, and its dilated ureter can often be traced distally to its insertion (Fig. 1.23B). CT and MR can also demonstrate the hydronephrotic upper moiety and its dilated ureter. If necessary, antegrade pyelography may be performed to delineate the anatomy

of the ectopic insertion. In some cases, the ectopic orifice can be identified and catheterized, to allow retrograde studies to be performed. Voiding cystourethrography should be performed in all cases of duplication in which pathology is suspected because it may demonstrate reflux into either moiety.

Ectopic Ureterocele

A ureterocele is a focal dilation of the submucosal portion of the distal ureter. Ureteroceles may be orthotopic (simple) or ectopic. An orthotopic ureterocele is associated with a single collecting system and is discussed in the next section. Virtually all ectopic ureteroceles are associated with ipsilateral complete duplication. The ureterocele is always associated with the ureter from the upper moiety. This dilation may extend to the bladder neck or even into the posterior urethra (Fig. 1.24). Approximately one-half of all ectopic ureteroceles terminate within the bladder, where they may be associated with vesicoureteral reflux into the lower-pole moiety. However, the majority have stenotic orifices that do not reflux but are associated with hydronephrosis of the upper pole. Ectopic ureteroceles may also course submucosally through the bladder neck and may terminate in the posterior urethra, where a widely patent orifice is common. This latter ureterocele often refluxes during voiding but is obstructed when the patient is not voiding because it empties into the normally closed urethra. Overall, almost one-half

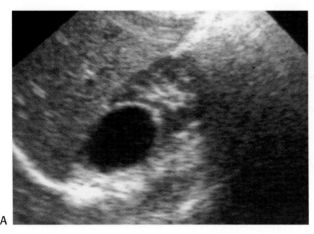 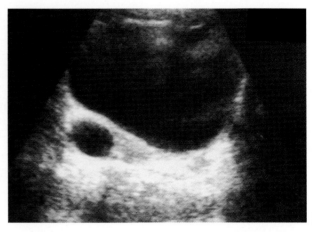

FIGURE 1.23. Ectopic ureteral insertion in a completely duplicated system. **A:** Sonography shows an echo-free mass in the upper pole of the right kidney. **B:** The dilated ureter can be seen coursing behind the bladder on the right in this transverse sonogram through the pelvis. (From Amis ES Jr, Newhouse JH. *Essentials of Uroradiology.* Boston, MA: Little, Brown & Co.; 1991:262, with permission.)

of ureteroceles may demonstrate reflux during cystourethrography, at least during voiding.

As with ectopic ureteral insertions, ectopic ureteroceles may be associated with little or no function of their associated ipsilateral upper-pole collecting systems, or obstruction by the ureterocele may be mild, allowing good opacification of the upper moiety in the pyelographic phase of CT urography. Because of their size and location, large ectopic ureteroceles may distort the ipsilateral lower-pole ureteral orifice and may increase the incidence of reflux into the lower moiety. Conversely, large ectopic ureteroceles may directly compress and obstruct the ipsilateral lower-pole orifice. An ectopic ureterocele may be large enough to extend across the midline and obstruct the contralateral ureteral orifice or prolapse into the bladder neck with subsequent bladder outlet obstruction.

An ectopic ureterocele typically presents as a smooth, rounded, or ovoid filling defect in the bladder (Fig. 1.25). Although ectopic ureteroceles tend to be laterally oriented, if large enough, they can be midline. Ectopic ureteroceles may range in size from 1 cm to several centimeters in diameter.

Urographic upper tract findings in completely duplicated systems complicated by either ectopic ureteral insertion or ectopic ureterocele tend to be identical, as both abnormalities affect the upper

moiety, often resulting in dilation and nonfunction. Therefore, ultrasonographic, MR, and CT (Fig. 1.26) findings will be similar to those described in earlier paragraphs for ectopic ureteral insertion. Pelvic sonography for ectopic ureterocele will demonstrate a thin septation in the bladder representing the distended ureterocele.

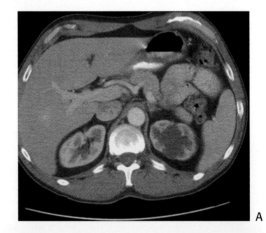

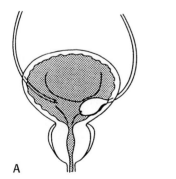 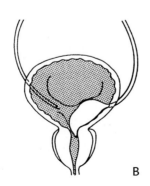

FIGURE 1.24. Diagram of types of ectopic ureteroceles. **A:** Approximately one-half of ectopic ureteroceles terminate in the bladder. **B:** The remainder of ectopic ureteroceles extends through the bladder neck and terminate in the proximal urethra. (From Amis ES Jr, Newhouse JH. *Essentials of Uroradiology.* Boston, MA: Little, Brown & Co.; 1991:263, with permission.)

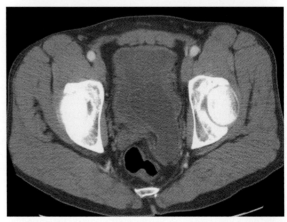

FIGURE 1.25. Ectopic ureterocele with obstruction. **A:** CT reveals atrophy of the left upper-pole moiety secondary to obstruction. **B:** The obstructing ureterocele is unopacified and clearly defined within the bladder.

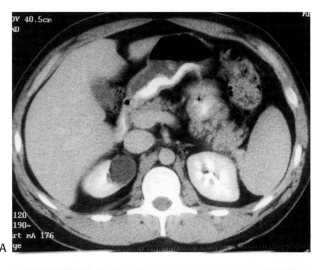

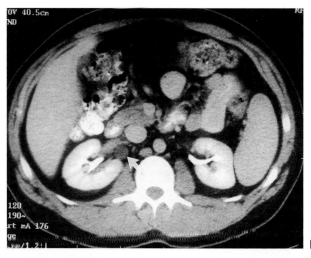

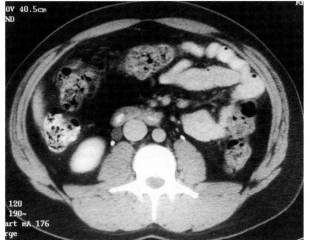

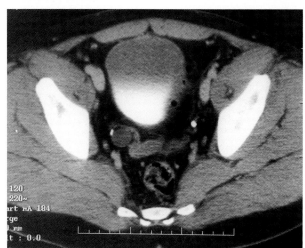

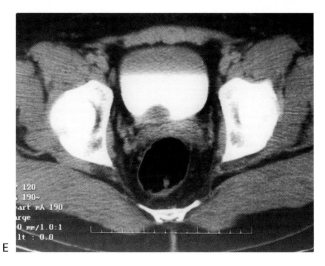

FIGURE 1.26. Complete duplication with obstructed upper moiety due to ectopic ureterocele. **A:** Section through kidney shows a cystic mass in the upper pole of the right kidney. **B:** Section through lower moiety shows the nonopacified and dilated upper moiety ureter (*arrow*) posterior to the renal pelvis of the lower moiety. **C, D:** Sections through the midabdomen and pelvis show the normal-size opacified lower moiety ureter. **E:** Section through bladder shows the ectopic ureterocele as a water attenuation bulge in the posterior portion of the opacified bladder.

Anomalous Termination of the Ureter

The anomalies involving the termination of the ureter have been discussed to large degree in the above sections on primary mega-ureter and ureteral duplications. However, orthotopic ureterocele, ectopic ureteral orifice, and reflux can occur in nonduplicated systems.

Ureterocele

Orthotopic ureteroceles occur in normal position on the trigone and are also known as simple or adult-type ureteroceles. An ortho-topic ureterocele is seen as a smoothly rounded, water density, distal ureteral mass protruding into the bladder lumen in the region of the trigone. If the ureter is opacified with contrast, the central portion of

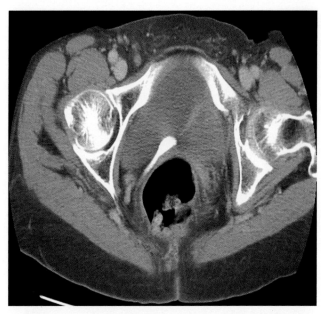

FIGURE 1.27. Ureterocele. A dilated distal right ureter is filled with contrast and easily distinguished from the unopacified urine in the bladder.

the ureterocele is also opacified in continuity with the remainder of the ureter but is surrounded by a lucent rim, representing the bladder mucosa around the ureterocele. On CT, the dilated ureterocele is easily seen if imaged when contrast opacifies the ureterocele before the bladder is filled with contrast (Fig. 1.27). There is typically very little or no obstruction, although on rare occasions, the ureterocele may cause rather severe upper tract dilation. "Pseudoureterocele" is a term that has been applied to a radiographic finding that mimics a true ureterocele but is not caused by an anomalous termination of

the ureter. Most causes of pseudoureterocele are acquired; the most common is a stone impacted in the distal ureter producing a zone of edema around the ureteral orifice, which mimics a true ureterocele when the bladder lumen contains contrast.

Ectopic Ureteral Insertion

An ectopic ureter does not terminate in the normal location on the trigone of the bladder. By convention, the term is used to define a ureter that opens outside the urinary bladder. Eighty percent of ectopic ureters are found in association with complete duplication of the ureter. The anomaly is more common in female patients by a 6:1 ratio. In male patients, however, most ectopic ureters drain single systems. With ectopic insertion of a nonduplicated ureter, an absent hemitrigone will be found in the bladder on the side of ectopic insertion. The possible sites of ectopic insertion have been previously discussed in the section on ureteral duplication. The more distal the insertion (e.g., into the seminal vesicle in the male), the more dysplastic the ipsilateral kidney will be (Fig. 1.28). In such cases, there will be minimal, if any, kidney function. For more proximal extravesical insertions, such as into the posterior urethra, obstruction and reduced function of the involved kidney will be the predominant findings.

Vesicoureteral Reflux

The normal ureterovesical junction acts as a one-way valve that allows urine to flow freely from the ureter into the bladder but prevents reverse flow. The ureter traverses the bladder wall at a slightly oblique angle and then courses submucosally for approximately 2 cm to the ureteral orifice. As the bladder fills, the intravesical pressure is exerted on the wall of the bladder equally in all directions; this results in pressure on the bladder epithelium overlying the submucosal ureter and subsequent flattening of this portion of the ureter against its muscular backing, preventing reflux. This flattening, however, does not prevent normal ureteral peristalsis from propelling a bolus of urine from the ureter into the bladder as long as bladder pressure remains within normal limits.

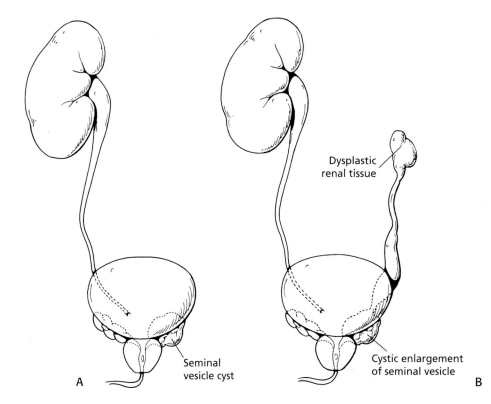

FIGURE 1.28. Diagram showing similarities between **(A)** seminal vesicle cyst associated with ipsilateral renal agenesis and **(B)** dysplastic kidney with ureter ectopic to the seminal vesicle.

If the course of the ureter through the bladder wall is more direct, and if the submucosal course is shortened, this valve mechanism fails to function properly, and vesicoureteral reflux occurs. The hydrostatic effect of reflux alone can result in reflux atrophy of the kidney. However, intrarenal reflux of urine can occur, resulting in reflux nephropathy, a combination of clubbed calyces and overlying parenchymal scarring. This is also known as chronic atrophic pyelonephritis and tends to occur in the renal polar regions. The presence of compound calyces in these areas is believed to facilitate reflux into the collecting ducts. Normally, duct orifices on the papillae have an antirefluxing configuration; but in compound calyces, this configuration is distorted, allowing the intrarenal reflux to occur.

PRUNE BELLY SYNDROME

Prune belly syndrome (Eagle–Barrett syndrome) is a rare congenital syndrome characterized by the classic triad of absent abdominal musculature, undescended testicles, and urinary tract abnormalities. Although absence of abdominal musculature has been described in females, the full syndrome, including the urinary tract abnormalities, develops only in males.

The syndrome is recognizable at birth because of the characteristic features produced by the absent abdominal musculature (Fig. 1.29). The deficiency typically affects the lower abdominal wall; the upper abdomen has a normal appearance. In some cases, the muscular defect is partial or asymmetric. The overlying skin has a wrinkled appearance reminiscent of a prune; in older children, the wrinkling tends to disappear and is replaced by a "potbelly" appearance. The urinary tract abnormalities affect the kidneys, the ureters, the bladder, and the urethra. Although the kidneys may be normal, renal dysplasia or hydronephrosis is often described. The findings in the kidneys may be asymmetric, with a normal renal unit on one side, whereas the opposite kidney is dysplastic. The ureters tend to be tortuous and dilated, most often in a segmental distribution. Vesicoureteral reflux is common. The ureteral abnormalities have been attributed to a deficiency of smooth muscle. The bladder is typically very large and may be associated with a patent urachus.

The prostatic urethra is characteristically dilated and tapers rapidly at the membranous urethra, occasionally resembling posterior urethral valves. The dilated posterior urethra is believed to be secondary to prostatic hypoplasia. The anterior urethra is usually normal, although an association with megalourethra has been described. The testes are cryptorchid, usually in an abdominal location.

LOWER URINARY TRACT ANOMALIES

Bladder

Anatomy

The bladder is a hollow pelvic viscus consisting of smooth muscle, lamina propria, submucosa, and mucosa. The muscle is the detrusor muscle, which has three layers: an inner longitudinal, a middle circular, and an outer longitudinal. The three muscle layers condense inferiorly to form the trigone, a muscular triangle with the apex extending to the bladder neck. The ureters enter the bladder at the lateral aspects of the trigone. The interureteric ridge, a muscular ridge between the two ureteric orifices, forms the base of the trigone. The internal sphincter is located in the bladder neck.

The bladder is extraperitoneal, with the exception of the dome and upper portions of the lateral walls, which are covered by peritoneum. The arterial supply to the bladder arises primarily from the hypogastric arteries. There is a rich venous plexus that drains into the internal iliac veins. Auxiliary veins connect this venous plexus to veins that drain into the intervertebral plexus and provide venous drainage when the IVC is obstructed.

Exstrophy

The most common congenital bladder lesion is exstrophy. It is the result of a deficiency in the development of the lower abdominal wall musculature, so that the anterior wall of the bladder is discontinuous so the lumen is open anteriorly and the mucosa of the bladder is continuous with the skin. There is associated epispadias in which the urethra is open dorsally and urethral mucosa covers the dorsum of a short penis. The condition occurs in approximately 1 in 50,000 births and has a male:female ratio of 2:1.

Skeletal and gastrointestinal anomalies are commonly associated with exstrophy. Separation of the symphysis pubis correlates directly with the severity of the exstrophy–epispadias complex. In full-blown exstrophy, the pubic bones are widely separated (Fig. 1.30). The exstrophy–epispadiac anomaly may be associated

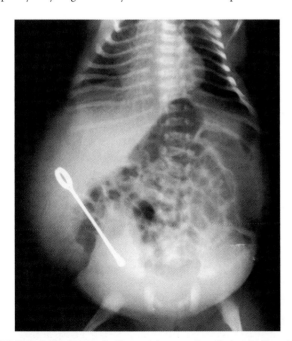

FIGURE 1.29. Prune belly syndrome. An abdominal radiograph of a newborn with prune belly syndrome shows bulging of the flanks as a result of the absence of abdominal musculature.

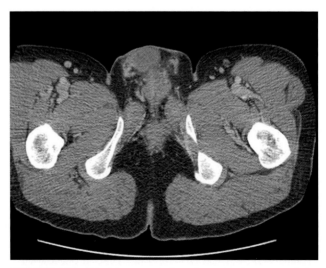

FIGURE 1.30. Bladder exstrophy. There is diastasis of the pubic symphysis.

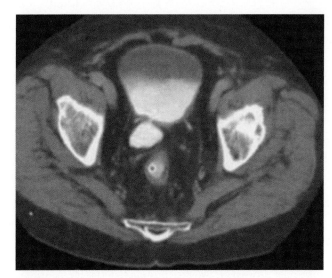

FIGURE 1.31. Hutch-type bladder diverticulum. CT scan showing a paraureteral bladder diverticulum.

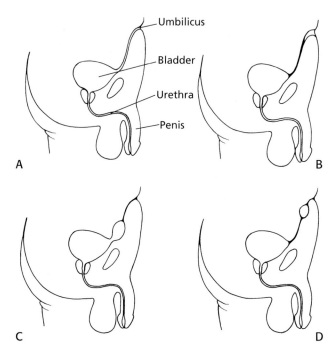

FIGURE 1.32. Urachal abnormalities. **A:** Patent urachus. **B:** Umbilical sinus. **C:** Urachocele. **D:** Urachal cyst.

with ureteric obstruction and unilateral or bilateral pelvicaliectasis due to fibrosis at the ureterovesical junction. However, in most cases, the upper tracts are normal, but there may be widening of the distal ureters. This widening has been likened to a "hurley," the stick used in the traditional Irish game of hurling. Umbilical and inguinal hernias are frequently present. Most children are treated with a primary closure of the bladder and subsequent bladder augmentation.

Agenesis of the bladder is usually incompatible with life; death results from obstruction and renal failure. A few cases of bladder agenesis have been reported in children who lived long enough for a diagnosis to be made. Most of these patients were female.

Congenital Bladder Diverticulum

A congenital diverticulum occurs in close relationship to the ureteral orifice (Fig. 1.31) typically opening just above and lateral to it. Such a finding is often called a "Hutch" diverticulum. Because of distortion of the valve mechanism at the ureterovesical junction by the diverticulum, vesicoureteral reflux may result.

Urachus

The allantois is the attachment of the bladder dome to the umbilicus. The bladder is initially an abdominal organ, but it then descends into the pelvis. As this happens, the bladder dome narrows to form the urachus, which elongates with bladder descent. This umbilical attachment of the bladder normally becomes a completely obliterated fibrous cord (umbilical ligament). Failure of this fibrous closure results in a patent urachus through which urine can flow from the bladder to the umbilicus (Fig. 1.32). The male:female ratio of patent urachus is 3:1. Segmental failure of closure of the urachus at the bladder attachment results in a urachocele, or diverticulum in the dome of the bladder. Failure of closure at the umbilical attachment results in a draining umbilical sinus. Failure of closure in any other part of the duct results in a urachal cyst (Fig. 1.33). Urachal cysts are usually clinically silent unless infection supervenes. Calculi have been reported within urachal cysts and may be seen on plain films as small punctate calcifications above the bladder outline.

Müllerian Duct Cyst and Dilated Prostatic Utricle

Anatomy

The male urethra consists of four parts. The prostatic urethra extends approximately 3.5 cm from the bladder neck to the superior aspect of the urogenital diaphragm. A longitudinal ridge of smooth muscle on the posterior wall of the prostatic urethra swells to form a 1-cm mound, the verumontanum (Fig. 1.34). The utricle is a small depression in the midportion while the ejaculatory ducts enter the urethra on either side of the verumontanum. The prostatic urethra is continuous with the bladder and lined by transitional cells.

The membranous urethra measures only approximately 1.0 cm in length and extends from the distal end of the verumontanum to the tip of the cone of the bulbous urethra. It is the narrowest part of the urethra. The Cowper glands lie on either side of the membranous urethra.

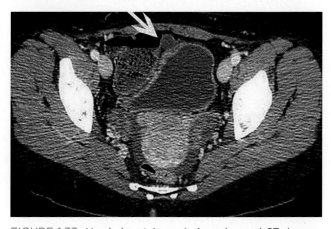

FIGURE 1.33. Urachal cyst (*arrow*). An enhanced CT demonstrates a small urachal cyst anterior and superior to the bladder.

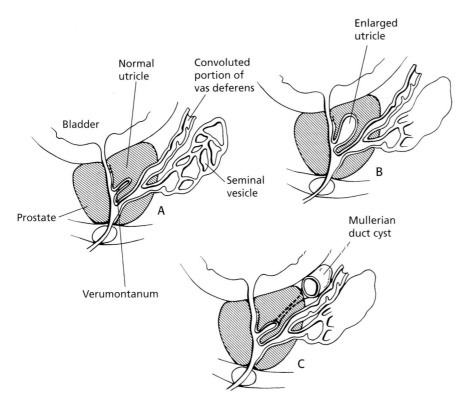

FIGURE 1.34. Müllerian remnant abnormalities in the male. **A:** The normal utricle is a small pocket in the verumontanum. **B:** Dilated utricle; this communicates with the urethra and will opacify during urethrography. **C:** Müllerian duct cyst—a cystic structure above the prostate and between the seminal vesicles. There is no communication with the urethra.

The bulbous urethra extends from the inferior end of the urogenital diaphragm to the angulated penoscrotal junction. The proximal portion has a conical shape with a narrow tip at the urogenital diaphragm. The two ducts draining Cowper glands enter the bulbous urethra, which is the widest portion of the urethra.

The penile urethra extends from the penoscrotal junction to the meatus. The fossa navicularis is the slightly dilated portion at the distal 2 cm of the penile urethra.

The bulbous and penile portions of the urethra comprise the anterior urethra and are lined by stratified columnar epithelium. The anterior urethra is lined with the submucosal glands of Littre, which secrete mucous into the urethra during sexual stimulation.

Urethral Sphincters

Three sphincters maintain continence of urine. The internal sphincter lies at the bladder neck and is the primary muscle of passive urinary continence. The second smooth muscle sphincter is the intrinsic sphincter, which lies below the verumontanum surrounding the membranous urethra. The external sphincter is comprised of striated muscle and lies below the verumontanum in the distal portion of the prostatic urethra.

Female Urethra

The female urethra is a straight tube approximately 4 cm long. The internal sphincter is at the bladder neck and the external sphincter is near the meatus.

Normal müllerian duct atrophy occurs in about the 6th week in the male fetus. The vestigial remnants of this ductal obliteration are the prostatic utricle and the appendix of the testis. Nonatrophy of the müllerian duct may produce cystic dilations along the route of the vas deferens from the scrotum to the ejaculatory ducts (Fig. 1.35). Müllerian duct cysts are rare but most commonly occur in the midline just above the prostate. They may occasionally become large enough to cause an impression on the posterior bladder wall or to obstruct the bladder outlet. If infection supervenes, suprapubic and rectal pain occur. Fluid aspirated from a müllerian

duct cyst may be serous, mucoid, purulent, or hemorrhagic but contains no spermatozoa. These cysts can be imaged with ultrasound, CT, or MRI (Fig. 1.36).

A dilated utricle may be an incidental finding but is associated with hypospadias and incomplete testicular descent, a complex of findings suggesting intersex. The normal prostatic utricle is 8 to 10 mm in length, narrow at its orifice (2 mm) in the verumontanum, and bulbous at its blind end. Because the dilated utricle communicates with the urethra, it can be imaged during antegrade or retrograde urethrography.

Seminal Vesicles

The vas deferens arises from the tail of the epididymis and enters the pelvis through the internal spermatic ring. The distal portions dilate to form the ampullae before joining the excretory duct of the seminal vesicles to form the ejaculatory ducts. The seminal vesicles are paired structures lying adjacent to the ampullae of the vas deferens.

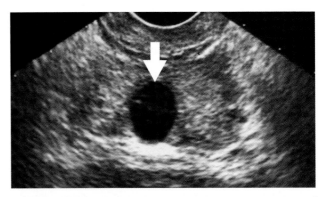

FIGURE 1.35. Müllerian duct cyst. A cystic mass is well defined in this transrectal ultrasound examination.

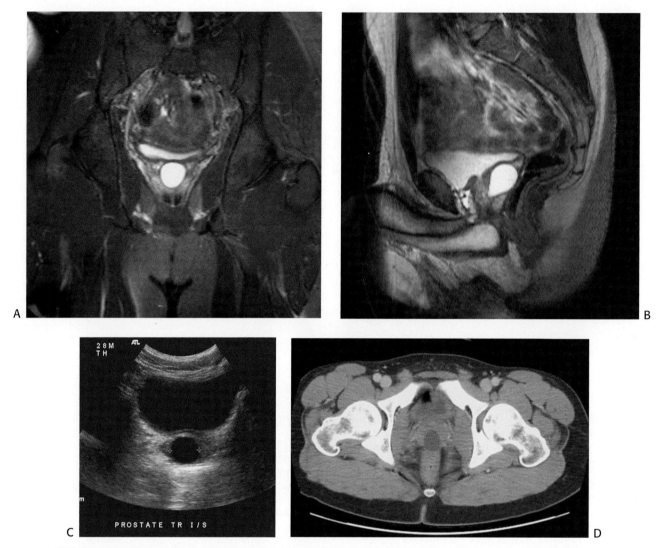

A

B

C

D

FIGURE 1.36. Müllerian duct cyst. **A:** Coronal. **B:** Sagittal: T2-weighted MR images show a cystic mass behind the bladder representing a müllerian duct cyst. **C:** Ultrasound. **D:** CT image.

Congenital seminal vesicle anomalies result from interruption or failure of the normal development of the mesonephric duct. The mesonephric duct develops ureteric buds dorsomedially after 5 weeks of gestation. The ureteric buds grow cranially and dorsally to meet the nephrogenic ridge and form the metanephros, which becomes the normal kidney. As fetal growth continues, the ureters derive separate openings into the bladder, and the mesonephric duct moves caudally and ends as the ejaculatory duct. Small buds develop in the distal mesonephric duct that become the seminal vesicles.

Any deviation in the development of the ureteric bud or the seminal vesicle bud results in a congenital anomaly. When both buds fail to develop, the ipsilateral kidney, ureter, hemitrigone, and seminal vesicle are lost. Failure to develop the normal ureteric bud results in renal agenesis and a normal seminal vesicle. Failure to develop a normal seminal vesicle bud results in a normal kidney, ureter, and hemitrigone and absent seminal vesicle. Abnormal development of the distal mesonephric bud may result in atresia of the seminal vesicle duct, resulting in seminal vesicle obstruction producing a seminal vesicle cyst (Fig. 1.37). Seminal vesicle cysts are commonly associated with ipsilateral absence of the kidney and ureter. Rarely, the anomaly involves delay in the origin of the ureteric bud such that the seminal vesicle bud gives rise to the ureteric bud, resulting in ectopic insertion of the ureter into the seminal vesicle. Seminal vesicle cysts rarely enlarge enough to be of clinical significance. They most commonly present in the third decade but have been reported in patients up to 60 years of age. When such cysts are large, patients present clinically with urgency, frequency, and dysuria. Pelvic and perineal pains are common.

Urethra

Many of the congenital urethral lesions discussed in the following paragraphs are obstructive and consequently produce vesical and ureteric dilation. Severe obstruction results in gross hydronephrosis with renal obstructive atrophy. Because the lower urinary tract has completely formed by the end of the 4th month of gestation and because fetal micturition also occurs at this time, complete obstruction may lead to intrauterine death. Incomplete obstruction may be compatible with a live birth, but failure to thrive and vomiting in the neonate or infant are symptoms of renal failure and raise the possibility of outlet obstruction from a urethral anomaly.

Posterior Urethral Valves

The continuation of the inferior aspect of the verumontanum is the urethral crest, which is a mucosal fold that is originally midline

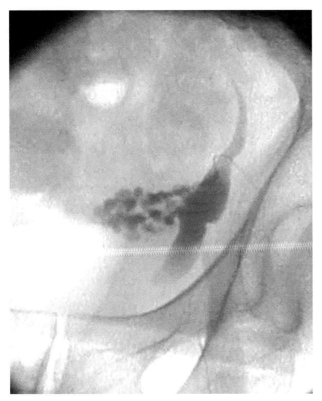

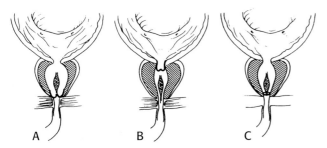

FIGURE 1.37. Seminal vesicle cyst. An ectopic ureter is seen entering a left seminal vesicle cyst.

but divides into two to four fins (plicae colliculi) that take a spiral course to end inferiorly in the membranous urethra, anteriorly and midline. These plicae colliculi are vestigial remnants of the migrating mesonephric duct orifices. When the origin of the mesonephric duct orifice is too far anterior, normal migration is altered, leading to abnormal fusion and insertion of the plicae colliculi and resulting in thick valve cusps.

In 1919, Young classified urethral valves into three types (Fig. 1.38). Type I is the most common and consists of valve leaflets extending from the distal verumontanum to the urethral walls. These valves balloon out during voiding and result in outlet

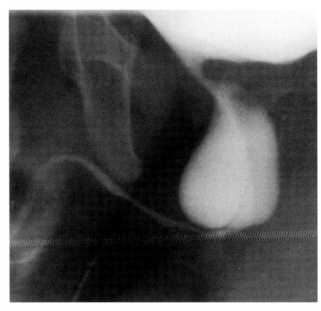

FIGURE 1.39. Voiding cystourethrogram in a 2-year-old boy. The posterior urethra is dilated down to the membranous urethra. The valves are visible. (Courtesy of A. Daneman, MD.)

obstruction (Fig. 1.39). Type II posterior urethral valves are mucosal folds extending proximally from the verumontanum to the bladder neck. These are rare and are probably caused by mucosal redundancy secondary to current or prior, more distal urethral obstruction. Thus, many authorities no longer consider type II valves to be true valves because they are acquired rather than congenital. A type III posterior urethral valve is also rare and is unrelated to the verumontanum. It occurs in the distal prostatic urethra as an iris-like membrane with a central pinhole orifice.

Posterior urethral valves are the most common cause of obstructive symptoms in infants and very young boys; they occur only in males. The condition may cause complete obstruction leading to renal failure, oligohydramnios, and intrauterine death. Vesicoureteral reflux (occurring in approximately 50% of patients) or high-intravesical pressure can result in massive hydrostatic pressure in the kidney, leading to calyceal rupture and resultant subcapsular or perirenal urinomas. Fetal or neonatal urine ascites may also occur. Neonatal clinical diagnosis includes palpable kidneys and bladder, abdominal distention, ascites, straining to void, and an absent or dribbling urinary stream. Elevated creatinine levels indicate renal impairment, which may return to normal after the obstruction is relieved, depending on the degree of renal damage. Occasionally, chronic renal failure may occur in spite of relief of the obstruction.

Young children may present with symptoms of urinary tract infection, whereas the degree of obstruction due to posterior urethral valves in older children or young adults may be so mild that investigation is delayed until superimposed infection occurs.

Posterior urethral valves are best demonstrated by voiding cystourethrography. There is no difficulty with the insertion of a catheter into the bladder in type I valves, but catheter insertion may be difficult in type III valves. Bladder filling demonstrates a large-capacity bladder, bladder trabeculation with diverticula, or vesicoureteral reflux in approximately one-half of the cases and a somewhat narrowed bladder neck due to hypertrophy of the bladder detrusor. The voiding study demonstrates a dilated posterior urethra with poor distention of the membranous and anterior urethra. The valves occasionally may be seen as lucent bands bulging distally across the prostatic urethra and impeding the flow of urine.

FIGURE 1.38. Classification of posterior urethral valves. **A:** Type I valves are leaflets extending from the distal verumontanum to the walls of the urethra. **B:** Type II valves are seen in the proximal prostatic urethra and probably represent redundant mucosal folds. **C:** A type III valve is a diaphragm extending across the distal prostatic urethra. The size of the opening in this diaphragm determines the degree of obstruction. (From Amis ES Jr, Newhouse JH. *Essentials of Uroradiology*. Boston, MA: Little, Brown & Co.; 1991:66, with permission.)

Fibroepithelial Polyp

Fibroepithelial polyps in the urethra are rare and usually originate in the prostate and project into the urethra. This condition presents at birth with difficulty in micturition or intermittent stream that may progress to retention. The polyp is connected to the verumontanum via a stalk, which allows it to rest in the prostatic urethra or even extend through the bladder neck into the bladder (Fig. 1.40); during the voiding phase of cystourethrography, they are typically seen as smooth filling defects extending into the midportion of the bulbar urethra.

Atresia Ani Urethralis

Anal atresia in the male may be associated with a fistulous tract between the bowel and posterior urethra, resulting in difficulty catheterizing the bladder. If the fistulous tract goes untreated, recurrent urinary tract infection may eventually result in renal failure. Treatment of the anal atresia by colostomy is insufficient, because urine passes along the fistulous tract into the bowel forming "bowel calculi," the result of urinary crystalloids combining with colonic mucus.

Meatal Stenosis

Congenital meatal stenosis can account for severe outlet obstruction in the male and can produce the same degree of hydronephrosis, bladder dilation, and trabeculation as urethral valves. Meatal stenosis of this degree is a much less common cause of hydronephrosis than posterior urethral valves. Catheter insertion through the external meatus is difficult or impossible. The stenosis is easily treated by a meatotomy. An associated, wide-necked diverticulum may arise from the dorsal urethra within the glans penis; this is referred to as a lacuna magna and can also be an isolated occurrence. Diagnosis of meatal stenosis is clinical.

Hypospadias

In hypospadias, the external urethral meatus is found on the ventral surface of the penis, anywhere from just proximal to its normal location to the perineum. Although clinically obvious on physical examination, hypospadias is usually asymptomatic

until bladder training has been completed, after which the urinary stream is found to be difficult to direct and may require sitting to void. Urethroplasty to construct a new distal urethra is required.

Epispadias

Epispadias is less common than hypospadias. The external urethral orifice opens onto the dorsum of the penis, and as for hypospadias, urethroplasty is required for correction. In patients with exstrophy, epispadias is complete with the entire urethra lying open along the dorsum of a foreshortened penis.

Anterior Urethral Diverticulum

Congenital urethral diverticulum occurs only in males and arises from the ventral surface of the anterior urethra. Urethral diverticulum in the adult female is thought to be acquired. In the male, anterior urethral diverticulum is the result of failure of closure of urethral folds or an abortive attempt at urethral duplication. The diverticulum has a somewhat narrow neck and fills during voiding. As the diverticulum fills, it increases in size and compresses the true urethra. This may result in significant obstructive voiding symptoms. At the end of micturition, the diverticulum empties, causing postvoid dribbling. Diagnosis is best accomplished by voiding cystourethrography. Removal of the diverticulum requires urethroplasty to repair the defect in the urethral floor.

Anterior urethral valves have also been described and result in a clinical and radiographic pattern difficult to distinguish from an anterior urethral diverticulum (Fig. 1.41). It is unclear whether such a valve is a true entity or is simply the anterior lip of a diverticulum.

A dorsal urethral diverticulum can occur in the region of the fossa navicularis. These diverticula are typically round and are known as lacuna magna. Their opening is obscured during retrograde urethrography but, if suspected, can usually be demonstrated by voiding studies.

Urethral Duplication

No satisfactory embryologic explanation has been suggested to explain urethral duplication, which may be complete or incomplete. In complete duplication in the male patient, there may be accompanying bladder or penile duplication or both. The two urethras lie one above the other in males, and the ventral channel usually proves to be the more functional and normal appearing. In female patients,

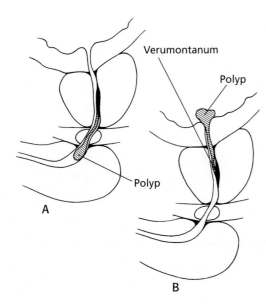

FIGURE 1.40. Diagram of congenital urethral polyp. **A:** During voiding, the polyp extends into the bulbar urethra. **B:** When resting, the polyp can coil in the posterior urethra and even extend through the bladder neck into the bladder.

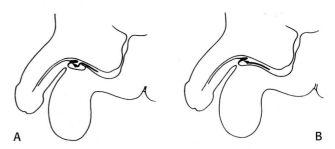

FIGURE 1.41. Diagram of anterior urethral diverticulum and anterior urethral valve. **A:** Note that the proximal portion of the diverticulum forms an acute angle with the urethra. Elevation of the distal lip of the diverticulum against the roof of the urethra acts as an obstruction as the diverticulum fills. **B:** An anterior urethral valve, if such an entity truly exists, has the same obstructive mechanism as a diverticulum. Note that there is no proximal angulation such as that seen with the diverticulum. (From Amis ES Jr, Newhouse JH. *Essentials of Uroradiology.* Boston, MA: Little, Brown & Co.; 1991:67, with permission.)

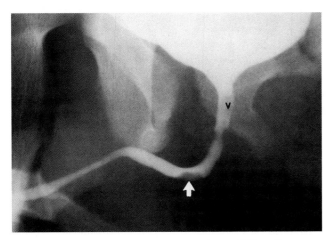

FIGURE 1.42. Cowper duct cyst. Voiding cystourethrogram reveals a well-defined indentation on the floor of the midbulbar urethra (*arrow*). There is no urethral obstruction in this case. The verumontanum is clearly seen (*v*).

duplicated urethrae lie side by side. When the anomalous urethra lies outside the control of the internal and distal sphincter mechanism, urinary incontinence is the presenting symptom. The anomalous urethra has an epispadiac or hypospadiac external meatus and is subject to recurrent infection. Indications for removal of the anomalous urethra are urinary incontinence and urethritis in the anomalous urethra.

In incomplete duplication, two external meatus may be found with two urethras joining near the bladder neck, or two urethrae may originate from the bladder neck and may join at some point distally to form a single urethra. Both retrograde and voiding urethrography may be necessary to completely define the extent of this anomaly.

Retention Cyst of Cowper Duct

Cowper glands are two pea-sized glands lying between the leaves of the urogenital diaphragm. The ducts of these glands are approximately 2 cm in length, extend from the urogenital diaphragm inferiorly, and enter the midportion of the bulbous urethra on both sides of the midline. Cowper glands secrete mucin that is a lubricator for semen and prevents coagulation of spermatozoa during ejaculation. Cowper duct cysts have been reported in newborn infants and are thought to be the result of a congenital malformation of the ostia, producing ductal obstruction resulting in retention cyst swelling. The retention cyst projects into the bulbous urethra and may cause minor urinary symptoms such as frequency or strangury; large retention cysts may cause obstructive symptoms.

On urethrography, a Cowper duct cyst is seen as an indentation on the floor of the mid- or proximal bulbar urethra (Fig. 1.42).

UNDESCENDED TESTICLE

The testis is 4 to 5 cm in length, 3 cm in width, and 2.5 cm in breadth. The epididymis lies along the posterolateral side of the testis. The appendix testis, a small ovoid, sessile body, lies at the upper end of the testis adjacent to the head of the epididymis.

Undescended testicle, also known as cryptorchidism, commonly occurs as an isolated phenomenon or may be associated with other urogenital anomalies, such as renal agenesis or ectopia, prune belly syndrome, and epispadias. Undescended testes are also found in patients with testicular feminization. In the complete form,

androgen insensitivity results in a female phenotype, with well-developed breasts and female external genitalia, but absent müllerian structures and a blind-ending vagina. Up to 20% of premature males are born with undescended testes. In most of these infants, normal descent into the scrotum occurs within the first few weeks to months of life. In term infants, the incidence of undescended testes is significantly lower and further decreases to approximately 1% by 1 year of age because of spontaneous descent.

The undescended testicle often is smaller than the normal descended testis. In a small number of patients, testicular agenesis occurs. The most common ectopic position for the undescended testicle is in the inguinal canal. However, arrested descent of the testes may occur in the abdomen, pelvis, or high in the scrotum after passage through the inguinal canal.

Complications of the undescended testicle include malignant change, sterility, and testicular torsion. A testis arrested in the inguinal canal is also subject to accidental injury. The incidence of malignant change in the undescended testicle is high. In the normal male population, the incidence of testis tumor is approximately 2:100,000. This increases to 10:100,000 in inguinally placed undescended testis, and the rate is even higher in arrested descent in the pelvis or abdomen.

In many centers, laparoscopy has become the procedure of choice for the nonpalpable testis. Imaging modalities that may be useful in the detection of undescended testicle include ultrasound, CT, and MR. Ultrasound is useful in the detection of the undescended testicle when the arrest is in the inguinal canal. However, ultrasound is of little value in detecting arrested descent in the abdomen or pelvis unless malignant change has occurred producing a mass. High-frequency transducers can successfully define the undescended inguinal testis in most cases. Both sides should be examined for symmetry. An asymmetric mass in the inguinal region with the echogenic characteristics of the normal testes is the most common finding. Malignant change in the undescended testis is seen on ultrasound as a mass of indefinable echogenicity in the inguinal canal.

CT accurately identifies the undescended testicle in and adjacent to the inguinal canal (Fig. 1.43). Normally, structures in this region are symmetric. In undescended testes, asymmetry occurs with a small mass on the affected side corresponding to the undescended testicle. An asymmetric mass larger than the expected testicular size raises the possibility of malignant change. Because an undescended testicle may be as small as 1 cm, it is necessary to opacify the bowel with oral contrast material. MR has similar spatial

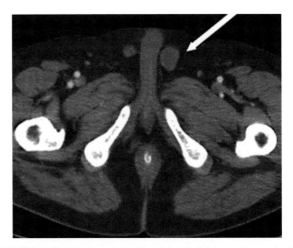

FIGURE 1.43. Undescended testicle. A CT scan through the level of the symphysis pubis demonstrates the left testis (*arrow*) in the inguinal canal.

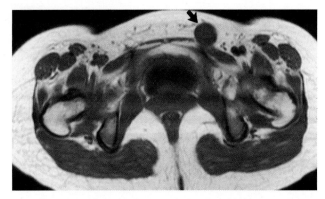

FIGURE 1.44. MRI of undescended testicle. A T1-weighted MR image clearly shows the medium–signal intensity testicle (*arrow*) in the left inguinal area.

resolution to CT. The undescended testis is seen as a medium-signal mass on T1-weighted images (Fig. 1.44) and as a high-signal mass on T2-weighted images.

IN UTERO ANOMALIES

Ultrasound is commonly used to screen the fetus in utero for anomalies. The urinary tract lends itself well to such evaluation, because the fetal kidneys are discernible at 13 to 14 weeks of fetal age using transabdominal techniques or a vaginal probe. The fetal bladder can be imaged as early as 11 weeks of gestation. Care must be taken in the diagnosis of hydronephrosis, because it is not uncommon for the renal pelvis to be distended to 1 cm when measured in anteroposterior diameter in the normal fetus. However, many anomalies can be diagnosed with confidence, although, to date, there has been no significant success in treating these conditions in utero. The ultrasonographic findings in these anomalies are generally the same as those described in the term infant after delivery.

FEMALE GENITAL TRACT

The ovaries lie on either side of the uterus and are attached to the back of the broad ligament of the uterus. The size of the ovary decreases with each decade of life; the mean ovarian volume diminishes from approximately 6.6 cubic cm in women under 30 years to <2 cubic cm in women more than 70 years of age.

Fallopian tubes carry the ova from the ovaries to the uterine cavity. Fertilization of an ovum takes place during its transit through the fallopian tube. The fallopian tubes are comprised of four portions. The interstitial portion is a short segment that traverses the myometrium. The isthmus is a narrow portion adjacent to the uterus. The ampulla is the dilated portion; the infundibulum has a fimbriated opening adjacent to the ovary. The epithelial lining of the tube is ciliated to facilitate passage of the ovum.

The uterus is a thick-walled, muscular organ lying between the bladder and the rectum. It measures approximately 8 cm in length and 4 cm in width and depth. After pregnancy, it is larger by about 1 cm in each dimension. The uterus decreases in size in postmenopausal women to approximately 7 cm by 3 cm by 2 cm. The body of the uterus is often anteflexed over the bladder while the cervix is relatively fixed in the midline.

The incidence of congenital uterine and vaginal anomalies ranges from 0.5% to 3%; the discrepancies probably have to do with whether some very mild uterine variants are considered anomalous. In general, they fall into three main categories, which are agenesis, duplication, and anomalies related to diethylstilbestrol (DES).

The clinical presentation of these congenital anomalies varies. If the anomaly involves vaginal atresia or uterine atresia, menarche is delayed. If the vagina is atretic but there is an endometrium, cyclic pain may appear with puberty even though menarche does not. Any form of obstruction may produce hematometra or hematocolpos. Infertility may be the first clue to the diagnoses of certain anomalies, or women who get pregnant may have spontaneous abortions or unusual fetal presentations. Patients whose menstrual flow is occluded but whose fallopian tubes are patent may extrude menstrual material into the peritoneal cavity and develop endometriosis.

The American Fertility Society has adopted a classification initially proposed by Buttram.

Class I constitutes müllerian agenesis or hypoplasia. There are various manifestations of this group, including hypoplasia of the vagina, cervix, uterus, and fallopian tubes or a combination of them. The Mayer–Rokitansky–Kuster–Hauser syndrome involves absence of the entire uterus, cervix, and vagina; in some types, there are normal fallopian tubes and kidneys, whereas in others, there are renal, ovarian, and fallopian tube anomalies as well. The vagina is usually short. The imaging findings are self-evident: there may or may not be normal ovaries and there may be unilateral renal agenesis; the uterus is not seen.

Class II anomalies involve the consequences of failure of development of one müllerian duct and comprise various forms of the unicornuate uterus. There may be complete agenesis of one side of the uterus, so that only one cornu and fallopian tube form. Alternatively, the abnormal cornu may be present but severely hypoplastic. The hypoplastic side may have no endometrial space or a hypoplastic one; the hypoplastic one may or may not communicate with the main portion of the endometrium.

Imaging findings depend on the details of the anomaly. If there is complete agenesis of one horn, hysterosalpingography may reveal a normal lower uterine segment but a small fundus with one cornu and one tube (Fig. 1.45); ultrasound may reveal an asymmetric uterus and fundal endometrium, and MRI may show only one cornu. If the abnormal side is hypoplastic but contains no endometrium, hysterosalpingography may appear no different from that of the first variety, but MR may reveal a stub of myometrium extending toward the abnormal side. If the abnormal side has an endometrial cavity that is very small but communicates with the main endometrial cavity, hysterosalpingography may fill it. If the endometrial cavity of the abnormal side exists but does not communicate, a local form of hematometra may appear that resembles a myometrial or adnexal mass; ultrasound will show it to be fluid-filled with internal echoes, and MR may reveal the mass to have characteristics of old blood.

Classes III, IV, V, and VI all involve uterine duplication, the degree of which is most severe in the lowest numbered classes.

Class III constitutes complete uterine duplication, often called uterus didelphys. There are two cervices; each endocervical canal connects with a fundus that has one cornu that extends to one tube. There may be one vagina or there may be a vaginal septum; often, the septum occludes one-half of the vagina, so that hematocolpos and hematometra appear. With unilateral vaginal atresia and uterus didelphys, unilateral renal agenesis is very common. Hysterosalpingographic demonstration of this anomaly requires that each cervical os be cannulated. Ultrasound and MR reveal the two uterine bodies; T2-weighted MR clearly reveals the separate endometrial cavities (Fig. 1.46) and cornua.

Class IV anomaly is a bicornuate uterus. In this condition, there is one cervix, but there are two upper uterine segments and two fundi, each of which has its own cornu. The external surfaces

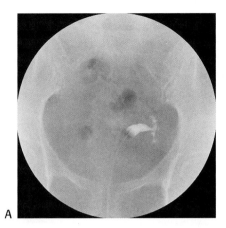

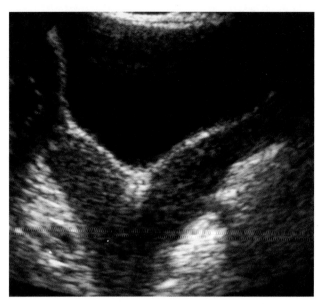

FIGURE 1.47. Bicornuate uterus. Ultrasound reveals two uterine horns, which are separated in the midline by a deep external cleft.

(Fig. 1.48). Because this condition may be treated with endoscopic surgery, it is important to be sure that the patient does not actually have a bicornuate uterus; MR is the most accurate noninvasive modality for demonstrating the external uterine configuration (Fig. 1.49).

Class VI is the arcuate uterus. In this condition, the fundal surface of the endometrial cavity, which normally is convex outward, bulges slightly into the endometrial space. This condition is only rarely associated with upper tract anomalies and may be considered a normal variant rather than an anomaly.

Class VII anomalies are those associated with in utero exposure to DES. This drug, when given to pregnant women, causes müllerian duct abnormalities in female fetuses. The drug was withdrawn from use in pregnant women in 1970, so that the cohort of affected patients is growing older, and diagnosis of their uterine anomalies is becoming less common.

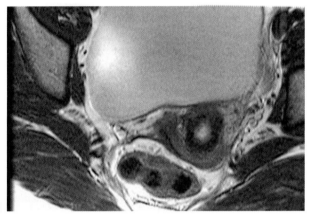

FIGURE 1.45. Unicornuate uterus. **A:** A single uterine horn is opacified on hysterosalpingography. **B:** MR confirms the presence of only one uterine horn.

of the two horns of the uterus can be demonstrated by surgical or laparoscopic inspection, MR, or ultrasound (Fig. 1.47).

Class V anomaly is a septate uterus. In this condition, the external surface of the uterus appears normal, but a septum of variable dimensions separates the left and right halves of the fundus

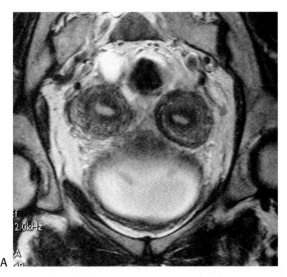

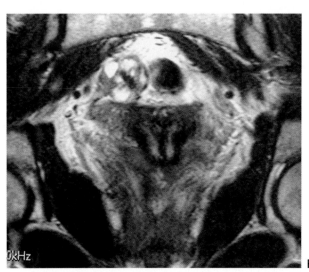

FIGURE 1.46. Uterus didelphys. **A, B:** Two separate endometrial cavities are seen on these coronal T1-weighted magnetic resonance images.

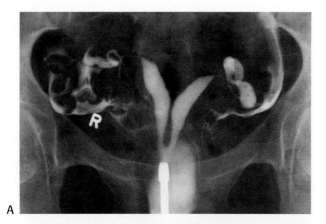

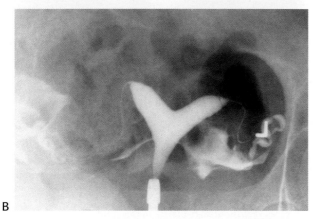

FIGURE 1.48. Two cases of septate uterus. **A:** A deep narrow septum almost completely divides the endometrial cavity. **B:** A wide, shallow septum separates the cornua of the fundus.

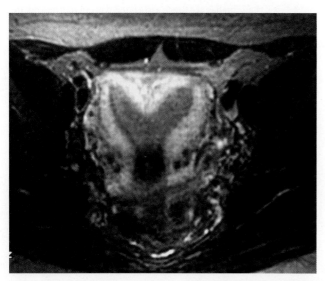

FIGURE 1.49. Septate uterus. T2-weighted MRI reveals a thick, shallow fundal septum; the external surface of the uterus reveals no cleft. (Courtesy of Tova Koenigsberg, MD.)

There are a variety of abnormalities that in utero exposure to DES cause, including morphologic abnormalities and adenosis of the vagina, which confers an increased risk of clear cell carcinoma of the vagina. There are cervical abnormalities, which include

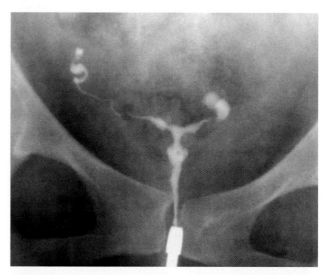

FIGURE 1.50. Uterus after fetal DES exposure. The uterine cavity is small and bizarre in configuration; the fundal cavity is T shaped.

transverse ridges, hoods, and stenoses. The uterus is often small and has a variety of hysterosalpingographically visible abnormalities. These include a small T-shaped cavity, shortened upper uterine segment, and irregular and narrow cervical canal (Fig. 1.50). Although the T shape is the classically described abnormality, a variety of peculiar endometrial cavity shapes have been reported. However, the cavities are virtually always diminished in size. MR and ultrasound simply display diminished uterine volume.

SUGGESTED READINGS

Upper Urinary Tract Anomalies

Amis ES Jr, Cronan JJ, Pfister RC. Lower moiety hydronephrosis in duplicated kidneys. *Urology.* 1985;26:82.

Claudon M, Ben-Sira L, Lebowitz RL. Lower pole reflux in children: uroradiologic appearances and pitfalls. *AJR Am J Roentgenol.* 1999;172:795.

Cronan JJ, Amis ES Jr, Zeman RK, et al. Obstruction of the upper pole moiety in renal duplication in adults: CT evaluation. *Radiology.* 1986;161:17.

Daneman A, Alton DJ. Radiographic manifestations of renal anomalies. *Radiol Clin North Am.* 1991;29:351.

Fernbach SK, Feinstein KA, Spencer K, et al. Ureteral duplication and its complications. *RadioGraphics.* 1997;17:109.

Smith SJ, Cass AS, Aliabadi H, et al. Unipapillary kidney: a case report and literature review. *Urol Radiol.* 1984;6:43–47.

Srinivasa MR, Adarsh KM, Jeeson R, et al. Congenital anatomic variants of the kidney and ureter: a pictorial essay. *Jpn J Radiol.* 2016;34:181–193.

Prune Belly Syndrome

Berdon WE, Baker DH, Wigger JH, et al. The radiologic and pathologic spectrum of the prune belly syndrome. *Radiol Clin North Am.* 1977;15(1):83.

Greskovich FJ, Nyberg LM. The prune belly syndrome: a review of its etiology, defects, treatment and prognosis. *J Urol.* 1988;140:707.

Lower Urinary Tract Anomalies and Undescended Testicle

Arora SS, Breiman RS, Webb EM, et al. CT and MRI of congenital anomalies of the seminal vesicles. *AJR Am J Roentgenol.* 2007;189:130–135.

Herman TE, McAlister WH. Radiographic manifestations of congenital anomalies of the lower urinary tract. *Radiol Clin North Am.* 1991;29:365.

Khati NJ, Enguist EG, Javitt MC. Imaging of the umbilicus and periumbilical region. *RadioGraphics.* 1998;18:314.

Nguyan HT, Coakley F, Hricak H. Cryptorchidism: strategies in detection. *Eur Radiol.* 1999;9:336.

Rowell AC, Sangster GP, Caraway JD, et al. Genitourinary imaging: part I, congenital urinary anomalies and their management. *AJR Am J Roentgenol.* 2012;199:W545–553.

Young HH, Frontz WA, Baldwin JC. Congenital obstruction of the posterior urethra. *J Urol.* 1919;2:298.

In Utero Detection of Genitourinary Anomalies

Hill MC, Lande IM, Larsen JW Jr. Prenatal diagnosis of fetal anomalies using ultrasound and MRI. *Radiol Clin North Am.* 1988;26:287.

Sanders RC. In utero sonography of genitourinary anomalies. *Urol Radiol.* 1992;14:29.

Female Genital Tract

Fedele L, Bianchi S, Agnoli B, et al. Urinary tract anomalies associated with unicornuate uterus. *J Urol.* 1996;155(3):847–848.

Hall-Craggs MA, Williams CE, Pattison SH, et al. Mayer-Rokitansky-Kuster-Hauser syndrome: diagnosis with MR imaging. *Radiology.* 2013;269:787–792.

Mueller GC, Hussain HK, Smith YR, et al. Müllerian duct anomalies: comparison of MRI diagnosis and clinical diagnosis. *AJR Am J Roentgenol.* 2007;189:1294–1302.

O'Neill MJ, Yoder IC, Connolly SA, et al. Imaging evaluation and classification of developmental anomalies of the female reproductive system with an emphasis on MR-imaging. *AJR Am J Roentgenol.* 1999;173:407–416.

Ozsarlak O, De Schepper AM, Valkenburg M, et al. Septate uterus: hysterosalpingography and magnetic resonance imaging findings. *Eur J Radiol.* 1995;21(2):122–125.

Robbins JB, Parry JP, Guite KM, et al. MRI of pregnancy-related issues: mullerian duct anomalies. *AJR Am J Roentgenol.* 2012;198:302–310.

Troiano RN, McCarthy SM. Mullerian duct anomalies: imaging and clinical issues. *Radiology.* 2004;233:19–34.

Woodward PJ, Wagner BJ, Farley TE. MR imaging in the evaluation of female infertility. *RadioGraphics.* 1993;13:293–310.

2 Functional Renal Anatomy, Renal Physiology, and Contrast Media

FUNCTIONAL RENAL ANATOMY

The kidney maintains the homeostasis of body fluids through the excretion of metabolic end products and toxins, the regulation of body fluid volume and blood pressure, and the regulation of mineral and acid–base balance. While the regulatory function of the kidney directly affects the one-third of the fluid that is located in the vascular compartment, because there is free movement of water between the intracellular and extracellular fluid (ECF) compartments, the latter containing two-thirds of the body fluid volume, renal function actually affects the composition of all body fluids.

The kidney consists of (1) an inner renal medulla and (2) an outer renal cortex (Fig. 2.1). The functional unit of the kidney is the nephron (Fig. 2.2). Each kidney contains approximately 1 million nephrons. Each nephron consists of a specialized capillary vascular network called the *glomerulus*, which is surrounded by Bowman capsule, a balloon-like structure into which the capillary tufts of the glomerulus protrude. Each glomerulus is connected to a series of specialized epithelial segments that collectively are known as the *renal tubule*.

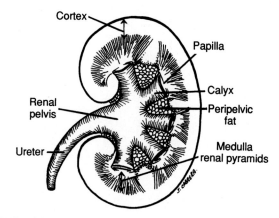

FIGURE 2.1. Bisected section of the kidney showing the relationship of the cortex, the medulla, and the renal collecting system. Fat in the renal sinus surrounds the calyces and the renal pelvis.

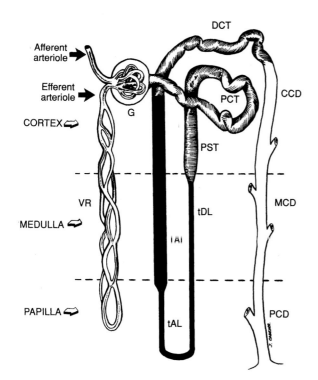

FIGURE 2.2. The nephron. G, glomerulus; TAL, thick ascending limb of the loop of Henle; tAL, thin ascending limb of the loop of Henle; PST, proximal straight tubule; PCT, proximal convoluted tubule; DCT, distal convoluted tubule; tDL, thin descending limb of loop of Henle; CCD, cortical collecting duct; MCD, medullary collecting duct; PCD, papillary collecting duct; VR, vasa recta.

The tubule is divided into several segments. The first segment, the proximal tubule, is subdivided into convoluted and straight portions; the second segment, the loop of Henle, is subdivided into the thin descending, the thin ascending, and the thick ascending limbs; and the third segment, the distal tubule, is subdivided into the distal convoluted tubule and the cortical, medullary, and papillary collecting ducts. The renal cortex contains the glomeruli, the proximal tubule, the distal tubule, and the cortical collecting duct. The renal medulla is made up of the loops of Henle, the medullary and papillary collecting ducts, and renal pyramids, the apices of which project into the minor calyces. The nephrons that are located close to the corticomedullary junction have larger glomeruli, and their loops of Henle descend deeper into the renal papilla than those located more superficially in the renal cortex.

The main renal artery branches into interlobar arteries that divide into the arcuate arteries located at the corticomedullary junction. These, in turn, become the interlobular arteries that finally divide into the afferent arterioles, each of which leads to a glomerulus. The glomerulus is drained by an efferent arteriole that subdivides to form a peritubular capillary network known as the vasa recta. The vasa recta then anastomose to form venous channels. This unique arrangement in the kidney, in which the glomerulus is located between two resistive capillary networks as opposed to the arteriole–capillary–venule arrangement of the other tissues of the body, helps to maintain constant hydrostatic pressure at the level of the glomerulus despite changes in blood pressure and is the driving force for glomerular filtration.

The *macula densa* is a distinctive portion of the tubule between the ascending loop of Henle and the distal convoluted tubule that courses between the afferent and efferent arterioles. It represents the tubular component of a specialized area of the nephron called the juxtaglomerular apparatus. The juxtaglomerular apparatus is the site of renin synthesis and plays a major role in blood pressure regulation.

BASIC RENAL PHYSIOLOGY

The homeostatic functions of the kidney are achieved through two simultaneous processes: (1) glomerular filtration and (2) tubular resorption/secretion. The net filtration pressure (NFP) is equal to the sum of the glomerular hydrostatic pressure and the colloid osmotic pressure in Bowman capsule (which favors fluid movement from the capillary space into Bowman space) minus the sum of the mean glomerular capillary oncotic pressure and the hydrostatic pressure in Bowman space (the principal forces opposing ultrafiltration). Because protein is not filtered by the glomerulus, the fluid of Bowman space is protein free; thus, the colloid osmotic pressure in Bowman space is negligible. The glomerular filtration rate (GFR) is determined by the NFP and the surface area available for filtration, as well as by the permeability of the glomerular capillary bed. The average GFR in a human with normal renal function is approximately 125 mL/min, which is equal to 180 L/day or approximately 12 times the volume of the ECF.

Although 180 L of fluid is filtered in a day, only 1 to 2 L of urine is produced per day in which wastes may be concentrated 100- to 200-fold above their plasma concentration. This concentration of the final urine product is the result of a combination of tubular secretion and reabsorption. Under normal conditions, approximately two-thirds of the ultrafiltrate volume is reabsorbed in the proximal tubule by a process linked to the active secretion of hydrogen ions and the active reabsorption of sodium, glucose, amino acids, and other solutes. Isotonicity of the fluid in the proximal tubule with the plasma is maintained because the cells of the proximal tubule are freely permeable to water.

In the loop of Henle, which begins at the corticomedullary junction, differential absorption of sodium chloride occurs so that the fluid in the tubular lumen, initially isotonic with the interstitium, becomes progressively more concentrated in the descending limb, reaching its maximum concentration at the bend of the loop and then becomes progressively more hypotonic with respect to plasma as it reaches the thick ascending limb of the loop. This differential absorption of sodium chloride occurs because the cells in the descending limb have a high permeability for water but a low permeability for salt, whereas in the thick ascending limb, the cells are impermeable to water but have a high permeability for salt, which is actively reabsorbed. This process, known as the *renal countercurrent mechanism*, results in progressive interstitial hypertonicity in the medulla and is required for final concentration of the urine by the distal tubules.

The distal tubule continues the water dilution of urine through the active transport of sodium and chloride coupled with relative water impermeability. The collecting ducts are the primary site of action of antidiuretic hormone (ADH). The final 15% of water absorption is achieved within the collecting ducts. The collecting ducts are virtually impermeable to water in the absence of ADH, but when ADH is present, water passes freely across the tubular wall, allowing the tubular fluid to achieve the same tonicity as the fluid in the surrounding interstitium. Thus, hypertonic urine is produced without the active transport of water. The distal nephron also reabsorbs sodium and secretes hydrogen ions and potassium under the influence of aldosterone. Parathyroid hormone also acts on the distal tubule to conserve calcium.

The rate at which a substance is removed from the plasma in a given period is termed the clearance of that substance. For a substance that is freely filtered and not reabsorbed or secreted by the tubule, the rate of clearance is equal to the GFR. The polysaccharide, inulin, meets this requirement and, therefore, can be used to determine GFR. Creatinine, an endogenous product of muscle metabolism, is produced in relatively constant amounts each day.

Creatinine is present in the plasma, and is excreted by glomerular filtration. Measurement of creatinine clearance is therefore convenient, although it is not as exact as the inulin clearance, because a small amount of creatinine is also secreted by the tubules. Because creatinine clearance tends to underestimate renal dysfunction, particularly with mild impairment, the National Kidney Foundation has suggested that the estimated glomerular filtration rate (eGFR) may be a better model for predicting renal dysfunction than relying solely on serum creatinine determinations. eGFR is generally calculated from the serum creatinine by either the Cockcroft–Gault formula or, more commonly, one of the modified diet in renal disease (MDRD) formulae. All of these formulae are calculated using a combination of the serum creatinine level, patient age, and patient gender. The Cockcroft–Gault formula also utilizes patient weight, while the MDRD formulae also accounts for patient race.

The most common of the abovementioned eGFR estimation formulae is the 4-variable MDRD formula, which is listed as follows: eGFR (mL/min/1.73 m^2) = 175 × [serum creatinine (µmol/L) × 0.0113]$^{-1.154}$ × age (years)$^{-0.203}$ (× 0.742 if female). There are many eGFR calculators available on the Internet.

CONTRAST MEDIA: HISTORICAL BACKGROUND

Although attempts at radiography of the urinary tract began shortly after Roentgen's discovery in 1895, the first report of opacification of the urinary tract was in 1923, when researchers at the Mayo Clinic discovered opacification of the bladder in patients being treated with sodium iodide. It is remarkable that in the more than 80 years since this discovery, no intravascular element other than iodine has proven suitable for imaging with x-rays.

Attempts at developing an injectable radiopaque iodinated contrast media were initially made in Germany under the direction of Moses Swick, an American urologist, who ultimately focused on linking the iodine to a 6-carbon benzene ring in an attempt to increase water solubility and decrease toxicity.

In 1955, Hoppe et al. at Sterling Winthrop Research Institute produced sodium diatrizoate (Fig. 2.3), a fully substituted derivative of 2,4,6-triiodobenzoic acid, which became the first modern iodinated contrast media. This agent was ionic in that the anionic benzene cation had to be conjugated with a positively charged sodium (cation), with the sodium diatrizoate molecule dissociating into two particles in solution (ratio of three iodine atoms to two particles in solution). This product and its derivatives, including sodium/meglumine diatrizoate and meglumine iothalmate, became the standard urographic contrast media for the next 30 years.

Although these ionic contrast media, which are still commonly used for enteric procedures today, including cystograms, some esophagograms, and some enemas, were safer than the previously used materials, much of the remaining toxicity of the compounds was related to their high osmolality (>1,500 mOsm/kg of water or approximately five times greater than plasma at standard contrast concentrations).

In 1968, Torsten Almen of Malmö, Sweden, theorized that the high osmolality of ionic contrast (with osmolality basically being a measure of the number of particles in solution) could be reduced by synthesizing a product that would be nondissociating. He demonstrated that the ionizing carboxyl group of conventional contrast media could be replaced with a nondissociating hydrophilic group such as an amide, resulting in a ratio of three iodine atoms per one particle in solution. This would theoretically decrease the osmolality by 50%, reducing the number of particles in solution without loss of iodine content. The first nonionic contrast media, metrizamide, was never used in the United States as a urographic agent, because of its considerable cost and the necessity to package it as a freeze-dried lyophilized powder that needed to be reconstituted with water immediately before use.

Several years after the introduction of metrizamide, second-generation low-osmolality contrast media were introduced into clinical practice. These products developed along two general lines. In the first group, hydrophilic nonionizing radicals were again introduced in positions one, three, and five of the benzene ring, whereas, positions two, four, and six remained the position of the iodine atoms. Because the radical at position number one did not dissociate, the number of iodine atoms relative to the number of particles in solution remained 3:1 rather than 3:2, as noted with ionic contrast media. Compounds in this category, which remain widely used today, include iohexol (Fig. 2.4; Omnipaque; GE Healthcare Inc., Princeton, NJ), iopamidol (Fig. 2.5; Isovue; Bracco Diagnostics Inc., Monroe, NJ), iopromide (Ultravist, Bayer Health Care, Wayne, NJ), and ioversol (Fig. 2.6; Optiray; Mallinckrodt Imaging, Hazelwood, MO). All of these products are generically known as *nonionic monomers*. Studies have demonstrated that the incidence of adverse events is greatly reduced (by a factor of about

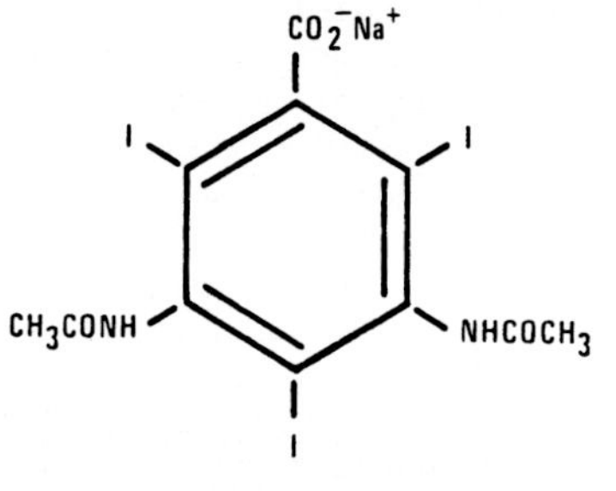

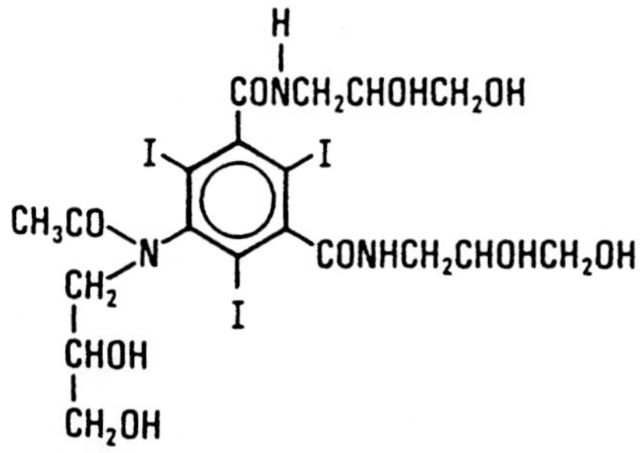

FIGURE 2.4. Iohexol (Omnipaque).

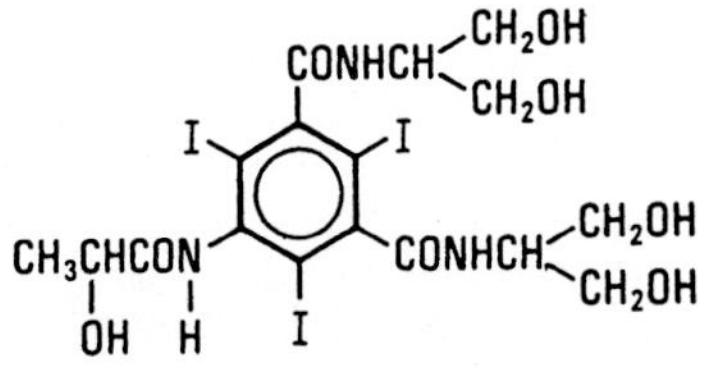

FIGURE 2.5. Iopamidol (Isovue).

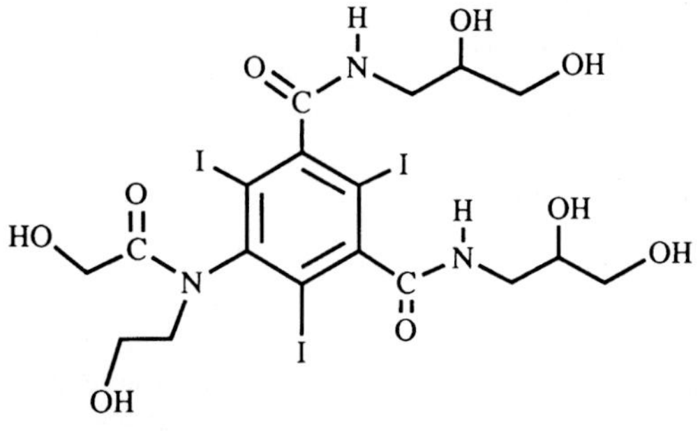

FIGURE 2.3. Sodium diatrizoate (Hypaque).

FIGURE 2.6. Ioversol (Optiray).

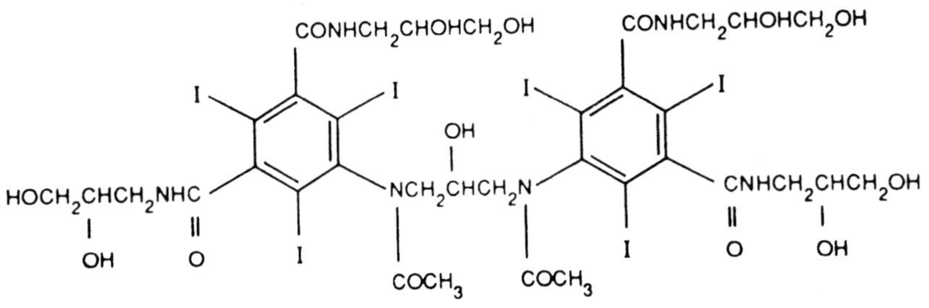

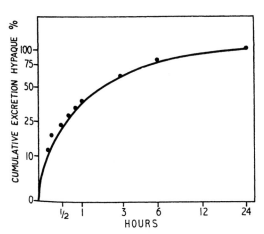

FIGURE 2.7. Iodixanol (Visipaque).

five) when nonionic monomers are injected intravenously, in comparison to ionic monomers, a difference that is likely the result of their lower osmolality.

The second line of development of low osmolality contrast was directed toward the linkage of two triiodinated benzene rings together sharing only one ionizing carboxyl group (at position one of one of the benzene rings). These compounds have a ratio of six iodine atoms to two molecules in solution and also produce a ratio of 3:1. These contrast particles are generally known as *ionic dimers* and have a similar osmolality to nonionic monomers.

Further development involved the linkage of two nonionic monomeric compounds to form a *nonionic dimer*, which has a ratio of six iodine atoms to one particle in solution, and, therefore, has a ratio of 6:1. This modification has further reduced the osmolality of the resulting contrast media, such that nonionic dimers have an osmolality equal to plasma. Iodixanol (Fig. 2.7; Visipaque; GE Healthcare, Princeton, NJ) is the only one of these agents to be approved for use in the United States. Interestingly, the incidence of acute adverse events after nonionic dimer injection has not been seen to be significantly lower than that encountered after nonionic monomer injection.

Another property of contrast media is viscosity. This property describes the relative adhesiveness of the molecules of the contrast media for one another and is important because the viscosity of the contrast determines how rapidly the contrast may be injected. In general, more concentrated solutions of contrast material are more viscous than less concentrated solutions. Also, larger molecules tend to have higher viscosity than smaller molecules at the same concentrations. So, it is not surprising that nonionic dimers are considerably more viscous than are nonionic monomers. The viscosity of contrast media decreases with increasing temperature. For this reason, warming of viscous contrast material makes injection easier.

PHYSIOLOGY OF CONTRAST EXCRETION

Principles

The currently used triiodobenzoic acid derivative contrast media are excreted by glomerular filtration without significant tubular secretion. After intravenous injection of contrast media, there is a rapid increase followed by a rapid decrease in plasma concentration of contrast media. Although most (88%) of the rapid decline is due to equilibration of the contrast material throughout the ECF, 12% of the decrease in contrast media concentration is due to excretion of the contrast media by the kidneys into the renal collecting systems and ureters. During this period, filtration of the contrast media is at its maximum. Therefore, it is within the first few moments after injection that the nephrogram, representing contrast media within the renal tubules, is at its peak intensity.

The degree of opacification of the urinary tract is not a function of the concentration of the contrast media in the urine alone, but it is the total amount of contrast media (urinary contrast concentration times the volume of urine produced) on which opaci-

fication depends. Thus, opacification depends on the total number of iodine atoms in the path of the x-ray beam rather than on their concentration in the urine. There is also a dose-related increase in the urine flow rate that occurs after contrast media administration, which is related to the fact that monomeric contrast media acts as an osmotic diuretic.

The rate of excretion of contrast media is greatest in the first 10 minutes after injection and falls logarithmically thereafter. With increasing time, the contrast media that had equilibrated with the ECF returns to the vascular space and is excreted. Approximately 24 hours is required to excrete 100% of the administered dose (Fig. 2.8).

The sequential change in the computed tomography (CT) attenuation value for the renal cortex that occurs after bolus administration of contrast media intravenously directly correlates with the amount of iodine administered. Indeed, a plot of CT number against time (Fig. 2.9) produces a curve similar in appearance to the plot of plasma contrast concentration against time. Therefore, the change in CT number in the renal cortex following contrast media administration accurately reflects the physiology of contrast media excretion.

Physiologic Considerations

In the past, overnight fluid restriction was often recommended to improve the diagnostic quality of excretory urography, by increasing the concentration and, thereby, the radiopacity of excreted contrast material in the renal collecting systems and ureters. The rationale of this approach was based on the physiologic principle that in a dehydrated state, ADH production is stimulated and results in more concentrated urine. Fluid restriction is not needed prior to performance of CT or MRI, however, and, in fact, is discouraged. Overhydration may have an adverse effect on pyelographic density

FIGURE 2.8. Graph demonstrating cumulative excretion of Hypaque. (From Cattell WR, Fry IK, Spencer AG, et al. Excretory urography 1-factors determining the excretion of Hypaque. *Br J Radiol.* 1967;40(476):561–571.)

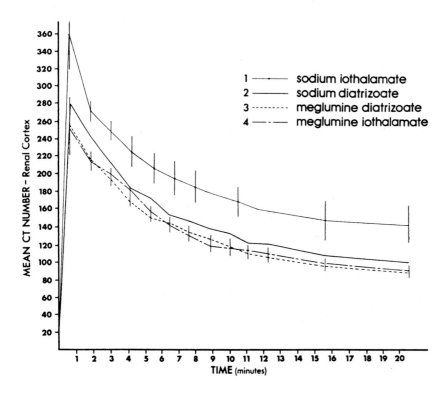

FIGURE 2.9. The sequential change in CT numbers measured in the renal cortex following an acute injection of contrast material shows a rapid decline. (From Brennan RE, Curtis JA, Pollack HM, et al. Sequential changes in the CT numbers of the normal canine kidney following intravenous contrast administration. I. The renal cortex. *Invest Radiol.* 1979;14(2):141–148.)

on CT or MRI in patients being hydrated with intravenous fluids. A "washout" of the pyelogram can occur if excretory phase CT is to be performed, although the quality of the nephrogram is usually unaffected. There is, however, no evidence that diagnostic accuracy is compromised by the reduced concentration of excreted contrast material in the renal collecting systems and ureters of these patients.

Phases of Contrast Enhancement on CT and MRI

On CT and MRI, four phases of contrast enhancement have been described: (1) an arterial phase, during which time abdominal arterial enhancement is highest, generally occurring at 20 to 40 seconds after initiation of contrast material injection; (2) a corticomedullary phase, at which time the arterial concentration decreases, but when there is a maximal difference in attenuation between hyperenhancing renal cortex and hypoenhancing renal medulla (peaking in most patients at 60 to 70 seconds after the contrast injection begins; (3) a nephrographic phase, during which time the renal cortex and medulla enhance similarly, resulting in renal parenchymal homogeneity, usually occurring at 90 to 120 seconds); and (4) an excretory phase, which begins with the appearance of excreted contrast material in the renal collecting systems, usually at about 120 seconds or longer.

Extrarenal (Vicarious) Excretion

In patients with normal renal function, <5% to 10% of injected low-osmolality contrast media is excreted via a nonrenal route. The primary routes of nonrenal excretion are through the biliary tract and the small bowel. In normal circumstances, this excretion is not detectable on plain radiographs, even when a high dose of contrast media is employed. Contrast media may be visible normally in the gallbladder, however, on CT scans obtained 15 to 48 hours after a large dose of contrast media is administered. This visibility is presumed to be related to the high contrast sensitivity of CT and is not a manifestation of renal or hepatic disease.

In patients with depressed renal function, however, excretion of the contrast material via the biliary and small bowel routes is increased and may be visible on plain films. Such excretion has been termed *vicarious excretion*. The exact mechanism for this phenomenon is not certain, but it is speculated that, in such patients, protein binding of the contrast media occurs and results in increased hepatic excretion. In addition to biliary excretion, there is evidence of direct transmural excretion of contrast media through the small bowel. Such excretion is usually not visible until the contrast media reaches the colon, where water absorption increases the concentration of the contrast media. Direct colon excretion of the contrast media is not thought to occur. There has been a concern that the administration of contrast media to patients with little or no renal function might have adverse hemodynamic effects, and therefore, immediate hemodialysis after contrast administration should be instituted. However, it has been shown that immediate postprocedure dialysis is not necessary and that even functionally anephric patients can be given nonionic contrast media with no discernible adverse effects. The contrast media so administered will eventually be excreted through biliary and small bowel routes and also removed at the time of subsequent dialysis.

CONTRAST MEDIA: PACKAGING

As can be seen, a variety of physical and chemical properties may be used to describe the contrast media in general use in the United States, the most important of which are ionicity and osmolality. With the older, ionic contrast media, the strength of the contrast media was frequently expressed in terms of percent contrast molecule concentration. This number represents the number of grams of the total contrast molecule per 100 mL of water. This designation does not, per se, describe the amount of iodine in solution, but in general, the higher the percent concentration, the more radiopaque the contrast media. Currently, many commonly used contrast media use a numerical designation to denote the amount of iodine in milligrams per milliliter of the contrast media. Thus, Conray 325 (Mallinckrodt Imaging, Hazelwood, MO), an ionic monomer, contains 325 mg of iodine per mL of solution. Isovue 370 (Bracco, Monroe, NJ), a nonionic monomer, contains 375 mg of iodine per mL of solution.

ACUTE ADVERSE REACTIONS TO CONTRAST MEDIA

Reactions to contrast media, although uncommon, continue to constitute a significant hazard to patients despite considerable research into their nature, incidence, and mechanisms. Fortunately, most adverse reactions are mild and self-limited, with symptoms including a metallic taste in the mouth, a sensation of warmth, and, occasionally, a few hives.

Adverse effects of contrast media can be divided into two groups: (1) allergic-like reactions, those which mimic an allergic response to contrast media, and (2) physiologic or chemotoxic effects, those thought to be secondary to a direct toxic effect of the contrast media. Because many of the allergic-like reactions to contrast media mimic those produced by true known allergens (i.e., urticaria or bronchospasm), but are not mediated by immunoglobulins, these reactions are sometimes referred to as "anaphylactoid" or "allergic-like" rather than anaphylactic.

ACUTE ALLERGIC-LIKE REACTIONS

Allergic-like reactions to nonionic contrast material are rare, in one series of more than 80,000 patients reported by Wang et al, occurring in 0.6% of patients injected for CT. Allergic-like reactions can be classified as (1) mild, (2) moderate, or (3) severe, with the vast majority of reactions being mild. Mild reactions are defined as those having only minor effects requiring no therapy. Moderate reactions are those that are transient and not life-threatening but usually requiring therapy. Severe reactions are defined as those that are life-threatening and that require intensive therapy. The more commonly encountered symptoms of these different types of allergic-like reactions are listed in Table 2.1.

Mechanism of Allergic-Like Contrast Reactions

There is no universally accepted mechanism that explains the diverse manifestations of allergic-like contrast reactions. Although an antigen–antibody-mediated mechanism has been suggested by some investigators, evidence indicates that, in the majority of cases, contrast reactions are not true allergic reactions. The fact that some patients react on their first exposure to contrast media (before any sensitization), that reactions are not consistent (upon reexposure), and that most repeat reactions are not progressive militates against the standard immune response theory. In addition, there are only occasional reports of circulating antibodies to contrast material having been identified. Some of these studies have shown, however, that a few patients manifesting anaphylaxis symptoms beyond simple urticaria have IgE-mediated reactions that can be detected through skin testing. Nonetheless, such testing has not been recommended as a routine procedure, as this will not detect the vast majority of patients for whom reactions occur unpredictably.

A variety of immune modulators appear to be involved in at least some contrast reactions. Contrast media can induce histamine release from mast cells and basophils without immunoglobulin mediation, but whether this can occur in sufficient quantities to produce the type of reaction seen with contrast hypersensitivity has been questioned. Activation of the complement system has also been shown to occur after contrast administration, and this mechanism is implicated by some, but whether a cause-and-effect relationship between complement activation and the clinical syndrome of con-

TABLE 2.1
Symptoms of Contrast Material Reactions

Mild

Physiologic

Dizziness
Headache
Heat sensation
Nausea
Mild vasovagal reaction (resolving quickly and without treatment)
Mild vomiting, retching
Arm pain

Allergic-like

Mild urticaria or edema
Limited cutaneous edema
Nasal congestion
Sneezing/stuffy nose/watery/red eyes

Moderate

Physiologic

Chest pain (angina)
Hypertension
Hypotension and bradycardia (vasovagal) requiring treatment
Protracted nausea or severe vomiting

Allergic-like

Generalized urticaria
Bronchospasm with mild or no hypoxia
Facial edema without dyspnea
Throat tightness or hoarseness without dyspnea

Severe

Physiologic

Arrhythmia
Cardiopulmonary arrest
Hypertensive crisis
Loss of consciousness
Pulmonary edema
Vasovagal reaction resistant to treatment
Seizures

Allergic-like

Bronchospasm resistant to treatment and/or with hypoxia
Loss of consciousness, including cardiopulmonary arrest
Laryngeal edema with stridor and/or hypoxia
Hypotension (systolic blood pressure <70 mm Hg) and tachycardia (rate > 100 bpm)
Pulmonary edema
Sustained cardiac arrhythmia

From ACR Manual on Contrast Media (v. 10.1)

trast sensitivity exists remains in doubt. Attention has also been directed to the contact system as a cause of reactions to contrast media. This system begins with activation of clotting factor XII (possibly by local disruption of the vascular endothelium as a result of the needle puncture and the introduction of the contrast media) and continues as a cascade involving the activation of kallikrein from prekallikrein and kinins from high molecular weight kininogens.

Risk Factors

Allergies and Asthma

A number of risk factors have been identified that place patients at increased risk for having an allergic-like contrast reaction (Table 2.2). A history of a previous reaction to the administration of contrast media is the greatest single predictor of an untoward reaction to a subsequent contrast media injection, increasing the risk of a subsequent reaction by a factor of about five. Fortunately, only a small minority of such patients will have an adverse reaction to a subsequent contrast injection. Thus, a history of prior mild or moderate reaction to contrast media should not be taken as an absolute contraindication to reexamination when a repeated study is based upon sound medical indications. A history of a severe reaction to contrast media, however, is considered a relative contraindication to reexamination in all, but the most urgent cases, due to the concern that should such a patient have another reaction, it could be equally, or even more, severe.

A history of prior exposure to contrast media without difficulty in the past does not confer immunity to a subsequent contrast reaction. Multiple cases have been reported in which patients suffered a contrast reaction after several prior studies that were performed without difficulty, or in which patients have reacted inconsistently to subsequent contrast material injections.

Patients with a history of allergy to food, drugs, and seasonal allergies (i.e., hay fever) or asthma also have an increased chance of having a contrast reaction, but the magnitude of this increased risk varies in the reported series (usually only doubling or tripling the risk of an adverse reaction in comparison to all exposed patients).

Shellfish

Although shellfish and contrast material both contain iodine, there is not believed to be any specific cross-reactivity. Therefore, patients with shellfish allergies are not felt to be at any significantly increased risk of having a contrast reaction, at least when compared to patients with other food or medication allergies. Contact allergy to iodine-containing products is also thought to be unrelated to contrast sensitivity. As such, sensitivity to such iodine-containing products such as povidone–iodine solution (Betadine; The Purdue Frederick Co., Norwalk, CT) should not be considered an absolute contraindication to the administration of iodinated contrast media.

Age

The incidence of mild, moderate, and severe reactions is approximately equal in all age groups. The data do not validate the commonly held notion that reactions are virtually unknown in the pediatric population. In fact, the large multicenter study by Katayama et al., published in 1990, found that there was a higher

TABLE 2.2
Risk Factors for Adverse Reactions to Contrast Media[a]
History of prior contrast reaction History of asthma History of allergy or atopy Cardiac disease Medications (interleukin-2)
[a]Modified from Morcos SK, Thomsen HS. Adverse reactions to iodinated contrast media. *Eur Radiol.* 2001;11: 1267–1275.

incidence of reactions in younger patients. However, most contrast reaction deaths occur in patients with significant preexisting cardiac or vascular disease.

Dose

The incidence of allergic-like reactions is unrelated to the dose for mild and moderate reactions; for severe reactions, the incidence may be slightly higher when larger doses (>20 g of iodine) are used, although the data with respect to severe reactions and dose are limited.

Type of Examination

Intra-arterial contrast injection appears to reduce the overall incidence of reactions by approximately one-half; however, it may be associated with a higher percentage of severe reactions than those occurring after intravenous injections. With nonvascular examinations (e.g., retrograde pyelography, cystography, or GI studies), the exact incidence of reactions is very difficult to determine. Although allergic-like reactions and deaths have been reported following nonvascular studies, these are extremely rare. In these cases, it is assumed that a small amount of contrast media has been absorbed into the vascular system across the urothelium or bowel mucosa.

Timing of Reactions

Most contrast reactions begin within the first 10 to 20 minutes after injection of the contrast media; some patients have symptoms almost immediately, whereas in others, the reaction is not noted until the end of the examination.

Miscellaneous

Patients receiving β-adrenergic blockers or those with severe underlying cardiovascular disease have been suggested to be at increased risk for developing respiratory allergic-like reactions, especially bronchospasm.

Prevention of Anaphylactoid Contrast Reactions

Attempts to predict or modify allergic-like reactions to contrast media have resulted in varying degrees of success. The use of an intravenous test dose has not been shown to predict a subsequent adverse reaction to the full dose of contrast media, and its use has been abandoned. Furthermore, since the likelihood of an allergic-like reaction is felt to be no less likely and the reaction no less severe with a small dose of contrast material than with a larger dose, it is an accepted fact that if a patient is going to have reaction, a reaction of identical severity would simply occur to the test dose. Similarly, the use of antihistamines alone, either mixed with the contrast media or administered immediately before the contrast study, has not modified the overall incidence of severe adverse reactions to contrast media.

Premedication with Corticosteroids

Because of the allergic-like nature of idiosyncratic reactions, the empirical use of corticosteroids to prepare "high-risk" patients for contrast studies has been used for many years. A multi-institutional randomized prospective double-blinded study reported by Lasser et al. (1987) showed that two doses of orally administered corticosteroids (methylprednisolone, 32 mg) at 12 and 2 hours prior to a contrast-enhanced examination (utilizing the previously employed ionic monomeric contrast agents) significantly reduced the incidence of contrast reactions of all types in a group of both low-risk and high-risk patients (when compared with placebo). There was no such protective effect in a group of patients who received a single dose of steroids 2 hours before examination.

Pretreatment with corticosteroids is also likely effective prior to administration of nonionic contrast material. In a subsequent randomized controlled study, Lasser et al. (1994) demonstrated that pretreatment with 32 mg of prednisolone beginning 6 or more hours prior to contrast material injection significantly decreased the incidence of mild reactions in premedicated patients receiving intravenous nonionic contrast examinations. Although there was also a decrease in the number of moderate and severe reactions, this difference did not reach statistical significance.

Although the "Lasser" premedication regimen is employed today by some radiologists, the more commonly used regimen has been that recommended by Greenberger and Patterson (1991), which has been shown to be effective in high-risk patients receiving nonionic contrast media. This regimen consists of administration of 50 mg of prednisone 13, 7, and 1 hour prior and 50 mg of diphenhydramine 1 hour prior to contrast material injection.

Breakthrough Reactions

Some patients who have had prior allergic-like contrast material reactions will have subsequent contrast reactions despite the use of premedication with corticosteroids. Mervak et al. (2015) found that of 626 patients who were premedicated due to a prior contrast material reaction, only 13 patients had a subsequent reaction. These reactions, which occurred despite premedication, are referred to as breakthrough reactions. The patients who were at highest risk of a breakthrough reaction were those who had had both prior contrast reactions and who had at least one severe allergy to another medication or to food. In this series, of 425 patients who were premedicated for reasons other than a prior contrast reaction (usually food or medication allergies), none had a breakthrough reaction.

Interestingly, if a breakthrough reaction is to occur in a patient who has been premedicated, it will be of similar severity to the initial index reaction about 80% of the time. The remaining breakthrough reactions are equally likely to be more or less severe than the index reaction. A recent study by Davenport et al. (2009) also found that repeat breakthrough reactions are uncommon and, if they occur, are also likely to be of similar severity to a prior breakthrough reaction. So, for example, if a patient had a previous reaction despite premedication, it is acceptable to reinject him or her in the future following additional premedication, as long as the previous breakthrough reaction was mild.

Risks of Premedication with Corticosteroids

There are a number of potential risks of premedication, most of which have been overstated. Theoretically, infections can be exacerbated, peptic ulcer disease can be made worse, steroid psychosis can be encountered, and tumor lysis syndromes can be precipitated (such as in patients with lymphoma). One of the more commonly encountered concerns relates to the transient hyperglycemia that can be produced by even a brief course of corticosteroids, a phenomenon which could be problematic in some patients, particularly those with diabetes mellitus. Recent studies by Davenport and colleagues (2010, 2011) have shown, however, that transient hyperglycemia following corticosteroid premedication is almost always mild (with a rise of serum glucose levels usually between 5 and 20 mg/dL) and is only rarely associated with any symptoms, even in diabetic patients. Interestingly, in Davenport et al's series, diabetic patients who did not receive corticosteroids also often developed hyperglycemia after imaging studies. The authors concluded that serum glucose elevations in imaged diabetic patients are, therefore, often at least partially related to underlying illnesses that precipitated the need for such imaging in addition to the premedication regimens.

Patients have rarely reported having allergic reactions to steroid premedication. Such allergies are likely due to the formulations of oral steroids, which are usually comprised of a steroid-succinate ester, or to other additives. If a patient has a history of a steroid allergy, it has been suggested that he or she be referred to an allergist prior to corticosteroid administration. There is some cross-reactivity to different steroid preparations. The allergist can perform skin testing to a variety of steroid compounds to determine which steroids can be administered safely prior to contrast material injection.

Perhaps the greatest risk of corticosteroid premedication relates to the delay in patient care that results from administration of a full 13-hour premedication regimen. In a recent study by Davenport and associates (2016), inpatients who received corticosteroid premedication prior to CT had a significantly longer median length of hospital stay (by 25 hours) and were at increased risk of adverse consequences, especially hospital-acquired infections. The authors concluded that it would cost approximately $159,000 (in additional inpatient stay charges) to prevent a contrast reaction of any severity by administering corticosteroid prophylaxis. The cost to prevent a severe reaction would be dramatically higher (at $131,211,100). Theoretically, inpatient premedication would result in 0.04 more hospital-acquired infection-related deaths (as a result of prolonged hospitalization) to prevent a reaction of any severity and 32 more hospital-acquired infection-related deaths to prevent a severe reaction.

As can be seen, there are both benefits and risks of corticosteroid premedication, all of which must be considered for patients on an individual basis. At the present time, as a recent survey by O'Malley et al. (2011) has shown, it is generally considered the standard of care to administer premedication to patients who have had prior moderate or severe urticarial or any respiratory or cardiac allergic-type reactions to contrast media in the past, with the safest alternative being avoidance of contrast material administration to patients who have had prior life-threatening allergic-like reactions to contrast media. In comparison, there is some variation in behavior with respect to whether premedication is needed in patients who have developed one or a few hives from contrast media or in patients who have allergies to other substances or asthma. In these cases, no standard of care has been established.

DELAYED REACTIONS

Delayed reactions to contrast media (defined as those beginning between 1 hour and 2 days after contrast administration) are usually self-limiting and most often are manifested by headache or a skin eruption (rash or hives). The mechanism of delayed reactions is not known, although there may be a delayed immunologic component. An atypical form of late reaction to contrast media has also been reported in patients receiving interleukin-2 for chemotherapy (usually occurring in patients who have had recent injections of interleukin-2 [within the past few weeks]). The majority of such reactions occur 1 to 8 hours after contrast exposure and consist of erythema, diarrhea, flulike symptoms, flushing, joint pain, pruritus, and other nonspecific symptoms. Such reactions mimic those produced by the chemotherapy itself. In an occasional patient, such symptoms may be sufficiently severe to require hospitalization.

ACUTE ADVERSE PHYSIOLOGIC/ CHEMOTOXIC EFFECTS

Chemotoxic effects are those effects of the contrast media thought to be due to direct organ toxicity of the contrast media. Most physiologic effects of contrast media are mild and include a metallic taste or a sensation of warmth. Some diseases can be made worse by contrast material injection, including underlying chronic kidney disease (CKD) (see section below on Postcontrast Acute Kidney Injury), arrhythmias, myasthenia gravis, and hyperthyroidism (when the latter is severe and poorly controlled). In humans, contrast media overdosage results in neurotoxicity, including the induction of seizures.

The exact dose in humans at which this occurs is not known, but systemic doses of contrast media of over 5 to 6 mL/kg should be exceeded only in special circumstances.

POSTCONTRAST ACUTE KIDNEY INJURY

Reports linking contrast media with the development of acute renal failure began to appear with increasing frequency in the early 1970s. The controversy in how often this occurs is related, in part, to varying definitions of what constitutes acute kidney injury (AKI). Traditionally, most authors have defined postcontrast AKI as an increase in serum creatinine levels of 50% or 0.5 mg/dL within 48 hours of contrast media injection. In comparison, the Acute Kidney Injury Network (AKIN) defines acute kidney injury as an increase in serum creatinine of 0.3 mg/dL or of 50% within 48 hours.

AKI associated with contrast material is usually nonoliguric, and in the typical case, the serum creatinine peaks in 3 to 5 days and then returns to baseline values within 7 to 10 days. In rare cases, the renal failure is oliguric. Renal damage in oliguric patients is more likely to be permanent. The clinical impact of postcontrast AKI can be significant. Levy compared the mortality of a group of patients in whom postcontrast AKI developed with a matched group who had received contrast media but did not develop AKI. The mortality rate of the group with AKI was 34% compared with 7% for the group in whom AKI did not develop.

In vitro experiments have, indeed, demonstrated that iodinated contrast media is nephrotoxic, likely as a result of several potentially detrimental effects: (1) hemodynamic effects caused by vasoconstriction and medullary ischemia, (2) direct toxicity of contrast material molecules on the proximal tubule cells, and also, possibly, (3) free radical formation.

Recent studies have suggested, however, that it is probable that the in vivo nephrotoxic effects of contrast media have been greatly exaggerated. This has resulted from the lack of control groups of patients who did not receive contrast material in the vast number of published studies on postcontrast AKI, a point that was emphasized by Rao and Newhouse in 2006. More recently, McDonald and colleagues have demonstrated that when controlled studies have been performed, the incidence of post-CT AKI is often found to be higher in patients who have had unenhanced CTs than in those who have had contrast-enhanced studies. Results in these studies suggest that AKI following CT is often unrelated to contrast material administration and is likely due to a variety of additional causes, including a patient's underlying disease. The identification of higher AKI rates in patients undergoing unenhanced CT probably reflects the fact that, in these nonrandomized studies, patients were preferentially selected to undergo unenhanced CT because of other risk factors that they had for developing AKI.

Even more recently, two seminal studies from the Mayo Clinic (McDonald et al., 2013) and the University of Michigan (Davenport et al., 2013) have utilized a statistical technique called "propensity matching" in an attempt to compare AKI rates in patients who did receive a contrast-enhanced CT to those in a group of patients who did not receive contrast material (who were selected and matched with the contrast-enhanced group on a 1:1 basis), with both groups of patients being equally likely to have received contrast material based upon a large number of preidentified risk factors for AKI. In the Mayo Clinic study, there was no significant difference in AKI rates between those patients receiving contrast enhanced and noncontrast CT, including in patients with severe CKD. In the University of Michigan study, the only significant difference in AKI rates was observed in patients with severe CKD (36% vs. 19% in patients with an eGFR < 30 mL/min/1.73 m²). While the authors in the Davenport et al. study also found post CT AKI to be slightly more common in patients with an eGFR of 30 to 44 mL/min/1.73 m² in patients receiving versus those not receiving contrast media (17% vs. 14%),

this difference was not significant. Both the McDonald et al. and the Davenport et al. studies indicate that postcontrast AKI due to the contrast material is rare and, if it exists at all, is only found in patients with severe kidney disease.

Risk Factors for Postcontrast AKI

Preexisting Renal Insufficiency

Preexisting renal insufficiency has been identified as risk factor for postcontrast AKI; however, as previously stated, most cases of postcontrast AKI are actually not due to the contrast material injection itself, but rather to other coexistent morbidities. If contrast material does cause AKI, it most likely does so only in patients with an eGFR < 30 mL/dL. It is also possible that patients who are currently having an episode of AKI are at higher risk for developing true contrast-induced nephrotoxicity.

Because of the evidence that links the development of postcontrast AKI with severe preexisting renal insufficiency, many radiologists believe that routine determination of a patient's renal function is necessary before contrast material is administered, at least in patients with suspected or known CKD. In the outpatient setting, in particular, this policy can lead to patient delays, increased costs, and patient discomfort. Choyke et al. (1998) showed that a routine patient questionnaire to determine whether the patient has a history of prior kidney disease or surgery, diabetes, proteinuria, gout, or hypertension successfully screens 99% of patients in whom the creatinine is sufficiently elevated that the contrast material might not be routinely administered. The authors concluded that patients without such histories did not need a serum creatinine level to be measured prior to imaging. The ACR recommends that renal function testing should be performed prior to contrast-enhanced studies only in patients with any of the following risk factors: age over 60 years, history of renal disease (including dialysis, kidney transplant, solitary kidney, renal cancer, or renal surgery), hypertension requiring medical therapy, diabetes mellitus, or metformin or metformin-containing drugs administration). While, in the past, serum creatinine levels were assessed to determine baseline renal function, it is now recommended that eGFR levels be calculated instead, as this allows for a more accurate estimation of renal function (Fig. 2.10).

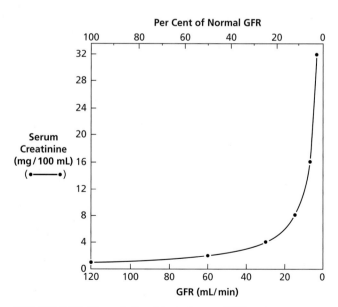

FIGURE 2.10. The relationship between GFR and serum creatinine. Serum creatinine rises slowly with early reductions in GFR. The rise in serum creatinine is most easily detected with a GFR of <60 mL/min.

Diabetes Mellitus

Although prior results have been conflicting, the recent propensity-matched analyses by McDonald and Davenport and associates have not found the incidence of AKI to be increased in patients with diabetes mellitus, at least in those patients who have an eGFR of 30 mL/min/1.73 m^2 or higher.

Dehydration

Some authors have speculated that dehydration from the contrast study or from the preparation for the study may play a role in the development of postcontrast AKI, at least in patients with severely compromised renal function.

Dose of Contrast

The dose of contrast material used has been felt by most authorities to be a factor in the development of postcontrast AKI, at least in susceptible patients. It is generally accepted that contrast-induced nephrotoxicity is more likely to occur in susceptible patients when higher doses of contrast material are administered.

Type of Contrast Media

Currently, there is no generally accepted advantage of nonionic dimers over nonionic monomers in terms of postcontrast AKI prevention.

Route of Administration

Postcontrast AKI may be more common after intra-arterial than intravenous contrast media injections. This is likely due to two factors: (1) with intra-arterial injections, the kidneys are exposed to the higher concentrations of contrast media in the arterial system, and (2) independent of contrast material injection, catheter manipulation in the arterial system can lead to dislodgement of atherosclerotic emboli from the aorta, some of which can enter the renal arteries and compromise renal function. For this reason, direct comparison of postcontrast AKI rates in patients receiving intra-arterial versus intravenous injections is likely not appropriate.

Other Factors

A multitude of other factors have been implicated in the past in the development of postcontrast AKI. These include advanced age, hypertension, peripheral vascular disease, congestive heart failure, proteinuria, and liver dysfunction. Multiple contrast studies within a short interval (72 hours or less) also have been implicated (probably because they expose the patient to a cumulatively high dose of contrast material in a short period of time). Patients with multiple myeloma have long been thought to be at increased risk for postcontrast AKI because of precipitation of myeloma proteins in the renal tubules. Most authorities now feel contrast-enhanced studies in patients with myeloma and normal serum creatinine can be performed with safety, provided dehydration is avoided. Several studies have shown that contrast media acts as a powerful uricosuric agent, and this mechanism has been implicated in the development of acute urate nephropathy in patients with hyperuricemia. This syndrome may also be encountered in patients with myeloproliferative disorders or leukemia after chemotherapy. It should be emphasized, however, that recent studies have failed to confirm the independent association of any of these factors with postcontrast AKI.

Prevention of Postcontrast AKI

Because treatment options are limited once oliguric renal failure has developed, much effort has been aimed at prevention of postcontrast AKI. Studies have suggested that IV hydration, preferably with isotonic fluids [normal saline or lactated Ringers]), is more effective than oral hydration. The best results seem to be achieved when intravenous hydration is performed (at a rate of about 125 mL/h) for a 24-hour period, beginning up to 12 hours before the procedure and continuing for up to 24 hours after the procedure.

In an initial study, Merten et al. showed that hydration with sodium bicarbonate was more effective than saline alone in preventing AKI. The authors postulated that bicarbonate might be more effective in reducing the number of free radicals compared with saline. This paper has been criticized by some because of the low number of "events" in the bicarbonate group and the fact that the trial was stopped early. Subsequent studies have had mixed results, and it remains unclear whether bicarbonate possesses any advantages over saline hydration. Vasodilators, including calcium channel blockers and low-dose dopamine, adenosine antagonists such as theophylline and dipyridamole, and the antioxidant N-acetylcysteine have all been recommended in the past, however, none of these pharmacologic interventions is now believed to be beneficial. Recent studies have suggested that the use of statins reduces the likelihood of AKI developing after cardiac catheterization. This likely reflects a reduction in AKI caused by multiple entities, including contrast material.

METFORMIN

Great attention has been drawn previously to the extremely uncommon development of lactic acidosis in diabetic patients taking the oral antihyperglycemic agent, metformin (Glucophage [Bristol-Myers Squibb, Princeton, NJ] or a large number of combination drugs) following iodinated contrast material administration. Because the kidneys excrete metformin, the continued use of this agent in the face of renal failure may be associated with metformin toxicity, the most feared manifestation of which is lactic acidosis, which can be fatal. Contrast material does not cause lactic acidosis in patients taking metformin; however, because it might cause AKI, patients on metformin could be at increased risk for developing lactic acidosis following contrast material administration.

It must be emphasized that the association between lactic acidosis and contrast administration is extremely rare. The package insert for Glucophage has stated that metformin can be continued up until the administration of contrast material but should be withheld after the contrast study until it has been determined that the patient has normal renal function. With the new knowledge that contrast-induced nephrotoxicity is much less common than previously thought, many have recommended that less strict criteria be utilized. Currently, the American College of Radiology Committee on Drugs and Contrast Media recommends that metformin need not be discontinued prior contrast material administration in patients with an eGFR of 30 mL/min/1.73 m^2 or more, and that there is also no need to retest a patient's renal function after contrast material is injected. This is because the likelihood of contrast-induced nephrotoxicity is exceedingly low in these patients. The committee does recommend, however, that metformin be discontinued in patients with an eGFR < 30 mL/min or in patients who are having an episode of AKI. Of course, metformin should not be used in these patients in the first place (due to the risk of lactic acidosis). In comparison, the Federal Drug Administration (FDA) now states that metformin need not be discontinued in patients with an eGFR of 60 or more mL/min/1.73 m^2. According to the FDA, metformin should be discontinued in any patient with an eGFR < 60 mL/min/1.73 m^2 and then only reinstituted once renal function is rechecked and found to be unchanged 48 hours after contrast material administration.

EXTRAVASATION OF IODINATED CONTRAST MEDIA

Subcutaneous or intradermal extravasation is an occasional complication of contrast material injection, nearly always encountered during attempted contrast material injection for CT, using a mechanical injector. The incidence of extravasations has been estimated to be 0.1% to 0.9% of contrast injections. Larger volume extravasations are more likely in children, the elderly, or other patients who may not be able to complain when the contrast material is extravasating. Extravasations occur more commonly when the injection is made in either the hand or the foot, with these cites likely chosen as a result of difficult venous access. Extravasations may result in local pain, erythema, and swelling, symptoms, which usually resolve without sequelae, even when amounts as large as 150 mL are extravasated.

Severe complications are extremely rare (<<1% of extravasations), with the most common severe complication being a compartment syndrome. Tissue necrosis and dermal sloughing can also occur following even small amounts of extravasation. Compartment syndromes can be difficult to identify initially, and if a patient's symptoms do not improve or worsen over time, consultation with a surgeon (plastic surgeon, vascular surgeon, or orthopedic surgeon) should be obtained. Features typical of a compartment syndrome include decreased capillary refill and paresthesias. Treatment of compartment syndrome is fasciotomy. Long-term sequelae (including the need for skin grafting) can result after extravasation, even if a fasciotomy is performed. These are more likely if surgery is delayed.

It is unclear whether there is any effective immediate treatment for most extravasation injuries or even whether such treatment is necessary in the vast majority of cases. Still, it is recommended that cold compresses be applied immediately. Elevation of the affected extremity above the level of the heart is also suggested. The injection of saline or water to achieve local dilution and/or the local injection of chemicals, including hyaluronidase, is not recommended. A protocol for the management of extravasations has been recommended by the ACR Committee on Drugs and Contrast Media and is summarized in Table 2.3.

RARE ADVERSE EFFECTS OF IODINATED CONTRAST MATERIAL

Hematologic Effects

The older ionic contrast media were noted to inhibit platelet aggregation and cause a prolongation of the thrombin time by inhibition of fibrin monomer polymerization. These anticoagulant properties had a potentially beneficial effect during angiography by helping to prevent thrombus formation in catheters and syringes. This antithrombogenic effect is not as pronounced with nonionic contrast media, however.

In patients with sickle cell anemia, older ionic contrast media is known to provoke sickling and occasional development of sickle cell crisis. This is not an acknowledged complication of nonionic contrast agents.

Chemical phlebitis may develop rarely after injection of contrast media, particularly when it is used for lower extremity venography. The likelihood of phlebitis, which is already low with use of low-osmolality contrast agents, can be further reduced using diluted contrast media and by other measures including use of a heparinized saline flush following the procedure. Phlebitis may also be rarely seen in patients in whom the contrast media has been injected in the upper extremity for other imaging studies.

Iodism

Iodism, which is an acute reaction to the iodine itself, is a syndrome characterized by sialadenitis, diarrhea, and occasionally pulmonary edema that has been reported rarely after contrast media administration. Such cases are referred to as "iodine mumps."

GADOLINIUM-BASED MAGNETIC RESONANCE CONTRAST AGENTS

Classification of Gadolinium-Based MR Contrast Agents

MR contrast agents are paramagnetic compounds that have chemically unpaired electrons and, as such, are associated with a magnetic moment much more powerful than a nuclear magnetic moment.

TABLE 2.3	
Recommended Protocol for the Treatment of Contrast Extravasation	
Initial Treatment	Subsequent Therapy
Elevation of affected extremity above the heart	Daily phone calls by nurse or radiologist until manifestations resolve to assess for the following:
Ice packs (15- to 60-min applications three times per day for 1–3 d)	Residual pain
Close observation for up to 2–4 h with release from department after physician evaluation of the patient	Blistering
	Redness or other skin color change
Clear instructions to the patient to seek immediate medical assessment if any signs of vascular or neurologic compromise develop or for worsening swelling or pain	Hardness
	Increased or decreased temperature of skin at extravasation site (compared with temperature of the skin elsewhere)
Surgical consultation if there is concern for a "significant" extravasation injury	Change in sensation distal to site of extravasation
All instructions and treatments must be clearly documented including the estimated amount and type of contrast involved.	Completion of a contrast material extravasation form (for departmental monitoring and quality assurance)
	Progress note (for medical record)

TABLE 2.4			
Approved GBCAs in the United States			
GBCA	Linear/Macrocyclic	Ionic/Nonionic	Stability
Gadodiamide (Omniscan—GE HealthCare)	Linear	Nonionic	Lower
Gadoversetamide (Optimark—Mallinckrodt)	Linear	Nonionic	Lower
Gadopentetate dimeglumine (Magnevist—Bayer)	Linear	Ionic	Higher
Gadobenate dimeglumine (MultiHance—Bracco)	Linear	Ionic	Higher
Gadoxetate disodium (Eovist—Bayer)	Linear	Ionic	Higher
Gadofosveset trisodium (Ablavar—Lantheus)	Linear	Ionic	Higher
Gadoteridol (ProHance—Bracco)	Macrocyclic	Nonionic	Higher
Gadobutrol (Gadavist—Bayer)	Macrocyclic	Nonionic	Higher
Gadoterate meglumine (Dotarem—Guerbet)	Macrocyclic	Ionic	Higher

From ACR Manual on Contrast Media v 10.1.

Gadolinium-based compounds, which are approved for use in the United States, are water soluble and therefore have a biologic distribution similar to iodinated contrast agents. There are currently nine FDA-approved gadolinium-based contrast agents (GBCAs) (Table 2.4). All but one agent are excreted primarily by the kidneys. One agent, gadoxetate (Eovist [Bayer Pharmaceuticals), has approximately 50% renal and 50% hepatic excretion.

Although all GBCAs contain a ligand that surrounds the gadolinium atom, some are classified as linear and others as macrocyclic (depending upon whether or not the molecule surrounds the gadolinium as an intact ring). Macrocyclic agents have greater stability than do the linear agents. GBCAs can also be classified as ionic or nonionic, although this distinction is thought to have less significance than it does for the iodinated contrast agents.

Acute Adverse Reactions to GBCAs

All of the gadolinium-based paramagnetic compounds have proven to be remarkably free of acute adverse effects. Acute reactions to all of the commercially available GBCAs occur with a much lower frequency than do reactions to iodinated media. For example, among 78,353 IV administrations of GBCAs, Dillman et al. found an adverse reaction rate of only 0.07%. The vast majority of reactions were mild; however, there were four severe reactions (but no deaths). Acute reactions most frequently manifest as nausea and vomiting (25% to 40%), pain at the injection site (13% to 25%), headache (18%), paresthesias (8% to 9%), and dizziness (7% to 8%). Urticarial reactions have also been reported. Life-threatening anaphylactoid and even fatal reactions are exceedingly uncommon but have been encountered.

Risk factors for adverse reactions to GBCAs are similar to those for iodinated contrast agents and include patients with prior adverse reactions to GBCAs, other food or medication allergies, and asthma. It should be noted that patients who have had prior allergic-like reactions to iodinated contrast agents are felt to be no more likely to have an allergic-like reaction to a GBCA than are patients with other medication or food allergies.

Nephrogenic Systemic Fibrosis

A systemic disorder most obviously manifested in the skin, nephrogenic systemic fibrosis (NSF), has been identified in some dialysis patients, end-stage renal disease patients not yet on dialysis, and occasional patients experiencing an episode of AKI, all of whom have also undergone contrast-enhanced MR examinations with GBCA, with the association between NSF and GBCAs first identified in 2006. NSF results in large areas of hardened skin with raised plaques and increased dermal deposits of mucin. In some cases, the patient is unable to flex or straighten their extremities. Complaints of muscle weakness are common. Death may occur in some patients as a result of parenchymal organ involvement. There is no known effective treatment.

NSF has developed in approximately 2% to 7% of patients with severe CKD (almost always on dialysis or near dialysis) or AKI who have been exposed to GBCAs, with the overwhelming majority of patients having received three of the less stable agents (gadodiamide, gadoversetamide, or gadopentetate dimeglumine). There have been only case reports of patients developing NSF who were exposed ONLY to the other GBCAs. Patients who have received high doses of the high risk GBCAs (such as for magnetic resonance angiography) or multiple repeated studies have been more likely to develop the disease.

The most widely held theory as to the cause of NSF is that in the presence of renal failure, clearance of GBCA from the blood is delayed, providing more time for dissociation of the gadolinium atom from the chelate molecule by a process known as transmetallation. The gadolinium then precipitates with other organic anions and is deposited in the skin, subcutaneous tissues, and many visceral organs. This is followed by a strong immune response that leads to thickening and fibrosis. Other factors, such as metabolic acidosis, other proinflammatory events, erythropoietin therapy, and immunosuppression have been implicated but have not been confirmed to play a role. Clearly, other unknown factors must be involved, however, as the majority of patients exposed even to the "high-risk" gadolinium agents do not get NSF.

The recognition of GBCA exposure and severe renal insufficiency as cofactors in the development of NSF has prompted radiologists to create guidelines to screen at risk patients prior to GBCA administration. Specifically, it is now recommended that GBCA administration be avoided when possible in patients with CKD who have eGFR levels of under 30 mL/min/1.73 m^2 or in patients with AKI; however, if GBCA injection is needed in these patients, then the three "high-risk" agents should be avoided. When GBCAs are required, the lowest dose needed to obtain a diagnostic study should be used. As a result of these modifications, the number of encountered cases of NSF has decreased substantially since 2006. At the present time, only isolated cases of NSF are being reported, with many of these possibly related to GBCA exposure that occurred years go.

Gadolinium Retention in the Brain and Bones

It has been known for many years that small amounts of gadolinium are retained in the bones following GBCA administration, with the retained amounts higher for linear nonionic than macrocyclic and ionic agents. A number of recent studies have demonstrated that there is also progressive gadolinium accumulation in the brains of patients who have been exposed to GBCAs, with the gadolinium producing areas of high T1 signal intensity in the dentate nucleus and globus pallidus (Kanda et al. 2015; McDonald et al. 2015). This accumulation is most pronounced in patients who have been exposed to the least stable GBCAs and is higher in patients who have had more GBCA exposures. It has occurred in all patients, including those with normal renal function. At the present time, gadolinium retention in the brain has not been associated with neurologic deficits, although it remains to be seen whether or not there will be any longer term complications of this accumulation.

TREATMENT OF ADVERSE REACTIONS TO CONTRAST MEDIA

Every physician using contrast media must be prepared to deal with contrast reactions, and all personnel involved in intravascular contrast administration must be familiar with the location of emergency drugs and equipment. A common sense approach to dealing with emergency contrast reaction should be used, because overtreatment may be as disastrous as undertreatment. Familiarity with the basic principles of cardiopulmonary resuscitation (now ordered as C, circulation; A, airway; and then B, breathing) is mandatory. The physician responsible for the contrast media injection must be immediately available after the injection. Equipment for resuscitation, including blood pressure monitoring equipment, pulse oximetry, drugs, oxygen, and appropriate tubing for administration of oxygen or suction, must be immediately available. Convenient access to other equipment including automated external defibrillators is also required. It is prudent to inject the contrast media through a secure intravenous line that is left in place for several minutes after the injection, so that immediate venous access is available.

While the radiologist should be prepared to deal with mild and moderate reactions, as well as the initial therapy of severe reactions, life-threatening reactions occur so infrequently in the career of an average radiologist, that, in inpatient settings, it is prudent to have available assistance of other physicians who deal with resuscitative emergencies on a more frequent basis. Only general principles for the initiation of therapy will be offered in the paragraphs that follow.

At the first sign of a significant reaction, the patient should be questioned promptly, so that a brief description of the patient's symptoms and his or her medical history can be obtained. The patient's pulse and blood pressure should be obtained. It may occasionally be necessary to perform chest auscultation to assess the adequacy of ventilation. Appropriate therapy for acute reactions to contrast media is summarized in Table 2.5.

Mild Reactions

For the most part, mild reactions do not require therapy. Nausea and vomiting are generally self-limited. Patients experiencing these symptoms should be closely monitored, however, because nausea and vomiting and other mild symptoms can be the precursors of a major reaction.

Most of the time, no treatment is needed for mild urticarial reactions. Occasionally, limited urticarial reactions may benefit from the administration of antihistamines, primarily for their antipruritic effects. Caution should be exercised when using many antihistamines, particularly in outpatients, because of the tendency of some, particularly the commonly used antihistamine diphenhydramine, to cause drowsiness.

More extensive dermal reactions usually respond to antihistamines (i.e., diphenhydramine 50 mg IV given over 1 or 2 minutes or, rarely, cimetidine 300 mg IV, diluted in 10 mL of 5% dextrose solution administered slowly). Epinephrine (1:1,000), 0.3 mL administered intramuscularly (usually via an injector [EpiPen—Mylan {Canonsberg, PA}]), may be necessary if the urticaria is so extensive that generalized edema is present.

TABLE **2.5**

Treatment of Acute Contrast Media Reactions

Type of Reaction	Drug	Dose/Route	Comments
Nausea and vomiting	None	—	Supportive measures; usually transient
Urticaria—mild	None	—	Self-limiting; supportive therapy only
Urticaria—generalized	Diphenhydramine	25–50 mg, PO slow IV or IM	Observe for drowsiness
Bronchospasm/wheezing			
Mild	Albuterol	Deep inhalations x2	β-Agonist inhaler
Moderate or severe	Epinephrine 1:1,000	0.3 mL IM	
	Epinephrine 1:10,000	1 mL IV	
Facial edema	Epinephrine 1:1,000	0.3 mL IM	May be repeated x3
laryngospasm/edema	Epinephrine 1:10,000	1 mL IV	If severe, may require intubation
Hypotensive bradycardia	Elevate legs		
	IV fluid (LR or NS)	Rapid infusion	
	Atropine	0.6–1 mg IV slowly	
Hypotensive tachycardia	IV fluids (LR or NS)	Rapid infusion	Place patient in Trendelenburg; O_2
	Epinephrine 1:10,000	1 mL IV	

Note: For all potential respiratory and hypotensive reactions, vital signs should be obtained. Administration of oxygen (6–10 L/min by mask) should be considered. Oxygen saturation should be monitored with a pulse oximeter. If respiratory or hypotensive symptoms deteriorate despite treatment, consider calling a code.

Respiratory Reactions

Bronchospasm is often treated effectively with a β-agonist metered dose inhaler (albuterol). The patient can be given two inhalations consecutively, with dosing repeated, as necessary. Bronchospasm that is unresponsive to a beta agonist inhaler and laryngospasm are often effectively treated with epinephrine (in a 1:1,000 concentration), 0.3 mL administered intramuscularly (usually via an injector) or epinephrine (in a 1:10,000 concentration) 1 mL intravenously. The dose of intramuscular epinephrine may be repeated in 15 minutes or more if no response is obtained or if symptoms recur. Intravenous administration of epinephrine should be slow, albeit titrated to the patient's symptoms. If intravenous administration is given at a rate of 1 mL every 5 to 10 minutes, the drug can be given as a constant infusion. Corticosteroids have no immediate impact on respiratory distress, but can be administered as a supplemental agent to prevent a recurrence of symptoms.

Hypotension

It is crucial to distinguish vasovagal (hypotensive bradycardia) from hypotensive allergic-like reactions, since treatment of these reactions is different; however, all patients who develop hypotension should be treated by raising the legs and with large volumes of isotonic intravenous fluid (500 to 1,000 mL of normal saline or lactated Ringers, administered rapidly). Supplemental oxygen should be administered (at high doses using a face mask rather than a nasal cannula).

Vasovagal reactions are characterized by sinus bradycardia and hypotension. When bradycardia is severe, atropine, 0.6 to 1 mg intravenously, should be administered. An additional dose of 0.5 mg may be administered every 5 minutes until a heart rate of 60 beats per minute is achieved or a maximum dose of 3 mg has been given.

In patients having hypotensive allergic-like reactions, tachycardia is usually present (unless the patient is taking β-blockers). In persistently symptomatic hypotensive patients, 0.3 mL of 1:1,000 epinephrine can be administered intramuscularly (usually via an injector), or 1 mL of 1:10,000 epinephrine can be administered intravenously.

Patients taking β-adrenergic blocking agents (i.e., propranolol) may present a special problem in diagnosis, should hypotension develop during the course of a contrast reaction. Beta-blockers produce a sinus bradycardia that may not vary in the face of shock, theoretically making the distinction of a vasovagal reaction from an anaphylactoid reaction difficult. However, bradycardia in vasovagal reactions tends to be more severe than that encountered in patients receiving β-blockers, so distinction is often possible.

Because epinephrine is both an α- and a β-adrenergic agonist, an administered β-blocker may successfully neutralize the β effects of epinephrine, leaving its α effects unopposed. This combination of circumstances can theoretically result in a precipitous increase in blood pressure. In such cases, fluid therapy alone should probably be used until more specialized help becomes available. This is much less of a problem in patients receiving cardioselective blockers, such as atenolol. Calcium channel blocking agents such as nifedipine and diltiazem are potent peripheral vasodilators and may also complicate the therapy of a contrast reaction.

Ventricular Arrhythmias

In the event that significant ventricular arrhythmias such as multiple premature ventricular contractions, couplets, or pulsatile ventricular tachycardia develop, immediate consultation with a qualified specialist should be obtained. A loading dose of 150 mg (in 100 mL of D5W) of amiodarone can be given over 10 minutes followed by 360 mg over 6 hours. If sustained ventricular tachycardia with hypotension or ventricular fibrillation develops, defibrillation will be necessary. If a full-scale cardiac arrest develops, cardiopulmonary resuscitation should immediately be instituted.

SUGGESTED READINGS

General

Almén T. Development of nonionic contrast media. *Invest Radiol.* 1985;20(suppl):S2–S9.

Bettmann MA. Frequently asked questions: iodinated contrast agents. *Radiographics.* 2004;24:S3–S10.

Dyer RB, Gilpin JW, Zagoria RJ, et al. Vicarious contrast material excretion in patients with acute unilateral ureteral obstruction. *Radiology.* 1990;177(3):739–742.

Lasser EC, Lang JH, Lyon SG, et al. Changes in complement and coagulation factors in a patient suffering a severe anaphylactoid reaction to injection of contrast material: some considerations of pathogenesis. *Invest Radiol.* 1980;15(suppl):S6–S12.

Sherwood T, Doyle FH, Breckenridge A, et al. Value of fluid deprivation in large dose urography. *Lancet.* 1968;2:754–755.

Siegle RL, Halvorsen RA, Dillon J, et al. The use of iohexol in patients with previous reactions to ionic contrast material: a multicenter clinical trial. *Invest Radiol.* 1991;26:411–416.

Trcka J, Schmidt C, Seitz CS, et al. Anaphylaxis to iodinated contrast material: nonallergic hypersensitivity or IgE-mediated allergy? *AJR Am J Roentgenol.* 2008;190:666–670.

Acute Adverse Reactions to Contrast Media

Caro JJ, Trindade E, McGregor M. The risks of death and of severe nonfatal reactions with high vs low osmolality contrast media: a meta-analysis. *AJR Am J Roentgenol.* 1991;156:825–832.

Cochran ST, Bomyea K, Sayre JW. Trends in adverse events after IV administration of contrast media. *AJR Am J Roentgenol.* 2001;176:1385–1388.

Curry NS, Schabel SI, Reiheld CT, et al. Fatal reactions to intravenous nonionic contrast material. *Radiology.* 1991;178:361–362.

Gomi T, Nagamoto M, Hasegawa M, et al. Are there any differences in acute adverse reactions among five low-osmolar non-ionic iodinated contrast media? *Eur Radiol.* 2010;20:1631–1635.

Katayama H, Yamaguchi K, Kozuka T, et al. Adverse reactions to ionic and nonionic contrast media: a report from the Japanese Committee on the Safety of Contrast Media. *Radiology.* 1990;175:621–628.

Morcos SK. Acute serious and fatal reactions to contrast media. Our current understanding. *Br J Radiol.* 2005;78:686–693.

Mortelé KJ, Oliva MR, Ondategui S, et al. Universal use of nonionic iodinated contrast media for CT: evaluation of safety in a large urban teaching hospital. *AJR Am J Roentgenol.* 2005;185:31–34.

Schabelman E, Witting M. The relationship of radiocontrast, iodine and seafood allergies: a medical myth exposed. *J Emerg Med.* 2010;39(5):701–707.

Somashekar DK, Davenport MS, Cohan RH, et al. Effect of intravenous low-osmolality iodinated contrast media on patients with myasthenia gravis. *Radiology.* 2013;267:727–734.

Premedication Prior to Contrast Media Injection: Efficacy and Risks

Davenport MS, Cohan RH, Caoili EM, et al. Hyperglycemic consequences of corticosteroid premedication in an outpatient population. *AJR Am J Roentgenol.* 2010;194:W483–W488.

Davenport MS, Cohan RH, Khalatbari S, et al. Hyperglycemia in hospitalized patients receiving corticosteroid premedication. *Acad Radiol.* 2011;18:384–390.

Davenport MS, Mervak BM, Khalatbari S, et al. Indirect cost and harm attributable to oral 13-hour inpatient corticosteroid prophylaxis prior to contrast-enhanced computed tomography. *Radiology.* 2016;279:492–501.

Greenberger PA, Patterson R. The prevention of immediate generalized reactions to radiocontrast media in high-risk patients. *J Allergy Clin Immunol.* 1991;87(4):867–872.

Lasser EC, Berry CC, Talner LB, et al. Pretreatment with corticosteroids to alleviate reactions to intravenous contrast material. *N Engl J Med.* 1987;317(14):845–849.

Lasser EC, Berry CM, Mishkin MM, et al. Pretreatment with corticosteroids to prevent adverse reaction to nonionic contrast media. *AJR Am J Roentgenol.* 1994;162:523–526.

O'Malley RB, Cohan RH, Ellis JH, et al. A survey on the use of premedication prior to iodinated and gadolinium-based contrast material administration. *J Am Coll Radiol.* 2011;8:345–354.

Breakthrough Reactions to Contrast Media

Davenport MS, Cohan RH, Caoili EM, et al. Frequency and severity of repeat contrast reactions in premedicated patients. *Radiology.* 2009; 253:372–379.

Freed KS, Leder RA, Alexander C, et al. Breakthrough adverse reactions to low-osmolar contrast media. *AJR Am J Roentgenol.* 2001;176:1389–1392.

Mervak BM, Davenport MD, Ellis JH, et al. Breakthrough reaction rates in high-risk inpatients premedicated before contrast-enhanced CT. *AJR Am J Roentgenol.* 2015; 205:77–84.

Delayed Reactions to Contrast Media

Choyke PL, Miller DL, Lotze MT, et al. Delayed reactions to contrast media after interleukin-2 immunotherapy. *Radiology.* 1992;183:111–114.

Christensen J. Iodide mumps after intravenous administration of a nonionic contrast media: case report and review of the literature. *Acta Radiol.* 1995;36(1):82–84.

Rydberg J, Charles J, Aspelin P. Frequency of late allergy-like adverse reactions following injection of intravascular nonionic contrast media. *Acta Radiol.* 1998;39:219–222.

Post-Contrast Acute Kidney Injury

Abujudeh HH, Gee MS, Kaewlai R. In emergency situations, should serum creatinine be checked in all patients before performing second contrast CT examination within 24 hours? *J Am Coll Radiol.* 2009;6:268–273.

ACT Investigators. Acetylcysteine for prevention of renal outcomes in patient s undergoing coronary and peripheral vascular angiography: main results from the randomized Acetylcysteine for Contrast-induced nephropathy Trial (ACT). *Circulation.* 2011;124:1250–1259.

ACR Manual on Contrast Media v. 10.1 Published by the American College of Radiologyww.acr.org/~/media/ACR/Documents/PDF/QualitySafety/Resources/Contrast/Contrast%20Manual/2015_Contrast_Media.pdf/#page=49. Accessed April 13, 2016.

Aspelin P, Aubry P, Fransson SG, et al. Nephrotoxic effects in high risk patients undergoing angiography. *N Engl J Med.* 2003;348(6):491–499.

Bruce RJ, Djamail A, Shinki K, et al. Background fluctuation of kidney function versus contrast induced nephrotoxicity. *AJR Am J Roentgenol.* 2009;192:711–718.

Choyke PL, Cady J, DePollar SL, et al. Determination of serum creatinine prior to iodinated contrast media: is it necessary in all patients? *Tech Urol.* 1998;4(2):65–69.

Davenport MS, Khalatbari S, Cohan RH, et al. Contrast-induced nephrotoxicity risk assessment in adult inpatients: a comparison of serum creatinine and estimated glomerular filtration rate-based screening methods. *Radiology.* 2013;269:292–100.

Davenport MS, Khalatbari S, Dillman JR, et al. Contrast material-induced nephrotoxicity and intravenous low-osmolality iodinated contrast material. *Radiology.* 2013;267:94–104.

Gleeson TG, Bulugahapitiya S. Contrast-induced nephropathy. *AJR Am J Roentgenol.* 2004;183:1673–1689.

Heinrich MC, Haberle L, Muller V, et al. Nephrotoxicity of iso-osmolar iodixanol compared with nonionic low-osmolar contrast media: meta-analysis of randomized controlled trials. *Radiology.* 2009;250(1):68–86.

Heinrich MC, Kuhlmann MK, Grgic A, et al. Cytotoxic effects of ionic high osmolar, nonionic monomeric, and nonionic iso-osmolar dimeric iodinated contrast media in renal tubular cells in vitro. *Radiology.* 2005;235: 843–849.

Herts BR, Schneider E, Poggio ED, et al. Identifying outpatients with renal insufficiency before contrast-enhanced CT by using estimated glomerular filtration rates versus serum creatinine levels. *Radiology.* 2008;248:106–113.

Katzberg RW, Newhouse JH. Intravenous contrast media-induced nephrotoxicity: is the medical risk really as great as we have come to believe? *Radiology.* 2010;256:21–28.

Kuhn MJ, Chen N, Sahani DV, et al. The PREDICT study: a randomized double blind comparison of contrast-induced nephropathy after low- or iso-osmolar contrast agent exposure. *AJR Am J Roentgenol.* 2008;191:151–157.

Levy E, Viscoli CM, Horwitz RI. The effect of acute renal failure on mortality. A cohort analysis. *JAMA.* 1996;275:1489–1494.

McDonald RJ, McDonald JS, Bida JP, et al. Intravenous contrast material-induced nephropathy: causal or coincident phenomenon? *Radiology.* 2013;267(1):106–118.

McDonald JS, McDonald RJ, Comin J, et al. Frequency of acute kidney injury following intravenous contrast media administration: a systematic review and meta-analysis. *Radiology.* 2013;267:119–128.

Morcos SK. Prevention of contrast media-induced nephrotoxicity after angiographic procedures. *J Vasc Interv Radiol.* 2005;16:13–23.

Newhouse JH, Kho D, Rao QA, et al. Frequency of serum creatinine changes in the absence of iodinated contrast material: implications for studies of contrast nephrotoxicity. *AJR Am J Roentgenol.* 2008;191:376–382.

Nguyen SA, Suranyi P, Ravene JG, et al. Iso-osmolality versus low-osmolality iodinated contrast media at intravenous contrast-enhanced CT: effect on kidney function. *Radiology.* 2008;248(1):97–105.

Pahade JK, LeBedis CA, Raptopoulos VD, et al. Incidence of contrast-induced nephropathy in patients with multiple myeloma undergoing contrast-enhanced CT. *AJR Am J Roentgenol.* 2011;196:1094–1101.

Rao QA, Newhouse JH. Risk of nephropathy after intravenous administration of contrast material: a critical literature analysis. *Radiology.* 2006;239(2):392–397.

Sandler CM. Contrast-agent-induced acute renal dysfunction—is iodixanol the answer? *N Engl J Med.* 2003;348(6):551–553.

Thompson HS, Morcos SK. Risk of contrast-media-induced nephropathy in high risk patients undergoing MDCT—a pooled analysis of two randomized trials. *Eur Radiol.* 2009;19:891–897.

Xie H, Ye Y, Shan G, et al. Effect of statins in preventing contrast-induced nephropathy: an updated meta-analysis. *Coron Artery Dis.* 2014;25:565–574.

Extravasation

Cohan RH, Ellis JH, Garner WL. Extravasation of radiographic contrast material: recognition, prevention and treatment. *Radiology.* 1996;200: 593–604.

Gadolinium Based Contrast Agents

Dillman JR, Ellis JH, Cohan RH, et al. Frequency and severity of acute allergic-like reactions to gadolinium-containing IV contrast media in children and adults. *AJR Am J Roentgenol.* 2007;189:1533–1538.

Li A, Wong CS, Wong MK, et al. Acute adverse reactions to magnetic resonance contrast media—gadolinium chelates. *Br J Radiol.* 2006;79:368–371.

Murphy KJ, Brunberg JA, Cohan RH. Adverse reactions to gadolinium contrast media. A review of 36 cases. *AJR Am J Roentgenol.* 1996;167(4):847–849.

Nelson KL, Gifford LM, Lauber-Huber C, et al. Clinical safety of gadopentetate dimeglumine. *Radiology.* 1995;196(2):439–443.

Perez-Rodriguez J, Lai S, Ehst BD, et al. Nephrogenic systemic fibrosis: incidence, associations and effect of risk factor assessment—report of 33 cases. *Radiology.* 2009;250:371–377.

Sena BF, Stern JP, Pandharipande PV, et al. Screening patients to assess renal function before administering gadolinium chelates: assessment of the Choyke questionnaire. *AJR Am J Roentgenol.* 2010;195:424–428.

Nephrogenic Systemic Fibrosis

Abujudeh HH, Kaewlai R, Kagan A, et al. Nephrogenic systemic fibrosis after gadopentetate dimeglumine exposure: case series of 36 patients. *Radiology.* 2009;253(1):81–89.

Cowper SE. Nephrogenic systemic fibrosis: an overview. *J Am Coll Radiol.* 2008;5(1):23–28.

Marckmann P, Skov L, Rossen K, et al. Nephrogenic systemic fibrosis: suspected causative role of gadodiamide used for contrast enhanced magnetic resonance imaging. *J Soc Nephrol.* 2006;17:2359–2362.

Thompsen HS. Nephrogenic systemic fibrosis: a serious late adverse reaction to gadodiamide. *Eur Radiol.* 2006;16:2619–2621.

Thompsen HS. How to avoid nephrogenic systemic fibrosis: current guidelines in Europe and the United States. *Radiol Clin North Am.* 2009;47(5):871–875.

Gadolinium Retention in Brain

Kanda T, Osawa M, Oba H, et al. High signal intensity in the dentate nucleus on unenhanced T1-wieghted MR images: association with linear versus macrocyclic gadolinium chelate administration. *Radiology.* 2015;275: 803–809.

McDonald RJ, McDonald JS, Kallmes DF, et al. Intracranial gadolinium deposition after contrast-enhanced MR imaging. *Radiology.* 2015;275: 772–782.

Ramalho J, Castillo M, AlObaidy M, et al. High signal intensity in globus pallidus and dentate nucleus on unenhanced T1-weighted MR images: evaluation of two linear gadolinium-based contrast agents. *Radiology.* 2015;276:836–844.

Treatment of Adverse Reactions to Contrast Media

Bush WH, Swanson DP. Acute reactions to intravascular contrast media: types, risk factors, recognition, and specific treatment. *AJR Am J Roentgenol.* 1991;157:1153.

Hamilton G. Severe adverse reactions to urography in patients taking beta-adrenergic blocking agents. *Can Med Assoc J.* 1985;133:122.

Segal AJ, Bush WH. Avoidable errors in dealing with anaphylactoid reactions to iodinated contrast media. *Invest Radiol.* 2011;46(3):147–151.

Wang CL, Cohan RH, Ellis JH, et al. Frequency, outcome and appropriateness of treatment of nonionic iodinated contrast media reactions. *AJR Am J Roentgenol.* 2008;191:409–415.

3

The Adrenal Gland

INTRODUCTION

The adrenal glands lie superior to the kidneys in the perinephric space. Since they are surrounded by fat, they are usually well visualized on computed tomography (CT) (Fig. 3.1) or MR examinations. Patients with abnormalities involving the adrenal glands may present with symptoms due to the adrenal disease, or the abnormality may be identified as an incidental finding on an examination performed for another indication. Because the adrenal gland is an active site of synthesis of a variety of hormones, patients may present with symptoms of hormone excess or, less likely, hormone deficiency. Thus, adrenal diseases are discussed as hyperfunctional disorders in which excess hormone is produced, as disorders of adrenal insufficiency, and as diseases in which adrenal function is normal. Because these hormones can be readily measured, there is seldom doubt as to which category a patient belongs.

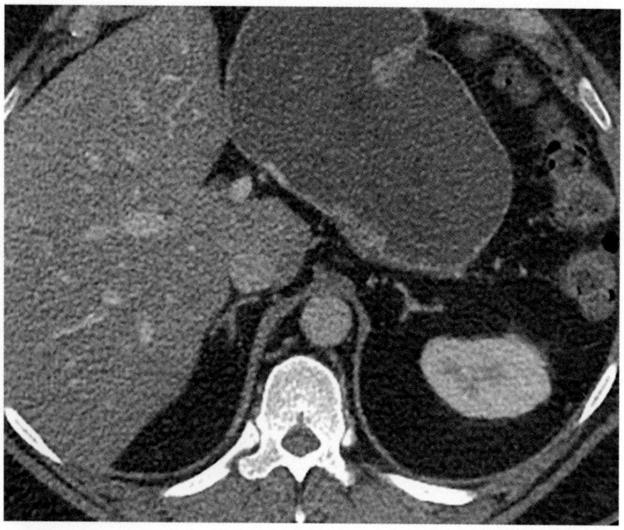

HYPERFUNCTIONAL DISEASES

Cushing Syndrome

Cushing syndrome is the clinical manifestation of excess glucocorticoids. These steroids may come from an exogenous or endogenous source. Exogenous Cushing syndrome is seen in patients treated with large doses of steroids. Endogenous Cushing syndrome is caused by overproduction of cortisol by the adrenal cortex. The characteristic appearance of a patient with Cushing syndrome includes truncal obesity, hirsutism, abdominal striae, and muscle atrophy. Hypertension and glucose intolerance are common findings. The diagnosis of Cushing syndrome may be confirmed by measuring urinary-free cortisol levels, which are elevated.

Patients may be further classified as having adrenocorticotropic hormone (ACTH)–dependent or ACTH-independent Cushing syndrome. Plasma ACTH levels are elevated in ACTH-dependent and depressed in those with ACTH-independent Cushing syndrome. In approximately 80% of cases, unregulated amounts of ACTH stimulate the adrenal cortex, which results in bilateral adrenal hyperplasia. This is referred to as *ACTH-dependent Cushing syndrome.* ACTH-independent causes of Cushing syndrome include adrenal adenomas, carcinomas, and two rare hyperplasia syndromes, primary pigmented nodular adrenal dysplasia (PPNAD) and ACTH-independent macronodular hyperplasia (AIMAH).

Among patients with ACTH-dependent Cushing syndrome, the pituitary gland is not always the source of ACTH. A variety of other tumors, such as oat cell carcinoma, bronchial adenoma, and tumors of the ovary, pancreas, thymus, and thyroid, may rarely secrete ACTH.

FIGURE 3.1. Normal adrenal glands. Both glands have an inverted "Y" configuration, with the tail pointed anteromedially.

The etiology of ACTH-independent Cushing syndrome includes an adrenal adenoma, adrenal carcinoma, and several inherited syndromes including multiple endocrine neoplasia type 1 (MEN1), McCune–Albright syndrome, familial adenomatous polyposis, and Carney complex. As many as 40% of patients with MEN1 may have adrenal lesions, usually bilateral nodular hyperplasia. The McCune–Albright syndrome, which usually presents in the first year of life, includes bony lesions, skin pigmentation, precocious puberty, and bilateral nodular hyperplasia. Patients with familial adenomatous polyposis have extensive colonic polyps as well as desmoid tumors, osteomas, retinal abnormalities, and adrenocortical lesions including adenomas, carcinomas, and hyperplasia. Carney complex includes myxomas of the heart, breast, and skin as well as psammomatous melanotic schwannomas and osteochondromyxomas. PPNAD is the most common adrenal lesion reported in these patients. A few patients with adrenal hyperplasia have macronodules that can be seen in the adrenal glands on CT examination. These macronodules usually measure <3 cm and may be <1 cm in diameter. Macronodular hyperplasia is caused by an ACTH-secreting pituitary microadenoma in the majority of cases. Macronodular hyperplasia with a dominant nodule may be distinguished from a cortisol-producing adenoma by the size of the contralateral adrenal gland. In patients with an adenoma, the contralateral gland and other limbs of the ipsilateral gland are atrophic, whereas they are enlarged (hyperplastic) in patients with macronodular hyperplasia.

Primary Aldosteronism

Primary aldosteronism, or Conn syndrome, is the result of excess aldosterone produced by the adrenal glands. Approximately 60% of cases of Conn syndrome are due to hyperplasia and 35% are caused by an adenoma. Rare causes include an adrenal cortical carcinoma and unilateral hyperplasia. Adrenal hyperplasia may be further subdivided into idiopathic hyperaldosteronism (IHA) and primary adrenal hyperplasia (PAH). IHA is far more common than PAH. Since bilateral adrenalectomy does not effectively control the hypertension and hypokalemia in patients with IHA, they are treated medically. Although morphologically PAH resembles IHA, PAH may be unilateral or bilateral, and adrenalectomy is an effective treatment for unilateral cases. Rarely does a primary adrenocortical carcinoma secrete enough aldosterone to cause a recognizable clinical syndrome. As diagnostic advances result in more cases of primary aldosteronism being found in hypertensive patients, a greater portion of these patients have IHA, which should be treated medically.

The syndrome Conn described in 1955 includes hypokalemia, hypertension, elevated serum aldosterone, but low serum renin levels. Excess levels of aldosterone cause sodium retention, an increase in the plasma volume, and hypertension. Because potassium is exchanged for sodium in the distal tubule, sodium retention creates hypokalemia. Aldosteronism occurs also in patients with renovascular hypertension. However, this form of secondary aldosteronism is distinguished from primary aldosteronism by measuring the serum renin level, which is low in patients with Conn syndrome.

Laboratory tests can also be used to help distinguish between hyperplasia and adenoma, as the etiology of primary aldosteronism. However, these tests are not entirely accurate, and radiographic confirmation is needed. Adrenal venous sampling (AVS) is the best method to identify a unilateral source of aldosterone secretion. Although technically challenging, in experienced centers, AVS is highly accurate. The combination of anatomic imaging with CT or MRI and a localizing AVS resulted in a cure rate of >95% after unilateral adrenalectomy.

Congenital Adrenal Hyperplasia

Congenital adrenal hyperplasia (CAH) is a group of autosomal recessive disorders that result in the absence or decreased synthesis of cortisol. The defect may lie in any of the five enzymatic steps necessary to convert cholesterol to corticosteroid, but >90% of CAH cases are due to a deficiency of 21-hydroxylase. The loss of normal feedback inhibition causes the pituitary gland to secrete excess ACTH, which overstimulates the adrenal glands and causes bilateral hyperplasia.

Because androgens do not require 21-hydroxylase for their synthesis, they are overproduced in response to high levels of ACTH. The clinical manifestation depends on the sex of the patient and the age at which the androgen excess appears. Ambiguous genitalia and subsequent virilization are seen in women, whereas precocious puberty is found in young boys.

Virilizing Tumors

Androgen-producing tumors are rare, may be benign or malignant, and occur in either males or females at any age. Patients whose virilization is the result of a tumor usually present at an older age than those with CAH.

The typical clinical manifestations include amenorrhea, hirsutism, enlargement of the clitoris, and deepening of the voice. Elevated testosterone levels are also frequently found in adrenal tumors, so a high testosterone level cannot be used to distinguish a gonadal tumor from an adrenal tumor.

Feminizing Tumors

Feminizing tumors are quite rare, and most are malignant. They are usually seen in men but have also been reported in prepubertal girls and postmenopausal women. Gynecomastia is the predominant clinical manifestation.

Adrenal Insufficiency

Adrenal insufficiency may be caused by tissue destruction of the adrenal glands (primary) or may result from inadequate stimulation by ACTH (secondary). Secondary adrenal insufficiency is more common than primary, and both are found more often in women. Because normal adrenal function depends on ACTH, any disorder that impairs the ability of the pituitary gland to secrete ACTH may lead to adrenal hypofunction. With decreased ACTH activity, cortisol and adrenal androgen secretion diminish, but aldosterone secretion remains relatively intact. Thus, patients with hypopituitarism can tolerate sodium deprivation better than patients with primary adrenal insufficiency. Furthermore, hypopituitary patients do not develop mucocutaneous hyperpigmentation, as this depends on excessive ACTH secretion.

Primary adrenal insufficiency, or Addison disease, occurs only after at least 90% of the adrenal cortex has been destroyed. Idiopathic adrenal atrophy, an autoimmune disorder, is the most common cause of Addison disease in the United States. The other common cause of Addison disease is destruction of the adrenal glands by a granulomatous disease, usually tuberculosis. Among the other causes of adrenal insufficiency, hemorrhage and destruction of adrenal tissue by metastatic tumor are reported most commonly.

The clinical onset of Addison disease usually is gradual and may be difficult to recognize. Manifestations are due to the deficiency of cortisol and aldosterone. Because cortisol deficiency results in increased pituitary secretion of ACTH and other melanocyte-stimulating hormones, patients with Addison disease develop a characteristic hyperpigmentation. Treatment includes cortisol and aldosterone replacement as well as saline to correct extracellular fluid depletion.

The radiographic manifestations of primary adrenal insufficiency depend on the cause of adrenal dysfunction. The plain abdominal radiograph may reveal adrenal calcification commonly seen in tuberculosis or histoplasmosis.

The most useful examinations are CT or MR, which define the size and shape of the adrenal glands. In patients with autoimmune disease, severe cortical atrophy is present, such that the adrenal glands may be difficult to detect.

Granulomatous involvement by tuberculosis or histoplasmosis is bilateral. The glands are enlarged but often maintain a normal configuration. Calcification is common.

If adrenal hemorrhage is acute, it may be recognized by the increased density of the recent hemorrhage. As the density of the hematoma decreases, it becomes indistinguishable from other adrenal masses. Although adrenal metastases are common, adrenal insufficiency infrequently occurs. This is because so much of the adrenal cortex must be destroyed before insufficiency ensues.

Radiology

Ultrasound

Although the normal adrenal gland may be difficult to image with ultrasound, tumors >2 cm often can be detected. The right adrenal gland usually is easier to study because the liver provides a good acoustic window. Ultrasound may be valuable in distinguishing a solid mass from an adrenal cyst.

Computed Tomography

The modality routinely used to evaluate the adrenal glands is CT. The perinephric fat present in most patients allows the adrenal glands to be clearly defined, and tumors as small as 5 mm can be detected. Intravenous contrast medium is seldom needed but may be helpful to distinguish an adrenal mass from the upper pole of the kidney.

The adenomas in Conn syndrome usually are the most difficult adrenal tumors to detect because they tend to be the smallest, averaging <2 cm in diameter (Fig. 3.2).

Patients with Cushing syndrome, conversely, are relatively easy to examine by CT. The tumors in these patients are larger than those causing Conn syndrome, and the adrenal glands are depicted clearly by the abundant retroperitoneal fat (Fig. 3.3). Tumors that are >4 cm in diameter or that demonstrate central necrosis are suspicious for malignancy.

Bilateral adrenal hyperplasia is seen as enlargement of the entire adrenal gland, but without a focal mass. The limbs of both adrenal

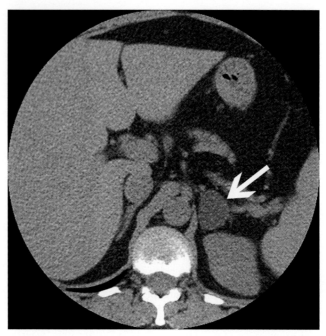

FIGURE 3.3. Adrenal adenoma. A cortisol-secreting adenoma (*arrow*) is seen in a patient with Cushing disease.

glands are thickened and elongated (Figs. 3.4 and 3.5). Patients whose hyperplasia is caused by an ectopic source of ACTH tend to have larger adrenal glands than those with a pituitary adenoma as the source of ACTH.

Enlargement of the adrenal gland usually is more obvious in patients with Cushing syndrome than in those with Conn syndrome. However, there is significant overlap with the appearance of normal adrenal glands, and hyperplasia should not be diagnosed by morphology alone.

A minority of patients with Cushing disease have macronodular hyperplasia in which one or more nodules may be seen (Fig. 3.6). Rarely, patients may have AIMAH in which the large size of the adrenal nodules suggests bilateral adenomas or metastases. PPNAD is another rare cause of ACTH-independent Cushing syndrome. PPNAD is transmitted as an autosomal dominant trait and is associated with the Carney complex. Histologically, pigmented nodules,

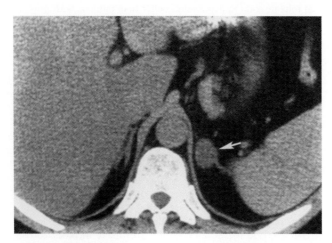

FIGURE 3.2. Adrenal adenoma. An aldosterone-secreting adenoma (*arrow*) is seen in the left adrenal gland.

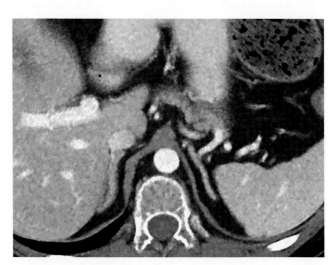

FIGURE 3.4. Bilateral adrenal hyperplasia. Both adrenal glands are elongated and thickened.

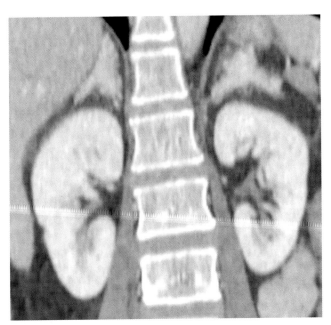

FIGURE 3.5. Bilateral adrenal hyperplasia. Both adrenal glands are seen as thickened on this coronal reconstructed CT image.

2 to 5 mm in diameter, are seen. Patients with AIMAH and PPNAD are treated with bilateral adrenalectomy.

Venous Sampling

Because each adrenal gland is drained by a central vein, the venous efflux of each gland can be sampled for hormone analysis. Adrenal venous sampling (ADV) can be valuable in patients with Conn syndrome because the aldosterone-secreting adenoma often is <1 cm and may be too small to be detected by CT. Furthermore, patients may have PAH or a nonhyperfunctioning adenoma, which cannot be distinguished from an adenoma secreting excess aldosterone. Localizing the side of excess hormone production by venous sampling guides surgical adrenalectomy. Venous sampling is needed rarely in evaluating patients with Cushing syndrome but may be applied to those patients suffering from masculinizing or feminizing tumors.

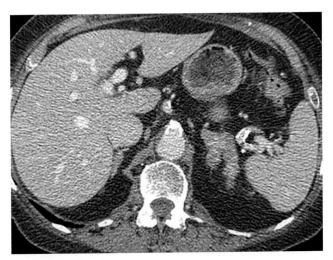

FIGURE 3.6. Bilateral macronodular hyperplasia. Multiple small nodules are seen in the left adrenal gland. Only the top of the right adrenal gland is shown, but it also contains multiple nodules.

AVS is technically difficult due to the small size of the adrenal veins. Since the left adrenal vein empties into the left inferior phrenic vein, it is easier to find and sample. The right adrenal vein empties directly into the inferior vena cava posteriorly in most patients but may have a common trunk with a hepatic vein in a significant minority of cases. Finely collimated CT scanning in the venous phase of contrast enhancement allows visualization of the right adrenal vein in most patients.

Magnetic Resonance

The perinephric fat provides excellent contrast for magnetic resonance imaging (MRI) as well as for CT. The spatial resolution of MRI is similar to that of CT, and the additional parameters available to distinguish benign from malignant lesions may be useful. For most patients with hyperfunction of the adrenal cortex, MRI does not provide additional information after a CT examination.

ADRENAL MEDULLA

Pheochromocytoma

Pheochromocytomas are tumors composed of chromaffin cells and usually are located in the adrenal medulla. They are rare tumors and account for <1% of patients with systemic hypertension. Extra-adrenal pheochromocytomas are called *paragangliomas* and may be divided into those that arise from parasympathetic tissues along the cranial or vagus nerves and those that arise from sympathetic chromaffin tissue. Thus, they may lie anywhere between the base of the brain and the epididymis but usually lie along the sympathetic chain in the retroperitoneum. Eighty-five percent of pheochromocytomas arise from chromaffin tissue in the adrenal medulla. Sporadic pheochromocytomas average 4 cm in diameter at presentation, while those associated with syndromes are often smaller.

Patients may complain of episodes of headaches associated with palpitation and diaphoresis. If the pheochromocytoma is located in the bladder wall, micturition may induce a symptomatic episode.

Hypertension is the most common finding and is present in >90% of patients. Hypertension from a pheochromocytoma may be difficult to distinguish from renovascular or essential hypertension; however, patients with a pheochromocytoma are more likely to have labile hypertension with discrete paroxysmal attacks. These patients are also prone to hypertensive attacks during anesthesia induction. Manipulation of the gland during surgery, percutaneous adrenal biopsy, or even selective adrenal angiography may also induce a hypertensive crisis.

Pheochromocytomas are associated with other endocrine tumors. The multiple endocrine neoplasia syndrome 2A (MEN2A) includes medullary carcinoma of the thyroid and parathyroid hyperplasia as well as pheochromocytoma. The MEN2B syndrome is rare and is composed of pheochromocytoma; medullary carcinoma of the thyroid; and the mucocutaneous manifestations of mucosal neuromas, intestinal ganglioneuromatosis, and a marfanoid habitus. The majority of patients with the MEN2A or the MEN2B syndrome have pheochromocytomas that are bilateral and usually intra-adrenal. However, all manifestations of the syndrome may not occur at the same time. Thus, a careful history of a previous endocrine abnormality should be obtained in evaluating patients who may fall into these categories. These syndromes are inherited in an autosomal dominant fashion.

MULTIPLE ENDOCRINE NEOPLASIA TYPE 2A

- Medullary carcinoma of thyroid
- Pheochromocytoma (usually bilateral)
- Parathyroid adenoma

MULTIPLE ENDOCRINE NEOPLASIA TYPE 2B

- Medullary carcinoma of thyroid
- Pheochromocytoma (usually bilateral)
- Mucosal neuromas
- Intestinal ganglioneuromatoses
- Marfanoid habitus

Pheochromocytoma is also associated with neurofibromatosis (type I) and von Hippel–Lindau syndrome (type II). Paragangliomas are also associated with tuberous sclerosis and Sturge–Weber syndrome.

A syndrome of familial pheochromocytomas not associated with other endocrine tumors has also been noted. Specific gene mutations have been identified involving the mitochondrial enzyme succinate dehydrogenase (SDH). The most common of these are SDHB mutations, where patients develop thoracic or abdominal paragangliomas with a propensity for malignancy. Patients with SDHD mutations develop paragangliomas in the head and neck.

In 1977, Carney et al. reported the association of a gastric leiomyosarcoma, a pulmonary chondroma, and a functioning extraadrenal pheochromocytoma. This rare combination of neoplasms often is termed *Carney triad*.

Although 85% of all pheochromocytomas are located in the adrenal medulla, there is a striking difference between sporadic tumors and those associated with the MEN syndromes. The sporadic pheochromocytomas are located outside the adrenal gland in as many as 25% of cases, whereas those associated with the MEN2 syndromes are almost always intra-adrenal. Pheochromocytomas found in patients with MEN2 syndrome are usually multicentric and involve both adrenal glands in >80% of cases.

The histologic appearance also differs in sporadic and MEN2–associated cases. In sporadic cases, the tumor is well encased with normal adjacent medulla. In patients with MEN2 syndrome, the medulla is hyperplastic and the tumor may be multicentric.

If a pheochromocytoma is suspected, the diagnosis can be made by measuring elevated levels of serum or urine catecholamines. Urinary metanephrine or vanillylmandelic acid (VMA) is elevated in >90% of patients when measured on 24-hour urine collections. Plasma-free metanephrine levels are elevated in 99% of patients. However, several separate determinations should be made because of the episodic hormone secretion found in these patients. Furthermore, patients taking medications such as methyldopa or methenamine may have falsely high catecholamine levels.

Approximately 15% of pheochromocytomas lie outside the adrenal gland. Those which arise from sympathetic paraganglia are called *paragangliomas*, whereas those which arise from the sympathetic tissue of the cranial or vagus nerves are glomus tumors, chemodectomas, or carotid body tumors. Although they may occur anywhere from the base of the skull to the epididymis, the most common locations are in the sympathetic chain in the retroperitoneum from the level of the adrenal glands to the aortic bifurcation, which includes the region of the organ of Zuckerkandl, which lies near the origin of the inferior mesenteric artery.

Pheochromocytomas usually are benign, but approximately 13% demonstrate malignant behavior. Extra-adrenal pheochromocytomas are more likely to be malignant than intra-adrenal tumors.

A small number of patients have a pheochromocytoma that does not produce sufficient catecholamine to cause clinical symptoms. These "nonfunctioning" pheochromocytomas are discovered as palpable masses or as incidental findings at surgery and at autopsy or on imaging studies such as CT or MR examinations. In a recent series by Motte-Ramirez et al., more than half of their series of pheochromocytomas were discovered incidentally. The nonfunctioning tumors tend to be larger than functioning pheochromocytomas whose hormone production brought them to attention earlier than patients with nonfunctioning pheochromocytomas.

The treatment for patients with pheochromocytoma is surgical resection. Biochemical confirmation of the diagnosis and accurate preoperative radiologic localization have made these operations much safer. Nevertheless, patients undergoing surgical resection still must receive adrenergic blockade before the induction of anesthesia as well as careful monitoring during the operation to treat any crises. Both an α-adrenergic blocker (phenoxybenzamine) as well as a β-blocker (propranolol) are advocated, whereas nitroprusside may be used to treat hypertensive episodes. This same regimen may be used in patients requiring invasive radiologic procedures.

Radiology

Ultrasound

Ultrasound may be used to localize an intra-adrenal pheochromocytoma, but also it may identify ectopic tumors lying in the para-aortic area. Pheochromocytomas tend to be more echogenic than normal adrenal tissue, possibly because of the hypervascularity they usually exhibit. Ultrasound is also often helpful in children, in whom the relative lack of retroperitoneal fat makes CT evaluation difficult.

Computed Tomography

CT is the primary imaging modality used to localize a pheochromocytoma (Figs. 3.7 and 3.8). Most intra-adrenal pheochromocytomas are detected, and a sensitivity of 95% can be expected. Care must be taken when examining patients with the MEN syndrome, however, because the tumors in these patients often are small (Fig. 3.9). Because most extra-adrenal pheochromocytomas (paragangliomas) lie in the para-aortic region, they are also demonstrated on an abdominal CT examination (Fig. 3.10).

The administration of intravascular contrast media is unnecessary for most patients. The adrenal glands are well visualized, and most tumors are large enough to be readily identified, measuring 2 to 5 cm in diameter at presentation. Areas of necrosis or

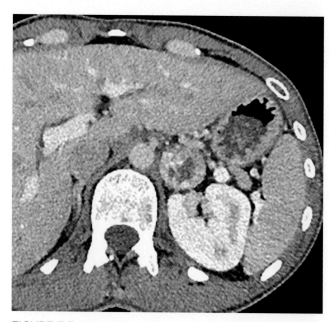

FIGURE 3.7. Pheochromocytoma. A 3-cm left adrenal mass just anterior to the kidney shows heterogeneous contrast enhancement.

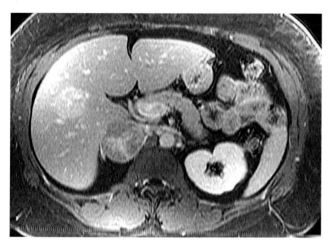

FIGURE 3.8. Pheochromocytoma. A 4-cm right adrenal pheochromocytoma demonstrates heterogeneous enhancement on this T1-weighted MR examination. An incidental hepatic hemangioma is present.

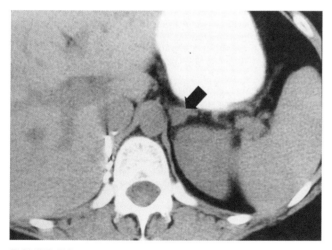

FIGURE 3.9. MEN syndrome. This patient with a history of medullary carcinoma of the thyroid had a right pheochromocytoma removed (surgical clips) 2 years earlier. A small left adrenal mass (arrow) is detected on this unenhanced CT scan.

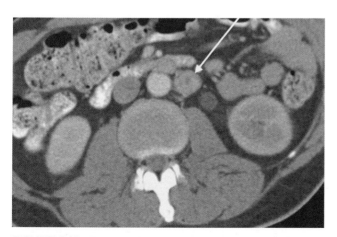

FIGURE 3.10. Paraganglioma. A 2-cm mass (arrow) is seen on this enhanced abdominal CT examination.

hemorrhage are common, especially in larger tumors. Although the intravenous administration of ionic contrast media in patients with a pheochromocytoma has been shown to stimulate sufficient catecholamine secretion to cause a hypertensive crisis, this does not appear to be the case with nonionic contrast media.

Magnetic Resonance Imaging

MRI has a high sensitivity for the detection of pheochromocytomas. The tumor is typically hypointense to the liver on T1-weighted images and may have a very high signal intensity on T2-weighted images. However, the most common appearance on T2-weighted images is an enhancing, heterogeneous mass with focal areas of high signal intensity (Fig. 3.11).

Nuclear Medicine

Radionuclide examinations using iodine-131–labeled metaiodobenzylguanidine (MIBG) or indium-111–labeled pentetreotide (Octreoscan) may be very useful in localizing pheochromocytomas or paragangliomas (Fig. 3.12).

The overall accuracy of MIBG is similar to that of CT and MRI; however, scintigraphy has several advantages. With a single injection of radionuclide, the entire body can be scanned. This is particularly helpful for ectopic tumors or for the detection of metastatic deposits. MIBG can also detect medullary hyperplasia, which is seen in patients with MEN syndromes and may be an early manifestation of a developing pheochromocytoma.

Positron emission tomography (PET) with 2-[fluorine-18] fluoro-2-deoxy-D-glucose (FDG) may also be used to localize pheochromocytomas. FDG is accumulated by the majority of both benign and malignant pheochromocytomas, including some that fail to concentrate MIBG.

Neuroblastoma and Ganglioneuroma

Neuroblastomas are primitive tumors that arise from sympathetic nervous system tissue. They may occur in the neck, thorax, abdomen, and pelvis, but no definite primary site can be found in a significant minority of patients. The most common location is the adrenal gland, which accounts for approximately 35% of patients.

Neuroblastomas usually occur in young children. Approximately 25% of cases occur in the first year of life, and as many as 60% occur by the age of 2 years.

Although neuroblastoma is the most common extracranial malignant tumor in childhood, its incidence is only 1 to 3 per

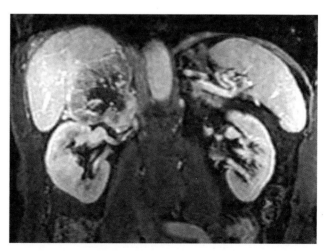

FIGURE 3.11. Pheochromocytoma. The right adrenal mass shows heterogeneous enhancement on this MR examination.

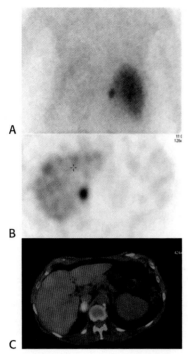

FIGURE 3.12. Pheochromocytoma. **A:** The posterior view of this 123-iodine MIBG scan demonstrates intense MIGB uptake in the right posterior abdomen and physiologic activity in the liver. SPECT **(B)** and fused SPECT/CT **(C)** scans demonstrate an MIBG-avid right adrenal nodule consistent with pheochromocytoma.

100,000 children per year. An increased incidence is seen in neurofibromatosis, and familial associations have been reported.

Some neuroblastomas spontaneously mature into benign ganglioneuromas. Histologically, neuroblastomas contain densely packed small round cells that may be difficult to differentiate from other tumors, such as Ewing sarcoma, lymphoma, or rhabdomyosarcoma. Tumors that contain more mature ganglion cells mixed with neuroblasts are classified as ganglioneuroblastomas. Ganglioneuroblastomas and ganglioneuromas are differentiated from neuroblastomas by a greater degree of cellular maturation. Ganglioneuroblastomas are malignant tumors but may be partially or totally encapsulated. Ganglioneuromas are benign tumors with an intact capsule, but careful evaluation of the entire tumor is necessary because there may be marked variation in different parts of the tumor.

Ganglioneuromas are benign, nonhyperfunctioning tumors composed of mature ganglion cells and Schwann cells in a fibrous stroma. They arise from the sympathetic nervous system and may be found in the neck, thorax, abdomen, or pelvis. In one series, 19 (41%) of 46 abdominal ganglioneuromas were found in the adrenal gland. Because they are not hormonally active, they are usually found as a large mass or as an incidental finding on CT or MRI examinations.

An adrenal ganglioma is seen as a well-defined, rounded, homogeneous mass with an attenuation slightly less than muscle on unenhanced CT images. With the administration of intravascular contrast media, mild heterogeneity may be seen, especially in larger tumors, but the attenuation still usually is less than muscle (Fig. 3.13).

A homogeneous tumor of relatively low signal intensity is seen on T1-weighted MR images. A heterogeneous high signal intensity has been reported on T2-weighted images.

The most common presentations of a child with a neuroblastoma are pain, abdominal distention, or an abdominal mass discovered by

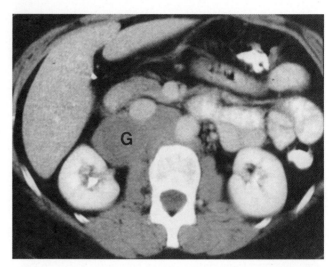

FIGURE 3.13. Ganglioneuroma. This retroperitoneal mass (*G*) was detected as an incidental finding on an enhanced CT examination.

a parent. Most patients have elevated urinary catecholamines when measured as catechol excretion per milligram of creatinine. More than 50% of patients excrete high levels of VMA, and up to 90% of patients have an elevation of VMA or homovanillic acid.

The International Neuroblastoma Staging System (Table 3.1) is based on clinical, radiologic, and surgical features. Stage I tumors are those that have no nonadherent positive lymph nodes or metastases and can be completely resected. Tumors that invade one side of the neural canal are stage II. Tumors that cross the midline to the opposite side of the vertebral body are stage III. Stage IV tumors are those with distant metastases, whereas stage IVs tumors are those in which the tumor cells represent fewer than 10% of all marrow cells; other metastases are limited to the liver and skin. Approximately 70% of patients have metastases at the time of presentation.

Radiology

Ultrasound

Ultrasound is valuable especially in small children who have a paucity of retroperitoneal fat. A mass of heterogeneous echogenicity usually is seen in the region of the adrenal gland (Fig. 3.14). The

TABLE **3.1**

Neuroblastoma Staging

Stage	Disease Extent
I	Confined to organ of origin
II	Contiguous extension beyond organ of origin, but not beyond midline. Regional ipsilateral lymph nodes may be involved
III	Contiguous extension beyond midline. Regional lymph nodes may be involved bilaterally
IV	Remote disease involving skeleton, parenchymal organs, soft tissues, or distant lymph nodes
IVs	Stage I or II disease and remote disease confined to one or more of the following sites: liver, skin, or bone marrow

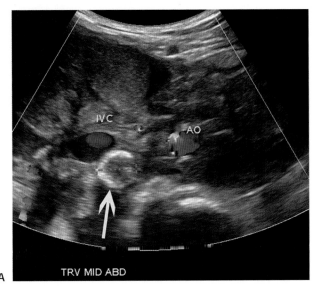
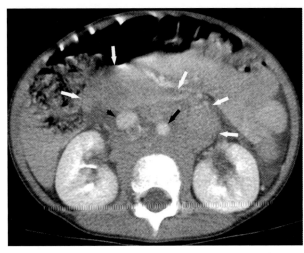

FIGURE 3.14. Neuroblastoma. **A:** Axial Doppler ultrasound demonstrates a retroperitoneal mass (*arrow*) displacing the inferior vena cava. **B:** Enhanced CT images demonstrate an ill-defined lobular mass (*white arrows*) encasing the inferior vena cava (*short black arrow*) and the aorta (*long black arrow*).

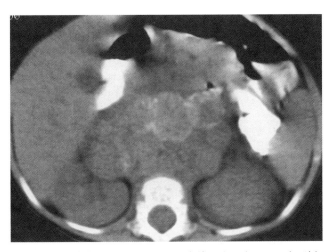

FIGURE 3.15. Neuroblastoma. Calcification is seen in this malignant tumor involving para-aortic lymph nodes.

margins are poorly defined, and a capsule is not present. A sonographic "lobule" of homogeneous increased echogenicity consisting of an aggregate of cells separated from the surrounding tumor by collagen deposition has been described in a minority of patients. Ultrasound can also be used to detect involvement of adjacent vascular structures, such as the inferior vena cava.

Computed Tomography

Unenhanced CT scans are more sensitive than plain radiographs in detecting the mottled calcification commonly seen in neuroblastoma (Fig. 3.15). Intravenous contrast medium commonly is used to distinguish a renal from an extrarenal mass (Fig. 3.16). CT may be used to identify neuroblastomas in the abdomen, pelvis, or chest. Involvement of adjacent organs or retroperitoneal lymph nodes can be detected.

Tumors are usually large and heterogeneous, with low-density areas representing hemorrhage or necrosis. Vascular encasement is common, but vascular invasion is rare. Invasion of paraspinal musculature and the neural foramina is common, although it may be better seen with MRI. Regional lymphadenopathy and liver metastases are usually readily detected.

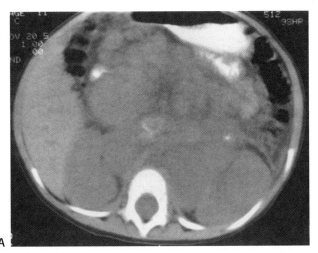
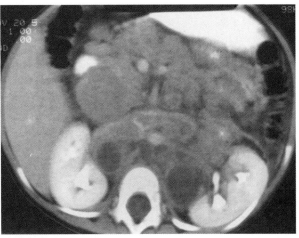

FIGURE 3.16. Neuroblastoma. **A:** Para-aortic masses are present but are difficult to distinguish on an unenhanced CT examination. **B:** After contrast injection, the kidneys and major retroperitoneal vessels are clearly defined.

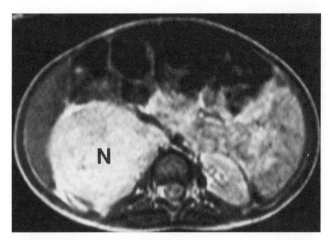

FIGURE 3.17. Neuroblastoma. A large right neuroblastoma (*N*) is easily seen on this T2-weighted MRI examination.

Magnetic Resonance Imaging

MRI is a useful study in children with neuroblastoma but generally requires sedation. The tumor has a signal intensity slightly lower than the liver or renal cortex on T1-weighted images. On T2-weighted sequences, the intensity is higher than the liver but similar to the kidney (Fig. 3.17). The signal often is heterogeneous as a result of tumor necrosis and hemorrhage.

The ability to scan in any plane is helpful to determine the organ of origin and to detect regional invasion. Using the coronal plane and T1-weighted sequences, the neuroblastoma can be distinguished from the kidney and liver. T2-weighted images have superior contrast differentiation and are used in differentiating the extent of the tumor from adjacent normal tissue.

MRI is especially valuable in defining intraspinal extension (Fig. 3.18). Tumor growth through the foramen with epidural expansion creates a "dumbbell"-shaped tumor seen in approximately 10% of abdominal tumors and is even more frequently seen in the thorax. Involvement of the bone marrow is seen as areas of low signal intensity on T1-weighted images and high signal intensity on T2-weighted images.

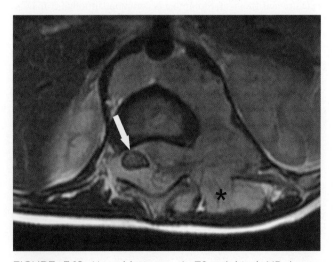

FIGURE 3.18. Neuroblastoma. A T2-weighted MR image shows a confluent retrocrural and paraspinal mass extending through the left neural foramen into the spinal canal, displacing the spinal cord (*arrow*) and extending into the left posterior paraspinal muscles (*asterisk*).

MR may also be useful in distinguishing residual or recurrent tumor from posttherapy fibrosis. Fibrosis has a decreased signal intensity on T2-weighted images, whereas tumor has a high signal intensity.

Nuclear Medicine

Because neuroblastomas commonly metastasize to bone, radionuclide bone scans are useful. In addition, many primary tumors demonstrate the uptake of a skeletal tracer. Either MIBG or Octreoscan is sensitive for the detection of neuroblastomas and may be useful in confirming neuroblastoma as the etiology of an abdominal mass.

Treatment

Surgical excision is the preferred treatment for patients with stages I and II disease. Patients in low- or intermediate-risk categories have a relatively good prognosis. Surgery followed by chemotherapy is used for higher-risk patients, but even with bone marrow transplantation, their prognosis is considerably worse. Radiation therapy in combination with chemotherapy improves the prognosis for selected patients.

NONHYPERFUNCTIONAL DISEASES

Adenoma

Benign, nonhyperfunctioning adrenal adenomas commonly are encountered on abdominal CT examinations and are more common among older patients and those with diabetes mellitus or hypertension. Nonhyperfunctioning adenomas are almost always detected as an incidental finding. Occasionally, they are large enough to cause pain or compress adjacent structures. Rarely, hemorrhage into an adenoma may occur.

Radiology

Although ultrasound can detect adrenal adenomas when they reach 2 to 3 cm in diameter, most adenomas are detected during a CT examination of the upper abdomen. Typically, the nonhyperfunctioning adenoma is a well-defined, rounded, homogeneous mass (Fig. 3.19). Calcification is uncommon and central necrosis

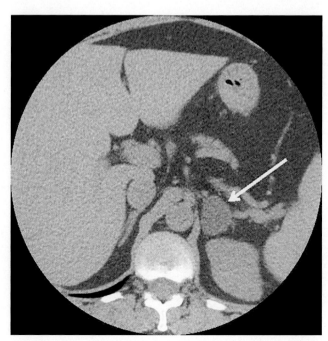

FIGURE 3.19. Adenoma. A left adrenal mass (*arrow*) is seen on this unenhanced CT examination.

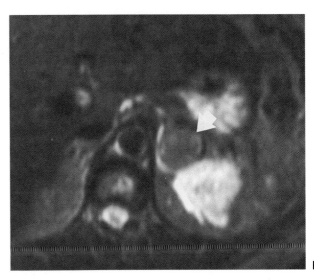

FIGURE 3.20. Adenoma. **A:** The left adrenal mass (*arrow*) is well defined on the T1-weighted image. **B:** The relatively low signal intensity on the T2-weighted image distinguishes this benign tumor (*arrow*) from an adrenal metastasis.

or hemorrhage is rare. Adrenal adenomas are distinguished from other adrenal masses, especially metastases and pheochromocytomas, by the presence of lipid. Approximately 80% of adrenal adenomas are "lipid rich" and contain abundant cytoplasmic lipid. The identification of this lipid on either an unenhanced CT or a chemical shift MR examination allows the confident diagnosis of an adenoma (Fig. 3.20).

Adrenal masses are demonstrated easily with MRI. Adenomas are well-defined, homogeneous masses with relatively low signal intensity on both T1- and T2-weighted images. MRI may also be useful in distinguishing a nonhyperfunctioning adenoma from metastatic tumor. Metastases typically have higher signal intensities than adenomas on T2-weighted sequences (Fig. 3.20), but loss of signal going from in-phase images to out-of-phase images is a more reliable method to identify an adenoma.

Carcinoma

Primary adrenal cortical carcinoma is an uncommon malignancy that occurs with a frequency of approximately 1 case per 1 million population. Men and women are affected equally, but functional tumors are more common among female patients. Although the median age at presentation is the fifth decade, patients ranging from 1 to 80 years of age have been reported. Most adrenal carcinomas are sporadic, but there are several genetic syndromes in which the incidence of adrenal carcinoma is increased, including the Beckwith–Wiedemann syndrome, MEN1, the Carney complex, familial adenomatous polyposis coli, and the Li–Fraumeni cancer syndrome.

Adrenal carcinomas usually are quite large at presentation, although a tumor as small as 1 cm has been reported. They have a nodular surface and are incompletely encapsulated. Central tumor necrosis and hemorrhage are common.

The microscopic appearance is variable. Some carcinomas are well differentiated such that differentiation from an adenoma is difficult. In more frankly malignant lesions, highly abnormal cells with giant nuclei, multinucleation, and atypical mitoses are found.

The most common presentation of patients with an adrenal carcinoma is abdominal pain or a palpable mass. Approximately 50% of these tumors produce a hormone in excess, which results in characteristic clinical manifestations. Cushing syndrome is most frequent, though signs of virilization and feminization may also be found. Hyperaldosteronism rarely is caused by carcinoma. Many of the "nonfunctional" carcinomas may produce hormones that do not cause a clinical syndrome. This may be demonstrated by measurement of urinary 17-ketosteroid levels. Nonfunctional carcinomas tend to be larger than those producing a recognizable hormone.

Surgical excision is the treatment of choice. Mitotane (OP'DDD), which affects adrenocortical cell mitochondria, both inhibits corticosteroid synthesis and destroys adrenocortical cells. Mitotane is the primary chemotherapeutic agent, but its use is limited by side effects that include gastrointestinal symptoms and adrenal insufficiency. Radiation therapy may be used for palliation, especially for bone metastases.

Radiology

Ultrasound can demonstrate a suprarenal mass. Smaller lesions, up to 6 cm, often are homogeneous, whereas larger tumors have a heterogeneous texture with scattered echogenic areas representing tumor necrosis or hemorrhage.

The typical CT appearance of adrenal carcinoma is a large mass with central areas of low attenuation representing tumor necrosis (Fig. 3.21). Coronal images (Fig. 3.22) can be helpful to

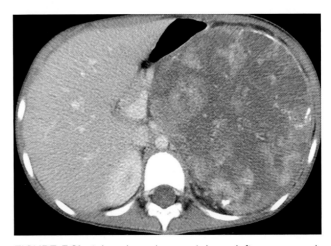

FIGURE 3.21. Adrenal carcinoma. A huge left upper quadrant mass is seen on this enhanced CT examination.

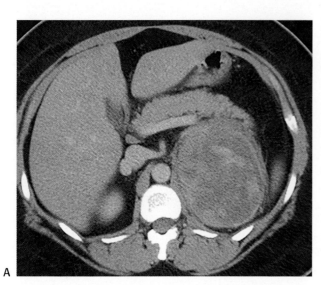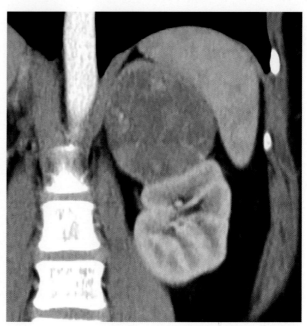

A   B

FIGURE 3.22. Adrenal carcinoma. The left upper quadrant mass on the axial image **(A)** is seen to displace the kidney inferiorly **(B)** on the coronal CT image.

confirm the adrenal origin of the mass. Calcification is seen in approximately 30% of cases (Fig. 3.21). Evidence of hepatic or regional lymph node metastases as well as extension of tumor into the left renal vein or IVC may be detected by CT (Fig. 3.23). If the extent of the tumor thrombus cannot be defined precisely, MRI may be needed.

The most difficult area for CT staging of adrenal carcinoma has been the detection of direct hepatic extension. If a fat plane exists between the tumor and the liver, there is no hepatic involvement. However, if there is no fat plane, it is impossible to accurately predict the presence or absence of liver invasion.

MRI often is used to evaluate a suspected adrenal carcinoma. The tumors usually are heterogeneous and hyperintense on both T1- and T2-weighted sequences (Fig. 3.24). The high signal intensity on T2-weighted images and heterogeneous enhancement on gadolinium-enhanced T1-weighted sequences further

support the malignant diagnosis (Fig. 3.25). The sagittal projection may be helpful in determining whether there is hepatic invasion. Venous extension often can be defined more clearly on MRI than with CT.

Adrenal carcinomas are usually FDG-avid and demonstrate hypermetabolic activity on 18 F-FDG PET/CT examinations (Fig. 3.26). These studies are useful in demonstrating the primary tumor, metastases, and local recurrence.

Arteriography is needed only infrequently for the evaluation of patients with suspected adrenal carcinoma. In patients with a huge mass in the region of the adrenal gland, it may be difficult to determine the tissue of origin. The adrenal gland may not be identified because of compression by the huge mass, and fat planes no longer separate it from adjacent organs such as the kidney and liver. Selective arteriography can identify the primary vascular supply and determine the organ of origin of the mass. Selective renal,

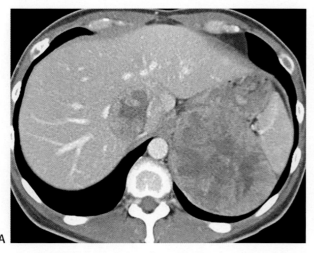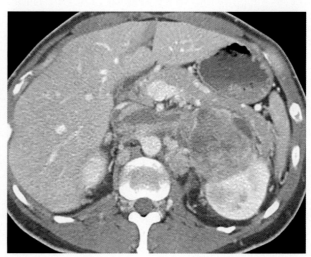

A   B

FIGURE 3.23. Adrenal carcinoma. **A:** A large left adrenal mass is seen as well as tumor in the inferior vena cava. **B:** The extension of the tumor into the left renal vein is clearly shown.

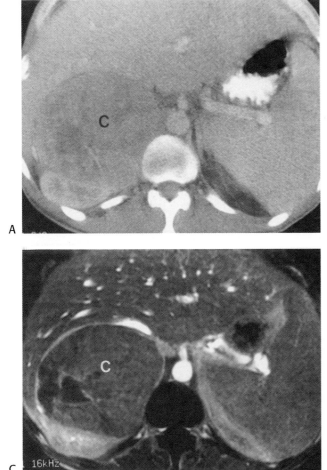

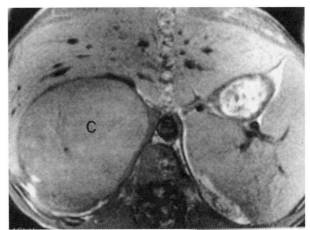

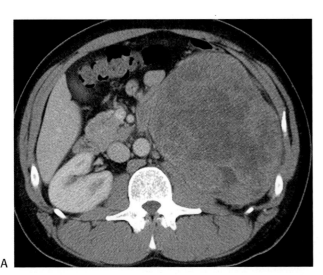

FIGURE 3.24. Adrenal carcinoma. **A:** A huge right adrenal mass (*C*) is seen on an enhanced CT examination. **B:** A moderate signal intensity of the tumor (*C*) is demonstrated on the T2-weighted image. **C:** There is heterogeneous enhancement of the tumor (*C*) on the gadolinium-enhanced, T1-weighted image.

inferior phrenic, and celiac or hepatic artery injections should be performed. If possible, selective injection of the middle adrenal artery may also be helpful.

Adrenal carcinomas are staged using a TNM system such as the one developed by the Union for International Cancer Control (UICC) (Table 3.2).

Myelolipoma

A myelolipoma is a benign tumor composed of mature adipose cells and hematopoietic tissue. The gross appearance resembles fatty tissue but may contain patchy red areas of blood-forming cells. Although considered an uncommon lesion, it often is recognized as

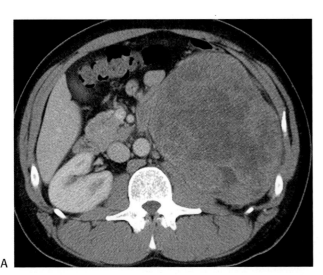

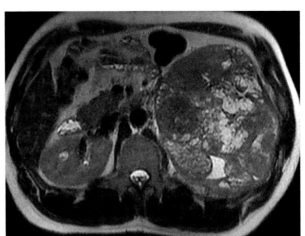

FIGURE 3.25. Adrenal carcinoma. **A:** A huge left upper quadrant mass is seen on this enhanced CT examination. **B:** Heterogeneous enhancement is demonstrated on the MR examination.

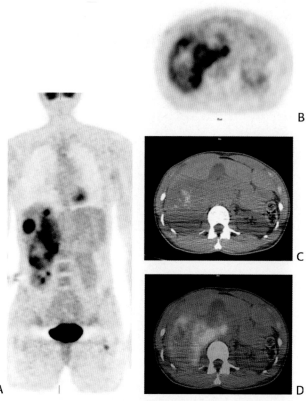

B

C

A

D

FIGURE 3.26. Adrenal carcinoma. 18F-FDG PET/CT scan. Multiple projection image **(A)** demonstrates a large hypermetabolic mass in the right abdomen and focal hypermetabolic lesions in the liver and proximal left femur indicating distant metastases. PET **(B)**, CT **(C)**, and fused PET/CT **(D)** images demonstrate a heterogeneous hypermetabolic right adrenal mass with calcification and central necrosis, as well as hypermetabolic activity in the retroperitoneal lymphadenopathy.

an incidental finding on an abdominal CT examination. Bilateral and extra-adrenal myelolipomas have been reported.

The tumors are functionally inactive and usually are detected as an incidental finding. Occasionally, large tumors may cause pain or present with displacement of adjacent organs. Retroperitoneal hemorrhage has been reported. The most common age at detection

TABLE 3.2			
Adrenocortical Carcinoma Staging (UICC)			
Stage I	T1	N0	M0
Stage II	T2	N0	M0
Stage III	T3	N0	M0
Or	T1 or T2	N1	M0
Stage IV	T3	N1	M0
Or	T4	N0	M0
Or	T3	N0	M1

T1 ≤ 5 cm
T2 ≥ 5 cm
T3 = infiltrating surrounding tissue
T4 = invasion or local organs or renal vein/IVC

is the sixth decade. There is no sex predilection, and both glands are equally affected.

Radiology

Ultrasound reveals a highly echogenic mass (Fig. 3.27). If the tumor is 4 cm or larger, a propagation speed artifact may be present. This appearance is suggestive of a myelolipoma; however, it cannot be distinguished clearly from a retroperitoneal lipoma or liposarcoma. If the tumor is small or the patient has abundant retroperitoneal fat, the myelolipoma may be difficult to distinguish from perirenal fat.

The most definitive radiographic examination is CT (Fig. 3.28), and unenhanced scans usually are adequate to make the diagnosis. A fatty adrenal mass is virtually diagnostic of a myelolipoma. However, rare cases of adrenocortical carcinoma, adenoma, and metastatic adenocarcinoma containing fat have been documented. An adrenal lipoma or liposarcoma could also mimic this appearance. The MR appearance of a myelolipoma reflects the variable amounts of fat and bone marrow elements in the tumor. Fat has a high signal intensity on both T1- and T2-weighted sequences, whereas bone marrow elements have a low signal intensity on T1-weighted sequences and a moderate signal intensity on T2-weighted images.

Treatment of myelolipomas usually is conservative. The clear diagnosis of this benign lesion does not require further confirmation, although diagnosis by fine-needle aspiration has been reported. Symptomatic lesions should be excised. Asymptomatic lesions larger than 4 cm sometimes are removed to avoid potential complications such as retroperitoneal hemorrhage.

Hemorrhage

Adrenal hemorrhage may be spontaneous, traumatic, or related to anticoagulation. Spontaneous adrenal hemorrhage often occurs in patients with septicemia, hypertension, renal vein thrombosis, or adrenal pathology, such as a tumor.

The relatively large size of the fetal adrenal gland may predispose it to hemorrhage during the stress of delivery or the neonatal period. Adrenal hemorrhage is more common in the newborn than in older children or adults. It may be because of the trauma of delivery, asphyxia, septicemia, or abnormal clotting factors. It is bilateral in only about 10% of cases. If the hemorrhage is large, a palpable mass, anemia, or prolonged jaundice may occur. Adrenal insufficiency is rare in the neonate. Hemorrhage usually can be distinguished from a tumor such as neuroblastoma and surgery avoided. Most adrenal hematomas will be resorbed, but some may liquefy and persist as an adrenal pseudocyst.

When adrenal hemorrhage occurs in the older child or adult, it often is a result of trauma or is associated with systemic illness or anticoagulation. It has been seen with hypertension, septicemia, renal vein thrombosis, seizures, surgery, or treatment with ACTH, insulin, or corticosteroids. When related to anticoagulation therapy, adrenal hemorrhage usually occurs during the first 3 weeks of therapy. However, it is not because of excessive anticoagulation, as associated hemorrhage does not occur in other areas.

Patients with the primary antiphospholipid syndrome have an increased frequency of thrombotic events, including deep venous thrombosis and strokes. Adrenal hemorrhage may occur in these patients, presumably resulting from adrenal vein thrombosis.

Adrenal hemorrhage may occur in up to 25% of severely traumatized patients, and approximately 20% of cases are bilateral. The right adrenal gland is involved much more commonly than the left. This may be from an acute rise in venous pressure, which is more directly transmitted to the right adrenal gland because the right adrenal vein enters the IVC directly while the left adrenal vein enters the inferior phrenic vein before entering the left renal vein and finally the IVC.

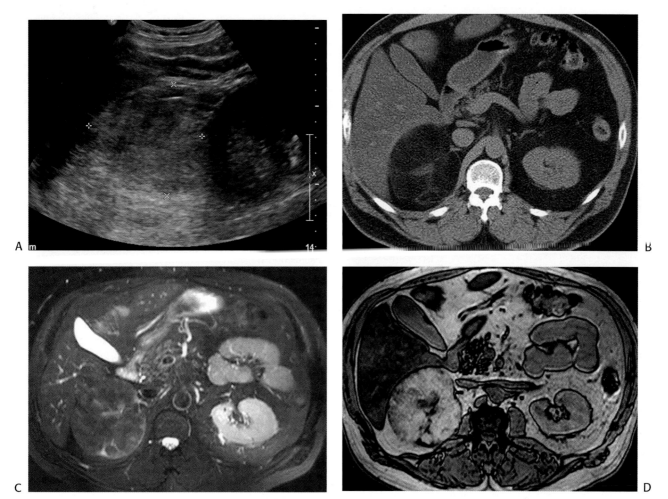

FIGURE 3.27. Myelolipoma. **A:** An echogenic adrenal mass suggests a myelolipoma. **B:** Fat density was confirmed on CT. **C, D:** The signal intensity is similar to fat on the T1-weighted MR exam **(C)** and the T2-weighted image **(D)**.

It is also suggested that the right adrenal gland may be crushed between the liver and spine. The hematoma usually is found in the adrenal medulla with stretching of the surrounding cortex.

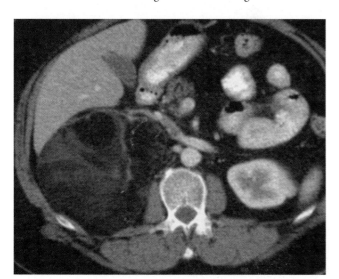

FIGURE 3.28. Myelolipoma. The fat density is clearly shown on this CT examination.

Most adrenal hemorrhage is clinically silent. Only rarely is the endocrine function of the gland sufficiently impaired to cause adrenal insufficiency, as both glands must be affected for this to occur.

Radiology

In children, adrenal hemorrhage usually is imaged with ultrasound. The echogenicity varies with the state of the hematoma and may be hypoechoic, mixed, or moderately echogenic. An acute hematoma may be difficult to distinguish from a solid mass. With lysis of the clot and liquefaction of the hematoma, the mass becomes progressively less echogenic.

The most common method of identifying adrenal hemorrhage in adults is CT (Fig. 3.29). Initially, the hematoma has a high density, 50 to 90 Hounsfield units (HU), reflecting the concentration of hemoglobin. Follow-up studies usually show resorption of the hematoma (Fig. 3.30) and a gradual decrease in density to near water.

The MR appearance of adrenal hemorrhage reflects the evolution from acute to chronic stages with hemoglobin breakdown. A heterogeneous signal intensity is seen on T1- and T2-weighted images of acute hemorrhage. The signal intensity often is quite low on T2-weighted images because of the intracellular deoxyhemoglobin. After a week, the ferrous hemoglobin is oxidized to ferric methemoglobin and the hematoma appears hyperintense on both T1- and T2-weighted images. If the hematoma is not resorbed, the imaging features resemble a cyst in the chronic phase. The central component is isointense on T1-weighted images and hyperintense

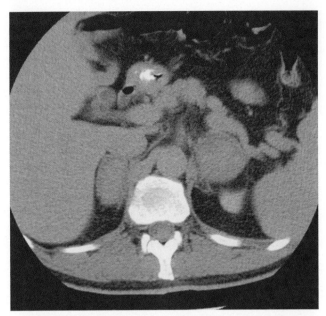

FIGURE 3.29. Adrenal hemorrhage. Bilateral adrenal masses representing hemorrhage are seen in this patient on heparin anticoagulation.

on T2-weighted scans. The periphery may demonstrate low signal intensity from intracellular hemosiderin. There is no enhancement after administration of gadolinium DTPA, but a peripheral rim may enhance if a vascular fibrous capsule has formed.

Cysts

Adrenal cysts are uncommon lesions that may occur at any age. They involve the right and left adrenal glands equally but have a 3:1 female predilection.

Most adrenal cysts are asymptomatic and are found either at autopsy or as incidental findings. Large cysts may cause dull pain or symptoms because of compression on the stomach or duodenum.

There are several recognized etiologies of adrenal cysts. Endothelial cysts are the most common, accounting for approximately

45% of all adrenal cysts. They have an endothelial lining and may be lymphatic or angiomatous in origin. Lymphangiomatous cysts are more common and probably develop from blockage of a lymph duct.

Epithelial cysts are quite uncommon because they comprise only 9% of adrenal cysts. They have a cylindrical epithelium and include cystic adenomas.

Parasitic cysts are the least common variety, comprising only 7% of the total. They are usually echinococcal in origin and are associated with widespread disease.

Pseudocysts are the second most common variety, as they comprise 39% of adrenal cysts. They are probably caused by adrenal hemorrhage into a normal or abnormal gland. The lining is not covered by epithelium. Pseudocysts are most commonly detected radiographically because they tend to be larger than endothelial cysts.

Radiology

Ultrasound demonstrates a cystic suprarenal mass (Fig. 3.31). Unlike renal cysts, adrenal cysts often exhibit a thick wall. Pseudocysts may also demonstrate internal septations. If a soft tissue masslike component is present, surgery may be required to exclude a neoplasm.

Similar findings are detected with CT (Fig. 3.31). The density of the fluid is near water density, and calcification has been reported in 60% of cases (Fig. 3.32).

The findings on MRI are similar to those of a renal cyst. The cyst fluid is hypointense on T1-weighted sequences and hyperintense on T2-weighted images. Wall enhancement is often seen in contrast-enhanced studies. Although cyst aspiration can be helpful if the fluid is clear and the cytology is benign, this is probably unnecessary, and the lesions can be followed with cross-sectional imaging studies.

Hemangioma

Adrenal hemangioma is a rare tumor of the adrenal cortex. They range in diameter from 2 to 22 cm and may undergo degenerative changes including thrombosis, hemorrhage, and necrosis. Patients have ranged from 25 to 79 years of age. The tumors more often involve the right adrenal gland and show a female preponderance. None of the hemangiomas reported have shown evidence of hyperfunction, although adrenal insufficiency has been seen.

Most patients are asymptomatic, and the tumor is found at autopsy or as an incidental finding during evaluation for another

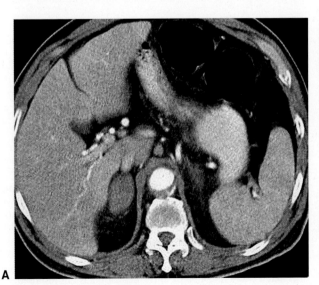
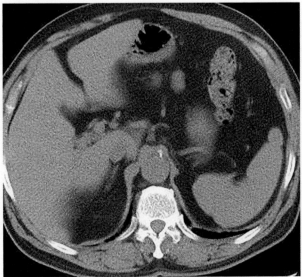

FIGURE 3.30. Adrenal hemorrhage. **A:** The high density of the right adrenal mass suggests it is hemorrhage. **B:** Follow-up scan demonstrates resolution of the hematoma.

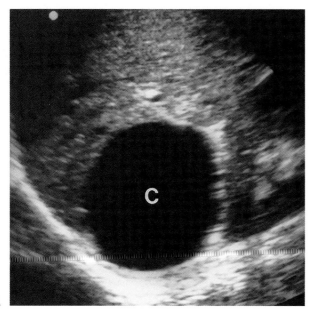 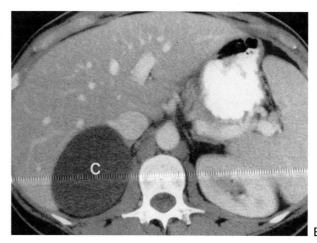

FIGURE 3.31. Adrenal cyst. **A:** Ultrasound demonstrates a huge cystic mass (*C*) above the right kidney. **B:** A water density mass (*C*) is confirmed on CT.

process. However, dull pain and vague upper gastrointestinal tract symptoms may be present in very large lesions.

Ultrasound demonstrates a complex mass and may reveal cystic areas. The CT appearance depends also on the tumor morphology. Typically, a large mass with a thick irregular wall and hypodense center is seen. There is patchy enhancement of the peripheral zone. Calcification is common due to either a phlebolith or prior hemorrhage. On MR, hemangiomas are hypointense to the liver on T1-weighted sequences; areas of increased signal intensity suggest hemorrhage. The tumors are hyperintense on T2-weighted images. Peripheral enhancement is common and is often persistent on delayed images.

The angiographic appearance of a hypovascular mass with contrast pooling and prolongation of the vascular stain is similar to hemangiomas in other organs. However, the radiographic findings are seldom sufficiently characteristic, and surgical resection often is performed.

Oncocytic Neoplasms

Oncocytic neoplasms arising in the adrenal gland are rare. They are composed of oncocytic cells with abundant granular eosinophilic cytoplasm. They are more common among women and may be benign or malignant. They are not hormonally active and are most often seen as an incidental finding.

The tumors are often quite large at presentation (Fig. 3.33). Those <5 cm in diameter are usually benign. They lack lipid and are easily distinguished from lipid-rich adenomas. Malignant oncocytic adrenal neoplasms are often large and indistinguishable from adrenal cortical carcinomas.

Metastases

The adrenal glands are a common site of metastatic disease. In a series of 1,000 consecutive postmortem examinations of patients with an epithelial malignancy, Abrams et al. found 27% to have adrenal metastases. The most common primary tumors are bronchogenic carcinoma, renal cell carcinoma, hepatocellular carcinoma,

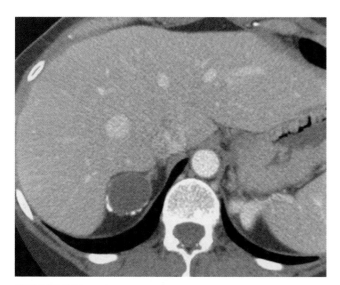

FIGURE 3.32. Adrenal pseudocyst. This water density right adrenal mass contains several peripheral calcifications.

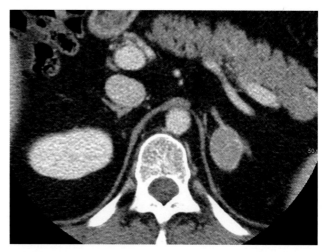

FIGURE 3.33. Oncocytic adrenal tumor. A small, benign oncocytoma is demonstrated in the left adrenal gland.

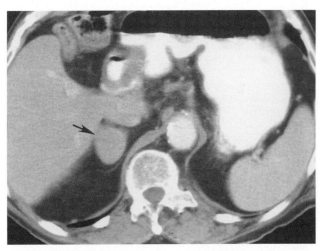

FIGURE 3.34. Adrenal metastasis. This right adrenal metastasis (*arrow*) from an underlying hepatoma is small, well defined, and homogeneous.

colorectal carcinoma, and melanoma. Adrenal metastases may be treated with chemotherapy, radiation therapy, or surgical resection. Recently, radiofrequency ablation has been shown to be a useful alternative, especially for patients who are poor surgical candidates.

The radiographic appearance of adrenal metastases is not specific. They may be large or small and unilateral or bilateral. A metastasis is a solid mass and, when <3 cm in diameter, is usually homogeneous (Fig. 3.34). Larger lesions may demonstrate central necrosis (Fig. 3.35) or areas of hemorrhage (Fig. 3.36). Thus, an adrenal metastasis can seldom be distinguished clearly from benign lesions such as adenomas, hematomas, pseudocysts, or inflammatory masses on the basis of morphology. However, if other metastases are present, it is unlikely that the presence of an adrenal metastases will alter therapy (Fig. 3.37).

Incidental Adrenal Lesions

An adrenal nodule detected on an imaging study performed for an indication other than tumor surveillance or evaluation of the adrenal glands is considered an incidental adrenal lesion (IAL) or "incidentaloma." These lesions are usually found on abdominal

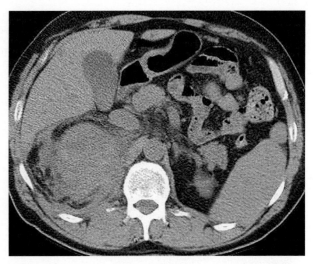

FIGURE 3.36. Hemorrhagic metastasis. The high-density right adrenal mass with soft tissue stranding indicates a hemorrhagic metastasis to the right adrenal gland.

CT examinations and range in size from small nodules measuring <1 cm to large adrenal masses.

IALs are seen in approximately 5% of patients, but the prevalence increases significantly with age. The majority of these lesions are benign, especially if there is no underlying malignancy.

Adrenal lesions are usually nonhyperfunctioning, but some may be unregulated and produce an adrenal hormone in excess. Thus, evidence of hypersecretion of cortisol, aldosterone, androgens, estrogens, or catecholamines should be sought. Elevated levels can be confirmed with urine or serum assays.

Most IALs are benign adenomas, though virtually any lesion can be detected in asymptomatic patients. The goal of imaging examinations in patients with an IAL is to characterize lesions that will affect patient treatment. The most common challenge is to distinguish an adrenal adenoma from a potential adrenal metastasis.

Distinguishing Adenoma from Metastasis

There are several clinical settings in which it is necessary to distinguish a benign adrenal mass from a malignant adrenal mass. In

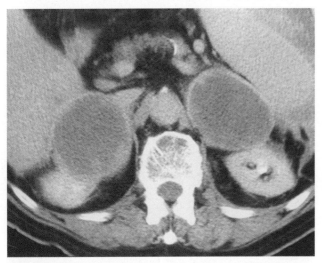

FIGURE 3.35. Adrenal metastases. Bilateral adrenal masses are seen with low-density central areas representing tumor necrosis.

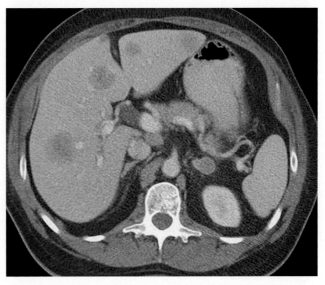

FIGURE 3.37. Multiple abdominal metastases. In addition to the right adrenal nodule, several liver metastases are present.

patients with a known underlying malignancy, an adrenal mass may be a metastasis but also could be an unrelated benign lesion such as an adenoma. If the patient has other evidence of metastatic disease, the presence of an additional metastasis to the adrenal gland may have no effect on staging or treatment. In such cases, little effort should be spent determining the nature of the lesion. On the other hand, if the adrenal mass is the only evidence of metastatic disease, it may be critical to confirm that it is a metastasis or to make a confident diagnosis of a benign etiology.

The second clinical setting where it may be important to clarify the nature of an adrenal mass is the patient in whom the mass is detected as an incidental finding. In these patients, the adrenal lesion most likely is benign; potential malignant etiologies include a

metastasis from an occult primary malignancy or a primary adrenal carcinoma.

An adrenal mass most often is detected on a CT or MR examination of the abdomen. These two modalities are often effective in distinguishing an adenoma from a metastasis, such that percutaneous biopsy is seldom needed.

Features that suggest a malignant lesion include a large size (>4 cm), poorly defined margins, invasion of adjacent structures, inhomogeneous attenuation, and a thick, irregular enhancing rim. A small ovoid lesion with a thin rim and homogeneous density is more likely to be benign. However, many metastases are small, well-defined homogeneous masses that are indistinguishable from adenomas (Fig. 3.38). Furthermore, some adenomas may be large and

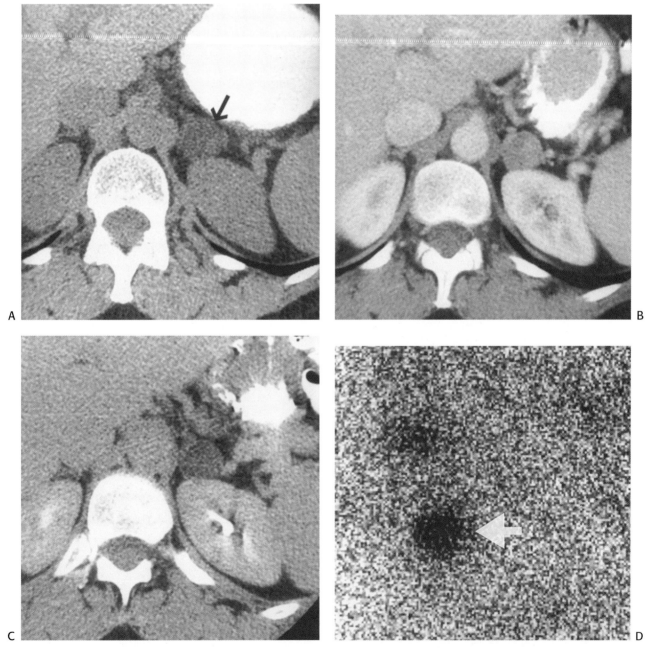

FIGURE 3.38. Adrenal adenoma. **A:** An unenhanced CT examination demonstrates a low-density (5 HU) mass in the left adrenal gland (*arrow*). **B:** After intravenous contrast injection, the density of the mass rises to 77 HU. **C:** A delayed image reveals contrast washout and a density of 15 HU. **D:** The radionuclide uptake (*arrow*) is concordant with the adrenal mass, indicating it is an adenoma.

undergo central necrosis or hemorrhage. Thus, these morphologic criteria are not sufficiently accurate to allow a confident diagnosis.

Nuclear medicine techniques can take advantage of differences in metabolic activity. Because malignant cells use more glucose than benign tissue, adrenal metastases would be expected to have increased uptake of the radiotracer FDG compared with adenomas.

One of the features that distinguish an adrenal adenoma from a metastasis is that the majority (approximately 80%) of adenomas contain abundant cytoplasmic lipid, whereas metastases do not. Thus, the detection of lipid in an adrenal mass allows a confident diagnosis of an adenoma, and further diagnostic testing is unnecessary. The absence of lipid does not have the same diagnostic accuracy, as some adrenal adenomas are lipid-poor and cannot be distinguished from other benign lesions or metastases, which do not contain demonstrable amounts of lipid.

Lipid may be detected either by a low-attenuation value on an unenhanced CT examination (Fig. 3.39) or by MR. An analysis of published reports found that with a CT threshold of 10 HU, the sensitivity and specificity for a diagnosis of adenoma were 71% and 98%, respectively. Lowering the threshold increases the specificity but at a significant decrease in sensitivity. Raising the threshold increases the sensitivity but diminishes the specificity. It is often more important to maintain a very high specificity at the cost of sensitivity, as a false-negative diagnosis of adenoma results in an unnecessary biopsy, whereas a false-positive diagnosis may place the patient in the wrong treatment protocol.

Since most adrenal incidentalomas are detected on contrast-enhanced CT examinations, patients must return for an unenhanced CT in order to use CT density to diagnose an adrenal adenoma. Initial reports using dual-energy CT suggest that virtual attenuation measurements of adrenal density are not significantly different from true unenhanced measurements.

Several investigators have used histogram analysis of adrenal masses on enhanced CT examinations. A plot of the pixel attenuation versus pixel frequency can be done on a standard workstation and the number of pixels that measure fat attenuation (<0 HU) determined. If more than 10% of the pixels measure fat, an adenoma can be confidently diagnosed. However, the low sensitivity of this technique limits its applicability.

Adrenal metastases and adenomas both show enhancement with intravascular contrast media administration, but adenomas "wash out" the contrast media faster and return to

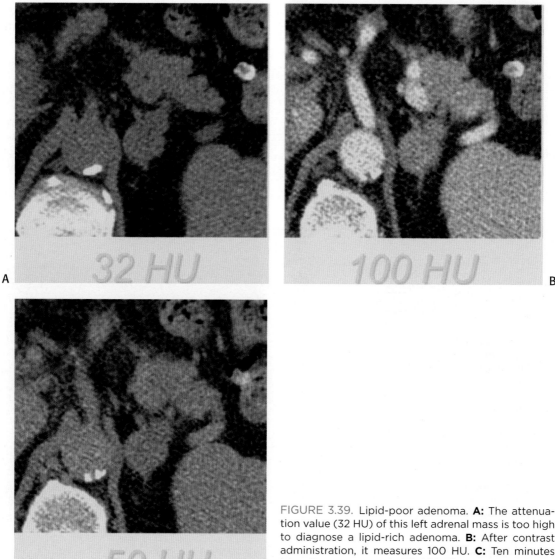

FIGURE 3.39. Lipid-poor adenoma. **A:** The attenuation value (32 HU) of this left adrenal mass is too high to diagnose a lipid-rich adenoma. **B:** After contrast administration, it measures 100 HU. **C:** Ten minutes later, it measures only 50 HU. The washout of 74% allows the diagnosis of benign adenoma.

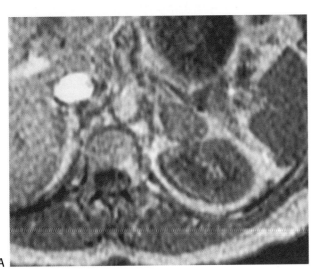 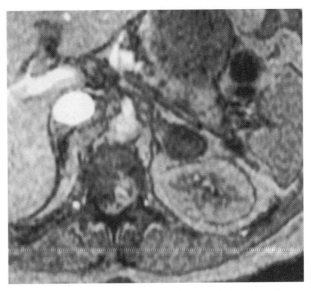

FIGURE 3.40. Benign adenoma. **A:** An in-phase gradient-recalled echo (GRE) image shows a left adrenal mass that is isointense to paraspinal muscles. **B:** The mass becomes hypointense to the paraspinal muscles on opposed-phase GRE images. (From Korobkin M, Lombardi TJ, Aisen AM, et al. Characterization of adrenal masses with chemical shift and gadolinium-enhanced MR imaging. *Radiology.* 1995;197:411–418, with permission.)

their precontrast levels of attenuation much faster than adrenal metastases. Furthermore, this rapid washout of intravascular contrast media is seen in both lipid-rich and lipid-poor adenomas (Fig. 3.39).

The percentage contrast washout can be calculated using the following formula:

$$\text{Percentage enhancement washout} = \frac{\text{Enhancement washout}}{\text{Enhancement}}$$

Enhancement is the difference between the enhanced attenuation value and the unenhanced attenuation value; enhancement washout is the difference between the enhanced attenuation value and the delayed contrast attenuation value.

If an unenhanced scan was not performed, a relative percent enhancement washout can be calculated using the following formula:

$$\frac{\text{Percentage relative}}{\text{enhancement washout}} = \frac{\text{Enhancement washout}}{\text{Enhancement attenuation value}}$$

Adrenal masses with a percentage enhancement washout >60% can be confidently diagnosed as adenomas. If the relative enhancement washout is >40%, the diagnosis of an adenoma is justified. These washout measurements can be applied to either lipid-rich or lipid-poor adenomas.

This technique of using contrast washout to distinguish a benign adenoma from a malignant lesion has potential pitfalls. Benign lesions including a myelolipoma with infarction, an angiomyolipoma with minimal fat, and a ganglioneuroma have all been reported with delayed contrast enhancement. Conversely, patients with adrenal metastases from renal cell carcinoma and hepatocellular carcinoma have been found with washout curves similar to benign lipid-poor adenomas.

The most accurate of the MR techniques for distinguishing an adenoma from a metastasis is chemical shift imaging (CSI). Because protons in water process at different frequencies than those in triglyceride when exposed to a magnetic field, even small quantities of lipid can be detected (Fig. 3.40).

Because both CT density measurements and MR CSI rely on the presence of lipid to diagnose an adrenal adenoma, it is assumed that CSI would not be useful in patients with an adrenal mass measuring >10 HU. However, more recent studies have demonstrated that CSI using a threshold of 20% signal intensity drop results in a higher sensitivity than CT histogram analysis.

Percutaneous aspiration biopsy is the most definitive method of confirming metastatic disease and may be performed with either CT or ultrasound guidance (Fig. 3.41). With experienced cytopathologists, the positive predictive value approaches 100%. A negative aspiration is not as diagnostic because sampling error or an inadequate specimen may preclude a confident diagnosis. The overall accuracy reported for percutaneous adrenal biopsy ranges from 80% to 100%. The results vary with the patient population and the

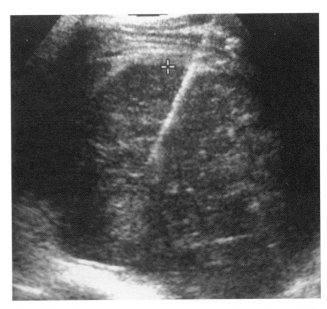

FIGURE 3.41. Adrenal biopsy. Ultrasound is used to guide the biopsy needle into the adrenal mass.

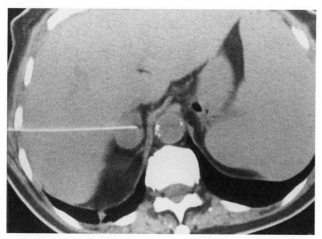

FIGURE 3.42. Adrenal biopsy. CT is the most useful modality for directing percutaneous adrenal biopsies into small tumors. (From Dunnick NR. The adrenal gland. In: Tavaras JM, Ferrucci JT, eds. *Radiology: Diagnosis, Imaging, Intervention.* Philadelphia, PA: JB Lippincott; 1991, with permission.)

types of lesions aspirated. Positive results indicate malignancy. A negative biopsy is much more reliable if normal adrenal cortical cells are present in the specimen and can be repeated to increase the confidence that the lesion is benign.

Adrenal biopsy is an invasive procedure, and complications may occur. The most common complication is pneumothorax. These pneumothoraces usually are small and resolve spontaneously. Large or symptomatic pneumothoraces should be treated with a small chest tube that can be placed by the radiologist under fluoroscopic guidance. Tumor seeding of the needle tract and bacteremia are rare. Right adrenal masses may be approached posteriorly or through the liver (Fig. 3.42). Left adrenal masses should be aspirated from a posterior approach. When biopsy of the left adrenal gland is attempted from an anterior approach, pancreatitis may occur and can be a serious complication. Thus, the pancreas should be avoided if possible. Many patients will have a small amount of bleeding, but this is seldom symptomatic. Welch et al. reported complications in 8 (2.8%) of their 277 adrenal biopsies.

The most worrisome complication of percutaneous needle biopsy of an adrenal mass is precipitation of a hypertensive crisis by a pheochromocytoma. This complication may be fatal despite regaining control of the blood pressure. Measurement of plasma metanephrines may be useful in hypertensive patients but may not be elevated in a nonfunctioning pheochromocytoma.

ADENOMA

- Low density (<10 HU) on unenhanced CT
- Rapid washout on enhanced CT
- Signal decrease on chemical shift MR
- Normal adrenal cells on percutaneous biopsy

METASTASIS

- High density (>20 HU) on unenhanced CT
- Slow washout on enhanced CT
- No change in signal on chemical shift MR
- Metastatic cells on percutaneous biopsy

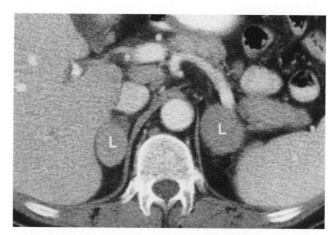

FIGURE 3.43. Lymphoma. The bilateral homogeneous adrenal masses (*L*) are consistent with lymphoma.

Lymphoma

Involvement of the adrenal gland is more common among patients with non-Hodgkin lymphoma than those with Hodgkin disease. Most patients have a diffuse rather than a nodular form of lymphoma. The adrenal glands are seldom an isolated site of disease, although other involvement may be distant. In most patients, however, retroperitoneal lymphoma is also present, although it may not be detected on imaging studies. Adrenal involvement is bilateral in approximately 50% of cases. Even with extensive disease, adrenal insufficiency is rare.

The modalities in which adrenal lymphoma can be identified are ultrasound, CT, and MRI. On ultrasound, lymphoma appears as a well-defined, relatively echogenic homogeneous tissue mass. If extensive retroperitoneal disease is present, it may be difficult to identify the adrenal glands. CT provides the best morphologic delineation. The adrenal glands are enlarged with a rounded mass (Fig. 3.43) or more symmetric enlargement, preserving the basic glandular configuration (Fig. 3.44). The tissue usually is homogeneous and demonstrates contrast enhancement. There is, however, no pathognomonic pattern to indicate lymphomatous involvement. On MRI, lymphoma appears hypointense to the renal cortex on T1-weighted images and hypointense to isointense on T2-weighted

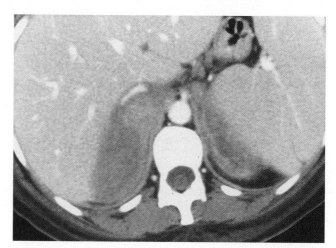

FIGURE 3.44. Lymphoma. There is diffuse involvement of the retroperitoneum and both adrenal glands by low-density tissue.

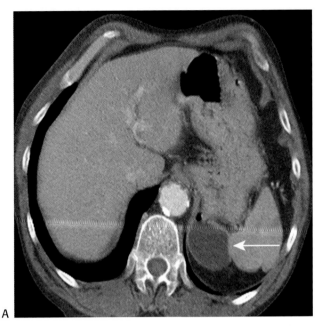
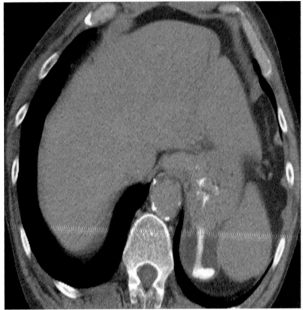

FIGURE 3.45. Pseudotumor. **A:** A mass (*arrow*) is seen in the region of the left adrenal gland. **B:** Subsequent barium study demonstrated this to be a gastric diverticulum.

sequences. Lymphoma enhances less than the renal parenchyma after intravenous contrast administration.

Pseudotumors

A number of abnormalities in the upper abdomen may simulate an adrenal mass. In addition to creating diagnostic confusion, percutaneous biopsy may be attempted. An appreciation of some potential etiologies of an adrenal pseudotumor may help avoid these pitfalls.

Lesions that may simulate an adrenal mass on either side include exophytic renal masses. A right-sided adrenal mass may be mimicked by a hepatic mass, interposition of the colon into the hepatorenal recess, or a dilated IVC.

Left-sided adrenal pseudotumors are more common. They include splenic lobulations, an accessory spleen, varices, tortuous splenic vessels, and a splenic artery aneurysm. The tail of the pancreas may extend to the adrenal area and mimic a left adrenal lesion. Although the stomach should be distinguished clearly by oral contrast medium, a gastric diverticulum may present a diagnostic problem (Fig. 3.45).

Careful attention to the adrenal glands and the use of oral contrast medium should distinguish most confusing structures. A bolus injection of intravenous contrast material should further delineate vascular structures. Volume rendering and coronal or sagittal image reconstruction may also help to elucidate the true nature of these lesions. If the diagnosis is still in doubt, however, an additional study such as ultrasound or MRI may be needed for a confident diagnosis.

Infections

The adrenal glands may be affected by fungal, mycobacterial, parasitic, bacterial, or viral agents. The most common infections to involve the adrenal glands are mycobacteria.

Tuberculosis is the most common infectious disease in the adrenal glands and, worldwide, is the most common cause of adrenal insufficiency. Spread to the adrenal glands is usually

hematogenous from a primary infection in the lung, though pulmonary involvement may not be apparent on imaging studies. Active adrenal involvement is manifest with bilateral enlargement and central necrosis. Later in the disease, the adrenal glands become atrophic and demonstrate only residual calcification (Fig. 3.46). Histoplasmosis is found in endemic areas and has imaging findings similar to tuberculosis.

Adrenal abscesses are rare and usually found after a surgical procedure or as a complication of adrenal hemorrhage. Immunocompromised patients are at increased risk of adrenal infection with *Pneumocystis carinii* and cytomegalovirus.

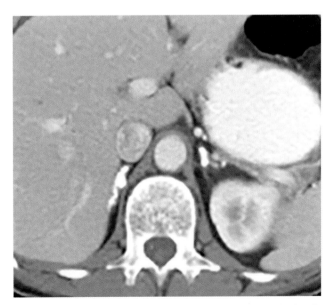

FIGURE 3.46. Granulomatous disease. The adrenal glands are normal in size but calcified. Prior infection with tuberculosis or histoplasmosis is the most likely cause.

SUGGESTED READINGS

General References

Adams SZ, Nikolaidis P, Horowitz JM, et al. Chemical shift MR imaging of the adrenal gland: principles, pitfalls and applications. *Radiographics.* 2016;36:414–432.

Johnson PT, Horton KM, Fishman EK. Adrenal mass imaging with multidetector CT: evidence-based protocol optimization and interpretative practice. *Radiographics.* 2009;29:1319–1331.

Johnson PT, Horton KM, Fishman EK. Adrenal mass imaging with multidetector CT: pathologic conditions, pearls and pitfalls. *Radiographics.* 2009;29:1333–1351.

Kawashima A, Sandler CM, Fishman EK, et al. Spectrum of CT findings in nonmalignant disease of the adrenal gland. *Radiographics.* 1998;18:393.

Lattin GE Jr, Sturgill ED, Tujo CA, et al. From the radiologic pathology archives. adrenal tumors and tumor-like conditions in the adult: radiologic-pathologic correlation. *Radiographics.* 2014;34:805–829.

Tirkes T, Gokaslan T, McCrea J, et al. Oncocytic neoplasms of the adrenal gland. *AJR Am J Roentgenol.* 2011;196:592–596.

Functional Diseases

Choyke PL, Doppman JL. Case 18: adrenocorticotropic hormone-dependent Cushing syndrome. *Radiology.* 2000;214:195.

Conn JW. Primary aldosteronism. *J Lab Clin Med.* 1955;45:661.

Doppman JL, Miller DL, Dwyer AJ, et al. Macronodular adrenal hyperplasia in Cushing disease. *Radiology.* 1988;166:347.

Doppman JL, Nieman L, Miller DL, et al. Ectopic adrenocorticotropic hormone syndrome: localization studies in 28 patients. *Radiology.* 1989;172:115.

Dunnick NR, Leight GS, Roubidoux MA, et al. CT in the diagnosis of primary aldosteronism: sensitivity in 29 patients. *AJR Am J Roentgenol.* 1993;160:321.

Galati S-J. Primary aldosteronism: challenges in diagnosis and management. *Endocrinol Metab Clin N Am.* 2015;44:355–369.

Nieman LK, Turner MLC. Addison's disease. *Clin Dermatol.* 2006;24:276–280.

Patel SM, Lingam RK, Beaconsfield TI, et al. Role of radiology in the management of primary aldosteronism. *Radiographics.* 2007;27:1145–1157.

Sohaib SA, Peppercorn PD, Allan C, et al. Primary hyperaldosteronism (Conn syndrome): MR imaging findings. *Radiology.* 2000;214:527.

Turcu AF, Auchus RJ. Adrenal steroidogenesis and congenital adrenal hyperplasia. *Endocrinol Metab Clin N Am.* 2015;44:275–296.

Adrenal Venous Sampling

Doppman JL, Gill JR Jr. Hyperaldosteronism: sampling the adrenal veins. *Radiology.* 1996;198:309.

Dunnick NR, Doppman JL, Gill JR, et al. Localization of functional adrenal tumors by computed tomography and venous sampling. *Radiology.* 1982;142:429–433.

Kahn SL, Angle JF. Adrenal vein sampling. *Tech Vasc Interv Radiol.* 2010;13:110–125.

Mailhot J-P, Traistaru M, Soulez G, et al. Adrenal vein sampling in primary aldosteronism: sensitivity and specificity of basal adrenal vein to peripheral vein cortisol and aldosterone ratios to confirm catheterization of the adrenal vein. *Radiology.* 2015;277:887–894.

Morita S, Nishina Y, Yamazaki H, et al. Dual adrenal venous phase contrast-enhanced MDCT for visualization of right adrenal veins in patients with primary aldosteronism. *Eur Radiol.* 2016;26:2073–2077.

Ota H, Seiji K, Kawabata M, et al. Dynamic multidetector CT and non-contrast-enhanced MR for right adrenal vein imaging: comparison with catheter venography in adrenal venous sampling. *Eur Radiol.* 2016;26:622–630.

Adrenal Insufficiency

Doppman JL, Gill JR, Nienhius AW, et al. CT findings in Addison's disease. *J Comput Assist Tomogr.* 1982;6(4):757.

Seidenwurm DJ, Elmer EB, Kaplan LM, et al. Metastases to the adrenal glands and the development of Addison's disease. *Cancer.* 1984;54:552.

Pheochromocytoma

Carney JA, Sheps SG, Go VL, et al. The triad of gastric leiomyosarcoma, functioning extra-adrenal paraganglioma and pulmonary chondroma. *N Engl J Med.* 1977;296:1517.

Lee KY, Oh Y-W, Noh HJ, et al. Extraadrenal paragangliomas of the body: imaging features. *AJR Am J Roentgenol.* 2006;187:492–504.

Motte-Ramirez GA, Remer EM, Herts, BR, et al. Comparison of CT findings in symptomatic and incidentally discovered pheochromocytomas. *AJR Am J Roentgenol.* 2005;185:684–688.

Mukherjee JJ, Peppercorn PD, Reznek RH, et al. Pheochromocytoma: effect of nonionic contrast medium in CT on circulating catecholamine levels. *Radiology.* 1997;202:227.

Saurborn DP, Kruskal JB, Stillman IE, et al. Paraganglioma of the organs of Zuckerkandl. *Radiographics.* 2003;23:1279–1286.

Scarsbrook AF, Thakker RV, Wass JA, et al. Multiple endocrine neoplasia: spectrum of radiologic appearances and discussion of a multitechnique imaging approach. *Radiographics.* 2006;26:433–451.

Walther MM, Herring J, Enquist E, et al. Von Recklinghausen's disease and pheochromocytomas. *J Urol.* 1999;162:1582.

Neuroblastoma

Lonergan GJ, Schwab CM, Suarez ES, et al. Neuroblastoma, ganglioneuroblastoma, and ganglioneuroma: radiologic-pathologic correlation. *Radiographics.* 2002;22:911–934.

Spottswood SE, Narla LD. Spectrum of adrenal lesions in children. *Acad Radiol.* 1999;6:433.

Adenoma

Hedeland H, Östberg G, Hökfelt B. On the prevalence of adrenocortical adenomas in an autopsy material in relation to hypertension and diabetes. *Acta Med Scand.* 1968;184:211.

Korobkin M, Giordano TJ, Brodeur FJ, et al. Adrenal adenomas: relationship between histologic lipid and CT and MR findings. *Radiology.* 1996;200:743.

Carcinoma

Agrons GA, Lonergan GJ, Dickey GE, et al. Adrenocortical neoplasms in children: radiologic-pathologic correlation. *Radiographics.* 1999;19:989.

Baudin E. Adrenocortical carcinoma. *Endocrinol Metab Clin N Am.* 2015;44:411–434.

Bharwani N, Rockall AG, Sahdev A, et al. Adrenocortical carcinoma: the range of appearances on CT and MRI. *AJR Am J Roentgenol.* 2011;196:W706–W714.

Dunnick NR, Heaston D, Halvorsen R, et al. CT appearance of adrenal cortical carcinoma. *J Comput Assist Tomogr.* 1982;6(5):978.

Fishman EK, Deutch BM, Hartman DS, et al. Primary adrenocortical carcinoma: CT evaluation with clinical correlation. *AJR Am J Roentgenol.* 1987;148:531.

Hamper UM, Fishman EK, Hartman DS, et al. Primary adrenocortical carcinoma: sonographic evaluation with clinical and pathologic correlation in 26 patients. *AJR Am J Roentgenol.* 1987;148:915.

Myelolipoma

Cyran KM, Kenney PJ, Memel DS, et al. Adrenal myelolipoma. *AJR Am J Roentgenol.* 1996;166:395.

Han M, Burnett AL, Fishman EK, et al. The natural history and treatment of adrenal myelolipoma. *J Urol.* 1997;157:1213.

Kammen BF, Elder DE, Fraker DL, et al. Extraadrenal myelolipoma: MR imaging findings. *AJR Am J Roentgenol.* 1998;171:721.

Rao P, Kenney PJ, Wagner BJ, et al. Imaging and pathologic features of myelolipoma. *Radiographics.* 1997;17:1373.

Hemorrhage

Hammond NA, Lostumbo A, Adam SZ, et al. Imaging of adrenal and renal hemorrhage. *Abdom Imaging.* 2015;20:2747–2760.

Kawashima A, Sandler CM, Ernst RD, et al. Imaging of nontraumatic hemorrhage of the adrenal gland. *Radiographics.* 1999;19:949.

Provenzale JM, Ortel TL, Nelson RC. Adrenal hemorrhage in patients with primary antiphospholipid syndrome: imaging findings. *AJR Am J Roentgenol.* 1995;165:361.

Rana AI, Kenney PJ, Lockhart ME, et al. Adrenal gland hematomas in trauma patients. *Radiology.* 2004;230:669–675.

Cysts

Johnson CD, Baker ME, Dunnick NR. CT demonstration of an adrenal pseudocyst. *J Comput Assist Tomogr.* 1985;9(4):817.

Ricci Z, Chernyak V, Hsu K, et al. Adrenal cysts: natural history by long-term imaging follow-up. *AJR Am J Roentgenol.* 2013;201:1009–1016.

Hemangioma

Derchi LE, Rapaccini GL, Banderali A, et al. Ultrasound and CT findings in two cases of hemangioma of the adrenal gland. *J Comput Assist Tomogr.* 1989;13(4):659.

Salup R, Finegold R, Borochovitz D, et al. Cavernous hemangioma of the adrenal gland. *J Urol.* 1992;147:110.

Ganglioneuroma

Johnson GL, Hruban RH, Marshall FF, et al. Primary adrenal ganglioneuroma: CT findings in four patients. *AJR Am J Roentgenol.* 1997;169:169.

Radin R, David CL, Goldfarb H, et al. Adrenal and extra-adrenal retroperitoneal ganglioneuroma: imaging findings in 13 adults. *Radiology.* 1997;202:703.

Oncocytic Neoplasms

Khan M, Caoili EM, Davenport MS, et al. CT imaging characteristics of oncocytic adrenal neoplasms (OANs): comparison with adrenocortical carcinomas. *Abdom Imaging.* 2014;39:86–91.

Metastases

Abrams HL, Spiro R, Goldstein N. Metastases in carcinoma: analysis of 1,000 autopsied cases. *Cancer.* 1950;3:74–85.

Casola G, Nicolet V, vanSonnenberg E, et al. Unsuspected pheochromocytoma: risk of blood-pressure alterations during percutaneous adrenal biopsy. *Radiology.* 1986;156:733.

Hasegawa T, Yamakado K, Nakatsuka A, et al. Unresectable adrenal metastases: clinical outcomes of radiofrequency ablation. *Radiology.* 2015;277:584–593.

Silverman SG, Mueller PR, Pinkney LP, et al. Predictive value of image-guided adrenal biopsy: analysis of results of 101 biopsies. *Radiology.* 1993;187:715–718.

Distinguishing Adenoma from Metastasis

Blodgett TM, Meltzer CC, Townsend DW. PET/CT: form and function. *Radiology.* 2007;242:360–385.

Boland GW, Blake MA, Hahn PF, et al. Incidental adrenal lesions: principles, techniques, and algorithms for imaging characterization. *Radiology.* 2008;249:756–775.

Caoili EM, Korobkin M, Brown RK, et al. Differentiating adrenal adenomas from nonadenomas using F-FDG PET/CT: quantitative and qualitative evaluation. *Acad Radiol.* 2007;14:468–475.

Caoili EM, Korobkin M, Francis IR, et al. Adrenal masses: characterization with combined unenhanced and delayed enhanced CT. *Radiology.* 2002;222:629–633.

Choyke PL. ACR appropriateness criteria on incidentally discovered adrenal mass. *J Am Coll Radiol.* 2006;3:498–504.

Dong A, Cui Y, Wang Y, et al. 18 F-FDG PET/CT of adrenal lesions. *AJR Am J Roentgenol.* 2014;203:245–252.

Elaini AB, Shetty SK, Chapman VM, et al. Improved detection and characterization of adrenal disease with PET-CT. *Radiographics.* 2007;27:755–767.

Ho LM, Marin D, Neville AM, et al. Characterization of adrenal nodules with dual-energy CT: can virtual unenhanced attenuation values replace true unenhanced attenuation values? *AJR Am J Roentgenol.* 2012;198:840–845.

Israel GM, Korobkin M, Wang C, et al. Comparison of unenhanced CT and chemical shift MRI in evaluating lipid-rich adrenal adenomas. *AJR Am J Roentgenol.* 2004;183:215–219.

Jhaveri KS, Wong F, Ghai S, et al. Comparison of CT histogram analysis and chemical shift MRI in the characterization of indeterminate adrenal nodules. *AJR Am J Roentgenol.* 2006;187:1303–1308.

Kebapci M, Kaya T, Gurbuz E, et al. Differentiation of adrenal adenomas (lipid rich and lipid poor) from nonadenomas by use of washout characteristics on delayed enhanced CT. *Abdom Imaging.* 2003;28:709–715.

Korobkin M, Brodeur FJ, Francis IR, et al. CT time-attenuation washout curves of adrenal adenomas and nonadenomas. *AJR Am J Roentgenol.* 1998;170:747.

Remer EM, Motta-Ramirez GA, Shepardson LB, et al. CT histogram analysis in pathologically proven adrenal masses. *AJR Am J Roentgenol.* 2006;187:191–196.

Sangwaiya MJ, Boland GW, Cronin CG, et al. Incidental adrenal lesions: accuracy of characterization with contrast-enhanced washout multidetector CT–10-minute delayed imaging protocol revisited in a large patient cohort. *Radiology.* 2010;256:504–510.

Song JH, Chaudhry FS, Mayo-Smith WW. The incidental indeterminate adrenal mass on CT (>10H) in patients without cancer: is further imaging necessary? Follow-up of 321 consecutive indeterminate adrenal masses. *AJR Am J Roentgenol.* 2007;189:1119–1123.

Pseudotumors

Berliner L, Bosniak MA, Megibow A. Adrenal pseudotumors on computed tomography. *J Comput Assist Tomogr.* 1982;6(2):281.

4

The Retroperitoneum

This chapter deals with those conditions that involve the urinary tract such as fluid collections, retroperitoneal fibrosis, and primary retroperitoneal tumors. It will not deal with the wide topic of lymphatic diseases; nodal metastases from urologic or gynecologic neoplasms will be dealt with in the chapters describing these tumors.

FLUID COLLECTIONS

Hemorrhage

The causes of retroperitoneal hemorrhage are numerous; clinical and imaging information usually reveals the source, but sometimes the reason for bleeding is initially obscure. Interventional procedures (Fig. 4.1) and other trauma are common causes of hemorrhage. Coagulopathies and anticoagulation therapy may cause hemorrhage with no associated underlying pathology and exacerbate the tendency of a number of kinds of retroperitoneal pathology to undergo spontaneous bleeding. Any tumor may bleed; in the kidney, angiomyolipomas (Fig. 4.2) and carcinomas are the commonest causes. In the adrenal gland, pheochromocytomas (Fig. 4.3), metastases, and adrenocortical carcinomas may hemorrhage. Vascular diseases may cause bleeding; any aneurysm, including those of the abdominal aorta (Fig. 4.4) and the extrarenal and intrarenal segments of the renal artery, may rupture. Arteriovenous malformations and fistulae may bleed, as may vessels affected by arteritis (Fig. 4.5). Severe shock may cause hemorrhage in normal adrenal glands. The psoas and iliacus muscles are particularly prone to undergo bleeding (Fig. 4.6), which may appear with anticoagulation, after arterial catheterization or following relatively mild trauma.

If an intrarenal or a perirenal hematoma appears spontaneously, and no underlying cause is visible at initial workup, repeat imaging after hematoma resolution may be advisable to exclude a small tumor.

Small hemorrhages may occur without symptoms; larger ones may produce pain, shock, and/or anemia. Rarely, an evolving perinephric or subcapsular hematoma will exert sufficient pressure on the kidney to produce the Page kidney phenomenon (Fig. 4.7), in which pressure-induced renal ischemia activates the renin–angiotensin system and causes hypertension. Most hematomas ultimately resorb completely, but some persist. These become encapsulated

and undergo resorption of hemoglobin, becoming chronic fluid collections known as seromas (Fig. 4.8).

CT is the first examination to employ if hemorrhage or hematomas are suspected. Noncontrast CT suffices to identify hematomas, but CT arteriography should be performed if active bleeding is suspected. MRI and MR arteriography are probably equivalent, but to date, there has not been extensive comparison of them in evaluating retroperitoneal bleeding, and CT is usually more quickly available, cheaper, and less prone to technically inadequate studies. Catheter arteriography may be necessary to demonstrate small vascular abnormalities, and permits embolotherapy.

Extravasated blood may infiltrate soft tissues to produce a contusion or may collect in a space containing only blood. Hematomas frequently appear in the perinephric space; anterior pararenal space hematomas may be caused by pancreatitis and pancreatic or duodenal trauma. Posterior pararenal space hematomas often originate

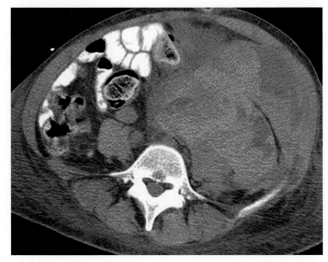

FIGURE 4.1. Retroperitoneal hematoma following biopsy of transplanted kidney (not shown). The denser portions of the hematoma are sites of concentrated hemoglobin.

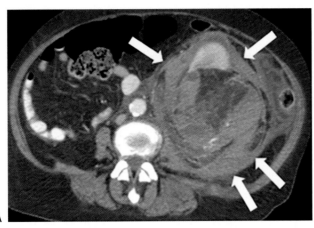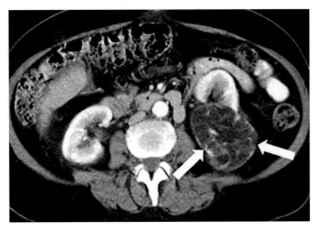

FIGURE 4.2. **A:** Large hematoma (*arrows*) surrounding spontaneously bleeding renal angiomyolipoma. **B:** The angiomyolipoma (*arrows*) several months prior to hemorrhage.

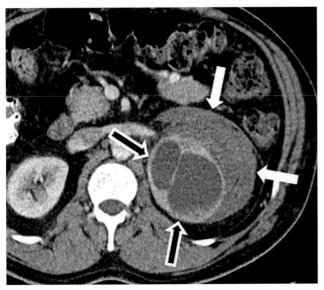

FIGURE 4.3. Cystic adrenal pheochromocytoma (*black* and *white arrows*) with spontaneous hemorrhage (*white arrows*).

in the psoas or iliacus muscles (Fig. 4.6). Hematomas may displace any retroperitoneal viscus or blood vessel.

Ultrasound delineates fatty contusion poorly but will reveal most discrete hematomas as regions hypoechoic compared to fat but still containing disorganized echoes and usually displaying enhanced through-transmission (Fig. 4.9); chronic seromas usually have very few internal echoes. CT is highly sensitive in detecting hemorrhage and provides a clear delineation of its location and extent. Acute hematomas usually display feathery margins (Fig. 4.3) unless they are contained by a smooth fascial sheet. The CT density of blood is directly proportional to hemoglobin concentration, so that when clots form, or red cells settle in the dependent portion of the hematoma, dense regions appear. These will be denser than any noncalcified tissue (albeit <100 Hounsfield units) on unenhanced scans. Intramuscular hemorrhage may present without remarkable increases in density and appear as nonspecific swelling.

When studied by MRI, extremely acute hematomas generally exhibit low to medium signal intensity on T1-weighted images and brighter signal on T2-weighted images. As the hematoma ages, the periphery increases in signal intensity on T1-weighted images (Fig. 4.10), and in the chronic phase, there may be a region of uniform high intensity on both T1 and T2 images.

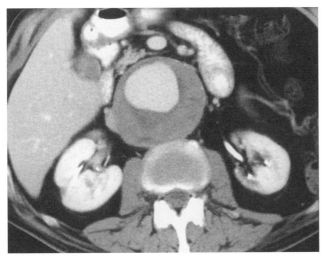

FIGURE 4.4. Hemorrhage from aortic aneurysm. High-density blood partially surrounds the aneurysm.

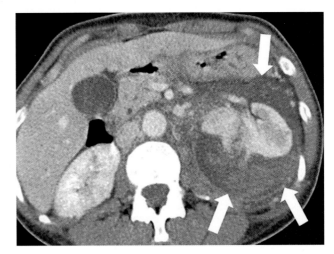

FIGURE 4.5. Arteritis. The kidneys are inhomogeneously enhanced, and a hematoma (*arrows*) from a bleeding vessel surrounds the left kidney.

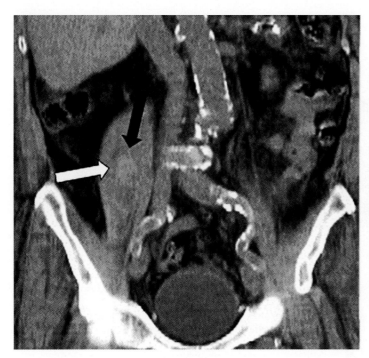

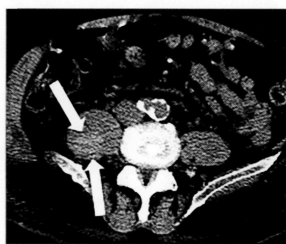

FIGURE 4.6. Noncontrast CT reveals hematoma as faint dense region (*arrows*) in enlarged right psoas muscle.

If a hematoma is treated conservatively, it may completely resorb and leave no more than thin linear fibrotic remnants. Sometimes, the hemoglobin will be resorbed but a fluid collection, termed a seroma, will remain. On CT, the fluid will ultimately approach water density. MRI may reveal a hemosiderin ring (low signal on all sequences) with fluid that is low to moderate signal on T1-weighted images and high signal on T2-weighted images.

Urinoma

Urine may escape from the collecting system or ureter into the retroperitoneum. If the urine leak is transient and of low volume, the fluid is usually resorbed. But a large volume leak may appear as a fluid collection while it is being resorbed, and occasionally, such a collection becomes encapsulated and remains as a chronic cystic lesion. A urinoma may be subcapsular in location (Fig. 5.6) or confined to the perirenal or pararenal spaces. Leaking urine occasionally tracks into the peritoneal cavity and becomes urinary ascites. Subcapsular urinomas, like hematomas, may compress the renal parenchyma and cause hypertension via the Page kidney phenomenon.

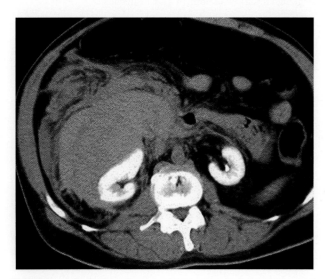

FIGURE 4.7. Perirenal hematoma producing Page kidney. Despite acute blood loss, patient became actively hypertensive.

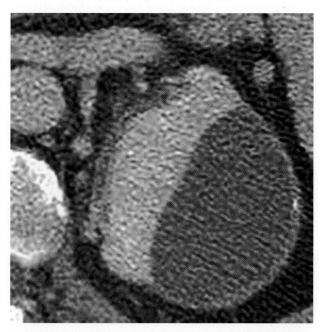

FIGURE 4.8. Subcapsular hematoma. The flattened surface of the kidney indicates that the fluid is within the renal capsule. The hemoglobin has been resorbed; the collection is now a seroma.

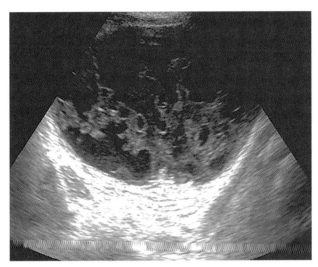

FIGURE 4.9. Ultrasound of supravesical hematoma. The anechoic spaces and enhanced through-transmission are characteristic of fluid; the network of echogenic material within the hematoma represents fibrinous material and clot.

Urine leaks may be caused by trauma (Fig. 4.11), including surgery, that interrupts the walls of the collecting system or ureter or causes a renal parenchymal laceration that extends into the collecting system. Ureteral obstruction may also produce a urine

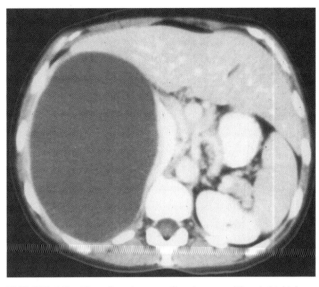

FIGURE 4.11. Chronic urinoma after trauma. The right kidney is distorted by a large fluid collection.

leak: a healthy kidney may generate very high urine pressure proximal to a stone or other cause of acute severe ureteral occlusion, which in turn causes a rupture where the wall of the calyceal fornix meets the surface of the medullary papilla. Leaked urine ("pyelosinus extravasation") then extends from the renal sinus through the renal hilum into the perinephric space (Fig. 4.12), where it may accumulate in a layer adjacent to the renal capsule, or flow along the outer surface of the ureter, sometimes forming urinomas. Leakage of sterile urine is seldom of concern, but, if infected, extravasated urine may produce perinephric abscesses.

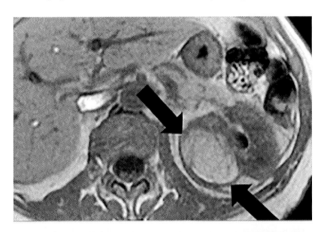

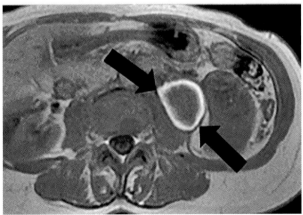

FIGURE 4.10. T1-weighted MR images reveal a renal angiomyolipoma (**top**, *arrows*), which had hemorrhaged a few weeks earlier. The resultant hematoma (**bottom**, *arrows*) is inferior to the tumor and displays a bright rim.

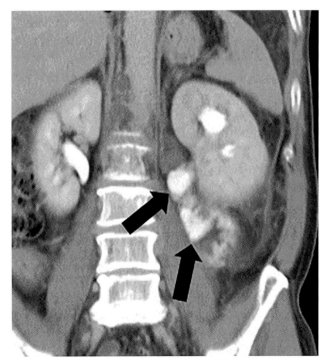

FIGURE 4.12. Urine leak caused by acute obstruction. The left renal calyces are dilated, and opacified urine (*arrows*) has tracked from the renal sinus into the perirenal space, demonstrating the origin of obstructive urinomas.

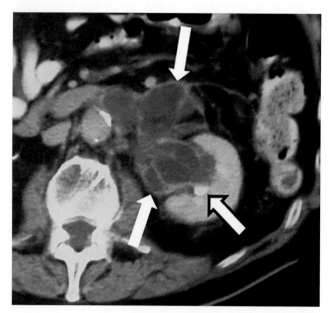

FIGURE 4.13. Multichambered urinoma. The left ureter had been acutely obstructed several times by stones; the consequent calyceal urine leaks have produced a chronic urinoma (*solid white arrows*). There is no current obstruction; a normally opacified calyx (*bordered arrow*) is demonstrated on this CT urogram.

Urinomas may be demonstrated by any cross-sectional imaging technique. Ultrasound will reveal an anechoic cystic region with enhanced through-transmission; the fluid will be of water attenuation on CT (Fig. 4.13) and have the signal characteristics of water (low signal on T1-weighted images, bright on T2-weighted images) on MRI. Acutely leaking urine may be opacified by excreted contrast if delayed images are obtained (Fig. 4.11).

Abscess

Retroperitoneal abscesses rarely occur spontaneously; they usually arise because of infection or perforation of a viscus within or adjacent to the retroperitoneum. Severe pyelonephritis, obstructive pyonephrosis, pancreatitis, spinal osteomyelitis and perforation of ulcers, and inflammatory or neoplastic disease of the ascending or descending colon, duodenum, or retrocecal appendix may all produce retroperitoneal abscesses. There is a tendency for duodenal and pancreatic disease to produce abscesses in the anterior pararenal space and for renal disease to cause abscesses in the perirenal space and osteomyelitis in the posterior pararenal space, but abscesses do not always respect the fascial planes that separate these compartments. Rarely, retroperitoneal fasciitis, which is like necrotizing fasciitis in any anatomic location, may be encountered.

Radiographically, abscesses may be identified since their walls are usually thicker and enhance more than those of sterile fluid collections (Figs. 4.14 and 4.15) and occasionally contain gas bubbles. These signs are not infallible: wall thickness and enhancement of infected and sterile collections may overlap, and air may appear from recent intervention and fistulae. There is often evidence of inflammation in adjacent tissue. Sonographically, pus is more likely than is sterile fluid to contain echo-producing debris; on CT, pus may be slightly denser than water, but absolute CT density is of little use in diagnosing infection.

Unless it is mixed with blood, pus has the same MRI characteristics as other fluid: low intensity on T1-weighted images and bright on T2-weighted images. CT is probably the best imaging technique

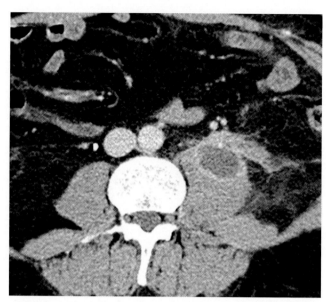

FIGURE 4.14. Psoas abscess. Thickening of the wall of the left psoas fluid collection suggests inflammation.

for initial searches for retroperitoneal abscesses. Retroperitoneal fasciitis may produce CT evidence of inflammation, including fatty edema or "stranding," fluid dissecting along fascial planes, and gas bubbles; these findings appear in a variety of conditions, but when encountered in a patient whose clinical picture is that of severe sepsis with pain and shock, retroperitoneal fasciitis should be considered.

Lymphocele

Lymphoceles are discrete collections of chylous fluid. They may occur as complications of pelvic or retroperitoneal surgery, particularly lymphadenectomy and renal transplantation. Typically presenting several weeks after surgery, they have been reported as occurring from as early as several days to as late as years after surgery. When quite large, lymphoceles may cause venous obstruction and lower extremity edema.

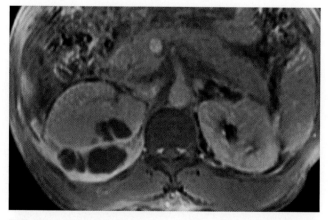

FIGURE 4.15. Retroperitoneal abscess. T1-weighted gadolinium-enhanced image shows right posterior perirenal multichambered fluid collection with a thick enhancing wall. This arose from severe pyelonephritis, which, after antibiotic treatment, evolved to a renal abscess.

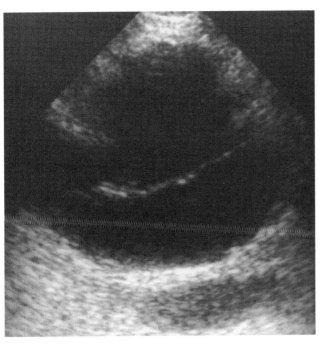

FIGURE 4.16. Lymphocele with septae.

Lymphoceles may be difficult to distinguish from other retroperitoneal fluid collections. Ultrasound evaluation of a lymphocele typically reveals a fluid-filled region with absent or faint echoes. Septations (Fig. 4.16) and dependent debris may be present, which may also occur in an abscess or resolving hematoma. On CT and MRI, the walls of lymphoceles are characteristically very thin (Fig. 4.17). Lipid within a lymphocele can be identified by negative CT numbers and on fat-sensitive MRI sequences.

Pancreatic Pseudocyst

The range of anatomic sites within which pancreatic pseudocysts have been found is wide and of course includes the retroperitoneum. Under most circumstances, they appear in patients with active pancreatitis or a known history of pancreatitis and are easily identified. Occasionally, however, they are chronic, and the prior pancreatitis is not recognized, so they appear as cystic collections

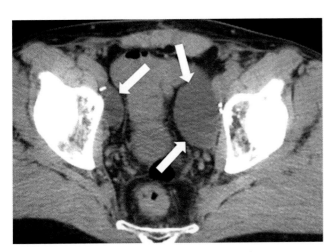

FIGURE 4.17. Bilateral pelvic lymphoceles (*arrows*) following prostatectomy with lymph node dissection.

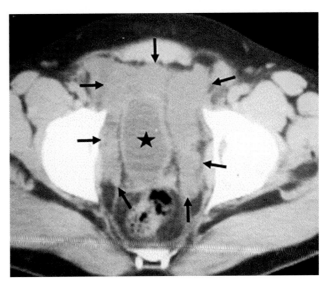

FIGURE 4.18. Extraperitoneal fluid collection formed by hemorrhagic effusion from severe pancreatitis. The collection (*arrows*) has the shape of a molar tooth and has compressed the bladder (*star*) to the center of the pelvis.

without known origin. These have the same appearance as pancreatic pseudocysts elsewhere: the fluid within them is usually not hemorrhagic and their walls are of variable thickness. The radiology of pancreatic inflammation has been extensively described but is outside the scope of this text.

Pelvic Fluid Collections

Fluid collections in the pelvis may be intraperitoneal or may lie in the prevesical extraperitoneal compartment. The prevesical space is directly contiguous with the retroperitoneal compartment below the cone of renal fascia. Fluid in the prevesical extraperitoneal space may have a "molar tooth" configuration on transverse CT or MRI images, with the "crown" portion of the "tooth" lying anterior to the urinary bladder and the "roots" of the tooth extending posteriorly on both sides of the bladder (Fig. 4.18). These roots are frequently asymmetric, resulting in bladder displacement away from the midline when the extraperitoneal pelvic fluid collections are large. As a rule, fluid collections (or masses) that displace any part of the bladder superiorly or medially are extraperitoneal; encapsulated fluid collections and masses within the intraperitoneal space tend to indent the bladder dome.

RETROPERITONEAL FIBROSIS

Retroperitoneal fibrosis is a condition of abnormal proliferation of fibrotic tissue in the retroperitoneum. When it was initially discovered seven decades ago, its tendency to obstruct the ureters, and the limitation of retroperitoneal imaging to urography, led to the conception that it was limited to the lower lumbar portion of the retroperitoneum, but more recently it has become apparent that the anatomic range of the abnormality may extend to any level of the retroperitoneum, along the mesentery and even into the chest.

Originally thought to be idiopathic, the disease is now known to be a group of conditions with multiple, and sometimes overlapping, causes. The immunoglobulin G4 (IgG4)-related conditions, which include autoimmune pancreatitis, cholangitis, and gallbladder inflammation, sometimes involve the retroperitoneum and cause retroperitoneal fibrosis. Vasculitis, especially aortitis, may involve perivascular tissues and ultimately produce fibrosis. Infection,

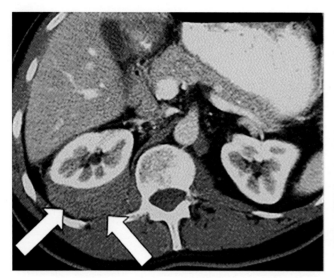 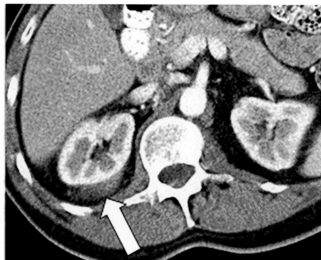

FIGURE 4.19. Retroperitoneal fibrosis after successful treatment of tumor. Pretreatment lymphoma (**left**, *arrows*) has produced a perirenal bulky mass, which has displaced the kidney anteriorly. A year after treatment, the tumor has changed to a much smaller fibrous plaque (**right**, *arrow*) that remained stable for many subsequent years.

like lumbar osteomyelitis, may do the same, as may retroperitoneal radiation. Certain drugs, including ergot alkaloid derivatives (methysergide, ergotamine) and dopamine agonists (methyldopa), have been associated with the condition. Retroperitoneal tumors, including metastatic carcinoma of the breast, stomach, colon, prostate, and lung, along with lymphoma and carcinoid tumors, may generate a desmoplastic reaction that becomes retroperitoneal fibrosis, and successfully treated tumor may resolve to a smaller volume of fibrosis (Fig. 4.19). Retroperitoneal bleeding may produce retroperitoneal fibrosis after the blood has been resorbed. Erdheim–Chester disease is a rare histiocytosis, which may appear in the retroperitoneum and progress to fibrosis.

Retroperitoneal fibrosis most often affects patients in their sixth decade; men are afflicted more often than are women. The disease often manifests clinically by obstructing the ureters (Fig. 4.20), producing hydronephrosis and renal failure. It can also compress and obstruct veins, including the inferior vena cava, iliac veins, and gonadal veins, producing edema of the corresponding anatomic regions. It may present with chronic abdominal or back pain.

The condition involves an initial inflammatory phase, followed by resolution to mature fibrosis, and its intrinsic imaging features reflect this transition. If the volume of the abnormal tissue is sufficient to be visible at ultrasound, the fibrotic mass is usually hypoechoic; it is usually hypovascular by Doppler imaging. At CT,

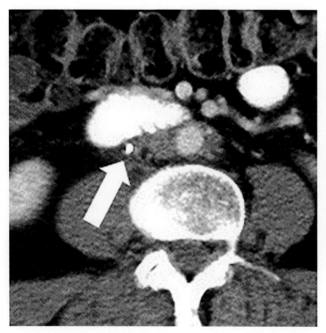 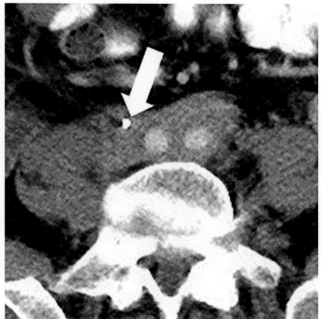

FIGURE 4.20. Retroperitoneal fibrosis. The process has enveloped and obstructed the right ureter, which has been treated with a stent (*arrows*).

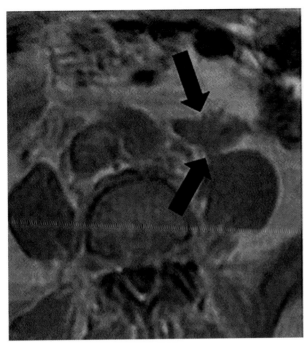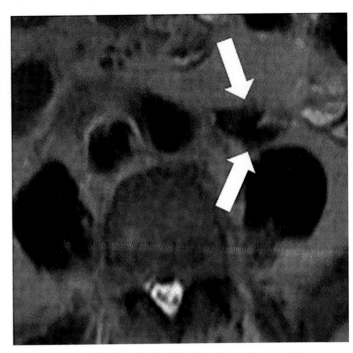

FIGURE 4.21. MRI of retroperitoneal fibrosis. T1-weighted image **(left)** reveals the fibrotic plaque (*arrows*) to be of intermediate intensity, equivalent to muscle. In a T2-weighted image **(right)**, the plaque (*arrows*) is of very low intensity, which is characteristic of mature fibrosis.

the tissue of all phases tends to be isodense to muscle; it reveals moderate enhancement in the inflammatory phase and minimal enhancement in the fibrotic phase. MRI shows it to be of low to intermediate intensity on T1-weighted images on all phases; it has high intensity on T2-weighted images in the inflammatory phase and low intensity in the fibrotic phase (Fig. 4.21), with enhancement patterns following those seen at CT; diffusion-weighted MRI shows that it causes little diffusion restriction. Neoplasm can often be differentiated from mature fibrosis demonstrating stronger signal on T2-weighted images and more pronounced diffusion restriction. Although PET scanning often reveals the inflammatory tissue to be FDG avid (Fig. 4.22), the subsequent fibrotic tissue is not; this feature may be useful to distinguish retroperitoneal fibrosis from malignancy.

The configuration of the abnormality is that of flat sheets or masslike accumulations of tissue. As mentioned above, it occurs in a number of locations but often appears in the retroperitoneum around the L4-L5 level. The tissue may envelop and obstruct the ureters at any level, frequently bilaterally; an occasional but classic finding is the retraction of the lumbar segment of the ureters toward the midline. Arteries and veins may be surrounded; the veins are often obstructed, but the arteries are not constricted. When the fibrosis is adjacent to or surrounds the aorta (Fig. 4.23), it does not displace the vessel; since periaortic malignancies often displace the aorta—specifically moving it anteriorly, away from the lumbar vertebrae, this feature may help in differential diagnosis.

The classic idiopathic form of retroperitoneal fibrosis often forms a plaque surrounding the great vessels and ureters.

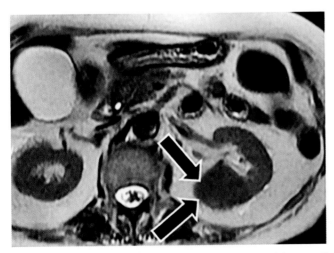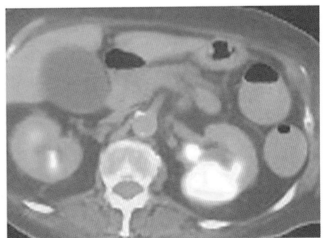

FIGURE 4.22. IgG4 disease. T2-weighted image **(left)** reveals an expansile process within the posterior aspect of the left kidney (*arrows*). PET-CT scan **(right)** shows the lesion to be FDG-avid.

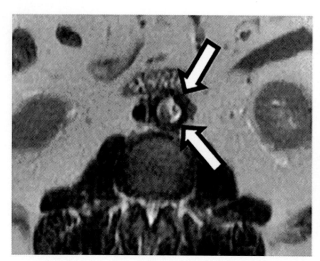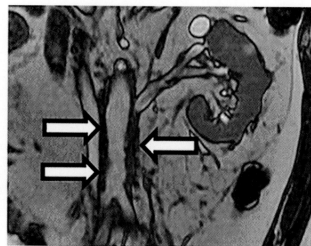

FIGURE 4.23. Periaortic retroperitoneal fibrosis. The enveloping rind of tissue (*arrows*) is low intensity.

IgG4-associated fibrosis has a more varied appearance: it may create masslike lesions in the retroperitoneum, surround the kidneys with mantles of tissue, or even infiltrate the kidneys to form peripheral tumor-like nodules or wedge-shaped poorly enhancing lesions. Erdheim–Chester disease is a rare histiocytosis, which often resembles retroperitoneal fibrosis; it characteristically surrounds the kidneys with a uniform mantle of soft tissue density histiocytes. Retroperitoneal fibrosis composed of desmoplastic reactions to tumors may display lumpy surfaces. It should not be surprising that distinction between benign retroperitoneal fibrosis and confluent neoplasm, especially lymphoma, may be difficult. Low intensity and lack of diffusion restriction on MRI, lack of FDG avidity, lack of aortic displacement despite large volumes of surrounding tissue and stable appearance over long surveillance periods all suggest retroperitoneal fibrosis, but biopsy is often required.

The mainstay of medical treatment of retroperitoneal fibrosis is corticosteroids. If there is ureteral obstruction, retrograde stenting or percutaneous nephrostomy may be necessary. Imaging plays a crucial role in documenting response to therapy, primarily by documenting any change in the volume of the abnormal tissue and by evaluating the degree of ureteral obstruction. If ureteral obstruction becomes chronic, surgical ureterolysis may be necessary.

PRIMARY RETROPERITONEAL TUMORS

The term primary retroperitoneal tumor refers to a neoplasm that originates in the retroperitoneum but not from a specific solid viscus like the pancreas, adrenal gland, or kidney. Retroperitoneal tissues that give rise to such tumors include muscle, fascia, connective tissue, fat, blood vessels, embryonic urogenital remnants, and nerve tissue. Given this plethora of sources, various tumors can be found arising de novo in the retroperitoneum. Lymphoma is the most common malignant tumor to arise in the retroperitoneal lymph nodes, and metastases from other tumors to retroperitoneal nodes are even more commonly encountered, but these conditions are not within the scope of this chapter.

Primary retroperitoneal tumors grow slowly and produce only vague symptoms, if any, before they attain significant size. Therefore, unless inadvertently discovered, the typical primary retroperitoneal tumor grows to be quite large before it produces pain or a palpable mass.

Very large tumors may occupy such a large volume of the abdominal cavity that it becomes difficult to determine the site from which they arise. As with fluid collections, they may be revealed to

be of retroperitoneal origin if they displace other retroperitoneal organs anteriorly.

Mesenchymal Tumors

Lipoma

A lipoma is a mesenchymal tumor composed of normal-appearing fatty tissue. It is uncommon in the retroperitoneum and may be hard to distinguish from a well-differentiated liposarcoma. They appear as homogeneous masses of any size that display fatty attenuation on CT and signal intensities of fat on MRI (Fig. 4.24). Although fine septations may be seen, nodularity or thickened septations suggest malignancy.

Lipoblastoma

This rare tumor is derived from fetal adipose tissue and is seen in infants and young children. They are usually superficial lesions that

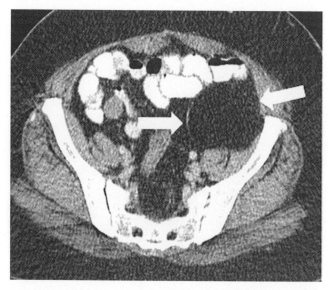

FIGURE 4.24. Retroperitoneal lipoma (*arrows*). The tumor is composed entirely of fat; the lack of soft tissue elements makes malignancy unlikely but not impossible. This lesion has been observed for over 4 years and has not enlarged.

occur most frequently in the extremities but may be found in the retroperitoneum.

Myelolipoma

A myelolipoma is a benign tumor composed of hematopoietic elements and mature fat. Most occur in the adrenal gland, but they may also arise in the retroperitoneum, especially the presacral space. They are usually incidental findings, but larger lesions are prone to hemorrhage. Like other fatty tumors, they are echogenic on ultrasound; CT often shows both fatty and nonfatty elements. On MRI, the fatty portions have the imaging characteristics of normal fat. These tumors may be impossible to distinguish from liposarcomas.

Liposarcoma

Liposarcoma is the most common primary retroperitoneal malignancy. Three subtypes of liposarcoma are recognized, well differentiated, myxoid, and pleomorphic; the well differentiated subtype is the most common. They are seen as fatty masses, with the CT and MR characteristics similar to normal fatty tissue (Fig. 4.25). Well-differentiated liposarcomas may be difficult to differentiate from benign lipomas.

Myxoid tumors have varying amounts of recognizable fat (Fig. 4.26). Pleomorphic liposarcomas are fully malignant tumors and may have no recognizable fat on imaging studies (Fig. 4.27). All types are usually large when initially diagnosed, and both displace and surround adjacent abdominal viscera. Treatment of retroperitoneal liposarcomas is primarily surgical. It is often impossible to resect the entire tumor, and portions remaining after surgery continue to enlarge.

Leiomyosarcoma

Leiomyosarcoma is an uncommon malignant neoplasm of smooth muscle; it occurs more commonly in women than in men. In the retroperitoneum, it arises from the vessel walls, often in the middle third of the IVC. Almost two-thirds of the tumors are completely extravascular, though many have both extravascular and intravascular components.

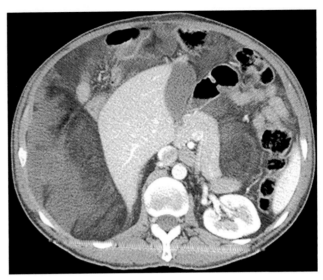

FIGURE 4.26. Myxoid liposarcoma. The large mass surrounding and displacing the liver is composed of regions of fatty tissue and regions of denser myxoid tissue.

On CT examination, leiomyosarcomas are usually large masses, often with areas of necrosis. Both extraluminal growth and intraluminal extension are well defined on contrast-enhanced images. Leiomyosarcomas show low to intermediate signal intensity on T1-weighted MR images and intermediate to high signal intensity on T2-weighted studies (Fig. 4.28). Surgical resection is the only effective therapy.

Undifferentiated Pleomorphic Sarcoma

This tumor was frequently called a malignant fibrous histiocytoma in the past. It is found more commonly in the extremities but is also seen in the retroperitoneum. The imaging features of undifferentiated pleomorphic sarcoma are those of a soft tissue mass with a CT density near that of muscle (Fig. 4.29). Calcification is more common in them than in other primary retroperitoneal tumors.

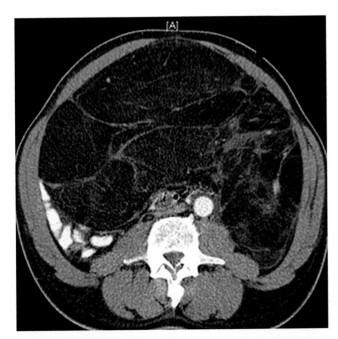

FIGURE 4.25. Well-differentiated liposarcoma. There is a huge mass composed nearly entirely of fatty tissue filling the abdomen.

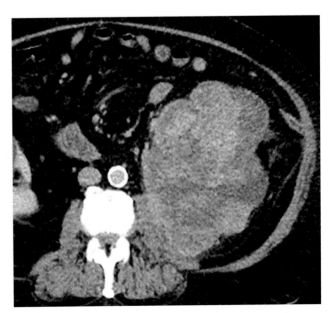

FIGURE 4.27. Pleomorphic liposarcoma. The mass has no visible fatty tissue.

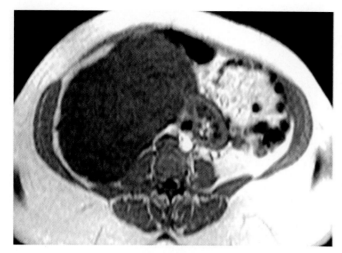 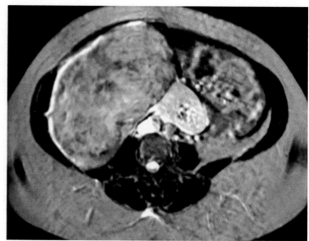

FIGURE 4.28. Retroperitoneal sarcoma. This large mass has displaced the right kidney across the midline. It is of low intensity on T1-weighted images **(left)** and high intensity on T2-weighted images **(right)**.

Neural Tumors

These include nerve sheath tumors (neurilemmomas or schwannomas, neurofibromas, and malignant nerve sheath tumors), ganglion cell tumors (ganglioneuromas, neuroblastomas, and ganglioneuroblastomas), and paraganglionic tumors (pheochromocytomas and paragangliomas). These of course can be found in a number of anatomic areas; when in the retroperitoneum, they tend to be paraspinal or to be clearly identifiable as of spinal origin by virtue of arising within the neural foramina. They often present difficult differential diagnostic problems and may be impossible to distinguish from each other.

Most neurilemmomas arise in the head and neck; they may also be found in the paraspinal region of the retroperitoneum. They are seen on CT as well-defined oval masses that are often low density, possibly due to the lipid myelin; they may contain areas of cystic degeneration and calcification (Fig. 4.30).

Like most peripheral neural tumors, these tend to be of relatively low intensity on T1-weighted MR images and to be bright on T2-weighted images (Fig. 4.31).

Neurofibromas may be seen as solitary tumors or as components of neurofibromatosis. Neurofibromas rarely undergo cystic degeneration and occasionally become malignant. Neurofibromas appear as well-defined ovoid masses with an attenuation of 20 to 25 HU on unenhanced CT examinations (Fig. 4.32).

Enhancement is modest and usually homogeneous. Neurofibromatosis, type I, predominantly affects the peripheral nervous system and skin, manifesting as café au lait spots and neurofibromatous nodules. These patients may develop numerous plexiform tumors arising from retroperitoneal nerves. These are elongated in appearance, have a relatively low density, and are frequently symmetrical (Fig. 4.33).

Malignant degeneration may occur in nerve sheath tumors. Imaging is not always a reliable method of distinguishing a benign from malignant tumor, but the malignant ones tend to be larger and more inhomogeneous with less distinct margins and grow faster (Fig. 4.34).

Ganglioneuromas tend to be relatively homogeneous and less dense than muscle and with occasional calcification on CT. MRI shows them to be of low intensity on T1-weighted images and high intensity on T2-weighted images. Extra-adrenal neuroblastomas

FIGURE 4.29. Undifferentiated pleomorphic sarcoma. CT shows a large heterogeneous mass arising in the pelvis.

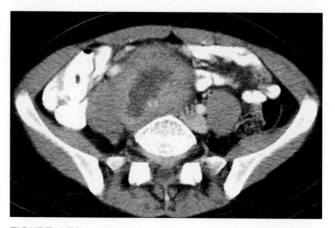

FIGURE 4.30. Schwannoma. The mass has a central region of cystic degeneration.

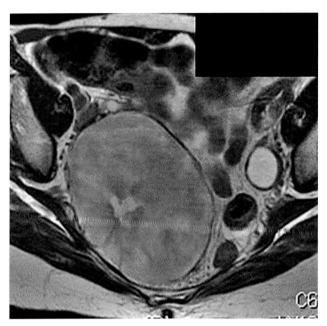

FIGURE 4.31. Schwannoma. This T2-weighted MRI reveals the mass to be of moderately high intensity. The small lesion on the patient's left is a physiologic ovarian cyst. Neurofibromas may be seen as solitary tumors or as components of neurofibromatosis. Neurofibromas rarely undergo cystic degeneration and occasionally become malignant.

are also of ganglion cell origin, are less common than are adrenal neuroblastomas, appear in the same age group, and have the same imaging characteristics.

Paragangliomas are extra-adrenal pheochromocytomas and may accompany MEN syndromes, neurofibromatosis, and von Hippel–Lindau disease. Although they may appear anywhere from the neck to the groin, they are most commonly found in the paraspinal regions not far from the adrenal gland and may involve the organ of Zuckerkandl. Occasionally, they arise in the wall of the bladder and produce manifestations of sympathetic activity during voiding. They have the same imaging characteristics as do adrenal pheochromocytomas. When solid, they often display intense enhancement with contrast media on both CT (Fig. 4.35) and MRI. They are of low-to-intermediate intensity on T1-weighted

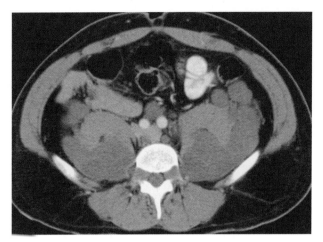

FIGURE 4.33. Neurofibromatosis. Multiple symmetrical low-density masses along the courses of the peripheral nerves have the classic appearance of neurofibromatosis.

MR images and are bright on T2-weighted images (Fig. 4.36). They are often cystic and then may be uniformly and strongly intense on T2-weighted images. If necessary, a radionuclide using metaiodo-benzylguanidine (MIBG) may serve to differentiate these from other retroperitoneal tumors.

Primitive Neuroectodermal Tumor

Peripheral primitive neuroectodermal tumors (PNETs) are uncommon tumors comprised of small round cells that occur in the thorax, abdomen, and soft tissues of the head and neck. Approximately 14% of PNETs occur in the abdomen where they have been reported in the kidney, adrenal gland, retroperitoneum, and pelvis. They may occur at any age but are more common in young adults. The tumors are often large, averaging more than 10 cm in diameter at presentation. Calcification is uncommon. Enhancement is heterogeneous, often with areas of tumor necrosis. Vascular invasion or direct extension is common, reflecting the aggressive nature of this tumor.

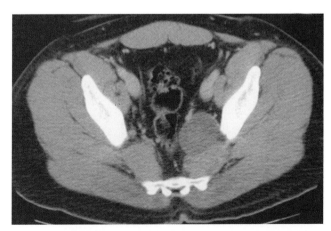

FIGURE 4.32. Nerve sheath tumor. This low-density mass adjacent to the left piriformis muscle lies along the course of the S1 nerve root.

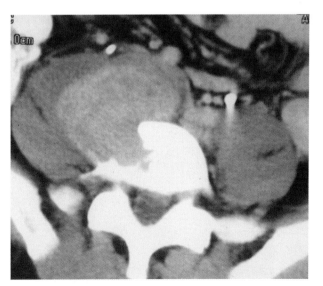

FIGURE 4.34. Malignant schwannoma. CT shows a large soft tissue mass arising posterior to the right psoas muscle and eroding the right side of the vertebral body.

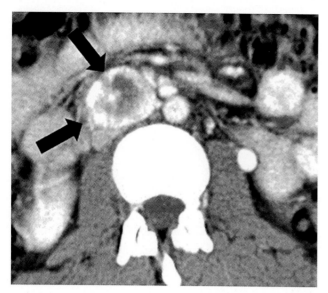

FIGURE 4.35. Retroperitoneal paraganglioma. The periphery of the tumor (*arrows*) displays characteristic intense enhancement.

Primary Vascular Tumors

Lymphangioma/Hemangioma

Rarely, these tumors appear as primary retroperitoneal tumors. Lymphangiomas are benign vascular lesions with lymphatic differentiation. Although most are found in the neck and axillae, they may also arise in the retroperitoneum where they are seen as thin-walled cystic masses. They tend to be anechoic on ultrasound but may contain echogenic debris. On CT, the cystic component has a low density that may be less than that of water due to the presence of chyle. MRI examinations reveal a low-signal intensity on T1-weighted images and high-signal intensity on T2-weighted

images. Hemangiomas sometimes display the same characteristics as do hepatic hemangiomas: they are well marginated, with relatively low density on CT, low intensity on T1-weighted MRI, and high intensity on T2-weighted images, and demonstrate slow peripheral contrast enhancement on both modalities.

Germ Cell Tumor

Teratoma

Teratomas constitute as many as 10% of primary retroperitoneal neoplasms. They can be found anywhere from the high retroperitoneum to the presacral area and typically are found in the first 6 months of life or in young adults. They are three times more common in females than in males. These usually are benign lesions, as <10% undergo malignant degeneration (Fig. 4.37).

Retroperitoneal teratomas may also exhibit imaging characteristics that allow a definitive diagnosis. They may be predominantly cystic or solid or may present as complex lesions containing fat or sebum/fluid levels.

DIFFERENTIAL DIAGNOSIS

The number of different kinds of retroperitoneal tumors, along with their overlapping radiologic features, leads to difficulty in differential diagnosis. Indeed, specific diagnoses are often not possible, but analysis of certain features often helps to reduce the possibilities. Most retroperitoneal malignancies are metastatic: nodal masses should always prompt a search for a primary tumor within the scope of the scan and for a history of any other malignancy. Whenever possible, it should be determined whether a tumor arises from a specific organ, such as the kidney, adrenal gland, pancreas, retroperitoneal intestine, or spine; if it does, the diagnostic possibilities are clearly different. Large heterogeneous tumors are often sarcomas. Fat-density tissue usually indicates liposarcoma or lipoma; liposarcomas are commoner and often have regions of denser tissue, whereas lipomas tend to look like pure fat. Myxoid tissue is more lucent than most nonfatty tissue and may be present in liposarcomas. Smaller well-defined fatty

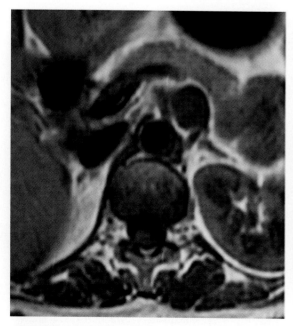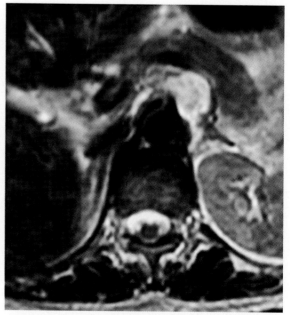

FIGURE 4.36. Paraganglioma. The lesion is low intensity on T1-weighted image **(left)** and bright on T2-weighted image **(right)**.

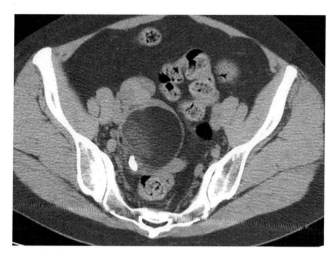

FIGURE 4.37. Teratoma. A mass with mixed soft tissue and fatty components, along with a toothlike calcification. This was originally thought to be ovarian but was found to be extraperitoneal at resection.

tumors may be teratomas or myelolipomas. Tumors that appear to arise from the walls of large vessels and to grow into vascular lumina are usually leiomyosarcomas. A tumor that enlarges a neural foramen is usually of nerve sheath origin; paragangliomas arise from the sympathetic chain. A positive MIBG scan may identify a pheochromocytoma, paraganglioma, or neuroblastoma. Nerve sheath tumors are usually smoothly marginated. Paragangliomas often show marked contrast enhancement. Almost any tumor may exhibit necrotic regions that become liquefied, but tumors that appear primarily cystic include schwannomas, paragangliomas, and lymphangiomas. Despite these clues, retroperitoneal tumors often defy specific imaging diagnosis and require pathologic examination, which more often depends upon resection than biopsy.

SUGGESTED READINGS

Fluid Collections

Aikawa H, Tanoue S, Okino Y, et al. Pelvic extension of retroperitoneal fluid: analysis in vivo. *AJR Am J Roentgenol.* 1998;171:671.

Bechtold RE, Dyer RB, Zagoria RJ, et al. The perirenal space: relationship of pathologic processes to normal retroperitoneal anatomy. *Radiographics.* 1996;16:841.

Korobkin M, Silverman PM, Quint LE, et al. CT of the extraperitoneal space: normal anatomy and fluid collections. *AJR Am J Roentgenol.* 1992;159:933.

Yang DM, Jung DH, Kim, H, et al. Retroperitoneal cystic masses: CT, clinical, and pathologic findings and literature review. *Radiographics.* 2004;24(5):1353–1365.

Retroperitoneal Fibrosis

Al Zahrani H, Kim TK, Khalili D, et al. IgG4-related disease in the abdomen: a great mimicker. *Semin Ultrasound CT MRI.* 2014;35(3):240–254.

Caiafa RO, Vinuesa AS, Izquierdo RS, et al. Retroperitoneal fibrosis: role of imaging in diagnosis and follow-up. *Radiographics.* 2013;33(2):535–552.

Kottra JJ, Dunnick NR. Retroperitoneal fibrosis. *Radiol Clin North Am.* 1996;34:1259.

Urban ML, Palmisano A, Nicastro M, et al. Idiopathic and secondary forms of retroperitoneal fibrosis: a diagnostic approach. *Rev Med Interne.* 2015;36(1):15–21.

Primary Retroperitoneal Tumors

Brennan C, Kajal D, Khalili K, et al. Solid malignant retroperitoneal masses—a pictorial review. *Insights Imaging.* 2014;5(1):53–65.

Craig WD, Fanburg-Smith JC, Henry LR, et al. Fat-containing lesions of the retroperitoneum: radiologic-pathologic correlation. *Radiographics.* 2009;29:261–290.

Kaushik S, Neifeld JP. Leiomyosarcoma of the renal vein: imaging and surgical reconstruction. *AJR Am J Roentgenol.* 2002;179:276–277.

Kim MS, Kim B, Park CS, et al. Radiologic findings of peripheral primitive neuroectodermal tumor arising in the retroperitoneum. *AJR Am J Roentgenol.* 2006;186:1125–1132.

Lane RH, Stephens DH, Reiman HM. Primary retroperitoneal neoplasms: CT findings in 90 cases with clinical and pathologic correlation. *AJR Am J Roentgenol.* 1989;152:83.

Levy AD, Cantisani V, Miettinen M. Abdominal lymphangiomas: imaging features with pathologic correlation. *AJR Am J Roentgenol.* 2004;182:1485.

Mingoli A, Feldhaus RJ, Cavallaro A, et al. Leiomyosarcoma of the inferior vena cava: analysis and search of world literature on 141 patients and report of three new cases. *J Vasc Surg.* 1991;14:688–699.

O'Sullivan PJ, Harris AC, Munk PL. Radiological imaging features of non-uterine leiomyosarcoma. *Br J Radiol.* 2008;81:73–81.

Pereira JM, Sirlin CB, Pinto PS, et al. CT and MR imaging of extrahepatic fatty masses of the abdomen and pelvis: techniques, diagnosis, differential diagnosis, and pitfalls. *Radiographics.* 2005;25:69.

Rha SE, Byun JY, Jung SE, et al. Neurogenic tumors in the abdomen: tumor types and imaging characteristics. *Radiographics.* 2003;23:29.

Sangster GP, Migliaro M, Heldmann MG, et al. The gamut of primary retroperitoneal masses: multimodality evaluation with pathologic correlation. *Abdom Radiol (NY).* 2016;41(7):1411–1430.

Scali EP, Chandler TM, Heffernan EJ, et al. Primary retroperitoneal masses: what is the differential diagnosis? *Abdom Imaging.* 2015;40(6):1887–1903.

Verstraete KL, Acten E, De Schepper A, et al. Nerve sheath tumors: evaluation with CT and MR imaging. *J Belge Radiol.* 1992;75(4):311–320.

Weiss SW, Enzinger FM. Malignant fibrous histiocytoma. *Cancer.* 1978;41(6):2250–2266.

Renal Cystic Disease

Renal cysts, cystic disease, and cystic masses are the most common abnormalities encountered in uroradiology. In some patients, renal cysts are part of a systemic process that also involves the kidneys. In most patients, however, one or several cystic masses are detected, and the radiologist must determine whether a particular cystic mass is benign or malignant. In most patients, the radiographic findings are sufficiently characteristic that further evaluation is not required. In some cases, however, an examination specifically designed to examine a renal mass may be necessary before a confident diagnosis can be reached.

CORTICAL CYSTS

Simple Cysts

The most common renal mass is a simple cortical cyst. Cortical cysts are uncommon in children or young adults but are detected routinely in the older population on computed tomography (CT), magnetic resonance imaging (MRI), and ultrasonography (US) examinations. In fact, renal cysts have been estimated to occur in 50% of the population older than 50 years of age. Thus, they are considered acquired lesions.

Simple cysts arise from the distal convoluted tubules or collecting ducts. The precise etiology of simple cysts is not known; it is proposed that they occur as a result of tubular obstruction such that the tubule no longer communicates with the nephron. They are composed of fibrous tissue and are lined by flattened cuboidal epithelium. They contain clear serous fluid and do not communicate with the collecting system.

Most patients with simple cysts are asymptomatic, and the cysts are detected as incidental findings. Hematuria is occasionally attributed to a benign cyst, but cysts bleed so infrequently that other lesions must be sought in patients with hematuria. Rarely, a large simple cyst may obstruct the collecting system or cause hypertension. Local pain may be attributed to distention of the cyst wall or spontaneous bleeding into the cyst; however, the vast majority of cysts are asymptomatic. Occasionally, a simple cyst may become infected.

Although simple cysts have been described in all age groups, they are unusual in children. A cyst in a child must be carefully examined to differentiate a benign cyst from a cystic Wilms tumor. A cyst in a child may also be an early sign of a cystic nephropathy.

A cortical cyst can occasionally be detected on an abdominal radiograph. The water-density cyst is seen as a cortical bulge projecting into the perinephric fat. Calcification is seen in the wall of a cyst in only approximately 1% of cases. If the calcification is thin and border forming, the lesion is likely to be a benign but complicated cyst.

Renal cysts are often detected as incidental findings during contrast-enhanced CT examinations of the abdomen, and there is no opportunity to test for contrast enhancement (Fig. 5.1). However, if the density of the cyst fluid is <20 HU and other criteria of a simple cyst are present, the lesion will almost certainly be benign.

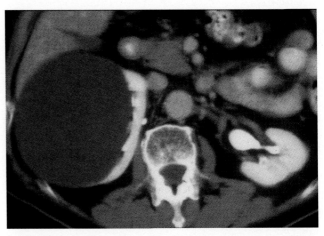

FIGURE 5.1. Large right renal cyst. The cyst has an imperceptibly thin wall and is sharply defined.

The wall of a benign simple cortical cyst is often too thin to be seen on CT, but a pencil-thin, smooth wall may be seen. When evaluating wall thickness with CT, it is important to evaluate the portion of the cyst that extends well away from the parenchyma so that a portion of adjacent renal tissue (beak) is not included in the section. If the cyst is completely intrarenal, wall thickness cannot be assessed.

Simple cortical cysts are readily detected with MRI (Fig. 5.2). The appearance of a homogeneous round mass with a thin, smooth wall and sharp interface with normal renal parenchyma is similar to that on CT. The long T1 values result in a low signal intensity on T1-weighted images. However, they have a very high signal intensity on T2-weighted images, which reflects the long T2 value of water.

Corresponding features are also seen on ultrasound examinations. A simple cyst is a round homogeneous mass with a sharp interface with the normal renal parenchyma. A simple cyst is echo-free with enhanced through transmission (Fig. 5.3). Thin septations that are too fine to be detected with CT may be seen with ultrasound.

Cysts may be seen with renal scintigraphy as photopenic regions because of the displacement of functioning parenchyma by the cyst. If the cyst is small or exophytic, scintigraphy may be normal.

Parapelvic cysts, or cortical cysts that extend centrally into the renal sinus, may cause photopenic regions in the renal sinus that mimic hydronephrosis. The correct diagnosis is reached if the isotope can be identified in the ureter, even though the photopenic region persists.

The accuracy of the radiographic diagnosis of a renal cyst depends on how well it is seen with each modality. When all of the criteria of a benign simple cyst are present, it is highly unlikely to be anything else and further evaluation is not warranted. Ultrasound is the most efficient method of diagnosing a simple cyst. Ultrasound is readily available, accurate, and relatively inexpensive. CT is the gold standard for the evaluation of renal masses, but it is a more expensive examination than ultrasound, requires intravenous contrast administration, and exposes the patient to ionizing radiation. It is indicated when an ultrasound examination is indeterminate or is technically inadequate due to the patient's obesity or overlying bowel gas. MRI is used in patients with a contraindication to the use of intravenous contrast medium, or if after the CT scan, the nature of the cystic mass is still in question. Although typically more expensive and not as widely available, MRI may also be utilized in lieu of CT, particularly in young patients in whom the desire to reduce radiation exposure is greater.

Rarely, renal cysts may regress in size or disappear completely, often silently. Although this phenomenon may be caused by resorption of a hematoma misdiagnosed as a cyst, most cases are probably due to spontaneous cyst rupture. An increase in pressure within the cyst relative to the collecting system or the perinephric space may result in rupture. Such a pressure increase could be caused by hemorrhage into the cyst or by a change in the composition of the cystic fluid.

When symptomatic, the most common manifestations of cyst rupture are hematuria and flank pain. The diagnosis can be made by CT or MRI if the cyst communicates with the collecting system. In most cases, the communication of the cyst with the collecting system closes spontaneously. Once the diagnosis is made, management is conservative.

Unilateral Cystic Disease

Unilateral or localized renal cystic disease is characterized by replacement of all or a portion of one kidney by multiple cysts (Figs. 5.4 and 5.5). It is sometimes referred to as *segmental cystic disease of the kidney*. Although sometimes described as unilateral polycystic kidney disease, it is not familial. The disease is not progressive, and there is no association with renal failure or cysts in other organs. The pathogenesis is obscure, but it is hypothesized to be developmental in etiology. The most common clinical presentation is flank pain with or without hematuria.

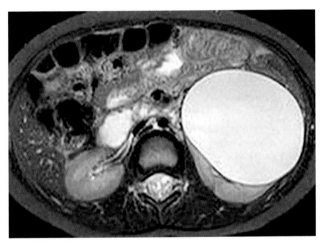

FIGURE 5.2. Large left renal cyst. A T2-weighted MR shows high signal intensity.

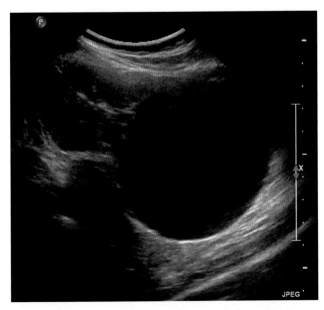

FIGURE 5.3. Large renal cyst. Ultrasound demonstrates an echo-free mass with enhanced through transmission.

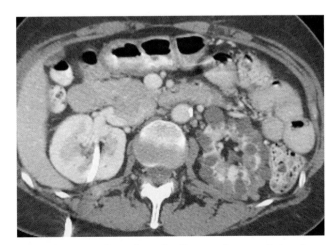

FIGURE 5.4. Unilateral cystic disease. An excretory phase CT image shows multiple left renal cysts and a normal right kidney. A right-sided percutaneous nephrostomy is present.

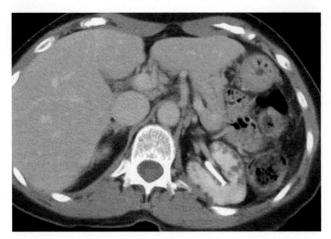

FIGURE 5.5. Unilateral cystic disease. Multiple small cysts are seen in the left kidney. The right kidney (not shown) was normal.

Complicated Cysts

Cystic masses that do not satisfy the criteria of a benign simple cyst must be further evaluated to exclude malignancy. Various morphologic features are now recognized that exclude the diagnosis of a simple cyst.

Septations

Cysts may develop septations; when they are thin, smooth, do not have localized areas of thickening or irregularity, and are few in number, the lesions are generally considered benign, complicated cysts. These thin septations are more easily detected by ultrasound or MRI than CT. When a cystic mass contains one or more thick septations, a malignant lesion is possible. If there is associated nodularity, the lesion must be considered malignant.

Calcification

The presence of calcification is also a nonspecific finding (Fig. 5.6). When evaluation of the kidney depended primarily on excretory urography, the presence of calcification, especially central calcification, was an ominous sign. However, CT has made the presence or absence of calcification almost irrelevant because wall thickening

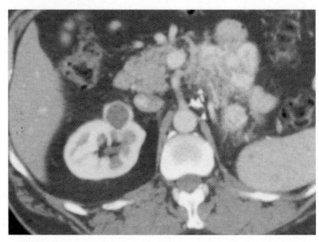

FIGURE 5.7. Bosniak type III cyst. A thick wall cyst is seen arising from the anterior surface of the right kidney in a patient who has already had a left nephrectomy for renal cell carcinoma. Pancreatic metastases are also present. Biopsy proved a second primary renal cell carcinoma.

and soft tissue masses can easily be detected without the help of calcification. Thin calcification in the wall or septum of a cyst is almost always benign and does not, in itself, warrant surgical exploration.

Thick Wall

A thick wall is incompatible with a simple cyst. It indicates that the lesion is another cystic mass or that the cyst has become complicated by some process such as infection, hemorrhage, or neoplasia. Inflammatory or infectious cystic masses may result in a thickened wall, typically associated with abundant perinephric stranding. A thick-walled cystic renal mass may also be a cystic renal cell carcinoma (see Chapter 6). These lesions are generally considered indeterminate, and unless an inflammatory or infectious diagnosis can be made clinically or via percutaneous needle aspiration, close-interval follow-up or surgical exploration is indicated (Fig. 5.7). The presence of a markedly thickened and irregular wall (Fig. 5.8) or an associated soft tissue tumor mass is an even more ominous finding and is highly suspicious for a malignancy.

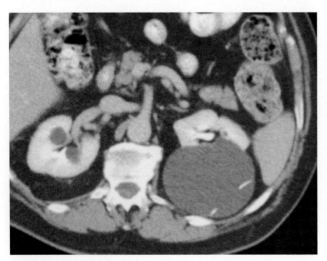

FIGURE 5.6. Bosniak type II cyst. Thin straight septal calcifications are present in this cyst. This is of minimal concern for malignancy.

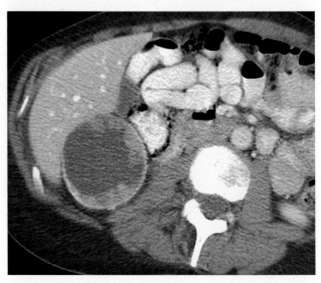

FIGURE 5.8. Cystic renal cell carcinoma. The cystic mass has a markedly thickened and irregular wall.

Increased Density

A cystic mass with a density above water must contain more than simple cystic fluid. Cystic renal masses with an attenuation above 20 HU are worrisome and may be proteinaceous cysts, hemorrhagic cysts, or solid neoplasms, and further evaluation is warranted. One category of an atypical renal cyst that has an increased attenuation is the *hyperdense* cyst. These lesions look like typical simple cysts on CT examination in that they are round, well-marginated, homogeneous masses that do not enhance with intravenous contrast material administration. Hyperdense cysts are typically small, peripheral lesions, measuring 3 cm or less in diameter (Fig. 5.9A,B). Instead of displaying an attenuation of water, they typically measure 50 to 90 HU. Those that are denser than the renal parenchyma are easily recognized on unenhanced CT examinations, but they may be masked by enhanced renal parenchyma. Thus, these lesions are probably more common than is appreciated, as most abdominal CT scans are performed after intravenous contrast medium administration. Hyperdense masses that are intrarenal are more problematic; care must be used to differentiate such lesions from hyperdense solid tumors. Almost all renal masses with an unenhanced attenuation above 70 HU are benign, hyperdense cysts.

There are several possible etiologies for a hyperdense renal cyst. The most common etiologies are hemorrhage and a high-protein content of the cyst fluid. However, a diffuse, pastelike calcified material has also been found. Most of these hyperdense cysts are benign, but they must be carefully examined for other atypical features. CT examination before and after intravenous contrast medium administration is often helpful. A cyst will not enhance, whereas a solid tumor will.

US may be useful in the evaluation of a renal mass with an attenuation higher than water on CT. It may enable the examiner to distinguish between a cystic lesion and a solid lesion. With ultrasound, blood elements can sometimes be seen floating within the cyst. However, if the lesion cannot be clearly evaluated with US, CT, or MRI examinations, percutaneous biopsy or surgical exploration may be needed.

Hyperdense cysts can also be evaluated with MRI. Simple cysts have low signal intensity on T1-weighted images, whereas hyperdense cysts due to hemorrhage or high-protein content may have high signal intensity on all pulse sequences. Because blood elements tend to settle out, the more intense signal of the paramagnetic methemoglobin can be seen in the dependent portion of the cyst on T1-weighted images. The relative intensity of the two cyst layers may reverse on T2-weighted sequences. With time, hemorrhagic or proteinaceous cysts show low to intermediate signal on T1-weighted images and have similar appearance on T2-weighted images (Fig. 5.9C). A renal cell carcinoma can often be distinguished

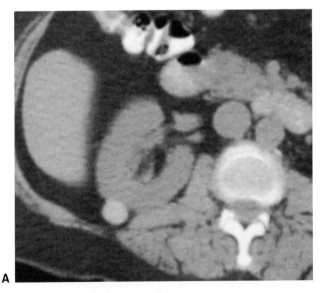

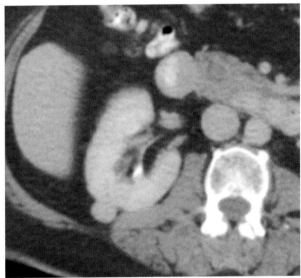

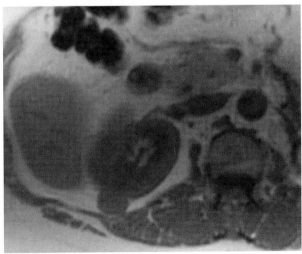

FIGURE 5.9. Hyperdense renal cyst. **A:** Unenhanced CT shows a hyperdense, exophytic mass arising from the right kidney. The left kidney has been removed. **B:** After contrast medium administration, the mass becomes isodense with enhanced renal parenchyma. **C:** An axial T1-weighted MR image shows intermediate signal intensity.

by its heterogeneity, indistinct or irregular margins, lack of a fluid-hemoglobin level, or enhancement.

Enhancement

The presence or absence of enhancement on CT or MRI after contrast medium administration is the single most important criterion for distinguishing benign cystic renal masses from vascular or solid lesions. Enhancement on MRI can be measured by determining the percentage change in signal intensity values of a renal mass after contrast material. Enhancement may be defined as an increase of 15% or greater. Subtraction MR imaging offers another method of determining whether enhancement is present in a cystic mass. With this method, unenhanced fat-saturated T1-weighted images are subtracted from T1-weighted gadolinium-enhanced images, and the corresponding images are displayed. Images must be obtained in the same phase of respiration to avoid misregistration artifacts. When there is no enhancement, the mass will display uniformly absent signal and appear black.

At CT, enhancement is determined by measuring the difference in attenuation of a mass or a region of a mass between the enhanced and unenhanced scans. If a region of a cystic mass enhances <10 H, it is considered nonenhancing. If a region enhances by 20 H or more, it is considered enhancing. If the difference is between 10 and 20, it is indeterminate and US or MRI may be used to determine if the mass is solid or cystic. With complex and heterogeneous lesions, multiple small attenuation measurements should be obtained while being certain that obvious sources of error like the renal sinus or perinephric fat are excluded from the measurement.

The term *pseudoenhancement* has been used to describe the spurious increase in enhancement after contrast medium administration. It is caused by the CT reconstruction algorithm that adjusts for beam-hardening effects. Pseudoenhancement is most pronounced with small (<1 cm), intrarenal lesions during the early phases of contrast enhancement when plasma contrast medium concentration is at its highest. When one is uncertain whether there is true enhancement or pseudoenhancement on CT, an alternate imaging modality such as US or MRI may be helpful.

Bosniak Classification

To clarify the need for further evaluation or treatment of complicated cystic lesions, Bosniak classified cystic renal masses into five categories.

Category I masses are cysts that fulfill all of the criteria for a benign, simple cyst (Fig. 5.1). No further evaluation is needed.

Category II masses are those with some atypical features but are reliably considered benign. Such features include few, thin, nonenhancing septa or thin, wall or septal calcifications (Fig. 5.6). Exophytic (at least a quarter of its circumference abutting fat) hyperdense cysts that fulfill all of the criteria described above are included in this category (Fig. 5.9).

Category IIF masses include a subset of patients with findings that are more worrisome. These lesions are considered Category IIF ("F" for follow-up). Such findings include more than a few thin septations with minimal, perceived enhancement (because the septa are too small to place a region of interest on them), or minimal wall or septal thickening (Fig. 5.10). Intrarenal or large (>3 cm) masses

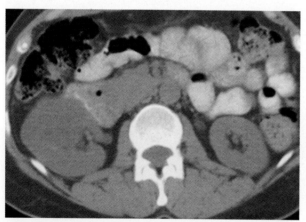

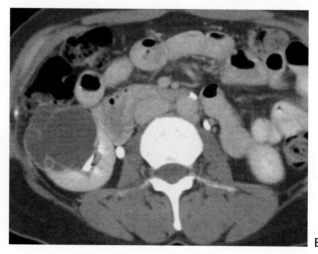

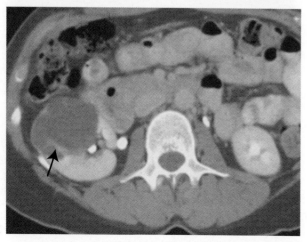

FIGURE 5.10. Bosniak IIF cyst. **A:** Unenhanced CT examination. **B, C:** Two excretory phase CT images show a septate right renal cyst. One of the septa (*arrow*) appears slightly thickened warranting follow-up.

that otherwise fulfill the criteria for a hyperdense cyst are placed in this category. Management recommendations include follow-up evaluation in 6 months and repeated at 1-year intervals to make sure the mass is not growing or, more importantly, not developing more worrisome morphologic features.

Category III lesions cannot be distinguished from malignancies and generally require surgical exploration. The overall risk of malignancy is probably >50%. Features of masses in category III include one or more thick or irregular septations, some thickened walls, or large, non–border-forming calcifications (Figs. 5.7 and 5.11). There may be measurable enhancement present. Although some will be benign, these masses generally should be removed because no additional imaging can unequivocally prove that they are benign. Lesions in this category are often mimicked by hemorrhagic, inflammatory, or infected cysts. As a result, it is important to consider nonneoplastic etiologies of a renal mass lesion before applying the Bosniak classification, particularly when the clinical presentation suggests an infections etiology such as focal bacterial pyelonephritis and abscess. If an infectious etiology cannot be diagnosed on the basis of the imaging findings and clinical presentation, percutaneous needle aspiration should be considered. If an infectious etiology cannot be demonstrated, surgery may be required to reach a diagnosis. If the patient is a poor surgical risk, percutaneous biopsy may be used. However, the solid portions of these masses are often difficult to sample, and unless a benign entity can be diagnosed confidently by biopsy, negative results should be viewed with caution.

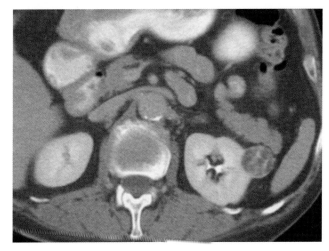

FIGURE 5.11. Bosniak III cyst. Excretory phase image shows a cystic left renal mass with enhancing septa. Proven renal cell carcinoma.

Category IV lesions have features that strongly suggest malignancy (Figs. 5.8 and 5.12). Although there may be a large cystic area, there is at least one enhancing nodule, particularly when it is apart from the wall. These are treated as presumed renal cell carcinomas.

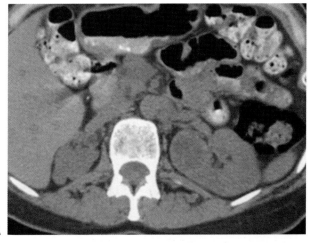

A

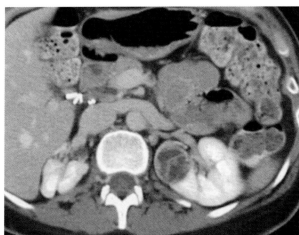

B

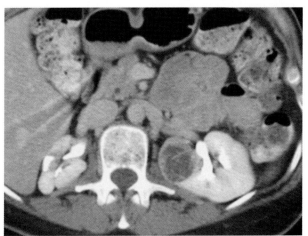

C

FIGURE 5.12. Bosniak IV cyst. **A:** Noncontrast CT examination. **B:** Nephrographic. **C:** Excretory phase CT images show a cystic mass with nodularly thickened walls and enhancing septa. Proven conventional renal cell carcinoma.

The Bosniak classification is a useful method by which the level of concern about a particular lesion can be expressed. Category I and IV lesions can generally be assigned with a high level of agreement among observers. The difficulty is in the assignment of lesions to categories II, IIF, and III and the markedly different management this assignment entails. In addition, other factors such as the patient's age and coexisting morbidity play a major role in how a lesion is managed. For example, a small cystic mass with a solid component may be followed in a patient with limited life expectancy or severe comorbidities, whereas it would be removed from otherwise healthy patients with similar imaging findings.

BOSNIAK CLASSIFICATION

Category I—uncomplicated simple cyst with no atypical features

Category II—minimally atypical features with little, if any, risk of malignancy

Category IIF—minimally concerning features requiring follow-up

Category III—indeterminate lesion with a significant concern for malignancy

Category IV—cystic appearing but frankly malignant features

Milk of Calcium Cyst

Milk of calcium is a collection of small calcific granules in the cystic fluid. The granules, usually calcium carbonate, are in suspension and layer out in the dependent portion of the cyst. They are seen most frequently in calyceal diverticula (see Chapter 12). Milk of calcium cysts have no sex predilection but are more common in the upper poles of the kidneys.

The milk of calcium nature of these calculi may not be appreciated on a supine radiograph, but the fluid calcium layer is easily detected on upright films or CT examinations (Fig. 5.13). A horizontal line of calcium density can also be detected using ultrasound, regardless of the patient's position. Most of these cysts are detected as incidental findings, and intervention is unnecessary.

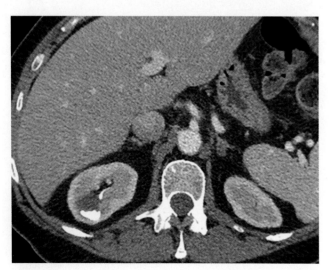

FIGURE 5.13. Calyceal diverticulum. A collection of small stones is layering out in the dependent portion of a right calyceal diverticulum.

MEDULLARY CYSTIC DISEASE

This disease complex includes medullary cystic disease and juvenile nephronophthisis. Extrarenal manifestations such as retinal degeneration, hepatic fibrosis, and skeletal abnormalities are associated with the juvenile form. The kidneys are small to normal in size and maintain a normal configuration and smooth contour. A variable number of small cysts, up to 2 cm in diameter, are located primarily in the medulla. The cortex is thin but does not contain cysts. Biopsy shows interstitial and periglomerular fibrosis as well as tubular atrophy. However, the diagnosis cannot be made if cysts are not included in the biopsy specimen, because the fibrotic changes are nonspecific.

The uremic medullary cystic diseases can be classified by the age of onset. The adult form is transmitted by autosomal dominant inheritance. Patients usually present as young adults with anemia, which may be severe, and have progressive renal failure. These patients have a salt-wasting nephropathy that is not corrected with mineralocorticoids. Other than a fixed low-specific gravity, the urine sediment is normal. Hypertension may develop near the end of the disease course.

Patients with juvenile nephronophthisis typically present at 3 to 5 years of age with polydipsia and polyuria. The clinical course with anemia and progressive renal failure is similar to the adult-onset variety, but progression is slower, with 8 to 10 years before terminal uremia. Juvenile nephronophthisis is transmitted by autosomal recessive inheritance.

Abdominal radiographs may demonstrate small kidneys without calcification. CT and MRI reveal a thin renal cortex. Linear contrast collections radiating from the renal pyramids may be seen. However, contrast medium-enhanced CT scans are not likely to be helpful and are seldom performed because of renal failure. Unenhanced CT or MRI demonstrates small, smooth kidneys and may reveal the small medullary cysts.

High-resolution ultrasound may be the examination of choice in these patients. The corticomedullary differentiation is lost, and the parenchyma appears isoechoic or hypoechoic with the liver or spleen. In patients with severe uremia, medullary cysts can usually be demonstrated, but they may not be detectable in milder cases. Examination with unenhanced MRI may be particularly useful when ultrasound is indeterminate. The problems with motion artifact due to breathing are decreased with fast spin echo breath-hold techniques.

POLYCYSTIC RENAL DISEASE

Autosomal Recessive Polycystic Disease

Autosomal recessive polycystic kidney disease (ARPKD) is the most common inherited disease that presents in infancy or childhood. It includes a spectrum of abnormalities ranging from newborns with grossly enlarged sponge kidneys to older children with medullary ductal ectasia. Both the kidney and liver are involved in ARPKD, though the severity of the involvement of one organ usually dominates.

In ARPKD, renal cysts develop from focal epithelial proliferation of the collecting ducts, which dilate and elongate. There is interstitial fibrosis. In the liver, the bile ducts are dilated and the portal tracts are fibrotic. This appearance of congenital hepatic fibrosis (CHF) is found in all patients with ARPKD. However, CHF is not diagnostic of ARPKD, as other entities are associated with CHF, including tuberous sclerosis, Caroli disease, and occasionally autosomal dominant polycystic kidney disease (ADPKD).

There is a broad spectrum of clinical manifestations, and patients are sometimes categorized into perinatal, neonatal, infantile, and juvenile based on their age at time of presentation, with the most severe disease in the youngest patients. Patients with severe forms of ARPKD have renal failure at birth and most die within the first few days of life. Patients with the less severe disease have a milder renal involvement characterized by tubular ectasia and renal cysts. Older patients (juvenile form) often present with symptoms arising from hepatic fibrosis with portal hypertension and varices rather than from renal failure. There is an inverse relationship between the renal and the hepatic manifestations of the disease; when the renal disease is present at birth, the hepatic manifestations are mild. When the disease presents in older children, the hepatic component dominates, whereas the renal manifestations are less severe. It appears as a single gene located on chromosome 6 for all forms of the disease.

The radiographic manifestations reflect the age of onset and the severity of renal involvement. In the neonatal form, there is a massive enlargement of the kidneys that maintain their reniform shape. The kidneys are enlarged but function poorly. The nephrogram is faint with blotchy opacification. Linear striations due to stasis of contrast medium in the dilated renal tubules have been described. The numerous small (1 to 2 mm) cysts in both the cortex and medulla result in increased echogenicity on sonography. However, with high-resolution scanners, a peripheral sonolucent rim can be seen representing compressed renal cortex (Fig. 5.14). A prominent renal pelvis and calyces may result in a sonolucent central zone.

Among older children, <10% of the renal tubules are affected and hepatic fibrosis dominates the clinical course. The clinical presentation is usually a result of portal hypertension with splenomegaly, gastric, and esophageal varices. The kidneys are only mildly enlarged but contain variably sized cysts that are predominantly medullary in location. The appearance of tubular ectasia in these children is similar to that seen in medullary sponge kidney in adults (see Chapter 12).

An increased echogenicity with loss of the normal corticomedullary junction is demonstrated on ultrasound. The sonolucent rim of compressed renal parenchyma may also be seen in the juvenile form. On CT, the kidneys have low attenuation, reflecting the dilated tubules. A striated pattern of enhancement is seen due to contrast collecting in the tubules.

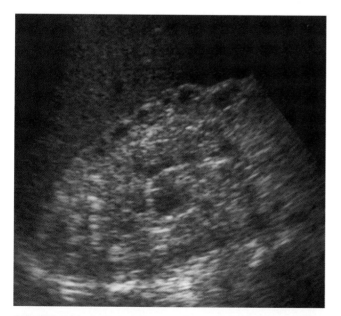

FIGURE 5.14. Autosomal recessive polycystic disease. The kidney is enlarged. Numerous small cysts create disorganized echogenicity and loss of corticomedullary differentiation on ultrasound.

Autosomal Dominant Polycystic Kidney Disease

ADPKD is the most common form of cystic kidney disease and is responsible for approximately 10% of patients on chronic dialysis. It is transmitted by autosomal dominant inheritance, with 100% penetrance. In most patients, the disease is inherited, but approximately 10% of patients develop the disease as a result of spontaneous mutation. There are two types of ADPKD. The gene (PKD1) for type I has been found on the tip of the short arm of chromosome 16 in approximately 85% of patients; the type II gene (PKD2) is located on the long arm of chromosome 4 and accounts for 15% of the cases. The type I gene codes for a protein known as *polycystin I*, which is involved in cell cycle regulation and calcium transport. The type II gene protein is known as *polycystin II*. Both proteins are found in the cilia of renal epithelial cells. The mechanism by which the cysts form appears to be related to a disturbance in the balance between cell proliferation and cell apoptosis under the influence of a protein called *epidermal growth factor*. Proliferation of tubular epithelial cells and increased fluid secretion into the tubules lead to cyst formation. Cysts develop in every part of the nephron and rapidly close off from the tubule of origin. Although only approximately 1% to 2% of nephrons develop cysts, the cysts enlarge and damage adjacent nephrons through ischemia.

Patients with ADPKD present most commonly in the third or fourth decades. Patients with type I ADPKD tend to have a younger age of onset of ESRD than patients with type II disease. However, ADPKD may also be seen in children or older adults. Patients with mutations in both genes have the worst prognosis. The initial complaint is usually lumbar, inguinal, or upper abdominal pain. The enlarged kidneys may be palpable as abdominal masses.

Patients with ADPKD often suffer from flank pain caused by a variety of etiologies. Acute pain may result from swelling of one of the cysts due to hemorrhage or infection. Colicky pain may arise from ureteral obstruction by stone, blood clot, or rarely a cyst. Chronic pain is more likely caused by progressive enlargement of the cysts with stretching of the renal capsule.

Hypertension, which occurs in almost two-thirds of patients with ADPKD, is caused by increased renin production by the kidneys. Hematuria may be caused by rupture of one of the renal cysts into the renal pelvis or by the presence of a stone.

All patients with ADPKD have progressive renal failure. The rate of progression of the azotemia is related to the age of onset; those patients whose symptoms begin after 50 years of age have a better prognosis. Although the incidence is variable, approximately one-half of patients with ADPKD have cerebral (berry) aneurysms in the circle of Willis, and stroke from rupture of a berry aneurysm is a significant cause of morbidity and mortality. Renal stones occur more frequently in patients with ADPKD than in the general population. Because more than one-half of these stones are predominantly uric acid, they may be radiolucent and may be overlooked on an abdominal radiograph. Using CT, Levine and Grantham (1985) found renal calculi in 36% of patients with ADPKD. Other abnormalities associated with ADPKD include hepatic cysts, mitral valve prolapse, and colonic diverticulosis.

Although a matter of dispute in the past, it is now recognized that there is an increased incidence of renal cell carcinoma in patients with ADPKD. Renal cell carcinoma in these patients occurs at a younger age, is often of the sarcomatoid variety, and is more commonly bilateral and multifocal than is seen in the general population.

The plain abdominal radiograph is remarkable for the poor visualization of the renal outlines. Three-fourths of the renal outline is seen in <10% of patients with ADPKD compared with 80% of patients with unilateral renal enlargement due to other causes.

Calcification in the cyst walls is common, and nephrolithiasis may be detected.

Sonography and CT have replaced nephrotomography as the standard methods of examination of patients with ADPKD. Innumerable renal cysts are seen with either modality. The kidneys are markedly enlarged but maintain their reniform shape.

CT has the advantage of clearly demonstrating the cysts and collecting systems of both kidneys. Unenhanced scans are needed to demonstrate renal stones and facilitate the diagnosis of hemorrhagic cysts (Fig. 5.15). Because the kidneys are typically riddled with innumerable cysts that abut each other, the cysts are not round in shape but assume various irregular contours.

Both CT and MRI are useful in demonstrating hepatic cysts, which are present in approximately 60% of patients with ADPKD. These liver cysts develop from dilatation of aberrant bile ducts that embryologically failed to establish communication with the biliary tree. The cysts gradually accumulate fluid secreted by the lining cuboidal epithelial cells. Associated cysts in other organs are much less common, although they have been reported in the pancreas, spleen, ovary, seminal vesicle, epididymis, testis, bladder, uterus, thyroid, esophagus, and brain.

Multiple renal cysts are easily identified on MRI. Uncomplicated cysts resemble simple cortical cysts with homogeneous low signal intensity on T1-weighted images and high signal intensity on T2-weighted images (Fig. 5.16). Complicated cysts may reflect infection or hemorrhage. Acute bleeding results in a hyperintense lesion regardless of the pulse sequence. However, the appearance varies with the age of the bleed. The high-protein content of an infected cyst results in a signal intensity between a simple cyst and one with acute hemorrhage.

Bleeding into renal cysts is common and may be the source of acute flank pain (Fig. 5.17). If the cyst ruptures into the renal pelvis, hematuria will occur. Cyst hemorrhage may be more common in patients with ADPKD because of the associated hypertension, the increased bleeding tendency of uremia or heparinization during dialysis. Hemorrhagic renal cysts may be seen in 70% of patients with ADPKD. Perinephric hemorrhage has been reported but is rare.

Both kidneys are affected in patients with ADPKD, but involvement may be asymmetric. Rare cases of unilateral ADPKD are reported, but these may represent localized renal cystic disease, which is not hereditary and has no cysts in other organs. Localized

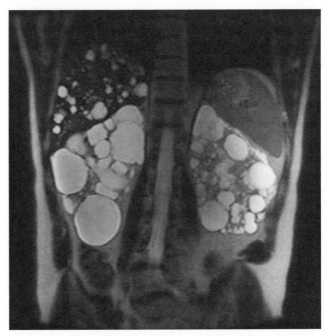

FIGURE 5.16. ADPKD coronal T2-weighted fat-saturated image shows large kidney bilaterally with multiple cysts.

renal cystic disease is not progressive and no treatment or follow-up surveillance is needed.

There is no treatment for ADPKD, and patients often must be sustained by dialysis or transplantation. By informing patients of the heritability of ADPKD, genetic counseling can help them with family planning. Thus, it is important for the diagnosis to be made before the patients reach childbearing age. Sonography is able to detect changes of ADPKD among children of affected families. Because ultrasound is less invasive, it is the preferred screening examination. The sensitivity of ultrasound in detecting evidence of ADPKD is virtually 100% among patients older than 30 years. When patients younger than 30 years are studied, the sensitivity remains very high for patients with type I disease but is significantly lower for type II disease.

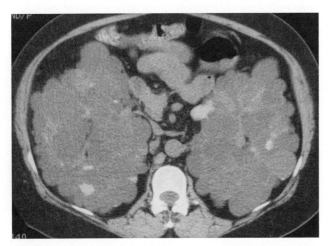

FIGURE 5.15. ADPKD bilateral renal enlargement due to numerous cysts is demonstrated on this enhanced CT examination. Several high-density cysts indicate hemorrhage.

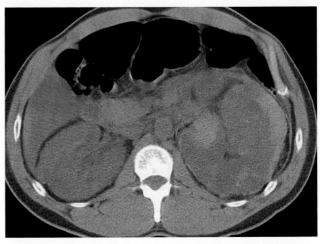

FIGURE 5.17. Subcapsular and intrarenal hemorrhage is seen in the left kidney in this patient with ADPKD.

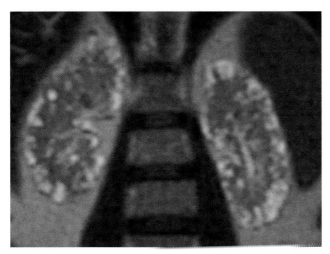

FIGURE 5.18. A 69-year-old man with mild renal insufficiency and innumerable, small cysts limited to the renal cortex on T2-weighted MR imaging, diagnostic of glomerulocystic disease. (Reprinted from Borges Oliva MR, Hsing J, Rybicki FJ, et al. Glomerulocystic kidney disease: MRI findings. *Abdom Imaging.* 2003;28:889–892, with permission of the author.)

GLOMERULOCYSTIC DISEASE

There is dilatation of Bowman space in patients with glomerulocystic disease. The disease is transmitted as an autosomal dominant trait but may be discovered during infancy in children suspected of having autosomal recessive polycystic disease.

On US, multiple minute cysts, smaller than those in patients with ADPKD (typically >2 cm), are found predominantly in the cortex, which helps to distinguish glomerulocystic disease from other renal cystic diseases such as ARPKD. Since patients are typically in renal failure, contrast is not given and unenhanced CT examinations show only small cortical cysts. Unenhanced MR imaging is the preferred if further imaging studies are needed (Fig. 5.18).

MULTICYSTIC DYSPLASTIC KIDNEY

Multicystic dysplastic kidney (MCDK) results from occlusion of the fetal ureters, usually before 8 to 10 weeks of gestation. The ureter fails to meet the metanephros and stimulate normal renal development. The kidney consists of a collection of irregularly sized cysts and fibrous tissue but no functioning renal parenchyma, giving the appearance of a "bunch of grapes." The cysts do not communicate, the renal collecting system is small or absent, and the ipsilateral renal vessels are atretic.

A variant, the hydronephrotic type of multicystic dysplasia, may result from incomplete ureteral obstruction later in gestation. In such cases, the cysts communicate with the renal pelvis. In rare cases, MCDK may be confined to one segment of the kidney. Most of these cases occur in the upper-pole moiety of a duplicated collecting system (Fig. 5.19).

Most renal dysplasias are detected as abdominal masses in infancy. MCDK is the second most common cause of an abdominal mass in the neonate, trailing only hydronephrosis in frequency. Males are more commonly affected than females, and there is a predilection for the left kidney.

Malformations including bilateral MCDK, ureteropelvic junction (UPJ) obstruction, contralateral ureterovesical reflux, hypoplasia of the opposite kidney, and horseshoe kidney are commonly associated with MCDK. These occurred in 41% of fetuses examined with ultrasound by Kleiner et al. (1986). Because some of these contralateral anomalies are fatal, less severe changes are more common,

and UPJ obstruction is the most common malformation seen in children or adults. If the MCDK is not detected in infancy, it may remain asymptomatic and be detected as an incidental finding in an adult.

Abdominal radiographs may demonstrate a soft tissue flank mass. In adults, calcification is common, usually in the cyst walls, and the lesion is usually small. There is no functioning renal parenchyma on the affected side, but imaging demonstrates compensatory hypertrophy of the contralateral kidney.

If retrograde pyelography is performed, an atretic ureter may be demonstrated. Atresia may be found at various levels, or there may be no ureter at all. Extravasation is common because cannulation of the small ureteric opening may be difficult.

The multiple cysts with thick septa can be demonstrated using CT or MRI. Mural calcifications can be seen in the cyst walls, but there is no evidence of contrast excretion.

Sonography is particularly valuable in assessing infants and demonstrates multiple cysts of varying sizes. There is no connection between adjacent cysts and the renal parenchyma surrounding the cysts. If angiography is performed, no ipsilateral renal artery will be seen.

Segmental multicystic renal dysplasia in an upper-pole moiety may be seen in patients with obstruction from an ectopic ureterocele. The dysplastic segment has the same features as the MCDK and causes compression of the normally functioning lower-pole moiety.

Focal multicystic renal dysplasia has also been reported. This presumably results from in utero infundibular obstruction. This entity is fortunately rare, because it cannot be distinguished from other renal cystic masses by imaging studies.

The classic MCDK must be distinguished from the "hydronephrotic" type of multicystic dysplasia. This hydronephrotic form probably results from incomplete obstruction of the ureter after the 10th week of gestation. In this form, a renal pelvis communicates with the multiple cysts. Function may be demonstrated by excretion of contrast medium during CT or by excretion of radionuclide during nuclear medicine studies. If the diagnosis is uncertain, percutaneous aspiration with antegrade pyelography may be required. Surgery is indicated in patients with the hydronephrotic type of disease, because significant renal function can often be preserved.

Our knowledge of the natural history of MCDK is increasing with the use of in utero ultrasound. As many as 41% of fetuses with MCDK have a contralateral renal anomaly, which is much higher than the 11% to 15% incidence seen in neonates. Many of these associated anomalies are fatal, and in some cases, there is involution of MCDK to what appears in the neonate as renal agenesis. Involution may also occur after birth. In a review of 30 patients with MCDK by Vinocur et al. (1988), 13.5% of the cystic masses decreased in size or disappeared, presumably due to leakage or reabsorption of cyst fluid. Most MCDKs (73%) did not change in size, and 13.5% increased in size. Surgery is needed if there is significant growth during the first year of life, if the diagnosis is inconclusive or if complications arise that require nephrectomy.

MULTICYSTIC NEPHROMA

Multicystic nephroma (MCN) is an uncommon lesion previously referred as multilocular cystic nephroma. It is a well-circumscribed lesion containing many cysts of variable sizes. The cystic mass is surrounded by a thick fibrous capsule that compresses adjacent renal parenchyma and may project into the renal pelvis. The cysts are lined by flattened, cuboidal, or hobnail epithelial cells that are typically devoid of prominent nucleoli and contain clear fluid. Hemorrhage and necrosis are uncommon.

The two forms of MCN in children are distinct histologically but not grossly. A cystic nephroma is a multiseptate cystic mass composed entirely of differentiated tissues, whereas cystic partially differentiated nephroblastoma also contains immature embryonal cells in the septations. These two subtypes of MCN cannot be distinguished radiographically and thus both are typically treated surgically.

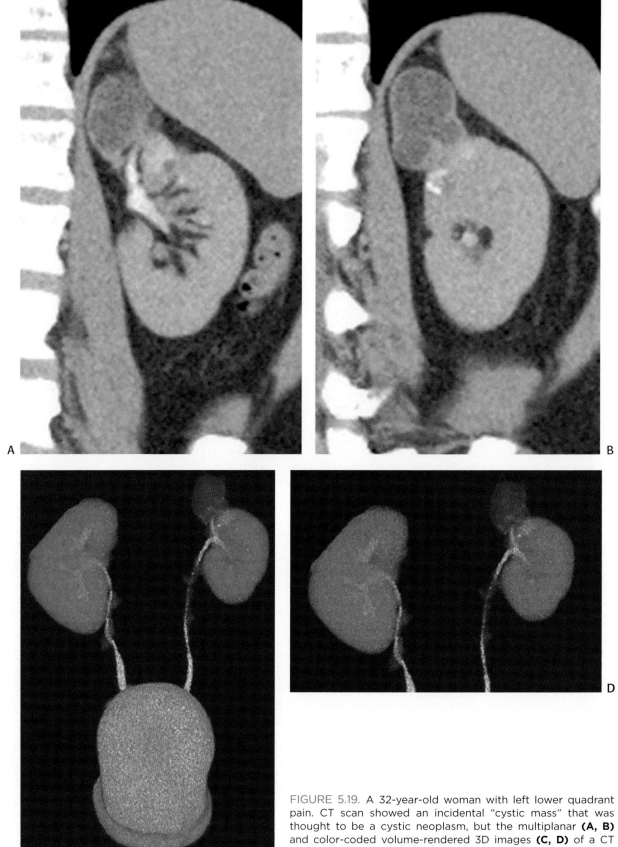

FIGURE 5.19. A 32-year-old woman with left lower quadrant pain. CT scan showed an incidental "cystic mass" that was thought to be a cystic neoplasm, but the multiplanar **(A, B)** and color-coded volume-rendered 3D images **(C, D)** of a CT urogram demonstrated a focal dysplastic upper pole of a non-duplicated system with distal hydronephrosis.

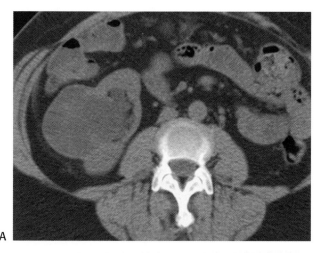

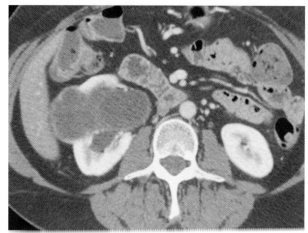

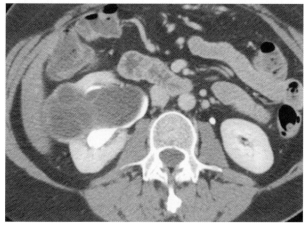

FIGURE 5.20. MCN. **A:** Unenhanced CT examination. Nephrographic **(B)** and **(C)** excretory phase images show a multicystic mass in the right kidney, which herniates into the renal pelvis.

In children, there are two discrete populations that are affected by MCN. The presenting signs and symptoms depend on the patient's age. Male patients with MCN are usually younger than 4 years and present with a palpable abdominal mass. Female patients typically present with symptoms between 4 and 20 years of age. Among children presenting younger than 4 years, 73% are male; of patients older than 4 years at presentation, 89% are female. In the adult, MCN may be found during examination of an unrelated complaint or during the investigation of pain, hematuria, or urinary tract infection. The differential diagnosis for middle-aged women (approximately 40 years of age) includes a mixed epithelial and stroma cell tumor, which is a multiloculated cystic tumor that contains ovarian-like stroma in lesion septa. A large renal mass is found on imaging examinations. The cystic mass occurs with equal frequency on either side but is more common in the lower pole. Projection of the mass into the renal pelvis is often demonstrated. The mass is hypovascular and mottled in appearance. Calcification in pediatric MCN is uncommon. However, radiographically detected calcifications were found in 7 of 12 adult patients reported by Banner et al. (1981). Such calcifications are usually found in the cyst walls or intervening stroma.

The multiple cystic spaces are best demonstrated using ultrasound. Large, multiple locules separated by echogenic stroma suggest the diagnosis of MCN. If the cysts are small, they may not be defined by ultrasound, and the echogenic stroma may suggest a complex or solid renal mass.

The CT appearance is usually characteristic. The masses are large, averaging approximately 10 cm in diameter. They are sharply delineated from the normal renal parenchyma. MCN is hypovascular, but the septations enhance after intravenous contrast administration. When large cysts are present, the internal septations are well defined. If the cysts are small, the mass may have a pitted appearance. A characteristic feature is herniation of the mass into the renal pelvis (Fig. 5.20). On MRI, signal intensities on both T1-weighted and T2-weighted images vary on unenhanced studies, reflecting differing proteinaceous or hemorrhagic components. Thin, enhancing septa are present and best appreciated on breath-holding sequences.

MCN must be differentiated from a cystic renal cell carcinoma. Although renal cell carcinoma arising in MCN has been reported, these cases may be multiloculated renal cell carcinomas, as the pathologic features of MLCN are not present.

Radiologic imaging studies are not adequate to exclude malignancy, and further evaluation is needed. Cyst aspiration is usually inadequate because the locules do not communicate and because an excessive number of punctures would be required to evaluate all portions of the lesion. Thus, surgical excision is generally indicated.

LITHIUM-INDUCED NEPHROTOXICITY

Patients on long-term lithium therapy may develop nephrogenic diabetes insipidus, which is reversible if lithium treatment is stopped. With long-term lithium therapy, patients may develop chronic renal disease. The kidneys are normal sized but have multiple small renal cysts measuring only 1 to 2 mm in diameter. The cysts can be appreciated on enhanced CT examinations but are better seen on unenhanced T2-weighted MR sequences showing multiple hyperintense foci (Fig. 5.21).

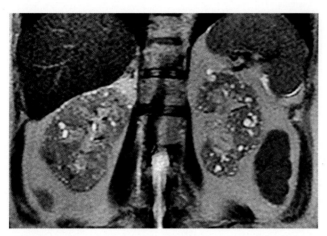

FIGURE 5.21. Lithium-induced renal cysts. Multiple small cysts are seen on a T2-weighted MR image.

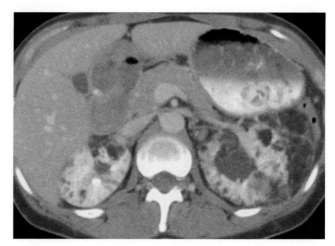

FIGURE 5.22. Tuberous sclerosis. Multiple fatty tumors, indicating angiomyolipomas, are present bilaterally along with multiple cysts.

CYSTS ASSOCIATED WITH SYSTEMIC DISEASE

The phakomatoses are a group of neurologic disorders that include congenital abnormalities of the skin and other organs. Two of these disorders, tuberous sclerosis and von Hippel–Lindau (VHL) disease, are associated with renal cysts.

Tuberous Sclerosis Complex

The complex of tuberous sclerosis (Bourneville disease) includes small cutaneous angiofibromas on the face (adenoma sebaceum) and hamartomas in various organs, such as the brain, eyes, heart, and kidneys. The disease is transmitted by autosomal dominant inheritance but with incomplete penetrance. Sporadic cases, presumably due to spontaneous mutation, occur in as many as 50% of cases. The disease is the result of inactivating mutations of the TSC1 gene located on chromosome 9 or the TSC2 gene located on chromosome 16.

Patients may present with mental retardation, seizures, or characteristic skin lesions. Approximately 80% of patients have renal angiomyolipomas, which may cause hematuria. Approximately one-third of patients also have renal cysts, which tend to be small and seldom exceed 3 cm in diameter. They have a distinctive microscopic appearance with hyperplastic epithelium. Severe renal involvement can lead to renal failure, which is second only to the involvement of the central nervous system (CNS) as a cause of death in these patients. Multiple enlarging renal cysts and retroperitoneal hemorrhage from an angiomyolipoma are the most common causes of renal failure. Cross-sectional imaging may demonstrate only angiomyolipomas (Fig. 5.22), angiomyolipomas and cysts, or only cysts.

Sonography clearly distinguishes the anechoic cysts from angiomyolipomas, which are typically echogenic. The appearance of the cysts is the same as that of simple cortical cysts. The appearance of an angiomyolipoma reflects the proportion of each tissue element within the tumor; some of the angiomyolipomas may contain little if any fat and are composed mostly of smooth muscle and vessels.

CT often is used to confirm the presence of an angiomyolipoma by demonstrating the fatty nature of the tumor. Angiomyolipomas without demonstrable fat may be indistinguishable from renal cell carcinomas without percutaneous biopsy or surgery.

von Hippel–Lindau Disease

This syndrome consists of cerebellar and retinal hemangioblastomas, renal cell carcinomas, pheochromocytomas, and various visceral cysts, including renal and pancreatic cysts. It is transmitted by autosomal dominant inheritance and has a high penetrance, which leads to manifestations of the disease early in life. VHL disease results from inactivating mutations of the VHL suppressor gene, which is located on chromosome 3. Increased levels of growth factors stimulate the development of hypervascular tumors.

Patients with VHL disease present most commonly with symptoms of a cerebellar hemangioblastoma. Capillary angiomas involve the retina and may cause progressive visual loss. Renal cysts occur in approximately three-fourths of patients, and renal cell carcinomas develop in 25% to 45% of patients (see Chapter 6). The renal tumors are often bilateral and are usually multifocal. Other manifestations include pheochromocytomas, neuroendocrine tumors, pancreatic cysts, and papillary cystadenomas of the epididymis.

Three distinct phenotypes of VHL disease are recognized. The most common pattern (type I) includes retinal and CNS hemangioblastomas, renal cysts and cancers, and pancreatic cystic disease (Figs. 5.23 and 5.24). The second most common pattern (type IIA) includes retinal and CNS hemangioblastomas, as well as pheochromocytomas and neuroendocrine tumors of the pancreas. Renal cysts and cancers are not present in type IIA. The least common phenotype of VHL (type IIB) includes retinal and CNS hemangioblastoma, pheochromocytoma, and renal and pancreatic disease.

The renal cysts, which usually range in size from 0.5 to 3 cm, are reported in approximately 60% of patients with VHL. However, if families with pheochromocytomas (type IIA) are excluded, the prevalence increases to 85%. They demonstrate a continuum from simple cysts to carcinoma manifesting as complex papillary projections into the cystic lumen. However, the hyperplastic epithelial lining may be a precursor of malignancy.

Radiographic evaluation of patients with VHL disease is difficult as the numerous cysts distort the normal renal architecture. Findings include simple cysts, cysts with atypical features, cystic tumors, and solid renal cell carcinomas, so careful evaluation is essential. Thin-section CT is useful for this purpose. Since follow-up examinations are recommended at least annually, MR imaging is often used to avoid the long-term effects of ionizing radiation. The growth of each tumor is followed carefully, as treatment is initiated before the tumor reaches 3 cm in diameter. Since multiple tumors are expected to occur, the emphasis is preservation of renal function. Thus, definitive treatment of larger tumors is by radiofrequency ablation or nephron sparing surgery.

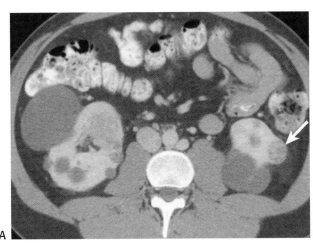
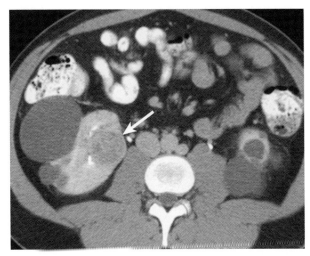

FIGURE 5.23. VHL type I. **A, B:** Axial images show both cysts and solid tumors (*arrows*).

ACQUIRED RENAL CYSTIC DISEASE

Since the initial description in 1977, many investigators have documented the progressive development of renal cysts and solid tumors in patients with renal failure. The mechanism of cyst formation is related to increased levels of growth factors as well as activation of protooncogenes. Fusiform dilations of the renal tubules with fluid accumulation result in cyst formation. After successful renal transplantation, the cysts involute.

Renal cysts occur in approximately 8% of patients at the initiation of dialysis and increase proportional to the duration of dialysis. After 3 years, 10% to 20% of patients have acquired renal cystic disease (ARCD). This increases to 40% of patients after 3 years of dialysis and to 90% after 5 to 10 years. ARCD is seen equally among patients receiving hemodialysis or peritoneal dialysis.

Solid tumors are also seen with increased frequency, up to 7%. These solid neoplasms include adenomas, oncocytomas, and renal cell carcinomas. From pathologic examination, it is not easy to determine the biologic behavior of these tumors, but the incidence of aggressively malignant renal cell carcinoma is small. Many of the tumors that are classified as malignant histologically do not demonstrate aggressively malignant behavior. In a review of 14 long-term dialysis series, Grantham et al. found that only 2 of 601 (0.33%) patients developed metastatic cancer. Prospective longitudinal studies indicate that the annual incidence of metastatic or locally invasive renal carcinoma among dialysis patients is three to six times that of the general population.

Although the renal cysts tend to regress after successful renal transplantation, the effect on the risk of developing renal cancer is less clear. Any carcinogenic factors associated with dialysis may not persist after successful transplantation, and the risk of renal cancer would then be reduced. However, transplant recipients have an increased risk of developing renal cell carcinoma, presumably due to immunosuppression. The net result is that these patients remain at increased risk for developing renal cell carcinoma, and those cancers may exhibit more aggressive behavior, even after successful transplantation.

The ultrasonographic examination of native kidneys is difficult because they are often small, distorted, and surrounded by highly echogenic fat. There is an increased incidence of hemorrhage into renal cysts and the perinephric space. Calcification frequently occurs in the cyst walls or in the renal interstitium, making ultrasonographic evaluation even more difficult. A renal mass with internal echoes, mural nodules, or no distal acoustic enhancement

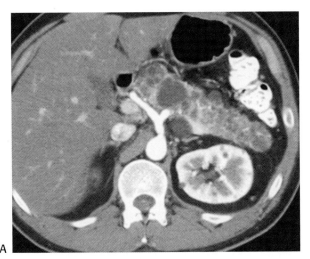
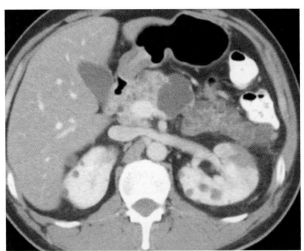

FIGURE 5.24. VHL type I. Arterial **(A)** and nephrographic **(B)** phase images show multiple pancreatic cysts and cysts in both kidneys. A solid tumor formerly in the anterior portion of the left kidney has undergone radiofrequency ablation.

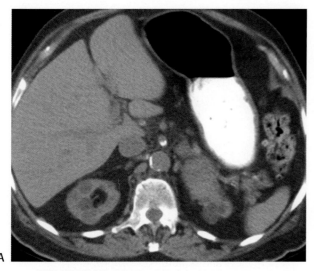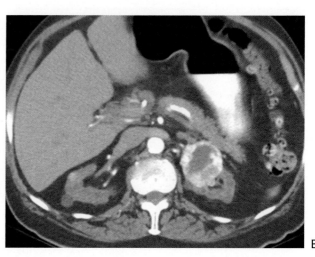

A   B

FIGURE 5.25. ARCD with renal cell carcinoma. Multiple small cysts in a patient on long-term dialysis with small kidneys bilaterally. Unenhanced **(A)** and enhanced **(B)** CT of the abdomen images demonstrate a large enhancing left renal tumor.

is likely to be a renal cell carcinoma. Tumor enhancement may be demonstrated with color flow Doppler.

It is easier to examine the native kidneys with CT (Fig. 5.25) and MRI than with ultrasound. Multiple small cysts are seen by CT or MRI in virtually all patients with ARCD. Dystrophic calcifications are common in the renal parenchyma or cyst walls. Bleeding is a common complication, so hemorrhagic cysts and subcapsular or perinephric hematomas are often found (Fig. 5.26). Carcinomas

are seen as masses with a density similar to the unenhanced parenchyma. If large (<3 cm), the masses may be heterogeneous on enhanced images (Fig. 5.27).

RENAL LYMPHANGIOMATOSIS

Renal lymphangiomatosis is a rare condition that refers to the presence of multiple cysts in both the renal sinus and the renal parenchyma (Fig. 5.28). It has been found in both adults and children. The etiology is unknown, but it is thought to be the result of lymphatic obstruction. Renin-dependent hypertension may be the presenting clinical complaint.

MISCELLANEOUS RENAL CYSTS
Orofaciodigital Syndrome

This rare X-linked inherited disorder includes malformations of the mouth, face, and digits. It is lethal in utero in males, and therefore, all patients are female. Multiple renal cysts may mimic autosomal dominant or autosomal recessive polycystic kidney disease. Many patients develop progressive renal insufficiency and eventually require dialysis.

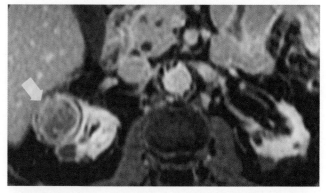

FIGURE 5.26. Acquired renal cystic disease. Multiple renal cysts and a perinephric hematoma are identified on this contrast-enhanced CT scan.

FIGURE 5.27. Acquired renal cystic disease. A small renal carcinoma was found (*arrow*) in the right kidney on this gadolinium-enhanced magnetic resonance examination using a T1-weighted, gradient echo, fat saturation technique.

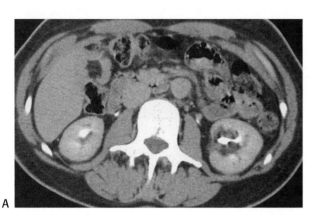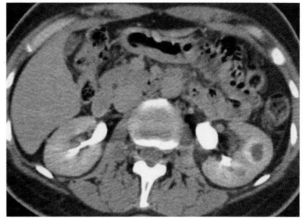

A
B

FIGURE 5.28. Renal lymphangiomatosis. **A, B:** CT axial images show renal parenchymal and renal sinus cysts in the left kidney of a middle aged woman with renal lymphangiomatosis.

Hydatid Disease

Hydatid disease in humans is usually caused by infection with either *Echinococcus granulosus* or *Echinococcus multilocularis*. The disease is endemic on all five continents and may be seen in nonendemic areas in patients who have traveled to endemic regions.

The adult worm lives in the intestine of a dog (definitive host) and discharges the egg-containing proglottid into the feces. The intermediate host is usually a sheep that ingests the eggs while grazing on contaminated ground. The protective chitinous layer is dissolved in the duodenum, and the hydatid embryo passes through the intestinal wall into the portal vein. Thus, the liver is the most commonly involved organ. The embryo develops into a slowly growing cyst. The cycle is completed when the intermediate host (sheep) dies and the larva are eaten by the definitive host (dog). The human being is infected as an accidental host by eating contaminated food.

Hydatid cysts are composed of three layers: (1) an outer protective pericyst, (2) an easily broken middle membrane, and (3) a thin inner germinal layer that produces the scolices. The organs most commonly involved in humans are the liver (75%) and lung (15%). Other organs, such as the brain, bone, and kidney, are infected in <10% of cases.

Although most cases are acquired in childhood, they are seldom detected until adulthood. The symptoms of renal hydatid disease are nonspecific, and many patients are asymptomatic. Flank pain, hematuria, or signs of urinary tract infection may be present. A serologic test is available for patients suspected of having hydatid disease, on the basis of contact or radiologic findings.

Curvilinear calcifications in the wall of the hydatid cyst may be detected on plain radiographs in 20% to 30% of cases. The appearance ranges from thin, eggshell-like calcification to a dense reticular appearance. A septate cystic mass is seen on ultrasound. Internal echoes may be seen and are caused by the presence of hooklets, scolices, and brood capsules within the hydatid fluid.

The thick wall of the cysts is well demonstrated by CT. If daughter cysts are present, they can be detected by a high-density component next to the clear, water-density cystic fluid. A rosette pattern may be seen as fluid within the daughter cyst as it has a lower density than fluid within the parent cyst.

Removal of hydatid cysts risks dissemination of daughter cysts into the peritoneal cavity or retroperitoneum. Allergic reactions ranging from cutaneous manifestations to anaphylactic shock and death may occur when cyst contents are spilled. However, successful treatment of patients with renal hydatid cysts has been reported.

Communicating Cysts

Occasionally, a renal cyst communicates with the collecting system and opacifies with intravenous contrast medium on CT or retrograde pyelography. Any cystic renal mass, such as a benign cortical cyst, inflammatory cyst, or even cystic renal cell carcinoma may rupture into the collecting system and produce this appearance. However, the most common etiology is a pyelogenic cyst or calyceal diverticulum (see Chapter 12).

A calyceal diverticulum is lined with transitional epithelium and communicates with the collecting system through a narrow isthmus. The connection is usually at the fornix but can be at any portion of the calyx. Most calyceal diverticula are small, usually <2 cm in diameter. They are usually asymptomatic but occasionally may contain calculi or milk of calcium, become obstructed or infected.

Because excreted contrast medium enters the calyces from the collecting ducts of Bellini, the calyces opacify before the calyceal diverticulum. This useful differentiating feature distinguishes the calyceal diverticulum from papillary necrosis or focal hydronephrosis. Communicating cysts are well demonstrated by CT, in which contrast accumulation can be clearly seen (Fig. 5.29).

EXTRAPARENCHYMAL CYSTS

Various investigators have used different terms to describe extraparenchymal cysts or cysts that arise in or just outside the kidney but project into the renal sinus. To minimize this ambiguity, we consider cysts in two anatomic locations. The term *parapelvic cyst* is applied to cortical cysts projecting into the renal sinus, and the term *peripelvic cyst* is used to describe those that arise in the renal sinus. Peripelvic cysts are thought to be lymphatic in origin and have been referred to as renal pelvic lymphangiectasia. Using this terminology, parapelvic cysts are usually large but solitary, whereas peripelvic cysts are typically small, multiple, and often bilateral.

Renal Sinus Cysts

These benign cysts lie in the region of the renal hilum and cause extrinsic compression on the collecting system. Smooth bowing or displacement of the infundibuli is seen on imaging (Fig. 5.30). The CT appearance is that of a benign cyst located in the hilar area rather than in the cortex of the kidney. Renal sinus cysts may not be renal in origin but could be lymphocytes or may arise from embryologic remnants in the renal hilum (peripelvic cysts). With increased use of CT and ultrasound, they are frequently recognized and are often multiple and bilateral (Fig. 5.31). Problems arise when renal sinus cysts are confused with other entities.

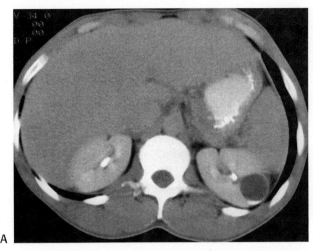 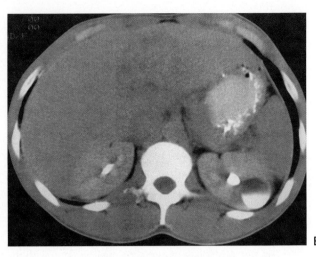

FIGURE 5.29. Communicating cyst. **A:** A small amount of contrast material is seen in the left renal cyst. The thick wall suggests it is most likely a calyceal diverticulum. **B:** Later images demonstrate further contrast accumulation.

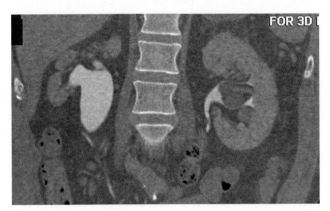

FIGURE 5.30. Parapelvic cyst. Reconstructed image from a CT urogram shows effacement of the left renal pelvis, secondary to a parapelvic cyst.

Ultrasound demonstrates their benign cystic nature. However, the multiple echo-free areas in the central portion of the kidney may suggest hydronephrosis. The same confusion may occur on unenhanced or early phase CT images. Excretory phase imaging usually clarifies the true nature of the cyst (Fig. 5.32).

Renal sinus cysts should not be confused with excess renal sinus fat (sinus lipomatosis). Both of these entities produce extrinsic compression on the renal collecting system but are easily distinguished on CT, MRI, or ultrasound examinations.

A perinephric cyst is renal in origin, but it is not a true cyst. It represents a collection of fluid, presumably extravasated urine, which is often formed after renal trauma, but trapped beneath the renal capsule. Perinephric cysts may also be seen in infants with congenital lower urinary tract obstruction. The cyst walls are composed of fibrous tissue and do not have an epithelial lining. They are seldom of any clinical significance but, if large, could result in hypertension due to the compressive force on the renal parenchyma (Page kidney).

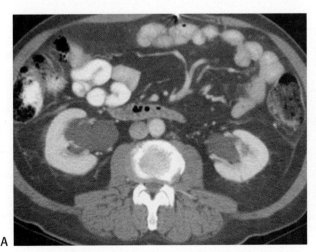 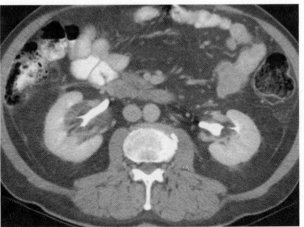

FIGURE 5.31. Bilateral parapelvic cysts. **A:** On a nephrographic phase image, the renal pelvis appears dilated simulating bilateral hydronephrosis. **B:** Excretory phase image shows the renal pelvis to be normal but surrounded by parapelvic cysts.

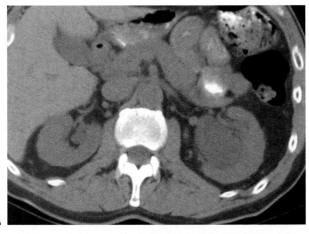

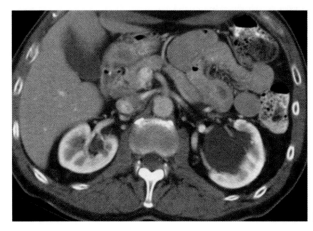

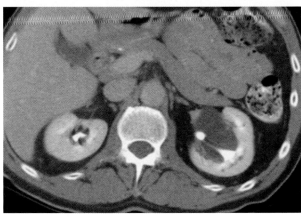

FIGURE 5.32. Parapelvic cyst. Unenhanced **(A)** and nephrographic phase **(B)** images suggest left hydronephrosis. **C:** An excretory phase image shows the apparent dilatation is secondary to a parapelvic cyst.

SUGGESTED READINGS

Cortical Cysts

Beer AJ, Dobritz M, Zantle N, et al. Comparison of 16-MDCT and MRI for characterization of kidney lesions. *AJR Am J Roentgenol.* 2006;186:1639–1650.

Berland LL, Silverman SG, Gore RM, et al. Managing incidental findings on abdominal CT: white paper of the ACR incidental findings committee. *JACR.* 2010;7:754–773.

Bosniak MA. Diagnosis and management of patients with complicated cystic lesions of the kidney. *AJR Am J Roentgenol.* 1997;169:819.

Bosniak MA. The Bosniak renal cyst classification: 25 years later. *Radiology.* 2011;202:781–785.

Coulam CH, Sheafor DH, Leder RA, et al. Evaluation of pseudoenhancement of renal cysts during contrast enhanced CT. *AJR Am J Roentgenol.* 2000;174:493.

Dunnick NR, Korobkin M, Silverman PM, et al. Computed tomography of high density renal cysts. *J Comput Assist Tomogr.* 1984;8(3):458.

Harisinghani MG, Maher MM, Gervais DA, et al. Incidence of malignancy in complex cystic renal masses (Bosniak category III): should imaging-guided biopsy precede surgery? *AJR Am J Roentgenol.* 2003;180:755–758.

Hartman DS, Choyke PL, Hartman MS. From the RSNA refresher courses: a practical approach to the cystic renal mass. *Radiographics.* 2004;24:S101–S115.

Hindman NM, Hecht EM, Bosniak MA. Follow up for Bosniak category 2F cystic renal lesions. *Radiology.* 2014;272:757–766.

Hindman NM. Approach to very small (<1.5 cm) cystic renal lesions: ignore, observe or treat? *AJR Am J Roentgenol.* 2015;204:1182–1189.

Israel GM, Bosniak MA. Calcification in cystic renal masses: is it important in diagnosis? *Radiology.* 2003;226:47–52.

Israel GM, Bosniak MA. How I do it: evaluating renal masses. *Radiology.* 2005;236:441–450.

Jonisch AI, Rubinowitz A, Mutalik P, et al. Can high attenuation renal cysts be differentiated from renal cell carcinoma at unenhanced computed tomography? *Radiology.* 2007;243:445–450.

Karabathina VS, Kota G, Dawyam AK, et al. Adult renal cystic disease: a genetic, biological and developmental primer. *Radiographics.* 2010;30: 1509–1523.

Levine E, Grantham JJ. High-Density renal cysts in autosomal dominant polycystic kidney disease demonstrated by CT. *Radiology.* 1985;154:477.

Nascimento AB, Mitchell DG, Zhang XM, et al. Rapid MR imaging detection of renal cysts: age based standards. *Radiology.* 2001;221:628–632.

Papanicolaou N, Pfister RC, Yoder IC. Spontaneous and traumatic rupture of renal cysts: diagnosis and outcome. *Radiology.* 1986;160:99.

Silverman SG, Mortele KJ, Tuncali K, et al. Hyperattenuating renal masses: etiologies, pathogenesis, and evaluation. *Radiographics.* 2007;27:1131–1143.

Silverman SG, Israel GM, Herts B, et al. Management of the incidental renal mass. *Radiology.* 2008;249:16–31.

Weber TM. Sonography of benign renal cystic disease. *Radiol Clin North Am.* 2006;44(6):777–786.

Wood CG III, Stromberg LJ, Harmath CB, et al. CT and MR imaging for evaluation of cystic renal lesions and diseases. *Radiographics.* 2015;35: 125–141.

Unilateral Cystic Disease

Curry NS, Chung CJ, Gordon B. Unilateral renal cystic disease in an adult. *Abdom Imaging.* 1994;19:366.

Medullary Cystic Disease

Garel LA, Habib R, Pariente D, et al. Juvenile nephronophthisis: sonographic appearance in children with severe uremia. *Radiology.* 1984;151:93.

Steele B, Lirenman DS, Beattle CW. Nephronophthisis. *Am J Med.* 1980; 68:521.

Wise SW, Hartman DS, Hardesty LA, et al. Renal medullary cystic disease: assessment by MRI. *Abdom Imaging.* 1998;23:649.

Polycystic Renal Disease

Alpern MB, Dorfman RE, Gross BH, et al. Seminal vesicle cysts: association with adult polycystic kidney disease. *Radiology.* 1991;180:79.

Bisceglia M, Galliani CA, Senger C, et al. Renal cystic diseases. A review. *Adv Anat Pathol.* 2006;13(1):26–56.

Borges Oliva MR, Hsing J, Rybicki FJ, et al. Glomerulocystic kidney disease: MRI findings. *Abdom Imaging.* 2003;28:889–892.

Levine E, Grantham JJ. Calcified renal stones and cyst calcifications in autosomal dominant polycystic kidney disease: clinical and CT study in 84 patients. *AJR Am J Roentgenol.* 1992;159:77.

Lonergan GJ, Rice RR, Suarez ES. Autosomal recessive polycystic kidney disease: radiologic-pathologic correlation. *Radiographics.* 2000;20:837–855.

Nicolau C, Torra R, Badenas C, et al. Autosomal dominant polycystic kidney disease types 1 and 2: assessment of US sensitivity for diagnosis. *Radiology.* 1999;213:273.

Wilson PD. Polycystic kidney disease. *N Engl J Med.* 2004;350(2):151–164.

Cysts Associated with Systemic Disease

Choyke PL, Glenn GM, Walther MM, et al. von Hippel–Lindau disease: genetic, clinical, and imaging features. *Radiology.* 1995;194:629.

Hough DM, Stephens DH, Johnson CD, et al. Pancreatic lesions in von Hippel–Lindau disease: prevalence, clinical significance, and CT findings. *AJR Am J Roentgenol.* 1994;162:1091.

Loughlin KR, Gittes RF. Urologic management of patients with von Hippel–Lindau's disease. *J Urol.* 1986;136:789.

Rabenou RA, Charles HW. Differentiation of sporadic versus tuberous sclerosis complex-associated angiomyolipoma. *AJR Am J Roentgenol.* 2015;205:292–301.

Shinohara N, Nonomura K, Harabayashi T, et al. Nephron sparing surgery for renal cell carcinoma in von Hippel–Lindau disease. *J Urol.* 1995;154:2016.

Acquired Renal Cystic Disease

Chandhoke PS, Torrence RJ, Clayman RV, et al. Acquired cystic disease of the kidney: a management dilemma. *J Urol.* 1992;147:969.

Grantham JJ, Levine E, Acquired cystic disease: replacing one kidney disease with another. *Kidney Int.* 1985;28:99.

Levine LA, Gburek BM. Acquired cystic disease and renal adenocarcinoma following renal transplantation. *J Urol.* 1994;151:129.

Levine E, Slusher SL, Grantham JJ, et al. Natural history of acquired renal cystic disease in dialysis patients: a prospective longitudinal CT study. *AJR Am J Roentgenol.* 1991;156:501.

Multicystic Dysplastic Kidney

Kleiner B, Filly RA, Mack L, et al. Multicystic dysplastic kidney: observations of contralateral disease in the fetal population. *Radiology.* 1986;161:27.

Pedicelli G, Jequier S, Bowen A, et al. Multicystic dysplastic kidneys: spontaneous regression demonstrated with US. *Radiology.* 1986;160:23.

Sanders R, Hartman D. The sonographic distinction between neonatal multicystic kidney and hydronephrosis. *Radiology.* 1984;151:621.

Cystic Nephroma

Agrons GA, Wagner BJ, Davidson AJ, et al. From the archives of the AFIP. Multilocular cystic renal tumor in children: radiologic–pathologic correlation. *Radiographics.* 1995;15:653–669.

Granja MF, O'Brien AT, Trujillo S, et al. Multilocular cystic nephroma: a systematic literature review of the radiologic and clinical findings. *AJR Am J Roentgenol.* 2015;205:1188–1193.

Kettritz U, Semelka RC, Siegelman ES, et al. Multilocular cystic nephroma: MR imaging appearance, current techniques, including gadolinium enhancement. *J Magn Reson Imaging.* 1996;6(1):145–148.

Madewell JE, Goldman SM, Davis CJ, et al. Multilocular cystic nephroma: a radiographic–pathologic correlation of 58 patients. *Radiology.* 1983;146:309.

Moch H, Cystic renal tumors: new entities and novel concepts. *Adv Anat Pathol.* 2010;17(3):209–214.

Sahni VA, Mortele KJ, Glickman J, et al. Mixed epithelial and stromal tumour of the kidney: imaging features. *BJU Int.* 2010;105:932–939.

Zhou M, Kort E, Hoekstra P, et al. Adult cystic nephroma and mixed epithelial and stromal tumor of the kidney are the same disease entity: molecular and histologic evidence. *Am J Surg Pathol.* 2009;33(1):72–80.

Orofaciodigital Syndrome

Curry NS, Milutinovic J, Grossnickle M, et al. Renal cystic disease associated with orofaciodigital syndrome. *Urol Radiol.* 1992;13:153.

Hydatid Disease

Akhan O, Üstünsöz B, Somuncu I, et al. Percutaneous renal hydatid cyst treatment: long-term results. *Abdom Imaging.* 1998;23:209.

Angulo JC, Sanchez-Chapado M, Diego A, et al. Renal echinococcosis: clinical study of 34 cases. *J Urol.* 1997;157:787.

Migaleddu V, Conti M, Canalis GC, et al. Imaging of renal hydatid cysts. *AJR Am J Roentgenol.* 1997;169:1339.

Turgut AT, Odev K, Kabaalioglu A, et al. Multitechnique evaluation of renal hydatid disease. *AJR Am J Roentgenol.* 2009;192:462–67.

Extraparenchymal Cysts

Amis ES Jr, Cronan JJ. The renal sinus: an imaging review and proposed nomenclature for sinus cysts. *J Urol.* 1988;139:1151.

Cronan JJ, Yoder IC, Amis ES Jr, et al. The myth of anechoic renal sinus fat. *Radiology.* 1982;144:149.

Hidalgo H, Dunnick NR, Rosenberg ER, et al. Parapelvic cysts: appearance on CT and sonography. *AJR Am J Roentgenol.* 1982;138:667.

Younathan CM, Kaude JV. Renal peripelvic lymphatic cysts (lymphangiomas) associated with generalized lymphangiomatosis. *Urol Radiol.* 1992;14:161.

6

Renal Tumors

INTRODUCTION

While there are many types of solid renal tumors; the most common solid renal masses are renal cell carcinomas (RCCs), angiomyolipomas (AMLs), and oncocytomas. Unfortunately, with the exception of the majority of AMLs, most solid renal tumors do not have a radiographic appearance sufficiently characteristic to allow for a definite diagnosis to be made. In some instances, however, combinations of imaging features can be used to suggest a likely diagnosis. Modern imaging techniques also play a major role in management and follow-up of many patients with renal tumors.

INDETERMINATE VERY SMALL RENAL MASSES (<1 TO 1.5 CM)

Continued improvement in cross-sectional imaging modalities has enabled detection of many very small renal lesions. Most masses <1 to 1.5 cm in maximal diameter appear to be of soft tissue attenuation but are usually too small to characterize as cystic or solid (Fig. 6.1). This is for two reasons: (1) volume averaging and (2) pseudoenhancement.

Volume averaging results from the unintentional averaging of pixels within a small renal mass with pixels in adjacent normal tissue. When a region of interest measurement is obtained in a small cystic mass, the obtained attenuation of the mass represents an average of the true attenuation of the mass itself and adjacent renal

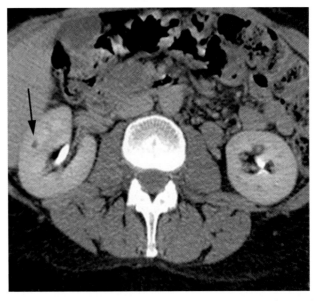

FIGURE 6.1. Indeterminate renal mass. Contrast-enhanced axial CT image demonstrates a tiny sub-cm indeterminate lesion in the right kidney (*arrow*). This mass is too small for accurate attenuation measurements to be obtained.

parenchyma. As a result, a cystic mass can be falsely assumed to be of soft tissue attenuation on unenhanced or enhanced CT images and can also be falsely identified as enhancing when both unenhanced and enhanced series are available. Volume averaging can be eliminated as a problem when CT image collimation is decreased to less than half of a renal mass's diameter. In this way, it can be assured that at least one image obtained through the mass does not contain any volume-averaged tissue.

Pseudoenhancement is an artifactual increase in attenuation of a renal cyst after contrast material administration, due to the reconstruction algorithm used for CT, even when the effects of partial volume averaging have been accounted for and eliminated. Thus, even when appropriately thinly collimated images are obtained on a contrast-enhanced CT, a small renal cyst can spuriously appear as solid. A number of factors have been identified that increase the likelihood of pseudoenhancement. Pseudoenhancement is more often present on multidetector CT examinations when masses are small. Thus, pseudoenhancement is seen in about one-third of renal masses <1 cm in maximal diameter (compared to about 10% of masses measuring 1 cm or larger). It is also more often present in masses that have a central location (as these are surrounded by brightly enhancing renal parenchyma), seen in about one-third of such masses (compared to only about 10% of masses that are peripheral). It should be emphasized that pseudoenhancement almost always results in attenuation increases of up to no more than 30 HU. Any measured enhancement exceeding this amount should, therefore, be considered to be true enhancement, providing that volume averaging has been accounted for.

The overwhelming majority of small renal masses are benign cysts. For this reason, nearly all small renal masses that cannot be characterized by CT can be ignored. In only a few settings, additional evaluation should be performed: (1) when a small renal mass is demonstrably heterogeneous (a feature that is unlikely to be encountered in a renal cyst) or (2) when a small renal mass is detected in patients with known renal cancer-causing syndromes, even if the mass is homogeneous. In these two instances, follow-up CT or MRI is suggested to assess these lesions for stability. It should be noted, however, that many benign and malignant renal masses grow at slow and comparable rates (of only 2 to 4 mm per year). So, the average rate of renal mass growth between two sequential 6-month CTs is actually close to the intraobserver and interobserver variability in measuring renal masses, even when they do not grow. For these reasons, follow-up studies should be compared to multiple previous examinations, and any detected renal masses should also be assessed for increasing complexity. Also, once an indeterminate mass enlarges above 1.5 cm in greatest dimension, it can be more reliably assessed as cystic or solid.

SOLID RENAL MASSES

Imaging Techniques

Two basic imaging characteristics of solid renal masses are encountered on cross-sectional imaging studies: those that contain macroscopic fat and those that do not. Nearly all of the former lesions represent benign AMLs, while the majority of the latter represent renal cancers. Pre- and postcontrast thin-section multiphasic CT or MRI are the methods of choice for evaluating a patient with a suspected renal mass. When a renal mass is identified on a CT scan performed for another purpose, it may be prudent to perform a dedicated renal CT in order to assess the vascularity of the lesion and its enhancement characteristics, as well as to assess the status of the inferior vena cava, regional lymph nodes, and adjacent organs.

Although ultrasound can be helpful in distinguishing solid from cystic renal masses, it is not nearly as sensitive in detecting small renal masses as is CT or MRI. In one study of patients with VHL followed with US and CT examinations US failed to identify 80% of masses smaller than 1 cm seen on CT. When detected on US, solid renal masses are usually identified as such, although cystic regions representing areas of hemorrhage or necrosis may be seen. Microbubble contrast ultrasound agents have been shown to enhance vascular elements within soft tissues, including the kidney, and may be useful in evaluating patients with known or suspected renal cancers when contrast agents cannot be administered for CT or MRI.

Isoechoic solid renal tumors may be difficult to detect with ultrasound, especially if they are small and do not displace the collecting system or produce a contour deformity. Less echogenic primary renal tumors can simulate more homogeneous tumors such as lymphomas or may be confused with renal cysts. However, these solid tumors usually have poorly defined margins and do not have the increased sound transmission seen with cysts. A few renal adenocarcinomas are primarily cystic. However, these cystic tumors can usually be distinguished from simple cysts by their irregularly thick walls and the presence of some internal echoes. Duplex and color Doppler ultrasounds provide a noninvasive measure of the vascularity of a renal mass. High-velocity signals, which are presumably due to arteriovenous shunting, are frequently seen in renal carcinomas.

Dedicated renal mass CT or MRI should be obtained as the study of choice in any patient with a known or suspected solid renal mass. At a minimum, a two-phase study that includes a noncontrast examination of the liver and kidneys and postcontrast study made during the nephrographic phase (NP) should be performed. In some instances, the addition of arterial phase (e.g., to evaluate the arteries prior to planned surgery), corticomedullary phase (CMP) (to evaluate the veins and other organs), and/or excretory phase (to evaluate the renal collecting systems) series may also be helpful. Arterial phase images (in which the arteries enhance briskly, the renal cortex enhances briskly, but the renal medulla demonstrates little enhancement) are usually acquired beginning at about 20 to 30 seconds following the initiation of intravenous contrast material administration. CMP images (in which the arterial enhancement is not as pronounced, but the renal cortex continues to enhance briskly and the medulla enhances, but to a much lesser extent) are routinely acquired beginning at about 60 to 70 seconds, NP images (in which the kidney now enhances homogeneously) beginning at about 90 to 100 seconds, and excretory phase (EP) images (when the nephrogram remains homogeneous but begins to fade and when excreted contrast material is detected in the renal collecting systems) beginning at 120 to 180 seconds.

CT is best performed by obtaining narrowly collimated thin-section images (no more than 2.5 to 5.0 mm in thickness) both before and after intravenous contrast material administration. A comparison of the density on the enhanced series to that of the unenhanced image allows for assessment of contrast enhancement. While all findings can be made on the axial images, coronal reformatted images are particularly helpful in identifying renal masses, especially those that are small or that have a polar location.

NP images are important for the detection of solid renal masses for several reasons. Firstly, some solid renal masses will not demonstrate definite enhancement on CT until the NP images occur. If only CMP images are obtained in these patients, a renal cancer might be falsely diagnosed as a high-density renal cyst. Secondly, the persistent differential enhancement of the renal cortex and renal medulla on CMP images may result in failure to diagnose some hypervascular cortical renal masses (enhancing similarly to normal renal cortex) or some hypovascular medullary masses (enhancing similarly to normal renal medulla) (Fig. 6.2).

There are a few problematic issues related to CT imaging of solid renal masses. It has recently been shown that just under 10% of

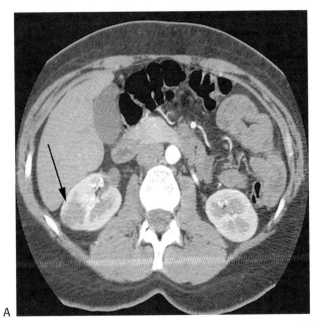
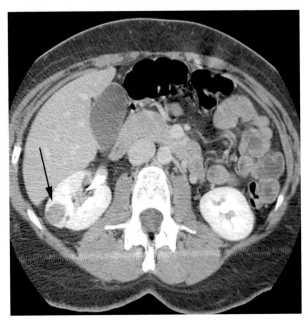

FIGURE 6.2. Advantage of NP or EP images over CMP images. A small renal cancer in the right kidney is less well seen on axial CMP images **(A)** than on EP images **(B)** (*arrows*).

renal cancers may measure water attenuation on noncontrast images (between −10 and 20 HU). This is problematic, as these lesions could be misdiagnosed as cysts if only unenhanced CT images are available (Fig. 6.3). The low attenuation of these lesions has primarily been seen in some patients with clear cell carcinomas, probably due to the fact that these tumors contain large amounts of intracellular lipid. While the vast majority of water attenuation masses seen on unenhanced CT are cysts, it is important to assess any such masses for even subtle heterogeneity, to minimize the likelihood that a renal cancer is not erroneously diagnosed as a benign lesion.

In general, a renal mass can be considered as being definitely solid (and enhancing) on CT if it increases in attenuation by 20 HU or more (between the unenhanced and enhanced series). Most investigators agree that an increase in attenuation of 10 to 20 HU should be considered equivocal, and follow-up (preferably with MRI, which is more sensitive in detecting enhancement) is warranted. In one recent study, 20 (17%) and 4 (3%) of 116 renal cancers did not enhance by 15 HU or more on CMP images alone and both corticomedullary and NP images, respectively. In this series, if the threshold was increased to 20 HU to define enhancement, the number of renal

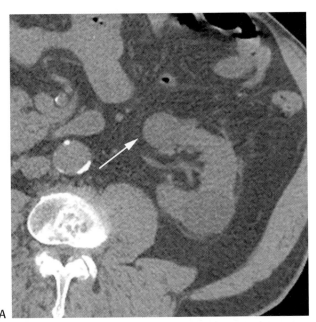
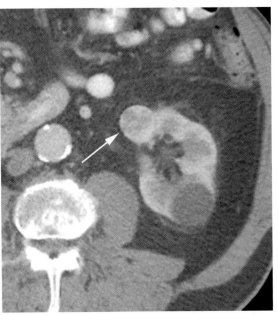

FIGURE 6.3. Renal cancer mimicking a cyst on noncontrast CT. **A:** Two left renal masses measure water attenuation on noncontrast axial images, one located posteriorly (4 HU) and the other located anteriorly (9 HU) (*arrow*). **B:** The posterior mass remains of water attenuation on the CMP contrast-enhanced images (12 HU); however, the anterior mass, which was subsequently diagnosed as a clear cell renal cancer (*arrow*), demonstrates brisk heterogeneous enhancement (up to 113 HU).

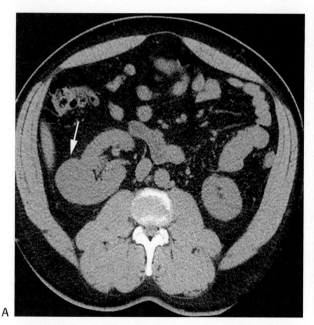
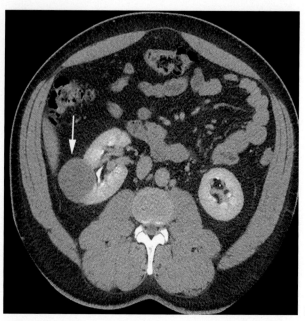

FIGURE 6.4. Nonenhancing papillary renal cancer. **A:** A homogeneous right renal mass measures 27 HU on precontrast axial images (*arrow*). **B:** After contrast material administration, the mass, which remains homogeneous, increases to measure 35 HU (*arrow*). This increment of 8 HU is not sufficient to diagnose this lesion as solid and enhancing.

cancers that did not enhance increased to 24 (21%) and 11(9%). Only masses that increase in attenuation by 10 HU or less should be considered as truly nonenhancing; however, even this threshold is not absolute. Some hypoenhancing renal cancers may increase in attenuation by <10 HU (Fig. 6.4). Once again, it is essential that any renal mass be assessed for heterogeneity on contrast-enhanced CT images. Most, but not all, nonenhancing or equivocally enhancing renal cancers will not be completely homogeneous. MRI is more sensitive for detecting enhancement. In some series, even those solid renal masses that did not demonstrate an increase in attenuation between nonenhanced and enhanced series on CT could be seen to enhance on subtraction MR images (Fig. 6.5).

Angiomyolipoma

Angiomyolipomas (AMLs) are tumors composed of a mixture of mature adipose tissue, thick-walled blood vessels, and sheets of smooth muscle. The amount of each component varies in each tumor. AMLs belong to a group of tumors classified as perivascular epithelioid cell tumors or PEComas. The vast majority of these tumors are benign. They are generally seen in two groups of patients: (1) as small isolated renal masses in middle-aged or older women and (2) in up to 80% of patients with tuberous sclerosis (in which case the tumors are often multiple and are equally likely to occur in men and women). The AMLs associated with tuberous sclerosis also occur at a younger age and tend to be larger in size than the sporadic lesions.

Manifestations of tuberous sclerosis include epilepsy, mental retardation, hamartomas (which may be cerebral), and retinal phakomas. Adenoma sebaceum may be seen in the malar areas of the face. Patients may also develop intrahepatic AMLs. In addition to renal AMLs, renal abnormalities in patients with tuberous sclerosis may also include the development of multiple renal cysts. Tuberous sclerosis is caused by an autosomal dominant inherited gene mutation, with variable expressivity. In some patients, the clinical syndrome is incompletely manifest.

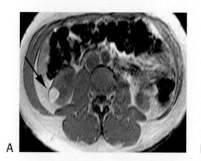
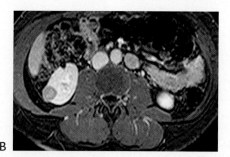
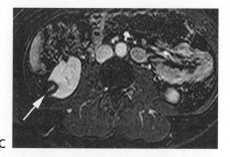

FIGURE 6.5. Minimal enhancement in a right renal mass seen only on subtraction MR images. **A:** T1-weighted axial image demonstrates a high T1 signal intensity mass in the posterolateral aspect of the right kidney (*arrow*). **B:** Following contrast material administration, the mass again has high signal intensity on this T1-weighted axial image; however, it appears slightly heterogeneous. It is difficult to determine whether the mass is enhancing, given its intrinsic T1 hyperintensity. **C:** A subtraction axial image reveals that the mass contains a thickened enhancing septation centrally (*arrow*).

Nonetheless, the presence of multiple AMLs with or without associated renal cysts on imaging studies should raise the possibility of tuberous sclerosis.

Renal AMLs are also found in approximately 15% of patients with lymphangiomyomatosis. Lymphangiomyomatosis, which is considered by many to be a *forme fruste* of tuberous sclerosis, is an idiopathic disease that occurs in young women. It consists of smooth muscle hamartomas along the lymphatic system. It most commonly involves intrathoracic lymphatics, but abdominal involvement can be extensive. The pulmonary findings are diffuse and include a reticular or reticulonodular pattern and multiple small cysts, with a honeycomb-like appearance.

Most patients with AMLs have no symptoms; however, patients with large tumors may present with abdominal fullness or pain. Patients who develop hemorrhage, the most common and potentially clinically significant complication, can present with sudden back or flank pain, hypotension, and/or hematuria. Hemorrhage is more likely to occur when AMLs exceed 4 cm in maximal diameter and/or in tumors that contain more and larger renal artery branch aneurysms.

About 95% of AMLs contain enough macroscopic fat to produce characteristic findings on imaging studies. On plain abdominal radiography, some large AMLs may contain enough fat to produce an area of increased radiolucency. Calcification is seldom seen with conventional radiography or on other imaging studies, but may rarely be present, usually as a result of previous hemorrhage.

On ultrasonography, most AMLs are very echogenic (Figs. 6.6 and 6.7). Hypoechoic areas are occasionally encountered within an echogenic mass, however, possibly resulting from prior hemorrhage. It should be noted, however, that small renal cancers may also be echogenic (Fig. 6.8). Therefore, hyperechogenicity cannot be used to establish a definite diagnosis of AML. Some AMLs may also demonstrate posterior shadowing, a finding not encountered posterior to renal cancers (Fig. 6.9). Conversely, an anechoic rim or halo is sometime present around hyperechoic renal carcinomas, but has not been seen surrounding AMLs.

Both CT and MRI can be used to make diagnoses of AML with certainty in most instances. On CT, the detection of any component of a solid renal mass that measures fat attenuation is considered to

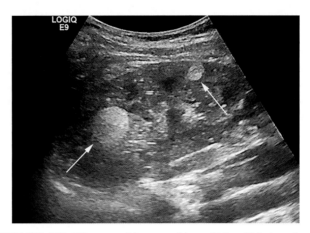

FIGURE 6.7. Ultrasound image of two AMLs. This longitudinal ultrasound image of a right kidney demonstrates two highly echogenic masses in this patient with tuberous sclerosis (*arrows*). Their appearance is characteristic, but not diagnostic of AMLs.

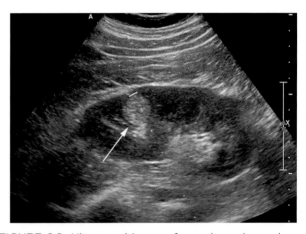

FIGURE 6.8. Ultrasound image of an echogenic renal cancer. This longitudinal image shows an echogenic renal mass (*arrow*). The appearance is suggestive of an AML; however, this lesion was subsequently diagnosed as a chromophobe renal cancer.

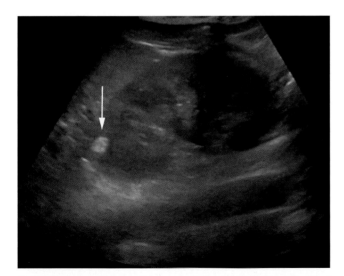

FIGURE 6.6. Ultrasound image of an AML. This longitudinal ultrasound image of the left kidney demonstrates a single echogenic mass in the upper pole in this middle-aged female (*arrow*). The appearance is characteristic but not diagnostic of a sporadic AML.

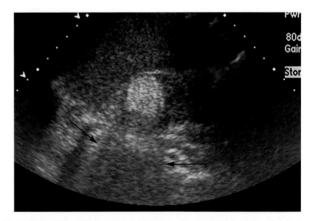

FIGURE 6.9. Ultrasound image of an AML with posterior shadowing. An echogenic mass in the lateral aspect of the upper pole of the right kidney demonstrates brisk posterior shadowing, a feature that has been described as being present only in AMLs (*arrows*).

be definitive. In general, macroscopic fat can be identified if any measured component of a solid renal mass measures −10 HU or less (Figs. 6.10 to 6.12). Examination of a small fatty renal mass by CT must be performed carefully to avoid volume averaging of a solid mass not containing any macroscopic fat with adjacent perinephric fat and a false low-density reading. Additionally, volume averaging of an AML containing macroscopic fat with adjacent normal renal parenchyma can create a false high density reading (Fig. 6.13). Other approaches for identifying small amounts of fat (such as counting individual pixels or pixel distribution) remain controversial and have not been widely accepted.

CT is occasionally performed in symptomatic patients with AMLs. Spontaneous hemorrhage can produce large acute perinephric hematomas or even active extravasation of blood if arterial phase contrast-enhanced images are acquired (Fig. 6.14). In some cases, the perinephric hematoma may be sufficiently large enough to obscure visualization of the bleeding tumor, in which case identification of the AML may require repeat imaging after the hematoma has resolved. For this reason, repeat 4- to 6-week follow-up imaging is recommended in any patient who has spontaneous subcapsular or perinephric hemorrhage if no cause of the hemorrhage can be visualized on the initial imaging study.

MRI can detect fat within an AML, also allowing for a definitive diagnosis to be made. The macroscopic fat in AMLs produces high signal intensity that is seen on both T1- and T2-weighted images. Most characteristic is the loss of signal intensity of components of macroscopic fat on fat-suppressed images (Fig. 6.15C). Chemical shift imaging may also be helpful, as a thin dark line, often termed "India ink" artifact, is usually seen at the interface between AMLs and adjacent renal parenchyma on opposed-phase images, with this line representing signal loss at a fat–fluid interface (Fig. 6.15A,B). While an entire AML may also lose signal on opposed-phase images, this feature is not as helpful for two reasons: (1) some AMLs do not lose signal (since they may contain a great deal of fat, but little fluid, with both of these components required for signal loss), and (2) some clear cell renal cancers can lose signal on these images (due to their containing a great deal of intracellular lipid) (Fig. 6.16).

Although macroscopic fat has occasionally been identified in other renal neoplasms, including renal cancer (often due to osseous metaplasia, in which case calcification is also often present), oncocytomas, Wilms tumor, and metastases, these are all considered to be case reportable exceptions (Fig. 6.17). For this reason, any

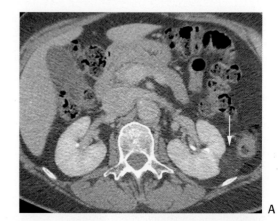

A

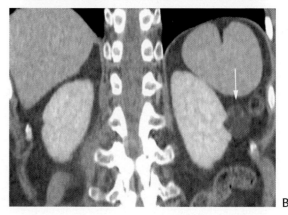

B

FIGURE 6.11. CT images of an AML. Axial **(A)** and coronal **(B)** reformatted contrast-enhanced CT images demonstrate a small mass in the lateral aspect of the left kidney, which is of homogeneous fat attenuation (*arrows*).

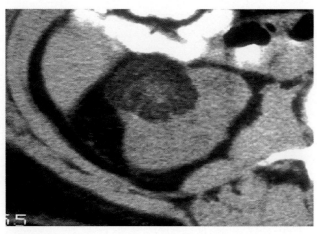

FIGURE 6.10. CT image of an AML. An axial unenhanced CT image shows a large mass in the right kidney, which is almost entirely of fatty attenuation (with most components measuring < −10 HU).

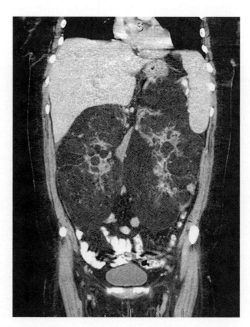

FIGURE 6.12. CT image of multiple AMLs in a patient with tuberous sclerosis. A coronal reformatted contrast-enhanced CT image demonstrates multiple lobulated fatty attenuation masses, which have almost completely replaced normal renal parenchyma.

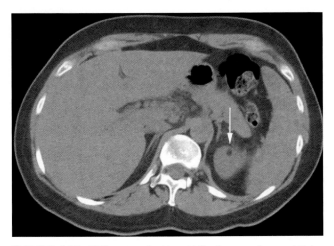

FIGURE 6.13. CT image of a tiny AML. An unenhanced thin-section axial CT image demonstrates a small AML in the upper pole of the left kidney (*arrow*). The macroscopic fat might not have been detected had thicker images been created or if contrast material had been administered.

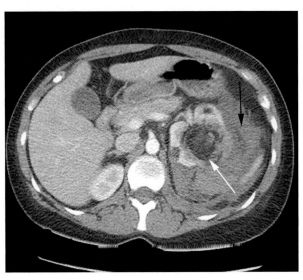

FIGURE 6.14. CT image of a hemorrhagic AML. A contrast-enhanced axial CT image shows a large fatty mass in the posterior aspect of the left kidney (*white arrow*). A large perinephric hematoma is also present (*black arrow*).

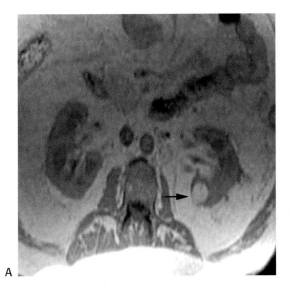

A

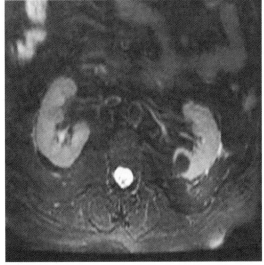

B

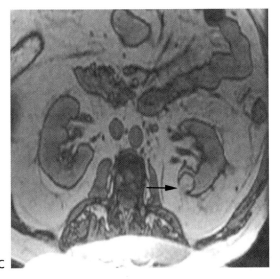

C

FIGURE 6.15. MR images of an AML. **A:** In phase T1-weighted axial image demonstrates a homogeneous hyperintense mass in the posteromedial portion of the mid left kidney (*arrow*). **B:** The mass loses signal on an axial fat-suppressed image, confirming the presence of macroscopic fat and a diagnosis of AML. **C:** The mass remains hyperintense on opposed-phase gradient-echo images (*arrow*), a feature that can be seen in some, but not all AMLs. There is a thin black line or "India ink" arti-fact between the hyperintense mass and the normal renal parenchyma, another feature diagnostic of AML.

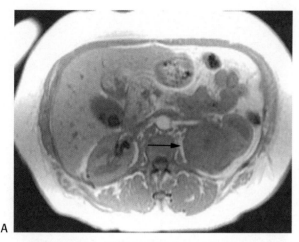
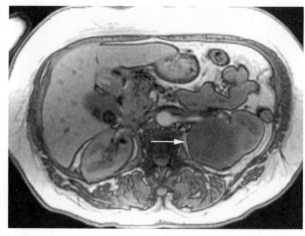

A   B

FIGURE 6.16. MR images of a renal cancer that loses signal on opposed-phase images. **A:** Phase axial MR image shows a solid appearing heterogeneous mass in the left kidney (*arrow*). **B:** The mass loses signal on an opposed-phase image obtained at the same level (*arrow*). This lesion was subsequently diagnosed as a clear cell renal cancer.

mass that contains macroscopic fat on CT or MRI should be considered an AML, unless that mass contains calcification (a feature that can only be detected on CT). Additionally, sometimes, solid renal masses can engulf perinephric or renal sinus fat, creating the impression that the mass itself contains the fat. Only rarely, does this create confusion on CT.

Both lipomas and liposarcomas usually also contain CT-detectable macroscopic fat. These neoplasms can usually be distinguished from AMLs, because the former create smooth impressions on the kidney, while the latter create a defect in the renal contour (indicating the site at which they originated) (Figs. 6.18 and 6.19). Also, AMLs are usually hypervascular lesions, demonstrating large enhancing vessels on contrast-enhanced CT, while lipomas and liposarcomas are hypovascular.

Several variants of AMLs have been described. Up to 5% of all AMLs contain little or no fat. For this reason, the absence of fat

does not exclude the diagnosis of AML. These tumors are referred to as lipid-poor or minimal fat-containing AMLs. On ultrasonography, lipid-poor AMLs are often isoechoic rather than echogenic (Fig. 6.20A). On CT, AML without detectable fat usually appear as homogenous tumors with attenuation higher than normal renal parenchyma (Fig. 6.20B). By definition, these lesions do not contain any identifiable macroscopic fat, as seen on either CT or MRI (Fig. 6.20C). They may demonstrate homogeneous enhancement after the intravenous administration of contrast material (Fig. 6.21). These lesions cannot be distinguished from other nonfat-containing renal masses, including renal cancers.

There are several rare histologic types of AML. Epithelioid AMLs are composed partially or entirely of epithelioid cells having abundant neoplasm. Most of these lesions behave as benign lesions; however, approximately one-third of these AML subtypes have aggressive features. On histology, these lesions contain two

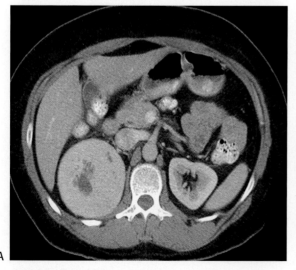
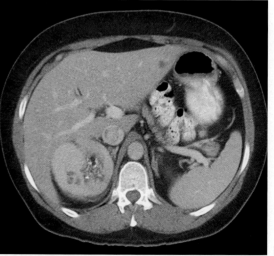

A   B

FIGURE 6.17. Macroscopic fat in a renal cancer. **A:** An axial contrast-enhanced CT image shows a large solid heterogeneous mass in the upper pole of the right kidney. **B:** A more caudally obtained axial image shows a small centrally located area of macroscopic fat, as well as several punctate calcifications. This combination of findings makes renal cancer with osseous metaplasia more likely than AML (since AMLs rarely contain calcification).

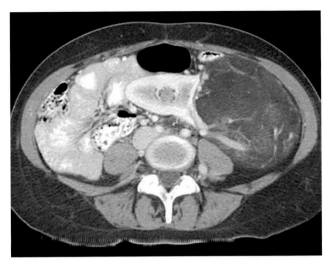

FIGURE 6.18. Large exophytic AML. A contrast-enhanced axial CT image demonstrates a large fatty mass intimately associated with the left kidney. There is a pronounced defect in the lateral aspect of the kidney, indicating the site of origin. The mass also contains several large vessels.

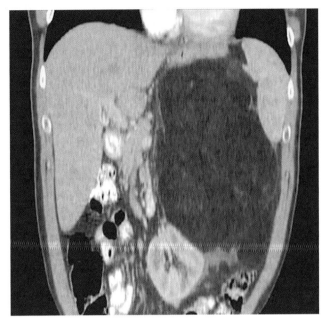

FIGURE 6.19. Large perinephric liposarcoma. A contrast-enhanced coronal reformatted CT image demonstrates a large fatty mass intimately associated with the left kidney. The mass has a smooth impression on the kidney, No renal cortical defect could be identified on this or other images.

or more mitotic figures per high-power field. Although epithelioid AMLs are probably less likely to contain identifiable macroscopic fat on cross-sectional imaging studies (Fig. 6.22), at least some of these tumors do have visible fat (Fig. 6.23), making distinction from other types of AML impossible. Clinically, these tumors can invade the renal veins or inferior vena cava and can even metastasize distantly. Thus, when a fatty mass appears to be behaving aggressively on CT or MRI (extending locally into other organs or growing into

the inferior vena cava), a diagnosis of epithelioid AML should be considered (Fig. 6.24).

Another AML variant is the AML with epithelial cysts (AMLEC). These tumors, which are benign, contain both solid and cystic elements, both of which can be visualized on cross-sectional imaging

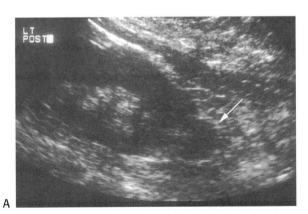

A

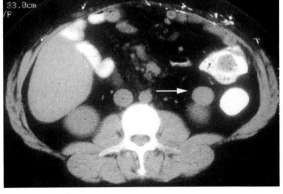

B

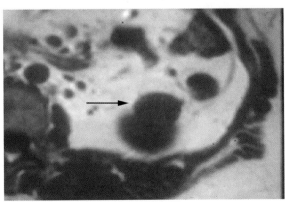

C

FIGURE 6.20. Lipid-poor AML. **A:** A longitudinal ultrasound image shows a small isoechoic exophytic mass in the lower pole of the left kidney (*arrow*). **B:** An unenhanced axial CT image shows the mass to be of soft tissue attenuation (*arrow*). There is no visible macroscopic fat. The mass also has higher attenuation than normal renal parenchyma. **C:** T1-weighted MR image shows the mass to be isointense to the normal renal parenchyma (*arrow*). There is no area of T1 hyperintensity, a feature characteristic of fat.

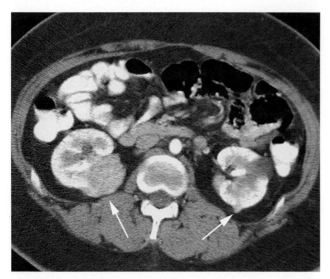

FIGURE 6.21. Lipid-poor AMLs in a patient with tuberous sclerosis. A contrast-enhanced axial CT image shows brisk enhancement of bilateral lipid-poor AMLs (*arrows*).

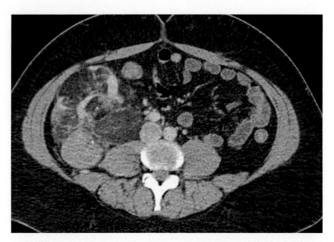

FIGURE 6.23. Epithelioid AML with macroscopic fat. A contrast-enhanced axial CT image demonstrates a large mass involving the lower pole of the right kidney. The mass, which contains both soft tissue and fatty components, is indistinguishable from any other AML.

studies. Macroscopic fat has not been described in these lesions. For this reason, AMLECs can be confused with cystic renal cancers.

Treatment of isolated/solitary AMLs is unnecessary in asymptomatic patients with lesions that measure up to 4 cm in maximal diameter. Partial nephrectomy is recommended by many urologists for AMLs exceeding 4 cm in diameter, due to their increased propensity to bleed. As an alternative, selective arterial embolization may be performed in patients with large tumors, if they are not considered amenable to partial nephrectomy. Should hemorrhage occur, prompt catheter embolization is often effective. Surgical treatment is much more problematic in patients with tuberous sclerosis, when many AMLs may be present. Recently, it has been found that some chemotherapeutic agents can be effective in reducing AML size in such patients. Specifically, mammalian target of rapamycin (mTOR) inhibitors, such as temsirolimus, have been used in this setting. These agents

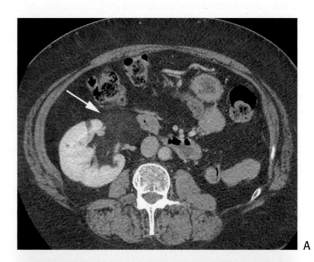

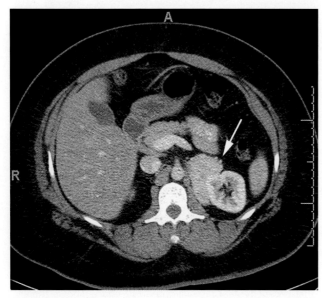

FIGURE 6.22. Epithelioid AML without macroscopic fat. A contrast-enhanced axial CT image demonstrates an exophytic homogeneous solid mass projecting medially from the upper pole of the left kidney (*arrow*).

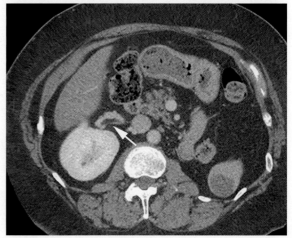

FIGURE 6.24. AML invading the renal vein. **A:** A contrast-enhanced axial CT image shows a relatively homogeneous fat attenuation mass growing exophytically into the renal sinus from the mid right kidney (*arrow*). **B:** An axial CT image obtained slightly more cephalically shows that there is a small amount of fatty attenuation tumor thrombus extending into the right renal vein (*arrow*).

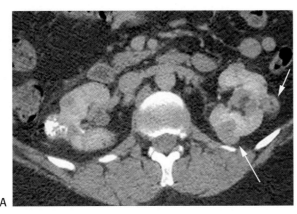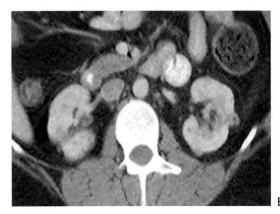

A   B

FIGURE 6.25. Response of AMLs to mTOR inhibitors in a patient with tuberous sclerosis. **A:** A contrast-enhanced axial CT image in a patient with tuberous sclerosis demonstrates multiple bilateral renal masses, all suspected to be AMLs, some containing macroscopic fat and others being lipid poor. This includes the two masses demarcated with *arrows*. The patient was started on the mTOR inhibitor everolimus. There is embolization material in one of the AMLs in the right kidney. **B:** Three months later, many of the AMLs have decreased in size, including the two previously annotated lesions.

have been observed to reduce tumor volumes by 50% or more in nearly half of the treated patients, with response being greatest during the first year of treatment (beginning at about 3 months) (Fig. 6.25). Of course, mTOR inhibitors are not without side effects, which include stomatitis, hyperlipidemia, amenorrhea, and increased susceptibility to infection.

Solid Renal Masses without Macroscopic Fat

Many renal masses do not contain any identifiable fat. Most of these non–fat-containing renal masses represent renal cancers; however, up to 20% of solid renal masses measuring 4 cm or less and nearly 50% of solid renal masses measuring 1 cm or less in size have been found to be benign. The odds that a large renal mass is a cancer are much higher, with nearly 95% of solid renal masses exceeding 7 cm in diameter being malignant.

While there have been a large number of studies attempting to analyze both CT and MRI features of non–fat-containing masses in an effort to identify imaging features, which allow for their differentiation from one another (including noncontrast attenuation or signal intensity, degree of enhancement, rate of enhancement, and pixel distribution on region of interest analysis), overall, these have not been very successful, due to overlap. Occasionally, however, some combinations of features may be suggestive, as will be discussed in the paragraphs that follow.

It should be emphasized that, to date, there is also no proof that differences in renal mass growth rate can be utilized to differentiate malignant from benign renal masses. Several studies have demonstrated that malignant and benign renal masses frequently enlarge at similar rates. Some researchers have recommended that growth of a renal mass should only be considered suspicious when it exceeds 5 mm within a 12 month period of time.

In recent years, there has been a concerted movement toward performance of percutaneous biopsy to determine the nature of small non–fat-containing solid renal masses. Biopsies can be performed safely in the vast majority of patients, with a low complication rate and little risk of significant bleeding or seeding along the tumor tract.

Renal Cancer

Renal cell carcinoma (RCC) is twice as common in men as in women. This tumor may occur at any age, but the incidence peaks in the sixth decade. No specific etiologic agents are recognized, but

there is an as much as 50% increased incidence in patients who use tobacco and an increased incidence in patients with obesity and uncontrolled hypertension. RCC has been increasing worldwide, partly owing to the more frequent detection by imaging, but also to an increase in the prevalence of risk factors. There is also a fourfold increase in the incidence of the disease in first-degree family members of patients with RCCs. This is largely because about 5% to 10% of renal cancers are believed to develop in patients with hereditary renal cancer syndromes, including von Hippel–Lindau (VHL) disease, hereditary papillary renal cancer, hereditary leiomyomatosis renal cancer syndrome, Birt–Hogg–Dube, hereditary succinate dehydrogenase-deficient renal cell cancer, and Lynch syndrome.

Also, patients on chronic hemodialysis or peritoneal dialysis nearly always eventually develop acquired renal cystic disease (see Chapter 8). These patients have an incidence of renal carcinoma of approximately 7%, although not all of these tumors behave in a biologically aggressive manner. Tumors in patients with acquired cystic disease of dialysis begin to appear in patients as early as 3 years after initiation of dialysis. They can be difficult to detect because these patients' kidneys are not functioning and usually contain multiple cysts and dystrophic calcifications. The incidence of renal tumors seems to parallel the development of acquired cystic disease, such that more tumors are seen the longer the patients are maintained on dialysis. The effect of renal transplantation on the development of renal cancer is unclear. Although it is likely that successful transplantation reduces the risk of renal carcinoma, this is counterbalanced by the increased risk of malignancy with immunosuppression.

The classic clinical presentation of renal cancer, of a flank mass, pain, and hematuria occurs in only a minority of patients. As abdominal computed tomography (CT) and ultrasound examinations are commonly performed for a variety of nonrenal indications, the vast majority of renal tumors are now discovered incidentally in patients who are asymptomatic.

Among symptomatic patients, hematuria is the most common sign, occurring in more than 50% of patients. Flank pain, present in more than one-third of patients, is probably caused by distension of the renal capsule. A flank mass is palpable at presentation in approximately one-third of patients with large tumors.

Occasionally, patients with large renal tumors may first complain of nonspecific symptoms such as weight loss, fatigue, or even gastrointestinal or neurologic symptoms. Less common presenting complaints include fever or a new left-sided varicocele (Fig. 6.26). Fatigue may be caused by a normochromic normocytic anemia. A variety of hormones may be secreted by

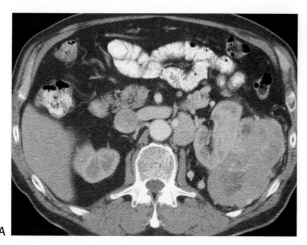
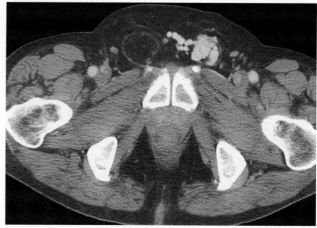

A   B

FIGURE 6.26. Renal cancer presenting as a varicocele. A patient with a large left renal tumor **(A)** presented with a varicocele of the left testes **(B)**.

RCCs in sufficient quantity to cause distinct clinical manifestations, including renin, erythropoietin, parathyroid hormone, adrenocorticotropic hormone, prolactin, and gonadotropin (Table 6.1).

It is difficult to predict the natural history of renal carcinoma. Some tumors demonstrate aggressive behavior by growing rapidly and metastasizing early. However, occasional patients may live for years with an untreated primary tumor. Small tumors, in particular, may show only minimal growth when followed over many years. Metastases generally occur when tumors are larger than 5 cm and are extremely rare when tumors are <3 cm in diameter. Metastases may be present at the time of initial presentation, but have also been reported to first appear as late as 31 years after nephrectomy. Spontaneous regression of metastases or the primary tumor may also occur.

Classification

Although it is now understood that renal cortical neoplasms are a family of differing neoplasms with distinct cytogenetic and molecular defects and differing prognoses and morbidities, assessment of histologic grade is similar for all primary renal cancers. The Fuhrman nuclear grading system is usually used to characterize renal cancer aggressiveness and has been shown to have an excellent correlation with staging and survival. The system ranges from grade 1 (small uniform nuclei) to grade 4 (severe nuclear anaplasia).

In recent years, the number of known distinct histologic types of renal cancers has expanded dramatically, particularly with the advent of genetic sequencing and multiple immunohistochemical stains. The 2016 World Health Organization classification is provided in Table 6.2. By far, the most common renal cancers are of the clear cell type, with these tumors accounting for nearly 70% of renal cancers. About 10% to 15% of renal cancers are then of the papillary type, with most papillary tumors behaving much less aggressively than most clear cell renal cancers. For this reason, in general, the majority of patients with papillary cancers have a better prognosis than do patients with clear cell cancers of similar size. Chromophobe renal cancers are the third most common type, accounting for 5% of renal cancer cases. There are many other rare types of renal cancers, including collecting duct carcinomas and renal medullary carcinoma (both of which behave very aggressively and which have a very poor prognosis), multilocular cystic renal neoplasms of low malignant potential, tubulocystic renal cancers, microphthalmia/TFE (MiT) gene family translocation renal cancers (which includes the Xp11 cancers), and unclassified tumors. As yet more genetic mutations in renal cancers are identified, there will likely be further modifications in the renal cancer histologic classification system.

TABLE **6.1**	
Endocrine Manifestations of Renal Adenocarcinoma	
Hormone	Manifestation
Renin	Hypertension
Erythropoietin	Erythrocytosis
Parathormone	Hypercalcemia
Prolactin	Galactorrhea
Gonadotropin	Gynecomastia
ACTH	Cushing syndrome

TABLE **6.2**
Classification of Renal Tumors
Type
Clear cell (67%)
Papillary (10%–15%)
Chromophobe (<10%)
Collecting duct (<2%)
Renal medullary (very rare)
Multilocular cystic neoplasm of low malignant potential (2%–3%)
MiT family translocation (Xp.11) (<1%)
Succinate dehydrogenase deficient
Mucinous tubular and spindle cell
Tubulocystic
Acquired renal cystic disease associated
Clear cell and papillary
Unclassified
Papillary adenoma
Oncocytoma

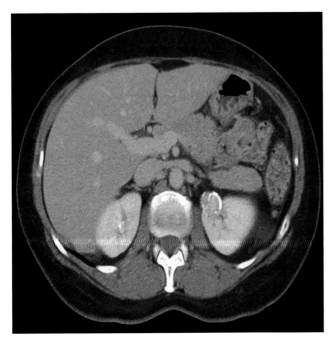

FIGURE 6.27. Solid renal cancer with dystrophic calcification. A contrast-enhanced axial CT image in a patient with a renal cancer demonstrates extensive dystrophic calcification within a minimally heterogeneous solid renal mass. Although some of the calcification is peripheral, some components are quite thick. Also, several calcifications are centrally located.

General Imaging Features of Renal Cancers

Most renal cancers appear as solid enhancing heterogeneous masses (with components measuring between 20 and 70 HU on unenhanced CT). Cystic renal cancers are not uncommon, however. In many instances, the correct diagnosis of a malignant rather than benign cystic renal mass can be suggested, because cystic cancers often demonstrate thickened enhancing walls or enhancing mural nodules. It is likely that there are pathologic mechanisms resulting in the unique cystic RCCs: intrinsic multiloculated growth, intrinsic unilocular growth (cystadenocarcinoma), cystic necrosis, and an origin from the epithelial lining of a pre-existing simple cyst. Three radiologic patterns of cystic RCC have been described: unilocular cystic mass, multiloculated cystic mass, and discrete mural nodule in a cystic mass.

Calcification can be detected on CT in many renal cancers. Calcification is not a specific finding, however, as it may also be seen in other renal masses, including benign cysts. The character of the calcification can be helpful in determining the etiology of a renal mass, however. Thin peripheral curvilinear calcification is more commonly seen in a cyst, whereas central or thick mural calcification means the lesion is more likely a renal carcinoma (Figs. 6.27 to 6.29). If a mass or component of a mass is partially located in the collecting system, the lesion is more likely to represent a urothelial carcinoma that has invaded the renal parenchyma rather than an RCC that invades the collecting system (Fig. 6.30), although in some instances, distinguishing a centrally located renal cancer from a urothelial cancer may be difficult (Fig. 6.31). On MRI, the T1 and T2 features and measured diffusion and contrast-enhanced signal characteristics of renal carcinomas vary with the vascularity of the tumor and the presence or absence of central necrosis, calcification, hemorrhage, and iron deposits, as well as the type of renal tumor that is present.

Perinephric hemorrhage may be the presenting sign of a renal tumor in some renal cancer patients (Fig. 6.32). While AMLs can bleed spontaneously, so can cancers. In fact, the most common

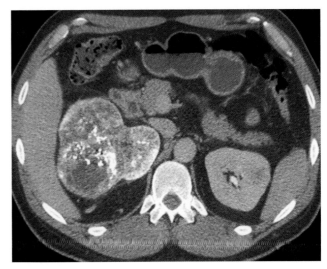

FIGURE 6.28. Solid renal cancer with dystrophic calcification. A contrast-enhanced axial CT image in a patient with a renal cancer demonstrates extensive dystrophic calcification within a large heterogeneous predominantly solid renal mass. Most of the calcification is centrally located.

cause of spontaneous perinephric hemorrhage in patients who are not being anticoagulated is one of these types of renal neoplasms.

CT FEATURES OF RENAL CANCER

- Typically exophytic but may be intrarenal or an infiltrative mass.
- May be hypervascular and heterogeneous (conventional) or homogeneous; poorly enhancing tumors are more likely to be papillary.
- Typically discovered as an incidental finding.
- Best characterized on nephrographic or excretory phase images.

MRI FEATURES OF RENAL CANCER

- Sensitivity similar to CT; but ability to detect enhancement superior to CT.
- Homogeneous tumors may be isointense with parenchyma on T1- and T2-weighted sequences (low T2 signal intensity should suggest papillary type).
- Opposed-phase signal loss should suggest clear cell type.
- May be hypervascular and heterogeneous (conventional) or homogeneous and poorly enhancing (papillary).

Imaging Features of Different Types of Renal Cancer

Clear Cell Renal Cancers

Histologically, clear cell renal cancers have abundant clear cytoplasm with a predominant alveolar architecture. On imaging studies, clear cell cancers are usually solid heterogeneous masses,

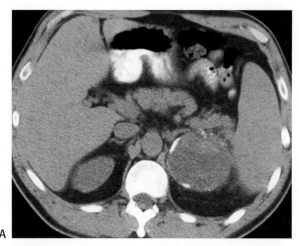
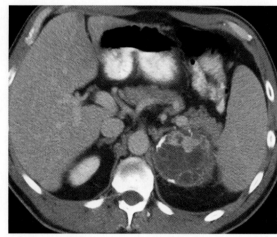

A

B

FIGURE 6.29. Cystic renal cancer with peripheral calcification. Noncontrast **(A)** and nephrographic phase **(B)** images show a cystic mass in the upper pole of the left kidney with thick mural calcification. Multiple enhancing tumor nodules are seen on a contrast-enhanced image.

although they can occasionally be homogeneous. Most clear cell cancers demonstrate brisk enhancement, due to the fact that the majority are very hypervascular. On CT and MRI, clear cell renal cancers tend to show much greater enhancement than other renal tumors on images obtained during the CMP phase (Fig. 6.33). As has been mentioned previously, clear cell renal cancers may demonstrate opposed-phase signal loss on chemical shift MR images, due to the extensive amount of intracellular lipid that is present in most tumors (Fig. 6.16).

Papillary Renal Cancers

On histologic examination, papillary renal cancers typically have a frondlike appearance and contain a central fibrovascular core on histologic examination. Papillary renal cancers often

demonstrate highly suggestive imaging features on CT and MRI. On unenhanced CT, papillary cancers often measure above the attenuation of normal renal parenchyma (a feature also seen with many lipid-poor AMLs). On contrast-enhanced CT or MRI, papillary cancers are often homogeneous. They frequently enhance less and on a more delayed basis than do other renal neoplasms (a feature which allows many of these tumors to be distinguished from briskly and rapidly enhancing lipid-poor AMLs) (Fig. 6.34). Papillary renal cancers do not enhance maximally until the nephrographic or excretory phases. On MRI, papillary cancers often are hypointense on T2-weighted images, a feature

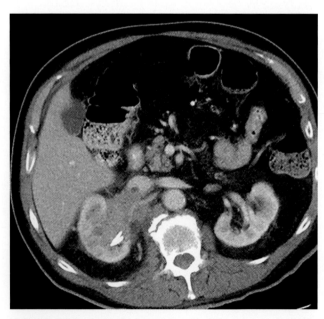

FIGURE 6.30. Centrally located urothelial cancer. A centrally located solid mass in the right renal sinus, seen on this cortico-medullary phase axial CT image, was subsequently confirmed to be a urothelial cancer. The high attenuation focus within the mass represents portion of the tip of a ureteral stent.

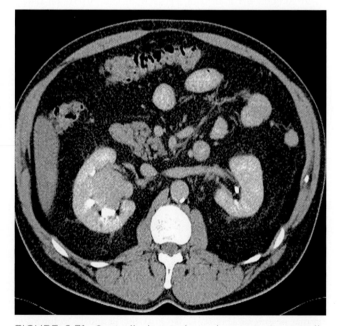

FIGURE 6.31. Centrally located renal cancer. A centrally located solid mass in the right renal sinus, seen on this excretory phase CT image, was subsequently confirmed to be a renal cancer. Differentiation from a urothelial cancer is difficult, although renal cancers can often be seen to displace, but not distort, the renal collecting system. They are also much more likely to invade the renal vein.

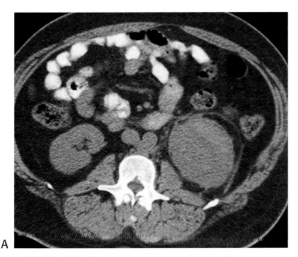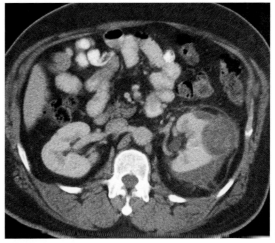

A   B

FIGURE 6.32. Renal cancer presenting with acute hemorrhage. **A:** An axial unenhanced CT image shows high attenuation acute perinephric hemorrhage surrounding the left kidney. **B:** The underlying renal mass is identified on this contrast-enhanced image obtained several centimeters more cephalad.

uncommonly seen in clear cell renal cancers (Figs. 6.35 and 6.36). Some papillary renal cancers can have predominantly cystic features (Fig. 6.37).

Some investigators divide papillary renal cancers into two major subtypes. Type 1 papillary tumors are of low grade (Fuhrman grade 1 or 2) and have a small amount of basophilic to clear cytoplasm. These are slow-growing tumors, which have a better prognosis than do clear cell renal cancers or type 2 papillary renal cancers (Figs. 6.35 and 6.36). Type 2 papillary tumors are higher-grade neoplasms (Fuhrman grade 3 or 4) and contain abundant eosinophilic neoplasm. Patients with type 2 papillary tumors have a much worse prognosis. It is controversial whether or not type 1 and type 2 papillary cancers can be differentiated from one another based upon their imaging appearance; however, a few studies have suggested that tumor heterogeneity, indistinct margins, and T2 heterogeneity are more commonly in MRI

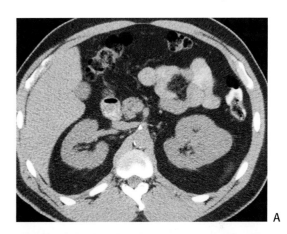

A

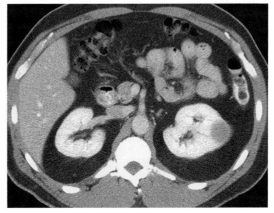

B

FIGURE 6.34. Renal cancer: papillary type. **A:** Unenhanced axial CT image shows an exophytic renal mass with an attenuation of 40 HU. While many papillary cancers have an unenhanced attenuation exceeding that of normal parenchyma, this mass is relatively isoattenuating to normal renal parenchyma. **B:** On the contrast-enhanced axial CT image, the mass is seen to be poorly enhancing. The mass increases to only 60 HU. Because of this low level of enhancement and the homogeneous appearance of the mass, confusion with a mildly hyperdense renal cyst may occur.

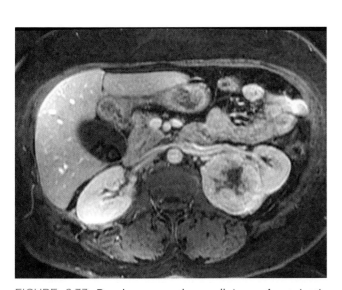

FIGURE 6.33. Renal cancer: clear cell type. A contrast-enhanced axial MR image obtained during the nephrographic phase shows a large briskly enhancing clear cell renal cancer in the posterior aspect of the mid left kidney.

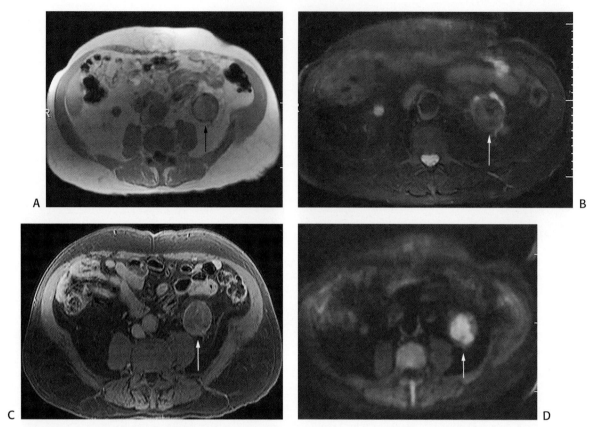

FIGURE 6.35. Renal cancer: papillary type 1. Axial MR images of a type 1 papillary renal cancer show the cancer to be mildly hyperintense on a T1-weighted image (**A**, *arrow*), to be characteristically hypointense on a fat suppressed T2-weighted image (**B**, *arrow*), to be relatively poorly enhancing on a fat suppressed T1-weighted image obtained after gadolinium-based contrast material administration (**C**, *arrow*), and to have restricted diffusion on diffusion-weighted images (**D**, *arrow*).

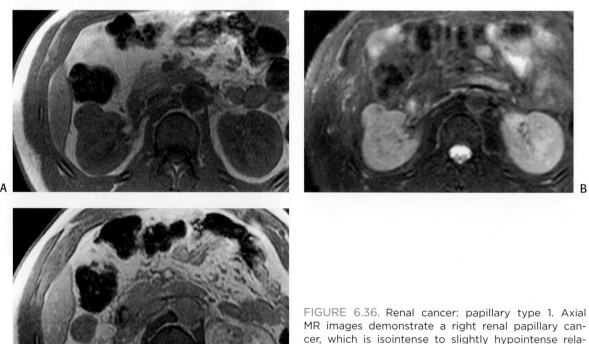

FIGURE 6.36. Renal cancer: papillary type 1. Axial MR images demonstrate a right renal papillary cancer, which is isointense to slightly hypointense relative to the adjacent kidney on T1-weighted **(A)** and fat suppressed T2-weighted **(B)** images and which is homogeneous and hypoenhancing on a T1-weighted nephrographic phase image obtained after contrast material administration **(C)**.

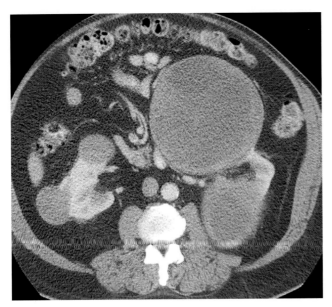

FIGURE 6.37. Renal cancer: cystic papillary type. Axial contrast-enhanced CT image in a patient with multiple cystic papillary cancers demonstrates near water attenuation central components. Most of the lesions have a thick enhancing rim of tissue.

examinations of patients with type 2 tumors than in patients with type 1 tumors (Fig. 6.38).

Unfortunately, up to one-third of papillary renal cancers cannot be classified as belonging to the type 1 or type 2 groups, due to the presence of confusing histologic features, including a more aggressive appearance and higher grade of tumors with otherwise type 1 histology, a less aggressive appearance and lower grade of tumors with otherwise type 2 histology, and/or the presence of clear and papillary cells. This has created some debate about whether this subtyping should be used at all.

Hereditary papillary renal cell carcinoma (HPRCC) is an autosomal dominantly inherited disease in which patients develop multifocal papillary renal cancers, usually classified as type 1 tumors (Fig. 6.39). As with other type 1 papillary renal cancers, HPRCC tumors metastasize less frequently than do clear cell tumors; however, when metastases occur, they may behave aggressively.

Chromophobe Renal Cancers

Chromophobe renal cancers arise from medullary collecting ducts. These tumors, which are the third most common cell type of renal cancer, generally show a much more favorable course than do the other types of renal cancer. Histologically, chromophobe renal cancers are characterized by the presence of large polygonal cells. Birt–Hogg–Dube syndrome is associated with inherited renal neoplasms also characterized by hair follicle hamartomas and frequent pneumothoraces from rupture of thin-walled lung cysts. Patients with this syndrome often develop chromophobe renal tumors or mixed chromophobe tumors and oncocytomas. No distinctive imaging features of chromophobe renal cancers have been identified (Figs. 6.40 and 6.41).

Clear Cell Papillary Renal Cancers

The fourth most common type of renal cancer is now believed to be the mixed clear cell papillary or clear cell tubulopapillary cancer. This cancer, which is generally slow growing and which rarely metastasizes distantly, can occur sporadically, but is often encountered in patients with end-stage renal disease. At the present time, no imaging features have been identified, which allow it to be differentiated from other renal cancers (Fig. 6.42).

Multilocular Cystic Neoplasms of Low Malignant Potential

There are several even more rare types of renal neoplasms. Multilocular cystic neoplasms of low malignant potential are very-low-grade tumors and have not been reported to metastasize. On cross-sectional imaging studies, these tumors tend to appears as complex cystic masses, with many being classified as Bosniak category III or IV lesions. Septal thickening and mural calcification are often present (Fig. 6.43).

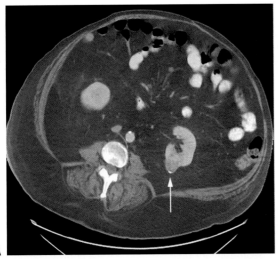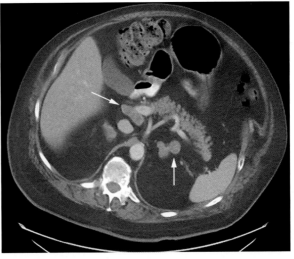

FIGURE 6.38. Renal cancer: papillary type 2. **A:** Axial contrast-enhanced CT images show type 2 papillary cancer projecting exophytically from the posterior aspect of the left kidney (*arrow*). This papillary cancer is heterogeneous and has indistinct margins, features more commonly seen in type 2 tumors. **B:** A CT image obtained several centimeters more cephalad shows both lymph node and left adrenal metastases (*arrows*), which have developed despite the relatively small size of the primary tumor.

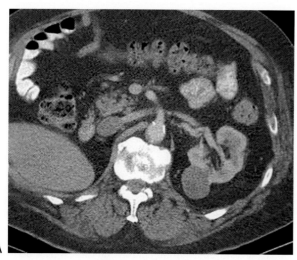
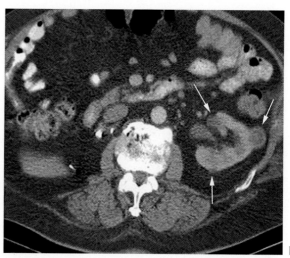

A

B

FIGURE 6.39. Hereditary papillary renal cancer syndrome (HPRCC). **A:** Axial contrast-enhanced CT image shows a large hypoenhancing papillary cancer in the posterior aspect of the left kidney in a patient who has already had a right nephrectomy for a papillary renal cancer. **B:** An image obtained slightly more caudally demonstrates three other papillary cancers (*arrows*) in the same kidney. Patients with HPRCC often present with multiple papillary tumors at the same time.

Renal Medullary Neoplasms

There are also a number of cancers that usually originate in the renal medulla. This includes collecting duct cancers, the microphthalmia (MiT) gene family translocation renal cancers (with one of the variants of these being the XP11.2 translocation cancers), and renal medullary cancer. None of these cancers has a distinctive imaging appearance, other than their usual central and sometimes infiltrative appearance. The differential diagnosis for centrally located renal masses also includes the other more common renal cancer cell types, urothelial cancers, and renal lymphoma. Renal aneurysms may also occasionally mimic centrally located solid renal masses (Fig. 6.44).

Collecting duct cancers frequently occur in older adults (Fig. 6.45), while renal medullary cancers are often encountered in young African American males with sickle cell trait. Collecting duct cancers tend to grow rapidly and patient prognosis is poor. Renal medullary carcinoma is an extremely aggressive tumor. Metastases, especially to regional lymph nodes, are present in most patients at presentation (Fig. 6.46). Treatment is surgical resection, but the mean survival after surgery is dismal. All reported cases have been fatal.

One of the most common MiT gene family translocation cancers is the XP11.2 cancer. This is usually encountered in young patients and, in fact, accounts for about one-third of pediatric renal

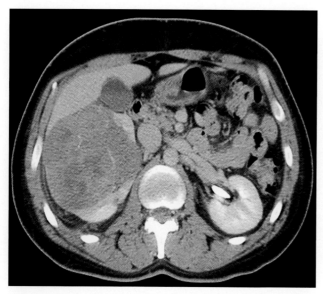

FIGURE 6.40. Renal cancer: chromophobe type. An axial excretory phase image from a contrast-enhanced CT shows a mildly heterogeneous mass in the right kidney. There are no definitive imaging characteristics that permit a specific diagnosis of chromophobe renal cancer to be made.

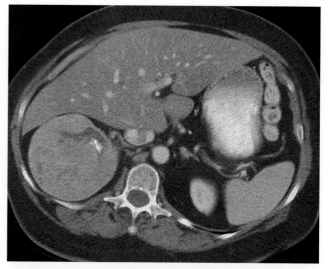

FIGURE 6.41. Renal cancer: chromophobe type. An axial corticomedullary phase image from a contrast-enhanced CT shows a mildly heterogeneous mass in the right kidney with a peripheral rim of enhancement. A small focus of dystrophic calcification is present as well. Again, the imaging features of this cancer overlap with those of many other types of renal cancer.

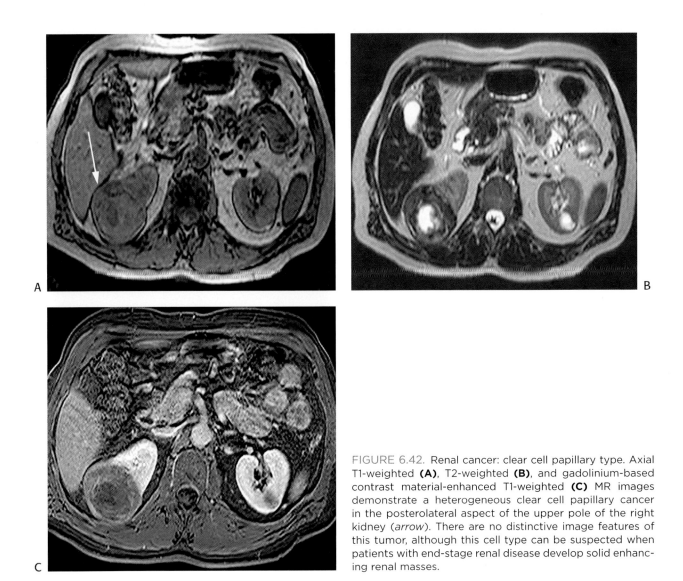

FIGURE 6.42. Renal cancer: clear cell papillary type. Axial T1-weighted **(A)**, T2-weighted **(B)**, and gadolinium-based contrast material-enhanced T1-weighted **(C)** MR images demonstrate a heterogeneous clear cell papillary cancer in the posterolateral aspect of the upper pole of the right kidney (*arrow*). There are no distinctive image features of this tumor, although this cell type can be suspected when patients with end-stage renal disease develop solid enhancing renal masses.

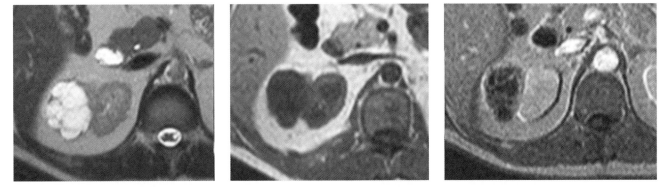

FIGURE 6.43. Renal cancer: multilocular cystic renal cancer. T2-weighted, T1-weighted, and gadolinium-based contrast material-enhanced T1-weighted axial MR images show a multiloculated cystic right renal cancer.

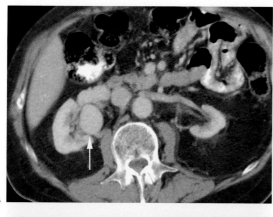

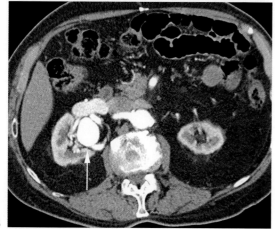

FIGURE 6.44. Renal artery aneurysm. **A:** A nephrographic phase contrast-enhanced axial CT image shows a homogeneously enhancing mass in the right renal sinus (*arrow*). This could be confused with a renal cancer on this image. **B:** The mass enhances even more briskly and similarly to the abdominal aorta on this earlier obtained arterial phase image (*arrow*). The vascular nature of this abnormality would be even more obvious on Doppler ultrasound images or MRI.

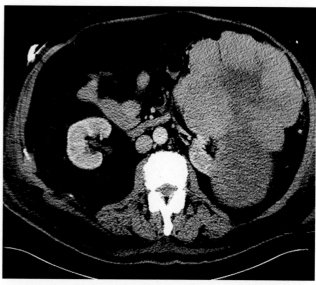

FIGURE 6.45. Renal cancer: collecting duct carcinoma. A contrast-enhanced axial CT image demonstrates a large heterogeneous collecting duct carcinoma in the left kidney.

cancers. In general, these cancers tend to have a medullary location, allowing for the diagnosis to be suspected in some cases. On imaging studies, Xp11.2 translocation tumors are heterogeneous briskly enhancing masses with necrotic or cystic components often involving both the renal cortex and medulla (Fig. 6.47). Unlike typical clear cell renal cancers, these cancers may demonstrate prolonged enhancement. Nevertheless, these imaging features are not distinctive enough to allow for definitive differentiation from clear cell or other types of renal cancer in any given case.

Sarcomatoid Dedifferentiation

Some renal cancers are described pathologically as having sarcomatoid features. Sarcomatoid renal cancers contain characteristic spindle-shaped cells but also include adenomatous and transitional elements. Sarcomatoid renal cancers are more often encountered in elderly patients. They are generally very aggressive and have a poor prognosis. Sarcomatoid features can occur

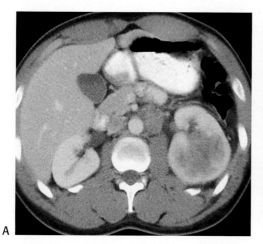

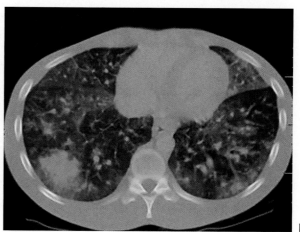

FIGURE 6.46. Renal cancer: renal medullary carcinoma. **A:** A contrast-enhanced axial CT image shows an infiltrative relatively centrally located mass in the mid left kidney. **B:** An axial CT image through the lung bases obtained at the same time shows that there is extensive pulmonary metastatic disease.

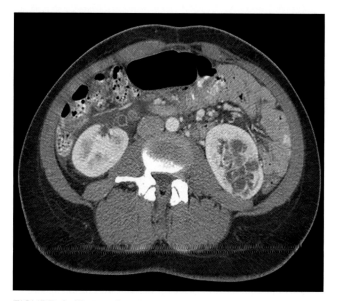

FIGURE 6.47. Renal cancer: Xp11.2 carcinoma. A contrast-enhanced corticomedullary phase image obtained in a young woman shows a heterogeneous mass in the left kidney, which extends from the medulla toward the cortex. The mass has a multiloculated appearance, containing cystic areas and many septations.

in different histologic types of primary renal cancer. They are not a distinct type of renal cancer in and of themselves. They cannot be distinguished from renal cancers that do not have sarcomatoid features on imaging studies (Fig. 6.48).

Multiple Renal Cancers

With the advent of routine cross-sectional imaging to follow patients with renal cancer, the incidence of multiple renal tumors being detected has increased. Multiple renal tumors are found in approximately 5% to 10% of patients with renal neoplasms, either as synchronous or metachronous tumors. Multifocality does not appear to be associated with larger or higher stage tumors.

In some patients, the presence of multiple solid renal masses indicates the presence of one of an increasing number of identified inherited renal cancer syndromes. A partial list of inherited renal cancer syndromes is provided in Table 6.3, with a few of the more common syndromes also mentioned in the paragraphs that follow.

VHL disease is an autosomal dominant disease in which patients can develop renal cysts, pancreatic cysts, and many hypervascular tumors, including cerebellar and spinal hemangioblastomas, retinal angiomas, pancreatic neuroendocrine tumors, and multiple bilateral clear cell renal cancers (Figs. 6.49 and 6.50). The renal cancers in these patients are often of low Fuhrman grade and tend to grow slowly when compared with sporadic clear cell renal cancers. Renal cancers are usually resected when they reach a threshold size of 3 cm. Thermal ablation can be performed as an alternative, but can make subsequent surgery problematic, due to the formation of extensive postprocedural scarring.

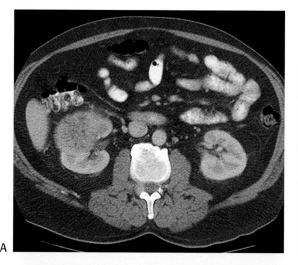

A

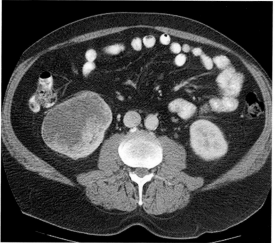

B

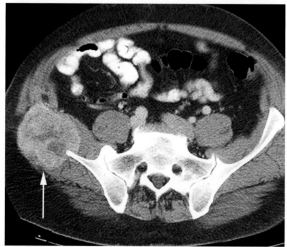

C

FIGURE 6.48. Renal cancer: sarcomatoid dedifferentiation of a clear cell cancer. **A, B:** Two contrast-enhanced corticomedullary phase axial images show a large mass in the right kidney. The mass is largely of low attenuation, due to extensive necrosis. **C:** A CT image obtained several centimeters more caudally demonstrates a large metastasis involving the right iliacus and gluteus musculature (*arrow*).

TABLE **6.3**	
Some Inherited Renal Cancer Syndromes, Type of Cancer, and Percentage of Patients Developing a Renal Cancer	
Von Hippel–Lindau	Clear cell (75%)
Tuberous sclerosis	Clear cell (2%–4%)
Hereditary papillary renal cancer	Type 1 papillary (90%)
Birt–Hogg–Dube	Chromophobe (and onco-cytomas) (10%–34%)
Hereditary leiomyomatosis renal cancer	Type 2 papillary (20%–30%)
Lynch syndrome	Urothelial (3%–5%)

Patients with tuberous sclerosis, which is also inherited in an autosomal dominant fashion, usually develop multiple renal AMLs (Figs. 6.21 and 6.25); however, there is now thought to be a slightly increased incidence of renal cancer in these patients. Renal cancers can be multiple and bilateral and, on imaging studies, are indistinguishable from lipid-poor AMLs (Fig. 6.51).

Hereditary papillary renal cancer is an autosomal dominant disease in which patients develop multiple papillary renal cancers. These tumors are usually low grade and are classified as type 1 papillary tumors (see Fig. 6.39).

Birt–Hogg–Dube syndrome is an autosomal dominant disease in which patients develop many skin lesions (fibrofolliculomas), pulmonary cysts with spontaneous pneumothorax, and renal neoplasms. The renal tumors tend to consist of chromophobe renal cancers and oncocytomas; however, clear cell and papillary renal cancers have also been encountered (Fig. 6.52).

Hereditary leiomyomatosis renal cancer syndrome is an autosomal disease in which patients develop skin and uterine leiomyomas, as well as papillary renal cancers. The renal cancers are often solitary rather than multiple. They may have a characteristic "papillary" appearance (with diminished enhancement on contrast-enhanced CT and MR images), but these are usually of high grade (classified by many pathologists as type 2 papillary cancers) and are considered to be very aggressive tumors, in spite of their indolent appearance (Fig. 6.53).

Lynch syndrome is another autosomal dominant disease in which patients develop colorectal and endometrial cancers, upper

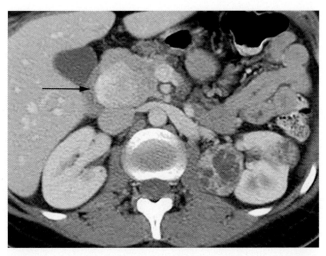

FIGURE 6.50. von Hippel–Lindau disease. Contrast-enhanced corticomedullary phase axial CT image in a patient with von Hippel Lindau disease shows two complex heterogeneous cancers in the left kidney, as well as a large hyperenhancing pancreatic neuroendocrine tumor (*arrow*).

tract urothelial neoplasms (which is the third most common malignancy in these patients), as well as malignancies at other sites.

Oncocytomas

Oncocytomas comprise approximately 5% of renal tumors. Oncocytomas most often are detected as an incidental finding. Occasionally, patients may complain of a flank mass, pain, or hematuria. The gross appearance of an oncocytoma is a well-defined tan to brown tumor. While some oncocytomas do not show necrosis or hemorrhage, they often contain a prominent central stellate scar, which can be seen on imaging studies. In contrast, renal carcinomas are orange-yellow and often have areas of hemorrhage and tumor necrosis. Unfortunately, on imaging studies, the central necrosis seen in renal cancers can have a similar appearance to that of central scars seen in oncocytomas. Although there are isolated reported cases of involvement of regional lymph nodes and tumor extension into the renal vein, the vast majority of oncocytomas behave in an indolent fashion and are considered to be benign.

On unenhanced CT, oncocytomas usually have similar attenuation to adjacent renal parenchyma, as do many renal cancers. On unenhanced MRI, oncocytomas may demonstrate low signal intensity on T1-weighted images, which may differ from the intermediate to high signal intensity often seen in RCCs (Fig. 6.54). On T2-weighted images, oncocytomas show high signal intensity, as is the case for many types of renal cancer (Fig. 6.54). Oncocytomas also demonstrate restricted diffusion on diffusion-weighted images, with considerable overlap in apparent diffusion coefficient values with those obtained many from renal cancers.

As with other hypervascular renal neoplasms, such as clear cell renal cancers, oncocytomas demonstrate at least some areas of brisk enhancement after administration of iodinated (for CT) (Figs. 6.55 and 6.56) or gadolinium-based (for MRI) contrast agents (Figs. 6.57 and 6.58). In one study, oncocytomas demonstrated less mean enhancement on CMP images than did many renal cancers; however, unfortunately, there was overlap with clear cell renal cancers. In another study, only oncocytomas demonstrated >50% washout on delayed phase images. In yet another review, oncocytomas more often demonstrated homogeneous enhancement and more pronounced enhancement during

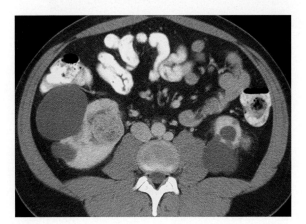

FIGURE 6.49. von Hippel–Lindau disease. Contrast-enhanced nephrographic phase axial CT image in a patient with von Hippel Lindau disease shows bilateral renal cysts and solid tumors.

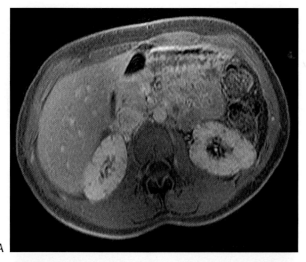

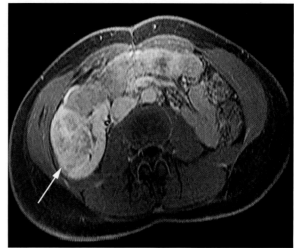

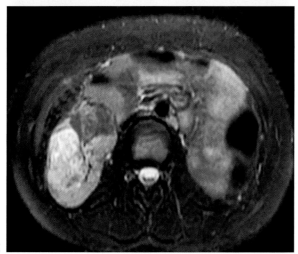

FIGURE 6.51. Tuberous sclerosis with renal cancer. **A:** Gadolinium-based contrast material-enhanced fat-suppressed axial T1-weighted MR image shows multiple tiny low signal intensity lesions scattered throughout both kidneys, corresponding to many tiny angiomyolipomas. **B:** A contrast-enhanced T1-weighted fat-suppressed axial image obtained several centimeters more caudally shows two large masses in the right kidney. A large hyperintense mass in the posterior portion of the right kidney (*arrow*) was subsequently confirmed to represent a renal cancer. This cannot be distinguished from a lipid-poor AML. A slightly more anteriorly located mass is not as briskly enhancing. This is a lipid-poor AML. **C:** An unenhanced T2-weighted fat-suppressed axial image at the same level demonstrates that the renal cancer is much more hyperintense than the adjacent AML.

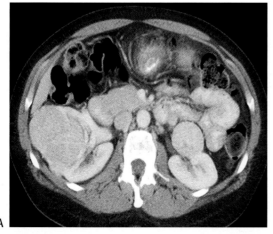

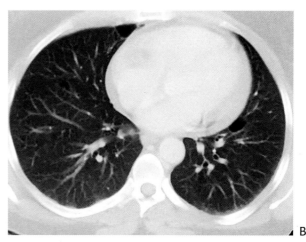

FIGURE 6.52. Birt–Hogg–Dube syndrome. **A:** Contrast-enhanced corticomedullary phase axial CT image shows bilateral solid renal masses, representing a combination of oncocytomas and chromophobe renal cancers. **B:** An axial image through the lung bases demonstrates several small bilateral lung cysts. These can rupture spontaneously in some patients and result in pneumothorax.

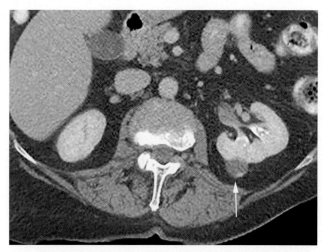

FIGURE 6.53. Hereditary leiomyomatosis renal cell carcinoma syndrome. A contrast-enhanced corticomedullary phase axial CT image in a patient with a history of fibroids shows a single primarily hypoenhancing solid attenuation mass in the posterior aspect of the mid left kidney (*arrow*). This was subsequently confirmed to be a papillary renal cancer. Despite the indolent appearance of the papillary cancers in these patients, they can behave very aggressively.

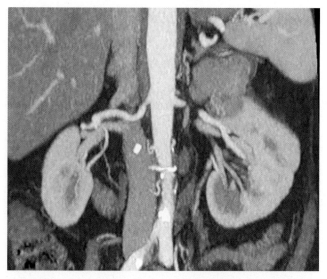

FIGURE 6.55. Oncocytoma. A contrast-enhanced corticomedullary phase coronal CT image shows a homogeneous oncocytoma in the upper pole of the left kidney. The oncocytoma has a distinct, well-defined interface with the renal parenchyma. It does not have a visible central scar.

the NP than did renal cancers, but, again, there was overlap. On contrast-enhanced CT and MRI, oncocytomas usually have a well-defined appearance and have a relatively sharp interface with the normal renal parenchyma (Fig. 6.55). The central stellate scar, if present, can often be seen (Figs. 6.56 and 6.58), but, as already mentioned, the appearance is not pathognomonic for an oncocytoma because it can have a similar appearance to the central necrosis seen in many renal cancers.

One recently described imaging feature that may occasionally be useful in differentiating oncocytomas from renal cancers is segmental enhancement inversion. In segmental enhancement inversion, two differently enhancing components are identified on CMP images, with the initially more brightly enhancing component becoming lower in attenuation on delayed enhanced images.

In comparison, an initially hypoenhancing component increases in attenuation on delayed enhanced images, such that its attenuation then exceeds that of the initially more brightly enhancing component. Thus, the hyperenhancing and hypoenhancing components demonstrate inversion of their enhancement characteristics when delayed enhanced images are compared to early enhanced images. Unfortunately, segmental enhancement inversion has been found inconsistently in oncocytomas, in at least some series, suggesting that this can be used as a suggestive feature in only some patients with oncocytomas.

Some researchers have recommended that several combinations of imaging features can be used to predict whether a solid renal mass is more likely to represent an oncocytoma or a renal cancer with a high degree of accuracy. In one series, for example, a mass that was over 4 cm in size and homogeneously enhancing and that

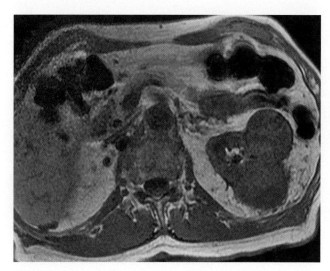

FIGURE 6.54. Oncocytoma. Unenhanced axial T1-weighted image shows two left heterogeneous enhancing renal masses, which have relatively low signal intensity.

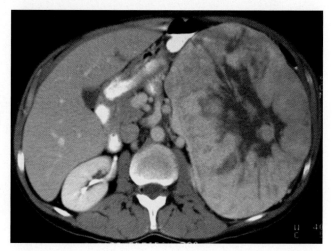

FIGURE 6.56. Oncocytoma. A contrast-enhanced excretory phase axial CT image shows a huge left renal oncocytoma. As is seen in many larger oncocytomas, this mass has a prominent central scar.

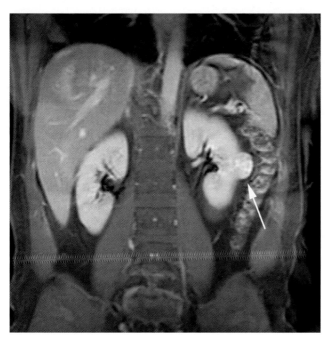

FIGURE 6.57. Oncocytoma. A contrast-enhanced nephrographic phase T1-weighted fat-suppressed coronal MR image shows a small exophytic oncocytoma projecting from the lateral aspect of the mid left kidney (*arrow*). The mass, which does not contain a central scar, enhances briskly and homogeneously.

demonstrated EP enhancement of 30 HU had a 99% probability of being malignant. Unfortunately, some of these combination models are complex, and it is questionable whether they will ever be widely adopted for clinical practice.

At the present time, it is believed that an oncocytoma cannot be consistently and reliably differentiated from a renal cancer. Thus, at many centers, biopsy is performed for further renal mass assessment. While, in the past, it has generally been believed that percutaneous biopsy could not be used to differentiate oncocytomas from renal cancer (due to the tendency for some renal cancers to contain

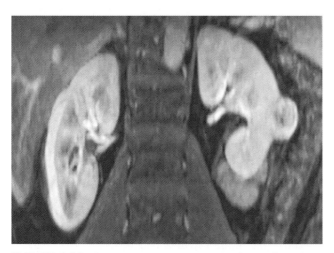

FIGURE 6.58. Oncocytoma. A contrast-enhanced nephrographic phase T1-weighted fat-suppressed coronal MR image shows a small exophytic oncocytoma projecting exophytically from the lateral aspect of the mid left kidney. This briskly enhancing mass contains a small central scar.

oncocytes), this is no longer felt to be the case in most instances. With newer immunologic stains, differentiation is frequently possible. It is still unclear, however, how a diagnosed oncocytoma should be treated. In the past, all such lesions were removed surgically or ablated (given the fact that differentiation from renal cancer could not be made prior to surgery). Currently, it is recommended that if a nonsurgical approach is to be considered (of a mass diagnosed as an oncocytoma by biopsy), the lesion should be followed by obtaining serial imaging studies, since it is not completely clear what the natural history of oncocytoma is (e.g., whether some might progress to oncocytic renal cancers).

Lipid-Poor Angiomyolipoma

As previously mentioned, up to 5% of AMLs may not contain enough lipid to permit diagnosis of AML to be made on cross-sectional imaging studies. In these cases, differentiation from renal cancer or oncocytoma may not be possible. While imaging features may be suggestive (such as attenuation exceeding that of normal renal parenchyma on unenhanced CT images), there is overlap with renal cancers (Figs. 6.20 and 6.21). Percutaneous biopsy may be helpful.

Staging and Nephrometry in Patients with Known or Suspected Renal Cancer

Staging

In the present day, the TNM staging system described by the American Joint Committee for Cancer Staging is utilized for staging of renal cancer (Table 6.4). This system has been found to correlate closely with patient outcomes and accurately allows comparison of data across different institutions.

CT and MRI are highly reliable in staging renal cancers, with overall accuracies exceeding 90% in some series. These modalities can correctly determine tumor size and can assess the renal veins, inferior vena cava, and adjacent organs for invasion (Fig. 6.59). They can detect enlarged involved regional lymph nodes and

TABLE 6.4	
Renal Carcinoma Staging	
2010 TNM Classification	
TX	**Primary tumor cannot be assessed**
T1	**Tumor ≤7 cm confined to kidney**
T1a	<4 cm
T1b	4–7 cm
T2	**Tumor >7 cm confined to kidney**
T2a	Tumor >7 cm but <10 cm confined to kidney
T2b	Tumor >10 cm limited to the kidney
T3	**Tumor extends into major veins or perinephric space but not ipsilateral adrenal**
T3a	Renal vein, perinephric of renal sinus but confined to Gerota fascia
T3b	Tumors extend to IVC below diaphragm
T3c	IVC above diaphragm
T4	**Extension into neighboring organs outside Gerota fascia or ipsilateral adrenal**
N0	**No nodal involvement**
N1	**Metastasis to a single regional node**
N2	**More than one node involved**
Mx	**Metastases cannot be assessed**
M0	**No distant metastasis**
M1	**Distant metastasis**

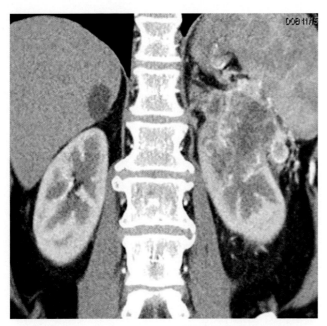

FIGURE 6.59. T4 renal cancer. A contrast-enhanced corti-comedullary phase CT image shows a large infiltrative renal cancer in the upper pole of the left kidney. The mass can be seen to be directly invading the left adrenal gland, a finding which is diagnostic of T4 disease.

distant metastases. Identification and precise delineation of venous extension is essential to plan the surgical approach and to gain vascular control of the kidney (Fig. 6.60). Both CT and MR may demonstrate blood flow within tumor venous thrombus and thus distinguish tumor from bland thrombus.

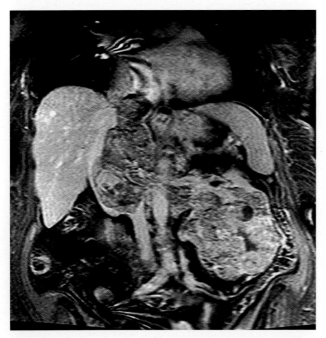

FIGURE 6.60. Stage T3c renal cancer. A contrast-enhanced T1-weighted fat-suppressed coronal MR image in a patient with a large left renal cancer demonstrates a large amount of heterogeneous tumor thrombus growing through the left renal vein and into the inferior vena cava to the level of the right atrium, findings diagnostic of stage T3c disease.

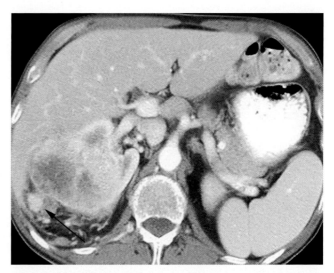

FIGURE 6.61 Stage T3b renal cancer. A contrast-enhanced corticomedullary phase axial CT image in a patient with a large right renal cancer shows an enhancing nodule in the right perinephric space (*arrow*). The presence of nodular masses such as these is strongly predictive of capsular invasion.

CT and MRI are most limited in their ability to evaluate the perinephric space for tumor infiltration through the renal capsule (T3a disease). False-positive and false-negative results can be encountered here. Increased linear soft tissue in the perinephric space can represent edematous changes, collateral vessels, or tumor strands. For this reason, it is suggested that renal capsular invasion should only be suggested when enhancing nodules are visualized in the perinephric fat (Fig. 6.61). Conversely, microscopic tumor invasion through the renal capsule may not produce any CT- or MRI-detectable abnormality (Fig. 6.62).

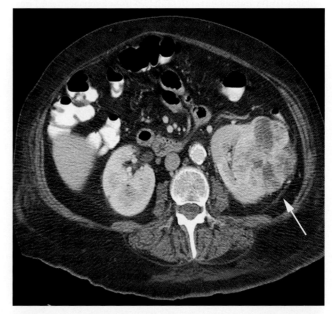

FIGURE 6.62. Stage T3b renal cancer. A contrast-enhanced corticomedullary phase axial CT image in a patient with a large left renal cancer shows soft tissue attenuation strands in the left perinephric space (*arrow*). This is a nonspecific finding and can indicate either tumor spread or merely perinephric edema or perinephric vessels.

RENAL Nephrometry

RENAL nephrometry is a system that is now employed by many urologists and radiologists to predict how amenable a renal mass would be to partial rather than radical nephrectomy and how likely it is that complications might be encountered should partial nephrectomy be performed. Some investigators have suggested that nephrometry can also be used to evaluate the likelihood of an effective and complication-free response to thermal ablation. As a result, at many institutions, patients with known or suspected renal cancers undergo both staging and RENAL nephrometry assessment of detected renal masses. The most commonly recommended nephrometry scoring system is listed in Table 6.5. In summary, the system evaluates six features of a renal mass, including its size, exophyticity (or approximately how much of the mass bulges away from the renal contour), nearness to the collecting system, anterior or posterior location, location with respect to the renal poles, and proximity to the renal arteries and veins. Masses are assigned higher scores when they are felt to be more problematic. Once the RENAL nephrometry score is determined, patients can be sorted into three groups. Those with nephrometry scores of 4 to 6 are felt to have favorable prognoses with respect to partial nephrectomy outcomes and those with scores of 7 to 9 to have moderately favorable prognoses. Masses with scores of 10 to 12 are felt to be unfavorable candidates for partial nephrectomy and will often require total or radical nephrectomy.

Treatment of Renal Cancer

The majority of patients with T1 renal cancers are treated with partial nephrectomy, a procedure generically known as *nephron-sparing surgery*. When the tumor is <4 cm in diameter, nephron-sparing surgery results in an outcome equivalent to treatment with radical nephrectomy. However, nephron-sparing surgery is technically more difficult than radical nephrectomy and can leave tumor behind in the occasional instances when the renal carcinoma is multifocal. Nephron-sparing surgery has been shown to offer similar, and in some cases improved, disease-free survival, a lower incidence of subsequent metastatic disease development, and with local recurrence of tumor being quite rare. Also, the incidence of progression to renal insufficiency is lower after partial nephrectomy, and there is a lower incidence of hypertension and proteinuria. Partial nephrectomy is now most often performed laparoscopically. Laparoscopic partial nephrectomy is associated with less patient perioperative morbidity and shorter hospital stays than is open partial nephrectomy.

Patients with larger tumors that encroach upon the renal sinus or renal collecting systems (with high RENAL nephrometry scores) are usually treated with total nephrectomy. In these procedures, the kidney is removed in entirety; however, the perinephric fascia is entered at the time of surgery, allowing for preservation of the ipsilateral adrenal gland.

Radical nephrectomy, which consists of complete surgical resection of the affected kidney, including the adrenal gland along with the entire perinephric space using a transabdominal approach that allows for early control of the renal pedicle, is no longer commonly performed. This procedure is now usually reserved only for very large tumors or tumors that have invaded the perinephric space, renal vein, and/or inferior vena cava. Indeed, tumor thrombus in the IVC can often be resected successfully, even when it extends cephalically to the level of the heart. This is because vascular tumor thrombus is usually well encapsulated and is not attached to the vessel wall. During radical nephrectomy, regional lymph nodes, para-aortic for left-sided tumors and paracaval for tumors of the right kidney, are also frequently resected.

On some occasions, patients with metastatic disease may be treated with nephrectomy. This may be done as palliation or to prevent complications such as hematuria, pain, or even congestive heart failure due to large arteriovenous fistulae. This procedure, termed *cytoreductive nephrectomy*, may offer an increase in survival in selected patients who present with metastatic disease, when compared with chemotherapy alone.

Occasionally, when renal cancers are very large, angiographic embolization may also have an ancillary therapeutic role. Presurgical embolization of a large hypervascular renal cancer dramatically reduces the vascularity of the tumor, thereby making resection easier (resulting in decreased surgical blood loss). Arterial embolization can also be used to treat complications from tumors in patients who are not surgical candidates. Hematuria can often be stopped with embolization.

As an alternative to partial nephrectomy, patients with T1a and, sometimes, T1b tumors may be offered thermal ablative therapy, (radiofrequency ablation (RFA) or cryoablation). Thermal ablation is usually performed percutaneously, thereby saving the patient from open surgery. In this procedure, the tumor cells are destroyed by either heating or cooling them sufficiently to cause tumor necrosis. While the zone of necrosis during RF ablation cannot be identified on imaging studies, during cryotherapy, the developing "ice ball" in the region of necrosis can be readily imaged with ultrasonography.

Given the many treatment alternatives that are now available, the choice of renal cancer treatment usually depends upon the patient's general condition, as well as upon the preoperative imaging characteristics of the cancer (as can be determined by the RENAL nephrometry score). Due to its less invasive nature, thermal ablation may be chosen preferentially in debilitated patients, who are more likely to have substantial morbidity from a surgical procedure.

TABLE 6.5

RENAL Nephrometry Scoring System

	1 point	2 points	3 points
Renal size	<4 cm	4–7 cm	> 7 cm
Exophyticity	≥50% exophytic	<50% exophytic	Endophytic
Nearness to collecting system	≥7 mm from	4–7 mm from	<4 mm from
Anterior or posterior	No points: assigned a letter: "a" for anterior, "p" for posterior, and "x" for neither		
Location with respect to renal sinus	Completely above or below the polar line (as best seen on coronal images)	Crosses polar line	More than 50% across polar line; or entirely between polar lines; or crosses midline or kidney

Also: Add "h" if touches renal artery or vein.

Avoidance of surgery with active surveillance of small renal masses (measuring <4 cm) is being performed more frequently, particularly in elderly patients who have shorter life expectancies, even when those detected solid renal masses are confirmed to be cancers by biopsy. This is because of the slow growth rate of most small renal cancers and the fact that the vast majority of small renal cancers (under 4 cm in maximal diameter) are unlikely to have metastasized. It is estimated that <5% of small tumors will have metastasized. Therefore, many older patients with small renal cancers are more likely to die with their cancers rather than of their cancers. They will die of other diseases before their cancer has spread.

As a result of the above observations, at some institutions, all small solid renal masses are now being biopsied, with active surveillance performed on renal cancers that have favorable histology (such as being low-grade [Fuhrman grade 1 or 2] papillary cancers or even low-grade clear cell or chromophobe renal cancers), especially in patients who are elderly or who have other comorbidity. Active surveillance of small renal cancers can be performed every 6 months for a year and then annually. Treatment would only be performed if the mass begins to grow rapidly (>5 mm in a 12-month time period) or exceeds a set maximal diameter in size (with 4 cm being the threshold at some centers).

Imaging after Partial or Total Nephrectomy

Following partial or total nephrectomy, 85% of renal cancer recurrences present within the first 3 years of surgery, with the risk of recurrence strongly correlated with the stage at presentation. The nuclear grade of the tumor (Fuhrman classification) is also strongly

associated with survival (Table 6.6). Interestingly, late renal cancer recurrences are also a known phenomenon, with metastases first appearing in some patients as long as 10 years after initial surgery. Recurrences may, obviously, be local, regional, or distant.

Both CT and MRI are used to evaluate patients for locally recurrent or metastatic disease or suspected complications after partial or total nephrectomy. The intervals at which follow-up imaging should be performed are not well defined; however, based upon the above-described observations, it has been recommended that asymptomatic patients be followed with chest radiography every 6 to 12 months and abdominal CT every 6 to 12 months for the first 2 to 3 years and then yearly for a total of at least 4 to 5 years. One possible follow-up scheme is presented in Table 6.7.

Normal postoperative changes after partial nephrectomy usually consist of a renal parenchymal defect and adjacent inflammatory soft tissue, which gradually decreases over time (Fig. 6.63). Tiny high attenuation foci at the resection site, representing suture material or mesh, are often identified. Hemostatic material is

TABLE 6.6

Five-Year Survival by Grade

Nuclear Grade	5-Year Survival (%)
1	89
2	65
3 or 4	46

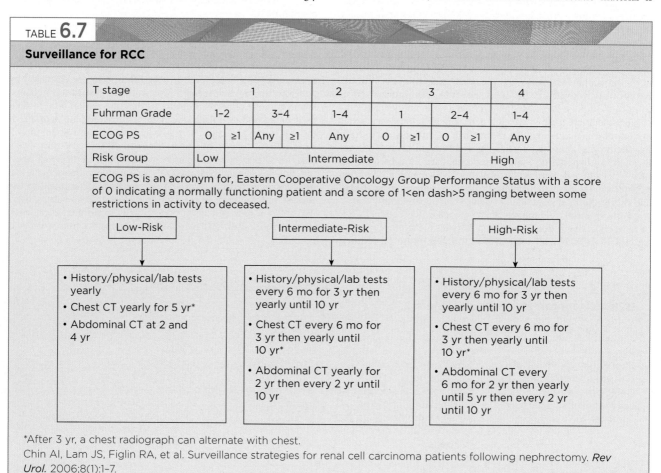

TABLE 6.7

Surveillance for RCC

T stage	1		2	3		4
Fuhrman Grade	1-2	3-4	1-4	1	2-4	1-4
ECOG PS	0	≥1 / Any / ≥1	Any	0 / ≥1	0 / ≥1	Any
Risk Group	Low	Intermediate			High	

ECOG PS is an acronym for, Eastern Cooperative Oncology Group Performance Status with a score of 0 indicating a normally functioning patient and a score of 1<en dash>5 ranging between some restrictions in activity to deceased.

Low-Risk
- History/physical/lab tests yearly
- Chest CT yearly for 5 yr*
- Abdominal CT at 2 and 4 yr

Intermediate-Risk
- History/physical/lab tests every 6 mo for 3 yr then yearly until 10 yr
- Chest CT every 6 mo for 3 yr then yearly until 10 yr*
- Abdominal CT yearly for 2 yr then every 2 yr until 10 yr

High-Risk
- History/physical/lab tests every 6 mo for 3 yr then yearly until 10 yr
- Chest CT every 6 mo for 3 yr then yearly until 10 yr*
- Abdominal CT every 6 mo for 2 yr then yearly until 5 yr then every 2 yr until 10 yr

*After 3 yr, a chest radiograph can alternate with chest.
Chin AI, Lam JS, Figlin RA, et al. Surveillance strategies for renal cell carcinoma patients following nephrectomy. *Rev Urol.* 2006;8(1):1-7.

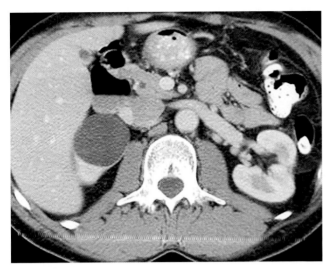

FIGURE 6.63. Imaging after partial nephrectomy. A contrast-enhanced corticomedullary phase axial CT image demonstrates a focal parenchymal defect in the lateral aspect of the left kidney. This is often associated with adjacent perinephric soft tissue attenuation fibrotic strands.

frequently utilized after partial nephrectomy and may appear as either small soft tissue masses or fluid collections, often containing gas (Figs. 6.64 and 6.65). The air can be present for long periods of time after surgery, leading to it being misdiagnosed as gas produced as a result of infection. The soft tissue components can take months to resorb and can be mistaken for recurrent tumor. Another occasionally reported complication following partial nephrectomy is the development of a fat–fluid level in the patient's urinary bladder, seen on CT as the result of the presence of asymptomatic chyluria (Fig. 6.66).

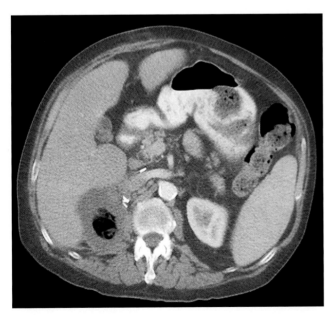

FIGURE 6.64. Hemostatic material following partial nephrectomy. A contrast-enhanced corticomedially phase axial CT image shows a collection of gas in a right-sided partial nephrectomy bed. This gas, which resides within surgically inserted hemostatic material, may remain visible for months after surgery and be misdiagnosed as indicating infection.

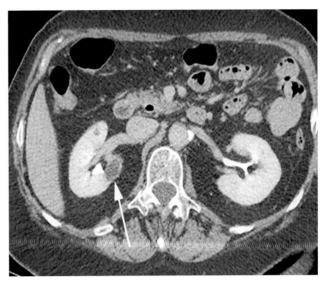

FIGURE 6.65. Hemostatic material following partial nephrectomy. A contrast-enhanced excretory phase axial CT image shows a small fluid attenuation collection in the posterior aspect of the mid right kidney, which corresponds to hemostatic material in a partial nephrectomy bed.

After total or radical nephrectomy, postoperative material may be identified in the renal fossa. Soft tissue stranding may be seen, which will, again, gradually decrease over time. Hemostatic material is less frequently utilized. Imaging studies can occasionally detect postoperative complications following surgery, such as pseudoaneurysms or renal collecting system leaks (Fig. 6.67).

After partial nephrectomy, renal cancer may recur in the surgical bed or regionally or distantly. Recurrences at the resection site may be difficult to detect early on, as they can be misidentified as postoperative scarring (Fig. 6.68). Of course, locally recurrent disease will be seen to increase in size on subsequent CTs, while

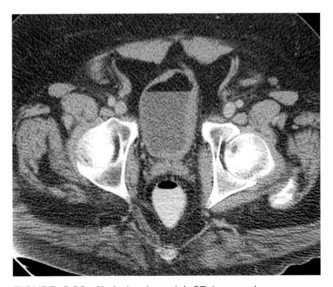

FIGURE 6.66. Chyluria. An axial CT image shows a nondependently located area of fat attenuation in the bladder, corresponding to layering lymphatic material. This finding, which is not clinically significant, can be seen in patients following partial nephrectomy and thermal ablation.

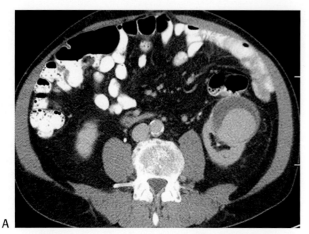

A

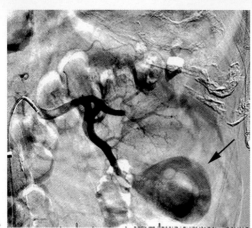

B

FIGURE 6.67. Pseudoaneurysm after partial nephrectomy. **A:** A contrast-enhanced excretory phase axial CT image obtained in a patient 6 months after left partial nephrectomy for renal cancer shows a large mass in the left kidney, which contains a central area that enhances similarly to the abdominal aorta. **B:** A subsequent selective renal arteriogram confirms that this represents a large pseudoaneurysm (*arrow*). This was successfully embolized.

postoperative changes generally decrease. It is also important to remember that, after laparoscopy, patients can also develop tumor implants by spread along the port sites, as well as along the mesentery and peritoneum (Fig. 6.69).

RCC metastasizes distantly via lymphatic spread as well as hematogenously. Renal cancer can spread via lymphatics into retroperitoneal lymph nodes and then travel into the thoracic duct. Hematogenous spread occurs via the renal vein, into the IVC and then throughout the body. The most frequent sites of distant metastases are (in decreasing order of frequency) the lung, bone, nephrectomy site, brain, liver, mediastinal lymph nodes, and contralateral kidney. Patients with only lung metastases have a better overall survival than do patients with multiorgan involvement. Metastasis to almost any other organ, including skeletal muscle, can occur.

Interestingly, renal cancer has an unusual proclivity to metastasize to the pancreas. It is the most common tumor to spread to this organ. Typically, pancreatic metastases are well-defined single or multiple hypervascular masses found anywhere in the pancreas (Fig. 6.70). Given its frequently hypervascular nature, renal cancer metastases to the pancreas can be confused with pancreatic neuroendocrine tumors.

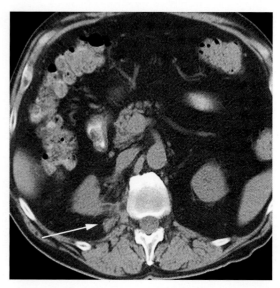

FIGURE 6.68. Locally recurrent tumor after partial nephrectomy. An unenhanced axial CT image obtained in a patient following right partial nephrectomy shows thickened linear areas of soft tissue attenuation at the surgical site (*arrow*). Since these were enlarging on successive CTs, a biopsy was performed, confirming the presence of recurrent tumor. This could easily be confused with postoperative scarring, when detected shortly after surgery.

Imaging after Thermal Ablation

Regular imaging follow-up of patients is required after thermal ablation. While a variety of follow-up protocols are used, one such algorithm includes obtaining CT or MRI at 1 month, 3 months,

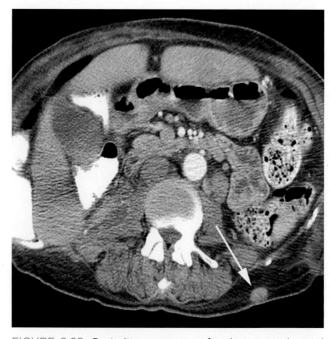

FIGURE 6.69. Port-site recurrence after laparoscopic total nephrectomy. A contrast-enhanced corticomedullary phase axial CT image obtained in a patient following left nephrectomy for renal cancer demonstrates a recurrent tumor nodule along the left posterolateral abdominal, at the site of a previous port (*arrow*).

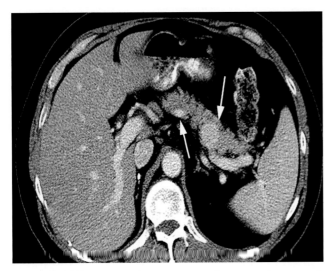

FIGURE 6.70. Pancreatic metastases from renal cancer. A contrast-enhanced corticomedullary phase axial CT image viewed at narrow windows shows two hyperenhancing metastases in the pancreas (*arrows*).

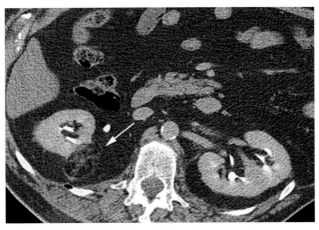

FIGURE 6.72. Normal appearance after thermal ablation. A contrast-enhanced excretory phase axial CT image shows a small defect in the posterior aspect of the right kidney, with adjacent invaginated fat surrounding a small area of low attenuation (*arrow*). This should not be confused with an AML.

6 months, 12 months, and then annually for 5 years. CT and MRI protocols should include precontrast and contrast-enhanced images, the latter obtained during both arterial and NPs. It has been shown that residual or recurrent tumor is sometimes best seen on arterial phase images.

Changes after successful renal mass radiofrequency or cryo-ablation generally have a distinctive evolution. The ablation site should be nonenhancing and initially appear larger than the original tumor (in order to ensure that the entirety of the tumor has been ablated) (Fig. 6.71). A thin rim of enhancement, likely representing granulation tissue, may be detected along a portion or the entirety of the periphery of the ablation site. This is seen more frequently on MRI examinations. On subsequent imaging studies, the ablation bed gradually decreases in size (although it rarely disappears completely). Adjacent peri-nephric fat eventually invaginates into the ablation defect and surrounds the ablation cavity (Fig. 6.72). The appearance should not be confused with an AML (which does not consist of a small soft tissue nodule completely surrounded by macroscopic fat).

Similar postprocedural complications can be visualized on imaging studies performed after thermal ablation as are encountered after partial nephrectomy. These again include posttreatment hematomas, renal collecting system leaks, and pseudoaneurysms. If thermal ablation inadvertently traverses bowel, bowel perforations may also occur.

Close imaging follow-up is required immediately after thermal ablation to ensure that there is no residual tumor present. Residual tumor, when detected in a patient with a hypervascular renal cancer, usually results in an enhancing rounded or crescent-shaped nodule, most commonly located at the interface between the ablation bed and the normal renal parenchyma. As previously mentioned, these tumor nodules are often most easily seen on early enhanced images (Fig. 6.73). Again, it is for this reason that postablation CT or MRI is best performed utilizing a protocol that includes an added arterial phase series (Fig. 6.74). As is the case after partial nephrectomy, in rare instances, residual or recurrent tumor may be encountered in the abdominal cavity or subcutaneous tissues along the access tract (Fig. 6.75).

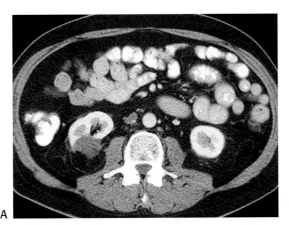
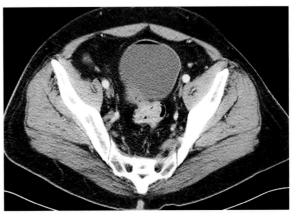

FIGURE 6.71. Normal appearance after thermal ablation. **A:** A contrast-enhanced corticomedullary phase axial CT image shows absence of perfusion in an ablation cavity shortly after radiofrequency ablation of a right renal cancer. The ablation cavity is considerably larger than the size of the ablated tumor. **B:** An image through the pelvis in the same patient also shows a fat–fluid level in the bladder due to chyluria.

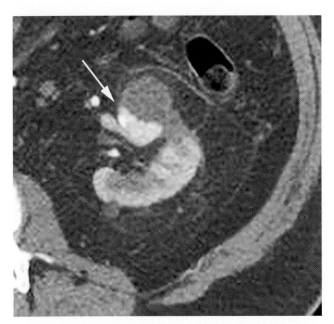

FIGURE 6.73. Recurrent tumor after thermal ablation. A contrast-enhanced corticomedullary phase axial CT image in a patient who has had a thermal ablation of a left renal cancer shows a crescent of abnormally enhancing tissue between the ablation cavity and adjacent renal parenchyma (*arrow*).

Imaging of Patients with Metastatic Disease after Chemotherapy

The Response Evaluation Criteria in Solid Tumors (RECIST) classification system has been the standard by which radiologists and oncologists have traditionally judged the effectiveness of therapy for treatment of unresectable tumors (including renal cancer) in patients receiving chemotherapy or radiation. RECIST, originally introduced in 2000 and revised in 2008 (RECIST 1.1), is based primarily on measurements of the maximal/long-axis diameters of the primary tumor and its metastases, with up to five lesions measured

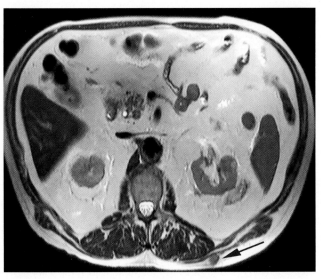

FIGURE 6.75. Tumor seeding along tract of percutaneous ablation. An unenhanced T2-weighted axial MR image demonstrates a small tumor nodule along the tract used for a prior thermal ablation (*arrow*). This is a very rare complication of thermal ablation.

(a maximum of two per organ). The only exception to the long-axis diameter measurements concerns lymph nodes, which are assessed in maximal short-axis diameter. Also, any obtained measurement must be at least 10 mm in length. According to RECIST, disappearance of metastases after treatment is considered to be a complete response. A decrease of 30% or more (without complete resolution) in the summed tumor measurements is considered to indicate a partial response. In comparison, a 20% or more increase is considered to indicate tumor progression, while measurements that fall between a 30% decrease and a 20% increase in size are considered to indicate stable disease. Until recently, RECIST has proven to be very useful in determining the effectiveness of nonsurgical tumor treatment.

With the recent introduction of targeted therapies, however, limitations in the RECIST criteria for many tumors have been

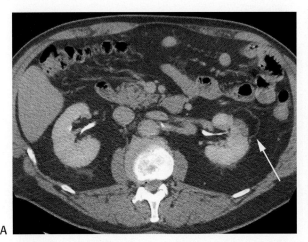
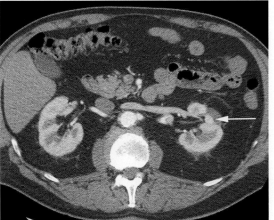

A   B

FIGURE 6.74. Recurrent tumor after thermal ablation. **A:** A contrast-enhanced excretory phase axial CT image in a patient who has had a thermal ablation of a left renal cancer demonstrates the ablation cavity (*arrow*). Residual tumor located at the junction of the ablation cavity with the normal renal parenchyma is not well seen. **B:** The tumor nodule is much more easily visualized on the arterial phase image obtained 90 seconds earlier (*arrow*).

encountered with increasing frequency. One of the chemothera-peutic agent groups of choice for treatment of unresectable/meta-static clear cell renal cancer is the multikinase inhibitors, agents which interfere with tumor angiogenesis. Early on, sunitinib was used preferentially; however, this agent has been supplanted by pazopanib, due to the latter agent having fewer side effects. Multikinase inhibitors have been much more successful than previously used chemotherapeutic agents in treating metastatic renal cancer. Firstly, they can be taken orally. Secondly, and more importantly, up to 75% of patients treated with these agents ini-tially demonstrate stable disease or a partial or complete response to therapy.

Patients responding to treatment with multikinase inhibi-tors may demonstrate posttreatment necrosis without a decrease in tumor size, a change that would not be considered a partial response according to RECIST. On imaging studies, many renal tumor masses responding to multikinase inhibitors do, indeed, demonstrate markedly diminished enhancement following treatment with or without decreases in tumor size (Figs. 6.76 and 6.77).

A number of modified tumor-imaging assessment systems have been advocated, which take into account changes in tumor mor-phology, as well as size. This includes the Choi and modified Choi criteria and the MASS (morphology, attenuation, size, and struc-ture) criteria. The Choi criteria consider metastatic lesions to have responded to treatment if they have decreased in size by 10% of more or if they have decreased in attenuation on contrast-enhanced CT by 15% or more (a feature that indicates decreased tumor per-fusion). The modified Choi criteria require both of these features to be present. To indicate a favorable response, the MASS criteria requires a decrease in tumor size of 20% or more or a decrease in size of 10% or more along with a decrease in contrast-enhanced CT attenuation of 40 HU in one or more target lesions, or interval development of pronounced central necrosis in one or more pre-viously predominantly solid lesions. To date, no one of these sys-tems has been universally accepted as superior to the others. It is clear, however, that further modification of the RECIST criteria is required.

Some investigators have recently attempted to also use assess-ment of tumor metastasis perfusion/enhancement prior to treat-

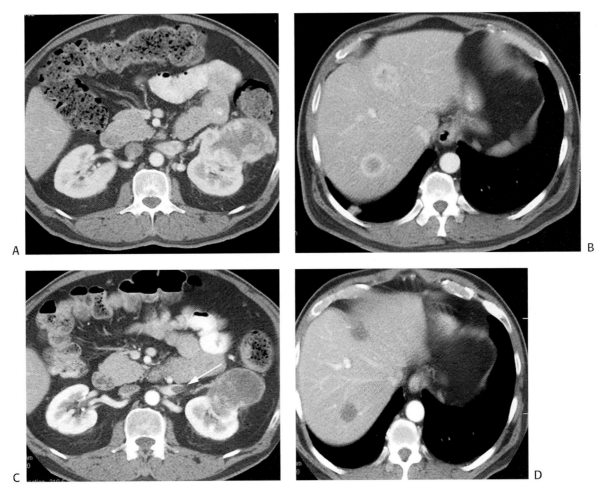

FIGURE 6.76. Metastatic renal cancer treated with a multikinase inhibitor. **A:** A contrast-enhanced cortico-medullary phase axial CT image shows a large heterogeneous clear cell renal cancer in the right kidney. **B:** An image obtained more cephalad shows two rim-enhancing metastases in the liver. The patient was treated with the multikinase inhibitor, pazopanib. **C, D:** One year after treatment was instituted, the renal and liver lesions are relatively similar in size, but have all become almost completely necrotic. There is a small amount of thrombus in the left renal vein (C, *arrow*). Although the patient has had a partial response from his treat-ment, the lesions have not decreased by more than 30% in size. This would not be considered a response according to RECIST.

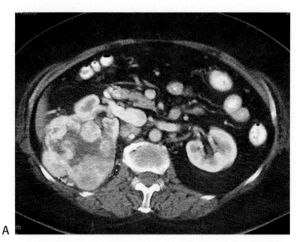 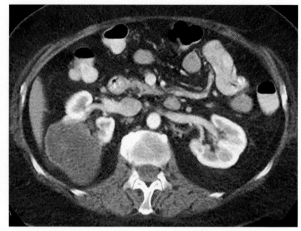

FIGURE 6.77. Renal cancer treated with a multikinase inhibitor. **A:** A contrast-enhanced corticomedullary phase axial CT image shows a large heterogeneous mass in the right kidney. The patient was started on the multikinase inhibitor pazopanib. **B:** Three months later, the mass has decreased in size and also markedly in attenuation.

ment in an attempt to predict the likelihood that a tumor will respond to therapy with multikinase inhibitors. Assessment of changes in perfusion or positron emission tomography activity has also been used to predict the effectiveness of an instituted treatment regimen soon after treatment is instituted. So, if tumor enhancement or PET activity has decreased after one cycle of chemotherapy, the remaining cycles can be administered with the knowledge that the treatment is being effective. Conversely, if, after one cycle of treatment, there has been no change in tumor mass perfusion/activity, then discontinuation of the treatment regimen can be considered prior to a patient's encountering any more serious side effects/toxicity. Studies in this area are promising, but still preliminary.

Multikinase inhibitors have toxicities in some patients. Many of these toxic effects are encountered on imaging studies. Some of the more commonly encountered complications include diffuse hepatic steatosis, cholecystitis, pancreatitis, and enteritis. Imagers should be aware of the potential complications of multikinase

inhibitor therapy and of other targeted agents and the appearance of these complications on imaging studies (especially on CT and MRI), so that the association is made promptly. Identification of a complication may warrant discontinuation of a treatment regimen (Figs. 6.78 to 6.79).

RARE PRIMARY RENAL NEOPLASMS

Juxtaglomerular Tumor

This tumor of the juxtaglomerular apparatus was first described in 1967. Although a rare tumor, it is a curable cause of hypertension, with the hypertension occurring because these tumors produce renin. Patients with juxtaglomerular tumors (reninomas) are usually younger than those with essential hypertension, and there is a marked female preponderance. The nature of the tumor can be confirmed by measuring selective renal vein renin levels.

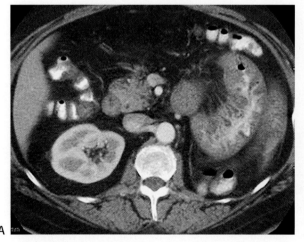 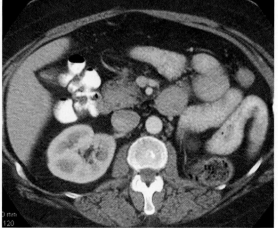

FIGURE 6.78. Complications from targeted chemotherapy. **A:** A contrast-enhanced corticomedullary phase axial CT image in a patient who was receiving the multikinase inhibitor pazopanib for treatment of metastatic renal cancer shows pronounced wall thickening in small bowel loops in the left upper quadrant. A presumptive diagnosis of pazopanib enteritis was made. Chemotherapy was discontinued. **B:** Three months later, the small bowel wall thickening had resolved completely.

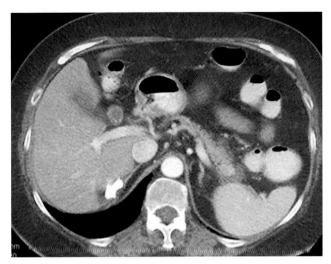

FIGURE 6.79. Complications from targeted chemotherapy. A contrast-enhanced corticomedullary phase axial CT image in a patient who was receiving the multikinase inhibitor pazopanib for treatment of metastatic renal cancer shows a small amount of peripancreatic fluid. The patient had no history of pancreatitis and no other risk factors for developing the disease. This was presumed to represent pazopanib pancreatitis.

Juxtaglomerular tumors are composed of small uniform cells with little nuclear pleomorphism or mitotic activity. Juxtaglomerular cells are similar to smooth muscle cells. Juxtaglomerular tumors range from 3 to 7 cm in diameter when they are detected. The tumors are benign. Local invasion and distant metastases have not been reported.

Patients usually present with symptoms of moderate to severe hypertension. Elements of secondary aldosteronism, such as hypokalemia, may also be present. Rarely, acute flank pain, hypotension, or anemia may reflect hemorrhage from the tumor.

The imaging appearance of these tumors is nonspecific. Sonography reveals an echogenic mass owing to the abundant small vascular channels within the tumor. On CT and MRI, these tumors appear as solid renal masses (Fig. 6. 80). They can be

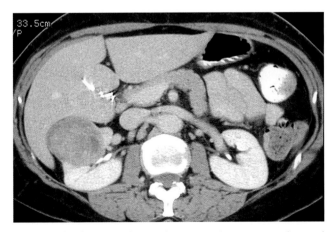

FIGURE 6.80. Juxtaglomerular tumor. A contrast-enhanced excretory phase axial CT image demonstrates a mildly heterogeneous mass in the anterior aspect of the mid right kidney. There are no known distinguishing imaging features of juxtaglomerular tumors. Differentiation from other solid renal neoplasms is not possible.

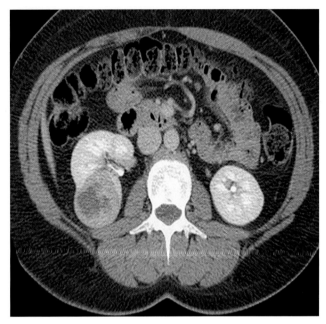

FIGURE 6.81. Metanephric adenoma. A contrast-enhanced excretory phase axial CT image shows a heterogeneous mass in the posterior aspect of the mid right kidney. The mass does not have a distinctive imaging appearance.

homogeneous or mildly heterogeneous. Treatment of juxtaglomerular tumors is surgical, with tumorectomy or partial nephrectomy performed.

Metanephric Adenomas

Metanephric adenomas are uncommon renal epithelial neoplasms derived from embryologic metanephrogenic tissue. These tumors, which are generally considered to be benign, can be diagnosed in individuals of any age. Patients are usually asymptomatic, so findings are often made on imaging studies performed for other reasons. There are only a few reports on the imaging appearance of these neoplasms. The few reported cases have described imaging features that are often similar to those of the more commonly encountered papillary renal cancers. Typical imaging features of metanephric adenomas include noncontrast CT attenuation exceeding that of normal renal parenchyma and only mild enhancement after IV contrast material administration, with the enhancement more pronounced on more delayed, EP, images (Fig. 6.81). Calcifications are occasionally encountered in these tumors. On MRI, the appearance is also similar to that of papillary renal cancers. Metanephric adenomas tend to be isointense or only mildly hyperintense on T2-weighted images, when compared to normal renal parenchyma. A differential diagnosis of metanephric adenoma can be offered when a hypoenhancing solid renal mass is encountered, with the knowledge that most such masses will be papillary renal cancers.

Mixed Epithelial and Stromal Tumors

Mixed epithelial and stromal tumors (MESTs) are rare renal tumors, which, as the name implies, contain both epithelial cystic and solid stromal components. These tumors are generally benign and are found in women the vast majority of the time. On cross-sectional imaging studies, they have a variable appearance but commonly appear as complex cysts or cystic masses, contain-

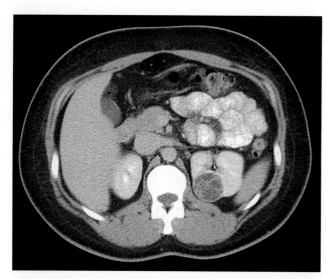

FIGURE 6.82. Mixed epithelial and stromal tumor. A contrast-enhanced excretory phase axial CT image demonstrates a small septated cystic mass in the left kidney, which also has a uniformly thickened wall. This would be classified by many as a Bosniak category III cyst. Although this lesion was eventually diagnosed as a mixed epithelial and stromal tumor, lesions with this appearance are more likely to be complex benign cysts or cystic renal neoplasms (including multilocular cystic neoplasms of low malignant potential).

ing enhancing septa and/or tumor nodules (Fig. 6.82). They cannot be differentiated reliably from other Bosniak category III and IV cysts.

SECONDARY RENAL NEOPLASMS

Renal Lymphoma

Because the kidneys do not contain lymphoid tissue, primary renal lymphoma is rare. However, the kidneys may become involved by hematogenous dissemination of lymphoma or by direct extension from adjacent retroperitoneal lymphomatous masses. Thus, renal lymphoma is almost always part of a generalized process, usually involving multiple sites at the time that it is identified. Secondary renal lymphoma is detected on imaging studies in fewer than 10% of lymphoma patients, but is seen in 30% to 60% of patients at autopsy. Patients who are immune compromised are more likely to develop lymphomas. This includes patients with human immunodeficiency virus (HIV) infections and the iatrogenic immunosuppression that occurs following organ transplantation. In fact, a solitary renal mass in a transplanted kidney is much more likely to be renal lymphoma than a primary renal cancer.

Renal involvement is much more common in non-Hodgkin lymphomas than in Hodgkin disease, and, among the non-Hodgkin types, it is more commonly seen in B-cell type and Burkitt lymphomas. When present, involvement more often is bilateral than unilateral.

Most patients with renal lymphoma have disease in other locations that dominates the clinical presentation. Fever, weight loss, and palpable enlarged lymph nodes are common complaints. Renal lymphoma is usually clinically silent and occurs late in the course of the disease. Rarely, diffuse involvement of both kidneys or ureteral obstruction by enlarged lymph nodes may compromise renal function.

Renal lymphoma often appears as single or multiple solid hypoechoic renal masses on ultrasonography (Fig. 6.83). Unlike

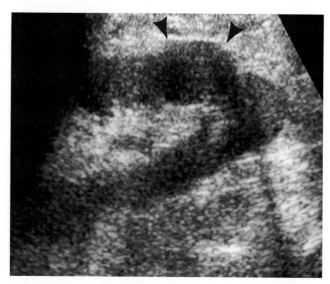

FIGURE 6.83. Renal lymphoma (ultrasound appearance). A relatively hypoechoic mass (*arrowheads*) is seen on this longitudinal image of the right kidney.

cysts, lymphomatous renal masses do not show enhanced sound through transmission. Ultrasound is also often helpful in identifying pelvocaliectasis (which may occasionally be present as a result of ureteral compression by enlarged retroperitoneal lymph nodes) and is the examination of choice in patients with renal failure or other contraindications to intravenous iodinated or gadolinium-based contrast media.

On CT, renal lymphoma may be difficult to detect on unenhanced examinations unless the masses are large, as they are usually of the same attenuation as normal renal parenchyma. The masses are usually easily seen following contrast material administration. The four encountered patterns of renal lymphoma are, in descending order or frequency, (1) multiple bilateral renal masses (Fig. 6.84), (2) a single mass within the kidney or growing into the kidney from the retroperitoneum (Fig. 6.85), (3) diffuse renal enlargement, and (4) infiltrative perinephric or renal sinus masses or nodules (Fig. 6.86). Lymphomatous masses tend to be rounded and homogeneous and hypoenhancing. Adjacent lymph node enlargement is well depicted (Fig. 6.87), although up to 50% of patients with renal lymphoma do not have enlarged retroperitoneal lymph nodes (Fig. 6.84).

RENAL LYMPHOMA

- Multiple renal parenchymal nodules
- Single mass
- Renal sinus involvement
- Diffuse infiltration with nephromegaly
- Perinephric disease

MRI is seldom needed in the evaluation of renal lymphoma; however, if it is performed, lymphomatous masses usually have low to medium signal intensity on T1-weighted and T2-weighted sequences. The masses are hypointense following contrast material administration. Lymphomatous masses also often demonstrate restricted diffusion. As with lymphoma elsewhere in the body, PET/CT is also very useful in detecting and characterizing renal or perirenal involvement. Renal lymphoma tends to be very FDG

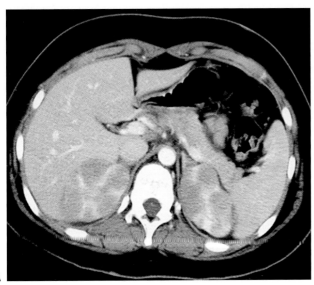 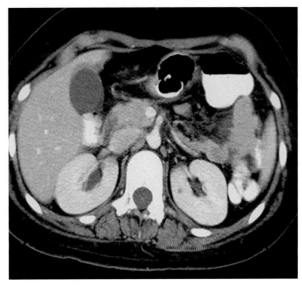

A   B

FIGURE 6.84. Renal lymphoma (multiple renal masses). **A:** A contrast-enhanced corticomedullary phase axial CT image shows multiple homogeneous hypoenhancing solid masses in both kidneys. This is the most common appearance of renal lymphoma. There is no retroperitoneal lymph node enlargement. **B:** A contrast-enhanced nephrographic phase axial image obtained 3 months after initiation of chemotherapy shows that nearly all of the masses have resolved.

avid (Fig. 6.87), while many renal cancers often do not demonstrate pronounced FDG uptake.

Leukemia

Kidney involvement in patients with leukemia is usually due to diffuse infiltration by leukemic cells. It occurs more often with the lymphocytic than granulocytic forms. Occasionally, a discrete mass, such as a chloroma, may be produced. Intrarenal hemorrhage and hematuria are common.

Renal abnormalities can be detected in the kidneys on imaging studies in leukemic patients with renal involvement. Both kidneys may be symmetrically enlarged (Fig. 6.88). The collecting systems are often attenuated. Filling defects occasionally may be seen within the collecting systems due to blood clots.

Multiple Myeloma

Multiple myeloma is a disorder of older adults characterized by proliferation of plasma cells and abnormal serum and urine proteins.

FIGURE 6.85. Renal lymphoma (single renal mass). A contrast-enhanced corticomedullary phase axial CT image shows a large mass extending from the retroperitoneum into the left kidney and diffusely invading the renal parenchyma. This is the second most common manifestation of renal lymphoma.

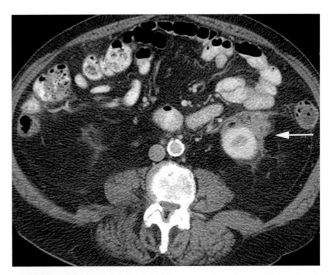

FIGURE 6.86. Renal lymphoma (perinephric disease). A contrast-enhanced corticomedullary phase axial CT image through the lower pole of the left kidney shows an infiltrative mass surrounding the kidney (*arrow*).

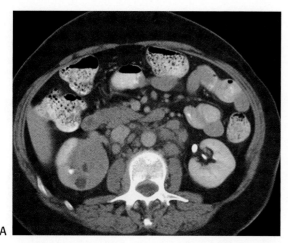
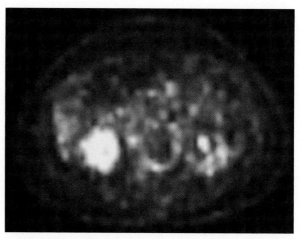

FIGURE 6.87. Renal lymphoma (CT and PET). A contrast-enhanced excretory phase axial CT image **(A)** and a FDG-PET image **(B)** show localization of FDG activity to a large lymphomatous right renal mass.

Renal failure results from precipitation of Bence-Jones proteins in the tubules that may cause mechanical obstruction or may damage tubular cells. Intravascular contrast media was reported in the past to cause in vitro precipitation of these proteins; however, since the adoption of the low osmolality contrast agents, this is no longer considered to be a concern. Hypercalcemia results from bone lesions and causes nephrocalcinosis. On imaging studies, the kidneys may be smoothly enlarged, and the renal collecting systems attenuated. On rare occasions, patients with multiple myeloma may develop focal renal masses (plasmacytomas), which may have an infiltrative appearance. These masses can extend into the renal sinus or the perinephric space (Fig. 6.89).

Metastases to the Kidney

Metastatic disease involving the kidneys is relatively common in autopsy series, where it may be seen in as many as 20% of patients. The most common primary tumors are carcinomas of the lung, breast, colon, and melanoma. At autopsy, approximately 50% of these patients have metastases to both kidneys, and the remaining 50% have involvement of only one kidney. Interestingly, metastases to the kidneys are not commonly seen clinically in living patients. When detected on imaging studies, most metastases are widespread, with multiple organs being

involved in addition to the kidneys. In one study, more than 50% of the patients with renal metastases died within 3 months of their demonstration.

The patient's symptoms are usually dominated by manifestations of the primary tumor, but hematuria and proteinuria can be present. Hypervascular renal metastases (such as from thyroid cancer or choriocarcinoma) may cause significant renal hemorrhage resulting in gross hematuria or a perinephric hematoma. Unless extensive metastases involve both kidneys, renal function is normal. Occasionally, urine cytology may be positive.

When multiple solid renal masses are detected on imaging studies, the differential diagnosis should include multiple renal cancers (such as is encountered in a hereditary renal cancer syndrome), renal lymphoma, and metastatic disease. If a patient with multiple renal masses has a known malignancy, metastatic disease is most likely. In contrast, if a solitary renal mass is detected in a patient with a known primary cancer elsewhere, a new renal mass is more likely to be a primary renal tumor, especially if the other cancer is in remission (Fig. 6.90).

In addition to renal parenchymal involvement, metastases from non-renal primaries may also spread to the perirenal space. Lymphatic connections may be responsible for this pattern of spread. Such metastases have been reported more frequently in patients with underlying melanoma (Fig. 6.91) and lymphoma, but

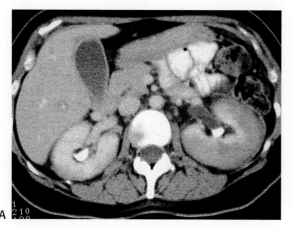
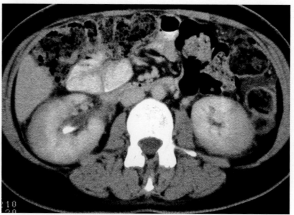

FIGURE 6.88. Leukemia. **A, B:** Two contrast-enhanced excretory phase axial CT images show low attenuation infiltrative soft tissue enveloping both kidneys, primarily along their periphery. The infiltrative tissue results in bilateral renal enlargement, often with attenuation of the renal collecting systems.

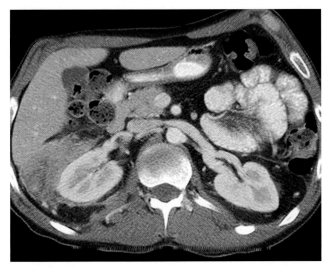

FIGURE 6.89. Multiple myeloma. A contrast-enhanced corticomedullary phase axial CT image in a patient with multiple myeloma shows a large infiltrative plasmacytoma surrounding the anterior and lateral aspects of the right kidney.

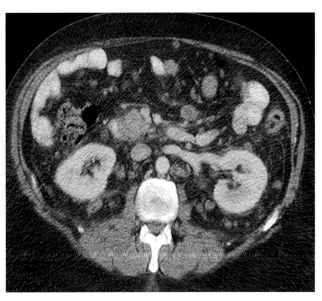

FIGURE 6.91. Metastatic melanoma to the perinephric space. A contrast-enhanced corticomedullary phase axial CT image shows a large number of metastatic tumor nodules in both perinephric spaces, as well as in the mesentery. Metastatic melanoma and lymphoma are more likely to produce perinephric nodules than are other neoplasms.

can also be encountered in patients with other common malignancies, including lung cancer.

On ultrasound, renal metastases are seen as solid renal masses. Echo-free areas may represent tumor necrosis or local hemorrhage. CT most commonly detects renal metastases, because this modality is most frequently used to monitor oncology patients during or after treatment (Figs. 6.90 and 6.91). Although tumor invasion of the renal vein and extension into the IVC is commonly seen in renal adenocarcinoma, it is rare in patients with renal metastases. On MRI, renal metastases demonstrate high signal intensity on T2-weighted images and restricted diffusion, an appearance that can be produced by other solid renal masses.

RENAL AND PERIRENAL MESENCHYMAL TUMORS

The renal capsule is composed of fibrous tissue, nerves, smooth muscle, blood vessels, and perirenal fat. A benign or malignant tumor may develop in any of these tissues or in other mesenchymal cells adjacent to the kidneys. On rare occasions, intrarenal masses may contain mesenchymal cells as well. Mesenchymal tumors may be benign or malignant. Such tumors include leiomyomas, lipomas, hemangiomas, lymphangiomas, and sarcomas. Malignant capsular tumors are often quite large at the time of diagnosis. Presenting complaints include a flank mass, abdominal pain, and weight loss. Unless the renal parenchyma is invaded, hematuria is uncommon. The prognosis for these patients is usually poor.

Lipoma and Liposarcoma

Lipomas or liposarcomas can develop in the renal capsule or in adjacent tissue. Because liposarcomas are more common than lipomas in the retroperitoneum, any retroperitoneal mass identified on CT or MRI that contains macroscopic fat should be considered a liposarcoma. On occasion, it can be difficult to distinguish an exophytic AML from a liposarcoma on imaging studies. This is obviously an important distinction. The former may not require any treatment, while the latter should be surgically resected, if possible. Several imaging features have been identified, however, which can be useful in differentiating AMLs from liposarcomas. Since AMLs originate from the kidney, there is usually a cleft or defect in the renal parenchyma revealing the area in the kidney from which the tumor arises (Fig. 6.18). In comparison, liposarcomas may compress the kidney, but do not produce such a parenchymal defect (Fig. 6.19). AMLs are almost always highly vascular neoplasms. Many demonstrate prominent vessels (some of which contain aneurysms) that enhance briskly. In comparison, liposarcomas tend to be hypovascular.

Intrarenal lipomas are very rare. These neoplasms are usually small and are seldom symptomatic. Most cases involve middle-aged

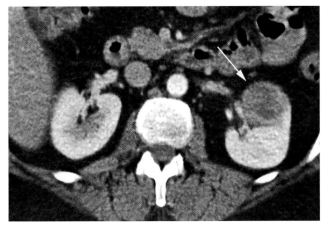

FIGURE 6.90. Metastasis to the kidney. A contrast-enhanced corticomedullary phase axial CT image shows a solitary metastasis in the left kidney (arrow) in a patient with endometrial cancer. The mass is indistinguishable from a primary renal neoplasm. Biopsy would be required for differentiation. In fact, a solitary solid renal mass in a patient with a known cancer elsewhere is actually more likely to be a second primary neoplasm.

women. They should be easily detected by CT as a well-defined fatty mass. They are not distinguishable from the much more common AMLs, although the inability to make such a distinction is usually not clinically relevant, since both entities are benign and usually do not require any treatment.

Leiomyoma and Leiomyosarcoma

Smooth muscle tumors may arise from vessel walls or scattered muscle fibers of the renal capsule. Most are found in the lower poles. There is a female preponderance and an increased incidence in patients with tuberous sclerosis. Most leiomyomas are small and asymptomatic. They are usually well-defined peripheral lesions and demonstrate homogeneous enhancement on CT. They are typically characterized by low signal intensity on both unenhanced T1- and T2-weighted MR images.

Leiomyosarcomas are usually large and locally invasive by the time they become clinically apparent. These tumors tend to metastasize widely, and the prognosis for affected patients is poor. On CT and MRI, leiomyosarcomas tend to be large and heterogeneous. They may envelop the kidney. Treatment is surgical resection, when possible. Local recurrence is common.

Solitary Fibrous Tumor

Solitary fibroma tumor is a rare spindle cell neoplasm found most frequently in the pleura. In the kidney, this tumor, which contains mostly fibrous tissue and collagen, may arise in the renal pelvis, cortex, or capsule. Most of these tumors are slow growing and behave in a benign fashion; however, malignant features (with local recurrence after resection or metastases) may be encountered in some patients. For this reason, these tumors, if diagnosed by biopsy, are usually resected.

On CT or MR imaging, the tumor, which is indistinguishable from other primary renal neoplasms, is usually well circumscribed and often large, measuring over than 5 cm in diameter. Enhancement is homogenous and usually pronounced, although areas of necrosis may be seen. On MRI, these tumors often have low T2-weighted signal, due to their fibrous components.

Hemangioma

Renal hemangiomas are extremely uncommon renal tumors of endothelial cells and capillary size vessels. They may be encountered in patients with tuberous sclerosis and in other conditions associated with hemangiomas in other organs, including Sturge–Weber syndrome. If the vessels are dilated, the tumor may be called a cavernous hemangioma. The tumors are usually small, but can range from several mm to 5 cm in diameter. They are most frequently located at the apex of the renal pyramids.

The most common presenting complaint is hematuria. Some patients may experience colicky pain due to passage of blood clots. Men and women are affected equally and present most often during the third or fourth decade.

Renal hemangiomas are often too small to be detected on imaging studies. Some, but not all, larger lesions demonstrate intense enhancement persisting into the venous phase. These tumors tend to have high T2 signal intensity on MRI examinations, a feature also seen with hepatic hemangiomas. Treatment has traditionally been surgical for symptomatic lesions. However, transcatheter ablation is an effective therapy and may minimize loss of renal tissue.

Lymphangioma

This rare renal lesion is also referred to as renal lymphangiectasia or lymphangiomatosis. It is seen most frequently in the renal

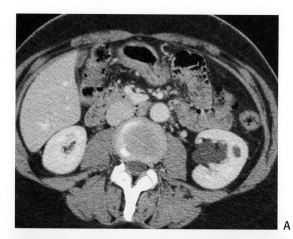

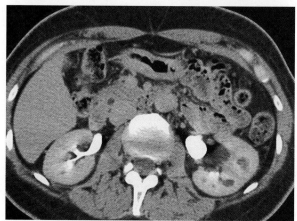

FIGURE 6.92. Lymphangiomatosis. **A:** A contrast-enhanced nephrographic phase axial CT image shows cystic masses in both the parenchyma and renal sinus of the left kidney. **B:** An excretory phase image shows that the cysts in the renal sinus are separate from the left renal collecting system.

sinus or perinephric space as a multiloculated cystic mass or masses (Fig. 6.92). Rather than a neoplasm, it is thought to be a developmental anomaly of the lymphatic system and is often bilateral. Most patients are asymptomatic and treatment is seldom needed.

Osteosarcoma

This tumor is rarely a primary renal neoplasm, but may arise from a fibrosarcoma undergoing metaplasia to tumor osteocytes. Diagnosis is based on the presence of formed bone. The main differential diagnosis is a metastasis to the kidney from a primary skeletal osteosarcoma. The age of the patient helps with this distinction, because patients with primary renal osteosarcoma are usually elderly, whereas primary skeletal osteosarcomas occur in adolescents and young adults.

RENAL PELVIC TUMORS

Most of the tumors arising from the renal pelvis are malignant, with urothelial neoplasms being most common. Less often, squamous cell carcinomas, undifferentiated carcinomas, or adenocarcinomas may occur. Papillomas comprise approximately 50% of the benign tumors, with the remaining 50% consisting of angiomas, fibromas, myomas, or polyps. These lesions are discussed in more detail elsewhere.

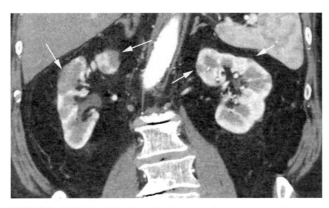

FIGURE 6.93. IgG4-related disease. A contrast-enhanced corticomedullary phase coronally reformatted CT image in a patient with autoimmune pancreatitis demonstrates multiple small bilateral renal masses (arrows), a known manifestation of the disease.

INFLAMMATORY DISEASES MASQUERADING AS RENAL TUMORS

A variety of benign inflammatory diseases can produce masses in the renal parenchyma and/or in the renal sinus or perinephric fat. These can be confused with renal or perirenal neoplasms when identified on imaging studies. In many instances, affected patients have histories indicating the diagnosis; however, on some occasions, the detected renal findings may represent the first manifestations of the disease. Inflammatory diseases that can result in renal, renal sinus, or perinephric abnormalities include IgG4-related disease (which is most commonly known to be associated with autoimmune pancreatitis) (Figs. 6.93 and 6.94), sarcoidosis (which, in the abdomen, more frequently affects the liver, spleen, and lymph nodes) (Fig. 6.95), amyloidosis (Fig. 6.96), Erdheim–Chester disease (Fig. 6.97), and extramedullary hematopoiesis (Fig. 6.98).

SOLID PEDIATRIC RENAL TUMORS

Wilms Tumor

Wilms tumor (nephroblastoma) arises from metanephric blastema and is most commonly found in young children. About half of all cases are diagnosed in patients younger than 2 years, and 75% of cases are diagnosed in patients younger than 5 years. There is no sex predilection, but there is a high association with several malformation syndromes.

Wilms tumor develops in approximately one-third of children with sporadic aniridia. Patients with aniridia and Wilms tumor present at an earlier age and more frequently have bilateral tumors than other patients with Wilms tumors. Patients with hemihypertrophy also have an increased incidence of nephroblastomas, along with adrenal cortical neoplasms, and hepatoblastomas. The side of hypertrophy and the side of the tumor are unrelated. An association of Wilms tumor with male pseudohermaphroditism and glomerulonephritis has also been reported (Drash syndrome). The different components of this syndrome may not occur at the same time. Thus, the development of any two should alert physicians to the possibility of the third component arising.

Wilms tumor is also encountered in patients with Beckwith–Wiedemann syndrome. This syndrome, comprising macroglossia, omphalocele, adrenal cytomegaly, and visceromegaly, often includes a proliferation of nephrogenic blastema (from which Wilms tumors develop). Other anomalies including microcephaly, malformed ears, a variety of genitourinary anomalies (e.g., horseshoe kidneys), and developmental retardation are also associated with Wilms tumor.

WILMS TUMOR ASSOCIATIONS

- Sporadic aniridia (WAGR syndrome, which also includes genitourinary tract abnormalities and mental retardation)
- Hemihypertrophy
- Denys–Drash syndrome
- Beckwith–Wiedemann syndrome
- Li-Fraumeni syndrome

Wilms tumor is usually a mixed tumor containing epithelial, blastemal, and stromal elements. The nonepithelial elements may differentiate into striated muscle, adipose, cartilage, or bone. This may explain the rare case in which the detection of macroscopic fat may cause confusion with an AML. There is usually a pseudocapsule that separates the tumor from the remainder of the kidney.

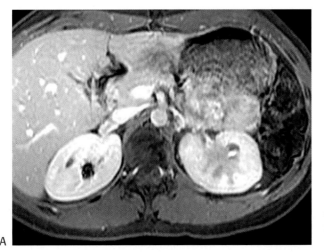
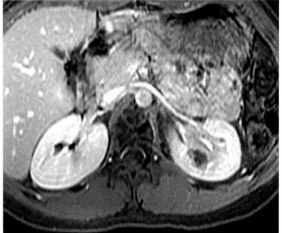

A   B

FIGURE 6.94. IgG4-related disease. **A, B:** Two contrast-enhanced T1-weighted fat-suppressed nephrographic phase axial MR images show an infiltrative mass in the left renal sinus, which has obliterated the normal renal sinus fat.

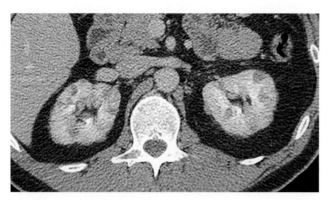

FIGURE 6.95. Renal sarcoidosis. A contrast-enhanced nephrographic phase axial CT image demonstrates multiple small bilateral renal masses in a patient with sarcoidosis.

Most children with Wilms tumor present with a palpable abdominal mass. Abdominal pain, anorexia, fever, and hypertension are also commonly present. Gross hematuria occurs in <10% of cases.

Prognosis, which is excellent in many patients with Wilms tumors and which has improved greatly in recent years, is based primarily upon the stage of the tumor at diagnosis (see Table 6.8), as well as on the histology. Wilms tumors are considered to have either favorable or unfavorable (anaplastic) histology. Prognosis is adversely affected by anaplastic tumor histology, especially when found in higher stage tumors.

Wilms tumors are usually large (averaging 12 cm) by the time they are detected. Because they develop in the renal cortex, tumor growth is often exophytic. Ultrasound has become the preferred examination for young children presenting with an abdominal mass (Fig. 6.99A). The solid nature and renal origin of the tumor mass can usually be determined. Most tumors will be hypo- to hyperechoic solid masses, are usually well defined, and may be separated from the normal parenchyma by a tumor pseudocapsule or compressed renal cortex. Hypoechoic areas within the tumor may represent regions of hemorrhage or tissue necrosis. Dystrophic calcification is uncommon, but may cause hyperechoic foci with shadowing when it occurs. Ultrasound is also useful in detecting tumor extension into the renal vein or IVC and for identifying hepatic metastases. The renal vein may be difficult to image, but identification of tumor thrombus in

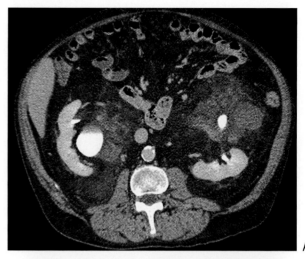

A

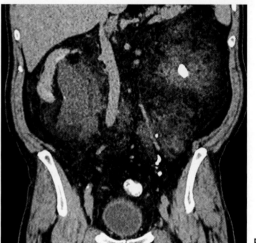

B

FIGURE 6.97. Erdheim–Chester disease. Contrast-enhanced excretory phase axial **(A)** and coronal reformatted **(B)** CT images show extensive soft tissue infiltration of both renal sinuses. Soft tissue surrounds portions of both renal pelves.

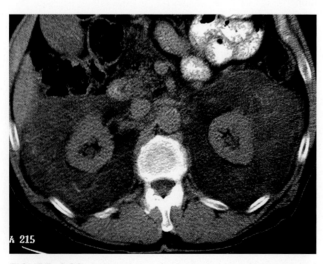

FIGURE 6.96. Perinephric amyloidosis. Unenhanced axial CT image shows diffuse infiltration and expansion of the perinephric spaces.

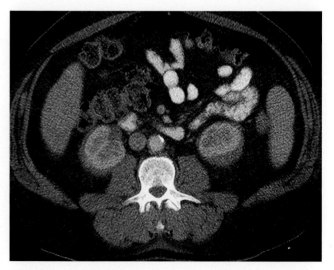

FIGURE 6.98. Extramedullary hematopoiesis. A contrast-enhanced corticomedullary phase axial CT image shows a small rind of soft tissue surrounding both kidneys.

TABLE 6.8

Staging of Wilms Tumors (from Children's Oncology Group)

Stage	Definition	% of Tumors at Presentation
I	Contained within renal capsule/no biopsy before surgery	40%–45%
II	Capsular invasion, but removed completely at surgery. No biopsy before surgery. No involved lymph nodes	20%
III	Incompletely removed, with one or more of the following: Invasion of adjacent organs; Involved regional lymph nodes; Spill of tumor before or during surgery (including during biopsy); Tumor removed in more than one piece	20%–25%
IV	Evidence of hematogenous spread (to distant lymph nodes, liver, lungs, brain, bones)	10%
V	Bilateral renal tumors	5%

Survival for stages: I, 83%–99%; II, 81%–98%; III, 72%–94%; IV, 38%–86%; V 55%–87%.

the IVC is of greater importance. The surgeon can examine the renal vein during surgery, but the extent of tumor thrombus determines the operative approach. Color-flow Doppler ultrasound is especially useful in detecting tumor thrombus in the IVC.

CT and MRI may add additional information to ultrasound in the local staging of Wilms tumors in up to 50% of patients (including by their ability to identify occasional contralateral tumors). The paucity of retroperitoneal fat in young children makes CT evaluation of Wilms tumor difficult in comparison to evaluation of renal tumors in adults, however. Furthermore, the ionizing radiation needed for CT makes this examination less desirable than ultrasound or MRI in children. Although ionizing radiation is spared with MRI, many children require sedation and monitoring to undergo an MRI examination (Fig. 6.99B,C). Nonetheless, MRI has played an increasing role in assessing patients with known or suspected Wilms tumor.

Contrast-enhanced CT and MRI can be very helpful in staging Wilms tumors (see Table 6.8). On contrast-enhanced CT or MRI, Wilms tumor is seen as a large mass that enhances less than the normal renal parenchyma. The degree of heterogeneity depends on the presence of tissue necrosis or hemorrhage. The tumor mass is usually large, causing compression of the remainder of the kidney. Patients with Wilms tumors should also be assessed for venous invasion and the extent of such invasion, as well as regional lymph node involvement, and distant metastases (with distant spread most frequently occurring to the liver and lungs, but with spread to

the peritoneum and mediastinum also encountered in occasional patients).

Approximately 5% of patients with Wilms tumors have bilateral renal involvement (stage V). These patients usually present at a younger age, and the tumors may be synchronous or metachronous. Patients at increased risk for bilateral involvement include those with a family history of Wilms tumor, multifocal lesions in the index kidney, nephroblastomatosis, and those with other associated congenital anomalies.

It must be stressed that imaging studies cannot distinguish Wilms tumors from other solid renal masses that may be encountered in children, including rhabdoid tumors, clear cell sarcomas, primitive neuroectodermal tumors, and, rarely, renal cancers.

Different approaches have been used to treat patients with resectable Wilms tumors, with some groups recommending surgery only and others recommending surgery following neoadjuvant chemotherapy.

Rhabdoid Tumor

Rhabdoid tumor of the kidney (RTK) is an uncommon childhood tumor. Originally considered a sarcomatoid variant of Wilms tumor, RTK is now recognized as a distinct pathologic entity. RTK, which originates in the renal medulla, is very aggressive. Patients with RTK have a median age at presentation of only 11 months, which is less than those with Wilms tumors. There is a strong association of RTK with a second primary malignancy of the central nervous system such as astrocytoma, ependymoma, or primitive neuroectodermal tumor. Metastases from RTK to the brain are common. On CT and MRI, RTK appears as an infiltrative centrally located renal mass invading the renal final hilum. Large fluid attenuation/signal intensity areas may be encountered, representing necrosis. Other solid pediatric renal masses, including the more common Wilms tumors and renal cancers, originate in the renal cortex and are most often better circumscribed.

Nephroblastomatosis

Nephroblastomatosis is a group of pathologic entities characterized by persistent nephrogenic blastema. It results from an arrest in normal nephrogenesis, with persistence of residual blastema. Although nephroblastomatosis is not malignant, it is associated with Wilms tumor and those conditions with a high incidence of Wilms tumor.

Nephroblastomatosis may be diffuse or, more commonly, multinodular. The radiographic features are dependent on the size and distribution of the embryologic remnants. The lesions in the multifocal form are usually microscopic nodules and are difficult to image. In the diffuse form, the kidneys are enlarged and the collecting system may be deformed by parenchymal nodules.

On ultrasound, the lesions are often hypoechoic, but may also be iso- or hyperechoic. Their subcapsular location suggests nephroblastomatosis and helps to distinguish this condition from polycystic renal disease or lymphoma. This distribution can also be seen on CT and MRI. Nephroblastomatosis is clearly distinguished from normal renal tissue by differences in contrast enhancement. Differentiation of nephroblastomatosis from Wilms tumor can be problematic.

Many patients with nephroblastomatosis are treated with antineoplastic drugs, which often decrease the renal size. However, such patients remain at risk and should be followed to detect any subsequently developing Wilms tumors.

Mesoblastic Nephroma

This benign tumor is usually present at birth and has been described as a congenital Wilms tumor or fetal mesenchymal hamartoma.

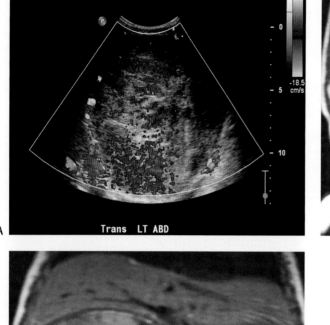

A

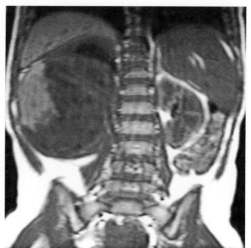

B

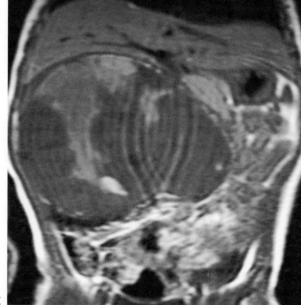

C

FIGURE 6.99. Wilms tumor. **A:** Color Doppler image of a large left Wilms tumor shows an area of increased flow in the left kidney. **B, C:** Two coronal T2-weighted MR images from a different patient show a large right-sided Wilms tumor.

Patients with mesoblastic nephroma typically present with a nontender abdominal mass detected either at birth or in the first few months of life. In fact, this represents the most common renal mass encountered in children under the age of 3 months. There is no sexual predilection. Mesoblastic nephromas are comprised of interlacing sheets of fibromatous cells. Small bundles of these fibromatous cells are characteristically found diffusely interspersed in the adjacent renal parenchyma.

Mesoblastic nephromas are usually large at presentation, averaging over 6 cm in diameter, and often replace almost the entire renal parenchyma. The cut surface has a whorled appearance resembling leiomyomas of the uterus. They are not encapsulated, and finger-like extensions of the tumors may extend into the adjacent kidney. Although these tumors may also penetrate through the renal capsule and may involve the perinephric space, they rarely extend into the renal vein or renal pelvis.

Ultrasound is the most commonly used modality in the evaluation of patients with mesoblastic nephromas. The most common pattern of a homogeneously isoechoic mass reflects the smooth mass of fibromatous cells. Occasionally, hyperechoic foci are seen. Although uncommon, areas of necrosis or hemorrhage may be

detected as hypoechoic regions. A fairly uniform, solid, intrarenal mass has been reported on CT and MRI, although cystic components may also be identified. T1- and T2-weighted MR signal intensity is variable. Restricted diffusion has been identified in these lesions on MRI. Although these neoplasms may extend to abut renal vessels and the IVC, vascular invasion does not occur.

Treatment of mesoblastic nephromas is by surgical excision, and cure is usually achieved with nephrectomy. In some patients, extensive tumor necrosis, extrarenal infiltration, and mesenchymal immaturity suggest more aggressive behavior. In these patients, who usually present beyond 3 months of age, adjunctive chemotherapy or radiation therapy may be given.

SUGGESTED READINGS

Indeterminate Renal Masses

Silverman SG, Israel GM, Herts BR, et al. Management of the incidental renal mass. *Radiology.* 2008;249(1):16–31.

Tappouni R, Kissane J, Sarwani N, et al. Pseudoenhancement of renal cysts: influence of lesion size, lesion location, slice thickness, and number of MDCT detectors. *AJR Am J Roentgenol.* 2012;198:133–137.

Angiomyolipomas

Bosniak M, Megibow AJ, Hulnick DH, et al. CT diagnosis of renal angiomyolipoma: the importance of detecting small amounts of fat. *AJR Am J Roentgenol.* 1988;151:497–501.

Catalano OA, Samir AE, Sahani DV, et al. Pixel distribution analysis: can it be used to distinguish clear cell carcinomas from angiomyolipomas with minimal fat? *Radiology.* 2008;247:738–746.

Davenport MS, Neville AM, Ellis JH, et al. Diagnosis of renal angiomyolipoma with Hounsfield Unit thresholds: effect of size and region of interest and nephrographic phase imaging. *Radiology.* 2011;260:158–165.

Davidson AJ, Davis CJ. Fat in renal adenocarcinoma: never say never. *Radiology.* 1993;188:316.

Farrelly C, Delaney H, McDermott R, et al. Do all non-calcified echogenic renal lesions found on ultrasound need further evaluation with CT? *Abdom Imaging.* 2008;33:44–47.

Halverson SJ, Kunju LP, Bhalla R, et al. Accuracy of determining small renal mass management with risk stratified biopsies: confirmation by final pathology. *J Urol.* 2013;189:441–446.

Hélénon O, Merran S, Paraf F, et al. Unusual fat-containing tumors of the kidney: a diagnostic dilemma. *Radiographics.* 1997;17:129–144.

Kim JY, Kim JK, Kim N, et al. CT histogram analysis: differentiation of angiomyolipoma without visible fat from renal cell carcinoma at CT imaging. *Radiology.* 2008;246:472–479.

Rabenou RA, Charles HW. Differentiation of sporadic versus tuberous sclerosis complex-associated angiomyolipoma. *AJR Am J Roentgenol.* 2015;205:292–301.

Rosenkrantz AB, Hecht EM, Taneja SS, et al. Angiomyolipoma with epithelial cysts: mimic of renal cell carcinoma. *Clin Imaging.* 2010;34:65–68.

Ryan MJ, Francis IR, Cohan RH, et al. Imaging appearance of renal epithelioid angiomyolipomas. *J Comput Assist Tomogr.* 2013;37:957–961.

Siegel CL, Middleton WD, Teefey SA, et al. Angiomyolipoma and renal cell carcinoma: US differentiation. *Radiology.* 1996;198:789–793.

Solid Renal Masses without Macroscopic Fat

Al Harbi F, Tabatabaeefar L, Jewett MA. Enhancement threshold of small (<4 cm) solid renal masses on CT. *AJR Am J Roentgenol.* 2016;206:554–558.

Bosniak MA, Birnbaum BA, Krinsky GA, et al. Small renal parenchymal neoplasms: further observations on growth. *Radiology.* 1995;197:589–597.

Cohan RH, Sherman LS, Korobkin M, et al. Renal masses: assessment of the corticomedullary-phase and nephrographic-phase CT scans. *Radiology.* 1995;196:445–451.

Orton LP, Cohan RH, Davenport MS, et al. Variability on computed tomography diameter measurements of solid renal masses. *Abdom Imaging.* 2014;39:533–542.

Pierorazio PM, Hyams ES, Mullens JK, et al. Active surveillance of small renal masses. *Rev Urol.* 2012;14:13–19.

Pierorazio PM, Hyams ES, Tsai S, et al. Multiphase enhancement patterns of small renal masses (<4 cm) on preoperative computed tomography: utility for distinguishing subtypes of renal cell carcinoma, angiomyolipoma, and oncocytoma. *Urology.* 2013;81:1265–1272.

Schieda N, Vakili M, Dilauro M, et al. Solid renal cell carcinoma measuring water attenuation (−10 to 20 HU) on unenhanced CT. *AJR Am J Roentgenol.* 2015;205:1215–1221.

Renal Cancers

Agarwal PP, Gross BH, Holloway BJ, et al. Thoracic CT findings in Birt-Hogg-Dube? syndrome. *AJR Am J Roentgenol.* 2011;196:349–352.

Ananthakrishnan L, Kapur P, Leyendecker JR. The spectrum of renal cell carcinoma in adults. *Abdom Radiol.* 2016;41:1052–1065.

Beer AJ, Dobritz M, Zantl N, et al. Comparison of 16-MDCT and MRI for characterization of kidney lesions. *AJR Am J Roentgenol.* 2006;186:1639–1650.

Blitman NM, Berkenblit RG, Rozenblit AM, et al. Renal medullary carcinoma: CT and MRI features. *AJR Am J Roentgenol.* 2005;185:268–272.

Choudhary S, Sudarshan S, Choyke PL, et al. Renal cell carcinoma: recent advances in genetics and imaging. *Semin Ultrasound CT MR.* 2009;30:315–325.

Choyke PL, Glenn GM, McClellan MW, et al. von Hippel-Lindau disease: genetic, clinical, and imaging features. *Radiology.* 1995;194:629–642.

Dang TT, Ziv E, Weinstein S, et al. Computed tomography and magnetic resonance imaging of adult renal cell carcinoma associated Xp11.2 translocation. *J Comput Assist Tomogr.* 2012;36:669–674.

Davidson AJ, Choyke PL, Hartman DS, et al. Renal medullary carcinoma associated with sickle cell trait: radiologic findings. *Radiology.* 1995;195:83–85.

Dilauro M, Quon M, McInnes MDF, et al. Comparison of contrast-enhanced multiphase renal protocol CT versus MRI for diagnosis of papillary renal cell carcinoma. *AJR Am J Roentgenol.* 2016;206:319–325.

Doshi Am, Ream JM, Kierans AS, et al. Use of MRI in differentiation of papillary renal cell carcinoma subtypes: qualitative and quantitative analysis. *AJR Am J Roentgenol.* 2016;206:566–572.

Egbert ND, Caoili EM, Cohan RH, et al. Differentiation of papillary renal cell carcinoma subtypes on CT and MRI. *AJR Am J Roentgenol.* 2013;201:347–355.

Frank I, Blute ML, Cheville JC, et al. Solid renal tumors: an analysis of pathological features related to tumor size. *J Urol.* 2003;170:2217–2220.

He J, Gan W, Liu S, et al. Dynamic computed tomographic features of adult renal cell carcinoma associated with Xp11.2 translocation/TFE3 gene fusions: comparison with clear cell renal cell carcinoma. *J Comput Assist Tomogr.* 2015;39:730–736.

Herts BR, Coll DM, Novick AC, et al. Enhancement characteristic of papillary renal neoplasms revealed on triphasic helical CT of the kidneys. *AJR Am J Roentgenol.* 2002;178:367–372.

Kawashima A, Young SW, Takahashi N, et al. Inherited renal carcinomas. *Abdom Radiol.* 2016;41:1066–1078.

Kim JK, Kim TK, Ahn HJ, et al. Differentiation of subtypes of renal cell carcinoma on helical CT scans. *AJR Am J Roentgenol.* 2002;178:1499–1506.

Kuroda N, Hess O, Zhou M. New and emerging renal tumor entities. *Diagn Histopathol.* 2016;22:47–56.

Leibovich BC, Lohse CM, Crispen PL, et al. Histological subtype is an independent predictor of outcome for patients with renal cell carcinoma. *J Urol.* 2010;183:1309–1316.

Moch H, Cubilla AL, Humphrey PA, et al. The 2016 WHO classification of tumours of the urinary system and male genital organs—part A: renal, penile, and testicular tumors. *Eur Urol.* 2016;70(1):93–105.

Outwater EK, Bhatia M, Siegelman ES, et al. Lipid in renal clear cell carcinoma: detection on opposed-phase gradient-echo MR images. *Radiology.* 1997;205:103–107.

Park SM, Cho SK, Lee JH, et al. Unusual manifestations of renal cell carcinoma. *Acta Radiol.* 2008;7:839–847.

Prando A, Prando D, Prando P. Renal cell carcinoma: unusual imaging manifestations. *Radiographics.* 2006;26:233–244.

Ruppert-Kohlmayr AJ, Uggowitzer M, Meissnitzer T, et al. Differentiation of renal clear cell carcinoma and renal papillary carcinoma using quantitative CT enhancement parameters. *AJR Am J Roentgenol.* 2004;183:1387–1391.

Sahni VA, Silverman SG. Biopsy of renal masses: when and why. *Cancer Imaging.* 2009;9:44–45.

Sandim V, Pereira DA, Ornellas AA, et al. Renal cell carcinoma and proteomics. *Urol Int.* 2010;84:373–377.

Sun MRM, Ngo L, Genega EM, et al. Renal cell carcinoma: dynamic contrast-enhanced MR imaging for differentiation of tumor subtypes—correlation with pathologic findings. *Radiology.* 2009;250:793–802.

Uppot RN, Harisinghani MG, Gervais DA. Imaging guided percutaneous renal biopsy: rationale and approach. *AJR Am J Roentgenol.* 2010;194:1443–1449.

Wang H, Cheng L, Zhang X, et al. Renal cell carcinoma: diffusion weighted MR imaging for subtype differentiation at 3.0 T. *Radiology.* 2010;257(1):135–143.

Yamanaka K, Miyake H, Hara I, et al. Papillary renal cell carcinoma: a clinicopathological study of 35 cases. *Int J Urol.* 2006;13:1049–1052.

Young JR, Margolis D, Sauk S, et al. Clear cell renal cell carcinoma: discrimination from other renal cell carcinoma subtypes and oncocytoma at multiphasic multidetector CT. *Radiology.* 2013;267:444–453.

Young JR, Zhu QQ, Wang ZQ, et al. The multislice CT findings of renal carcinoma associated with XP11.2 translocation/TFE gene fusion and collecting duct carcinoma. *Acta Radiologica.* 2013;54:355–362.

Oncocytomas

Bird VG, Kanagarajah P, Morillo G, et al. Differentiation of oncocytoma and renal cell carcinoma in small renal masses (<4 cm): the role of 4-phase computerized tomography. *World J Urol.* 2011;29:787–792.

Choudhary S, Rajesh A, Mayer NJ, et al. Renal oncocytoma: CT features cannot reliably distinguish oncocytoma from other renal neoplasms. *Clin Radiol.* 2009;64:517–522.

O'Malley MW, Tran P, Hanbidge A, et al. Small renal oncocytomas: is segmental enhancement inversion a characteristic finding at biphasic MDCT? *AJR Am J Roentgenol.* 2012;199:1312–1315.

Pano B, Macias N, Salvador R, et al. Usefulness of MDCT to differentiate between renal cell carcinoma and oncocytoma: development of a predictive model. *AJR Am J Roentgenol.* 2016;206:764–774.

Woo S, Cho JY, Kim SY, et al. Segmental enhancement inversion of small renal oncocytoma: differences in prevalence according to tumor size. *AJR Am J Roentgenol.* 2013;200:1054–1059.

Staging and Nephrometry of Renal Cancer

Hedgire SS, Elmi A, Nadkarni ND, et al. Preoperative evaluation of perinephric fat invasion in patients with renal cell carcinoma: correlation with pathological findings. *Clin Imaging.* 2013;37:91–96.

Kutikov A, Uzzo RG. The R.E.N.A.L. nephrometry score: a comprehensive standardized system for quantitating renal tumor size, location and depth. *J Urol.* 2009;182:844–853.

Ng CS, Wood CG, Silverman PM, et al. Renal cell carcinoma: diagnosis, staging, and surveillance. *AJR Am J Roentgenol.* 2008;191:1220–1232.

Imaging after Treatment of Renal Cancer

Chae EJ, Kim JK, Kim SH, et al. Renal cell carcinoma: analysis of postoperative recurrence patterns. *Radiology.* 2005;234:189–196.

Cowey Cl, Fielding JR, Rathmell WK. The loss of radiographic enhancement in primary renal cell carcinoma tumors following multitargeted receptor tyrose kinase therapy is an additional indicator of response. *Urology.* 2010;75:1108–1116.

Davenport M, Caoili EM, Cohan RH, et al. MR and CT Characteristics of successfully ablated renal masses status-post radiofrequency ablation. *AJR Am J Roentgenol.* 2009;192:1571–1578.

Fournier LS, Oudard S, Thiam R, et al. Metastatic renal carcinoma: evaluation of antiangiogenic therapy with dynamic contrast-enhanced CT. *Radiology.* 2010;256:511–518.

Ghavamian R, Klein KA, Stephens DH, et al. Renal cell carcinoma metastatic to the pancreas: clinical and radiological features. *Mayo Clin Proc.* 2000;75(6):581–585.

Howard SAH, Karjewski KM, Thornton E, et al. Decade of molecular targeted therapy: abdominal manifestations of drug toxicities—what radiologists should know. *AJR Am J Roentgenol.* 2012;199:58–64.

Kawamoto S, Solomon SB, Bluemke DA, et al. Computed tomography and magnetic resonance imaging appearance of renal masses after radiofrequency ablation and cyroablation. *Semin Ultrasound CT MR.* 2009;30:352–358.

Lall CG, Patel HP, Fujimoto S, et al. Making sense of postoperative CT imaging following laparoscopic partial nephrectomy. *Clin Radiol.* 2012;67:675–686.

McGahan JP, Ro KM, Evans CP, et al. Efficacy of transhepatic radiofrequency ablation of renal cell carcinoma. *AJR Am J Roentgenol.* 2006;186:S311–S315.

Ng CS, Loyer EM, Iyer RB, et al. Metastases to the pancreas from renal cell carcinoma: findings on three-phase contrast enhanced helical CT. *AJR Am J Roentgenol.* 1999;172:1555–1559.

Sirous R, Henegan JC, Zhang X, et al. Metastatic renal cell carcinoma imaging evaluation in the era of anti-angiogenic therapies. *Abdom Radiol.* 2016;41:1086–1099.

Smith AD, Lieber ML, Shah SN. Assessing rumor response and detecting recurrence in metastatic renal cell carcinoma on targeted therapy: importance of size and attenuation on contrast enhanced CT. *AJR Am J Roentgenol.* 2010;194:157–165.

Smith AD, Shah SN, Rini BI, et al. Morphology, attenuation, size and structure (MASS) criteria: assessing response and predicting clinical outcome in metastatic renal cell carcinoma on antiangiogenic target therapy. *AJR Am J Roentgenol.* 2010;194:1470–1478.

Thian Y, Gutzeit A, Koh DM, et al. Revised Choi imaging criteria correlate with clinical outcomes in patients with metastatic renal cell carcinoma treated with sunitinib. *Radiology.* 2014;273:452–461.

Tsivian M, Kim CY, Caso JR, et al. Contrast enhancement on computed tomography after renal cryoablation: an evidence of treatment failure? *J Endourol.* 2012;26:330–335.

Rare Primary Renal Neoplasms

Dunnick NR, Hartman DS, Ford KK, et al. The radiology of juxtaglomerular tumors. *Radiology.* 1983;147:321–326.

Hua F, Shao QQ, Li HZ, et al. The clinical characteristics of metanephric adenoma: a case report and literature review. *Medicine.* 2016;95:1–3.

Raman SP, Hruyban RH, Fishman EK. Beyond renal cell carcinoma: rare and unusual renal masses. *Abdom Imaging.* 2012;37:873–884.

Secondary Renal Neoplasms

Choyke PL, White EM, Zeman RK, et al. Renal metastases: clinicopathologic and radiologic correlation. *Radiology.* 1987;162:359–363.

Cohan RH, Dunnick NR, Leder RA, et al. Computed tomography of renal lymphoma. *J Comput Assist Tomogr.* 1990;14:933–938.

Ganeshan D, Iyer R, Devine C, et al. Imaging of primary and secondary renal lymphoma. *AJR Am J Roentgenol.* 2013;201:W712–W719.

Sheth S, Alis S, Fishman E. Imaging of renal lymphoma: patterns of disease with pathologic correlation. *Radiographics.* 2006;26:1151–1568.

Wilbur AC, Turk JN, Capek V. Perirenal metastases from lung cancer: CT diagnosis. *J Comput Assist Tomogr.* 1992;16:589–591.

Renal and Perirenal Mesenchymal Tumors

Israel GM, Bosniak MA, Slywotzky CM, et al. CT differentiation of large exophytic renal angiomyolipomas and perirenal liposarcomas. *AJR Am J Roentgenol.* 2005;179:769–773.

Katabathina VS, Vikram R, Nagar AM, et al. Mesenchymal neoplasms of the kidney in adults: imaging spectrum with radiologic-pathologic correlation. *Radiographics.* 2010;30:1525–1540.

Mohler JL, Casale AJ. Renal capsular leiomyoma. *J Urol.* 1987;38:853–854.

Park SM, Park YS, Kim JK, et al. Solitary fibrous tumor of the genitourinary tract. *AJR Am J Roentgenol.* 2011;196:W132–W137.

Radvany MG, Shanley DJ, Gagliardi JA. Magnetic resonance imaging with computed tomography of a renal leiomyoma. *Abdom Imaging.* 1994;19:67–69.

Rumancik WM, Bosniak MA, Rosen RJ, et al. Atypical renal and pararenal hamartomas associated with lymphangiomyomatosis. *AJR Am J Roentgenol.* 1984;142:971–972.

Westphalen A, Yeh B, Qayyum A, et al. Differential diagnosis of perinephric masses on CT and MRI. *AJR Am J Roentgenol.* 2004;183:1697–1702.

Renal Pelvic Tumor

Dillman JR, Caoili EM, Cohan RH. Multi-detector CT urography: a one-stop renal and urinary tract imaging modality. *Abdom Imaging.* 2007;32:519–529.

Pediatric Renal Cancers

Cox SG, Kilburn T, Pillay K, et al. Magnetic resonance imaging versus histopathology in Wilms tumor and nephroblastomatosis: 3 examples of noncorrelation. *J Pediatr Hematol Oncol.* 2014;36:e81–e84.

Farmakis SG, Siegel MJ. Rhabdoid tumor: an aggressive renal medullary tumor of childhood. *J Comput Assist Tomogr.* 2015;39:44–46.

Kembhavi SA, Qureshi S, Vora T, et al. Understanding the principles in management of Wilms' tumour: can imaging assist in patient selection? *Clin Radiol.* 2013;68:646–653.

Ko SM, Kim MJ, Im YJ, et al. Cellular mesoblastic nephroma with liver metastasis in a neonate: prenatal and postnatal diffusion-weighted MR imaging. *Korean J Radiol.* 2013;14:361–365.

McDonald K, Duffy P, Chowdhury T, et al. Added value of abdominal cross-sectional imaging (CT or MRI) in staging of Wilms' tumours. *Clin Radiol.* 2013;68:16–20.

Renal Inflammatory Disease

7

Inflammatory disease involving the kidney can be divided into two broad groups: (1) glomerulonephritis, which involves an immunologic injury of the glomerulus, and (2) interstitial nephritis, which is the effect of an infectious or toxic agent on the renal parenchyma. Radiologic studies play a limited role in the diagnosis and management of glomerulonephritis (see Chapter 8). Interstitial nephritis is divided into two major subgroups: (1) noninfectious interstitial nephritis, which is usually caused by the action of toxic agents on the kidney, and (2) infectious interstitial nephritis, which is the result of the action of a pathogen. In most cases, infectious interstitial nephritis is caused by a bacterial organism and is called *acute pyelonephritis*. This chapter will concentrate on renal infections.

BACTERIAL INFECTIONS

Pathophysiology

Urinary infections are extremely common. Most are limited to the bladder, but in a minority of cases, bacterial infection involves the renal parenchyma, causing acute pyelonephritis. In patients younger than 50 years of age, bacterial infections of the kidney are much more common in women than in men, presumably because of the relatively short length of the female urethra. Beyond this age, however, the incidence of urinary tract infection in men increases, often as a result of urinary stasis caused by bladder outlet obstruction from benign prostatic hypertrophy. Bacteria in the urine are not completely evacuated during micturition and remain in the bladder where they cause cystitis.

Bacteria most commonly reach the kidney through the ureter as a result of ascending infection from the lower urinary tract. In children, this usually occurs as a result of vesicoureteral reflux; in adults, however, frank reflux is uncommon, and bacteria are thought to ascend to the kidney through the ureter against the antegrade flow of urine. Much less commonly, bacterial infections are spread to the kidney hematogenously. Gram-negative enteric pathogens, including *Escherichia coli*, *Proteus mirabilis*, *Pseudomonas aeruginosa*, and *Klebsiella* spp., are responsible for the vast majority of bacterial renal infections.

Patients often present with fever, flank or abdominal pain, chills, and other systemic symptoms such as nausea, vomiting, and malaise. These symptoms occur in patients with upper urinary tract infection and help to differentiate them from those infections involving only the lower urinary tract. In most cases, symptoms, clinical signs, and laboratory studies permit a confident diagnosis, and imaging is not needed. There is usually a prompt response to appropriate antibiotic therapy.

Acute bacterial pyelonephritis involves infiltration of the renal interstitium with neutrophils. The kidney becomes edematous; and small microabscesses may form. The process may be unilateral or bilateral and focal or widespread; its distribution is usually patchy, so that involved areas are interspersed with zones of unaffected renal tissue. Although most cases of renal infection produce changes in the renal parenchyma, occasionally just the walls of the ureter and collecting system are involved (pyelitis or pyeloureteritis), producing edema, inflammation, and radiologically visible thickening. Uncommonly, there may be coalescence of the small microabscesses with consequent tissue liquefaction, so that an acute renal abscess appears. During abscess formation, fibroblasts migrate into the area of inflammation to build a wall between the normal parenchyma and the necrotic tissue. This "walling-off" process is characteristic of chronic abscesses, and the remainder of the renal parenchyma returns to normal. If the abscess breaks through the renal capsule, a perinephric abscess is formed. In patients with pyelonephritis and ureteral obstruction sufficiently severe that the affected kidney is oliguric or anuric, the collecting system becomes filled with pus (obstructive pyonephrosis). If pyelosinus extravasation occurs, a perinephric abscess may be formed by this mechanism as well.

Imaging Approach to Renal Inflammatory Disease

In most cases of urinary tract infection, imaging is not indicated. But if there is incomplete or slow response to therapy, multiple repeated infections, immune compromise (especially due to diabetes mellitus), or history of any condition, which may have altered urinary tract anatomy (surgery, vesicoureteral reflux, stones), renal imaging studies are often required for diagnosis and management. The rationale for performing an imaging study is not only to diagnose acute pyelonephritis but also to look for an underlying anatomic abnormality that may have predisposed the patient to the infection, to search for a calculus or an obstruction that may prevent a rapid therapeutic response, or to diagnose a complication of the infection such as a renal or perinephric abscess. If the investigation is confined to those patients whose fever does not lyse within 72 hours of appropriate antibiotic therapy, the proportion of patients with findings that have immediate clinical significance increases significantly.

Contrast-enhanced computed tomography (CT) or CT urography (CTU) is the imaging study of choice for the diagnosis of acute pyelonephritis or to look for a potential complication of the infection such as a renal or perinephric abscess or emphysematous pyelonephritis.

Conventional gray scale ultrasound detects most instances of abscess, obstruction, and stones in infected patients and sometimes can suggest pyonephrosis by detecting small particles in infected urine but may fail to detect these abnormalities if they are minor or if the patient is difficult to examine. Sonography is less sensitive than CT in revealing foci of inflamed renal parenchyma, although its accuracy can be improved with ultrasound contrast agents. The modality is safe and relatively inexpensive and can diagnose most of the abnormalities that require specific treatment and thus remains a commonly used technique for patients with renal infection.

Other imaging studies are of value in selected patients. Magnetic resonance imaging (MRI) may demonstrate infected regions of the renal parenchyma to enhance abnormally and to have restricted diffusion and can demonstrate obstruction and abscesses but often fails to reveal small stones; the technique should be reserved for patients who cannot undergo contrast-enhanced CT examinations. Retrograde pyelography may serve as both diagnostic and planning maneuvers in patients with obstructive pyonephrosis who are to be treated with ureteral stents or percutaneous nephrostomy tubes, respectively. Voiding cystourethrography is used to demonstrate vesicoureteral reflux but is performed only rarely in adults.

In children with multiple urinary tract infections, the classic imaging approach involves searching for reflux and other bladder and urethral abnormalities with voiding cystourethrography. Demonstration of reflux often leads to a search for renal infection and scars with renal scintigraphy (usually with technetium-99m

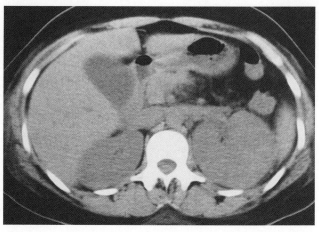

FIGURE 7.1. Acute pyelonephritis. An unenhanced CT demonstrates diffuse parenchymal swelling.

dimercaptosuccinic acid [99mTc-DMSA]) and/or renal gray scale and Doppler ultrasound. There is a growing tendency to use a "top-down" approach to imaging, in which renal abnormalities are sought with ultrasound or scintigraphy, and efforts to diagnose reflux are reserved for patients with renal findings that suggest it. Professional society guidelines are not unanimous on this issue.

Acute Pyelonephritis

The imaging examination providing the most complete information regarding the nature and extent of the inflammatory process is contrast-enhanced CT. Unenhanced scans may be normal or show only renal enlargement (Fig. 7.1); there may be perinephric stranding from inflammation or edema (Fig. 7.2), and Gerota's fascia may be thickened. After intravenous contrast administration, areas of decreased contrast enhancement appear (Figs. 7.2 and 7.3). These regions may be inhomogeneous or striated and their distribution is variable. They may be solitary or multiple and unilateral or bilateral and may involve little or most of the renal parenchyma. The distribution is typically patchy. Diffuse homogeneous involvement of the renal parenchyma is rare and is likely to appear only when there is ureteral obstruction. If delayed scans are obtained, the abnormal areas may reveal a dense nephrogram, which persists

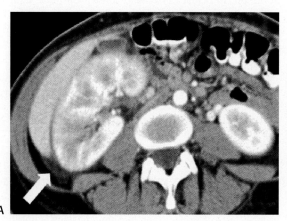

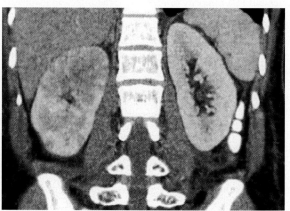

FIGURE 7.2. Acute pyelonephritis. **A:** There is inflammation in the fat posterolateral to the right kidney (*arrow*); the right kidney is enlarged, and there are patchy regions of diminished and heterogeneous enhancement of the cortex. **B:** A coronal projection from an enhanced CT in another patient. Patchy opacification is seen in the right kidney.

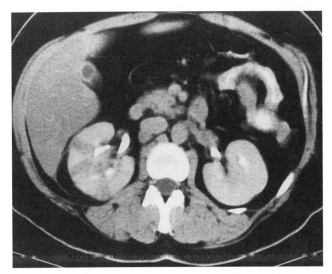

FIGURE 7.3. Acute pyelonephritis. Relatively narrow striated areas of decreased enhancement are seen in the right kidney.

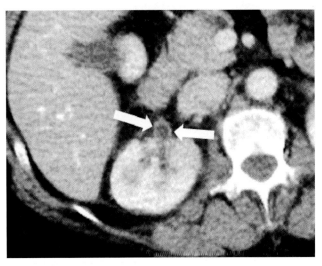

FIGURE 7.5. Pyelitis. The wall of the right renal pelvis (*arrows*) is thickened.

after the normal parenchyma has lost its enhancement (Fig. 7.4). Differential diagnosis of regions of diminished or inhomogeneous enhancement may include acute ischemia or contusion; if there is focal swelling, a focus of acute pyelonephritis may resemble an infiltrating tumor (tumefactive pyelonephritis). Clinical data often permit a specific diagnosis. Acute ischemia may be indicated by the peripheral rim sign or visible vascular abnormalities and produce fewer changes than pyelonephritis in the perinephric fat. The pyelitis which sometimes accompanies renal infection may be reflected by thickening of the walls of the collecting system (Fig. 7.5).

The appearance of pyelonephritis on CT may be modified by antibiotic therapy. Partially treated patients may demonstrate a rounded or ovoid area of decreased enhancement with poorly defined margins (Fig. 7.6). Long-term follow-up studies in patients with mild disease may show a return to normal renal morphology and enhancement (Fig. 7.7). With more severe disease, focal atrophy may appear at the sites of previous infection

(Fig. 7.8) and there may be focal calyceal clubbing, suggestive of papillary necrosis. The etiology of these morphologic changes has been postulated to involve ischemic insult to the kidney as a result of the inflammatory process. Ultrasound in patients with acute uncomplicated pyelonephritis may be normal or show diffuse or focal renal enlargement with regions of increased or decreased echogenicity of the renal parenchyma (Fig. 7.9). Perinephric inflammation may produce a thin layer of extracapsular fluid adjacent to the infected portions (Fig. 7.10). The normal corticomedullary differentiation may be lost. Doppler ultrasound may reveal focal regions of abnormal perfusion (Fig. 7.9); although there is hyperemia of the affected regions, the normal renal parenchymal flow is so high that the infected regions may have less flow than surrounding normal tissue, perhaps due to elevated interstitial pressure from edema.

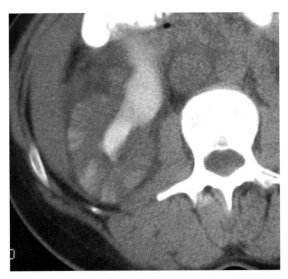

FIGURE 7.4. Acute pyelonephritis; delayed CT. The abnormal regions are revealed by wedge-shaped regions of retained parenchymal contrast.

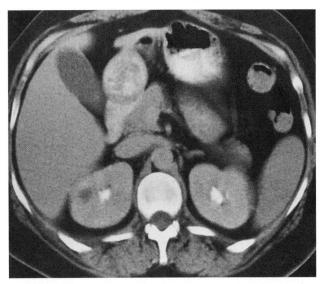

FIGURE 7.6. Atypical appearance produced by treated pyelonephritis. CT shows a rounded area of decreased enhancement in the right kidney without significant mass effect; this is in contrast to the striated areas more typical of untreated acute pyelonephritis.

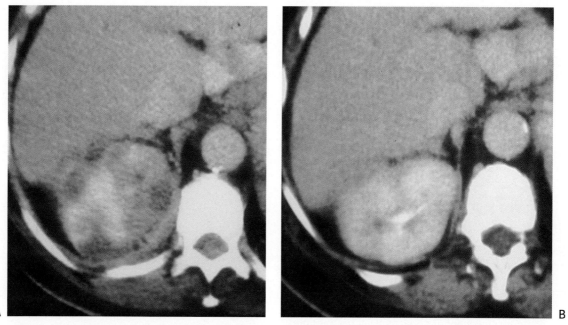

FIGURE 7.7. Acute pyelonephritis. **A:** Before treatment, the kidney is severely affected, with regions of markedly reduced enhancement. **B:** After treatment, morphology and enhancement are normal.

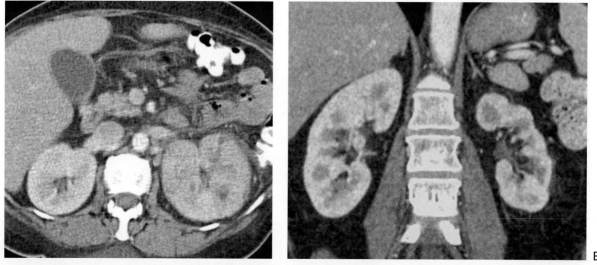

FIGURE 7.8. Acute pyelonephritis. **A:** Before treatment, the left kidney is swollen and has a diminished inhomogeneous nephrogram. **B:** Several months after treatment, the left kidney is smaller than normal and has focal cortical scars.

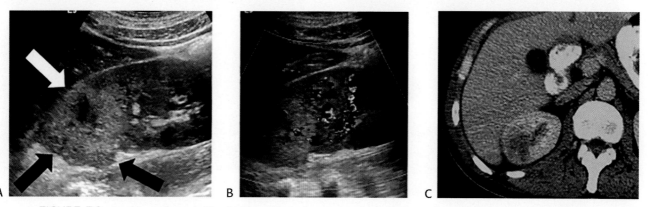

FIGURE 7.9. Acute pyelonephritis. **A:** The affected upper pole is abnormally echogenic (*arrows*). **B:** The abnormal region reveals diminished Doppler flow when compared to the normal parenchyma. **C:** CT confirms focal pyelonephritis.

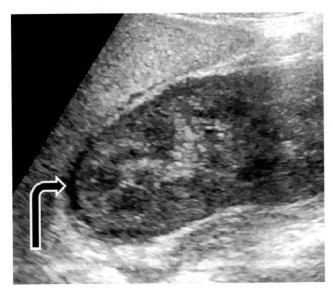

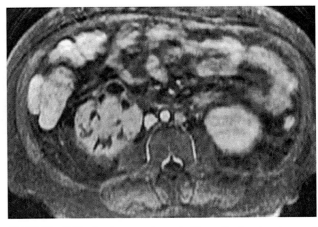

FIGURE 7.12. Acute pyelonephritis. Contrast-enhanced T1-weighted image with fat saturation reveals regions of poor or absent perfusion in the right kidney.

FIGURE 7.10. Acute pyelonephritis. There is a thin layer of pericapsular fluid (*arrow*).

The MRI findings are morphologically similar to those seen on CT and reflect swelling, altered perfusion, and focal areas of diminished enhancement (Fig. 7.11). Diffusion-weighted images reveal restricted diffusion in the affected portions (Fig. 7.11) and may be more sensitive than either T2-weighted or contrast-enhanced T1-weighted images (Fig. 7.12) for detecting regions of pyelonephritis.

Radionuclide imaging in patients with acute pyelonephritis has been reported using renal cortical imaging agents, such as 99mTc-DMSA, and agents that image inflammation, such as gallium (67Ga) citrate. Renal cortical imaging studies may show an inhomogeneous distribution of the radionuclide within the affected kidney or polar defects with asymmetric tracer uptake.

Chronic Pyelonephritis

The term *chronic focal atrophic pyelonephritis* applies to renal parenchymal scarring in which the cortex and medulla are focally thinned and the underlying calyces are blunted. This appearance may have a number of causes, including vesicoureteral reflux, calyceal stones, or severe focal pyelonephritis (Figs. 7.8B and 7.13). Once the scars have appeared, the gross pathologic and radiologic appearance of the affected kidney does not allow determination of the cause; microscopy reveals focal fibrosis in all cases. If the etiology is known to be vesicoureteral reflux, the term *reflux nephropathy* is used. It is thought that as urine refluxes during bladder contractions, the hydrostatic pressure in the collecting system rises transiently, and the urine, which is often infected, flows retrograde into the collecting tubules of the kidney (pyelotubular backflow or reflux). Such intrarenal reflux occurs in a patchy distribution, possibly because of local differences in the papillary openings of the collecting ducts of the renal medullae, which in turn is probably responsible for the focal nature of the resultant scarring. Within the scarred regions, dense fibrous tissue replaces normal nephrons (Fig. 7.14).

Calyceal stones, possibly by causing elevated calyceal pressure due to infundibular obstruction or by acting as foci of infection, frequently cause calyceal clubbing and scars that are indistinguishable from reflux nephropathy (Fig. 7.15). When chronic pyelonephritic scarring is found in middle-aged or elderly patients, stones are most likely to be the cause; in children, reflux has usually produced the

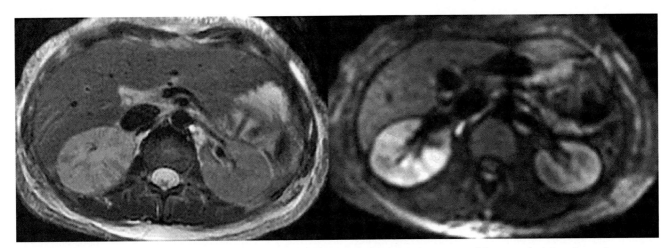

FIGURE 7.11. MRI of acute pyelonephritis. T2-weighted image **(left)** shows overall increase in intensity and a striated pattern in the infected right kidney. Diffusion-weighted image **(right)** reveals restricted diffusion in the same distribution.

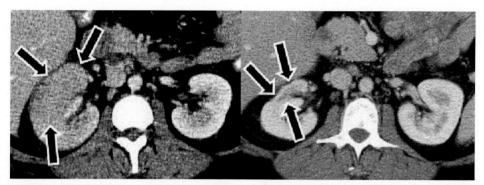

FIGURE 7.13. Acute pyelonephritis. The *arrows* indicate the affected region, which is swollen and displays diminished enhancement. Scar after treatment **(left)**. The renal parenchyma in the affected region (*arrows*) is atrophic and enhances less than normal parts of the kidneys **(right)**.

scars. Focal infarction may produce similar scars; however, calyceal blunting is less likely to be found in this condition. Trauma, including surgery, and radiation therapy, which includes portions of the kidney (Fig. 7.16), may also produce scars.

The radiologic findings of chronic pyelonephritis on CT, CTU, and MRI include the demonstration of one or more parenchymal scars (Fig. 7.17) overlying a deformed calyx. If parenchymal loss has been severe, focal areas of compensatory hypertrophy may be seen adjacent to the areas of cortical scarring. These may mimic solid parenchymal tumors but can be distinguished from tumors by observing that when contrast is administered, they enhance to the same degree as adjacent normal parenchyma.

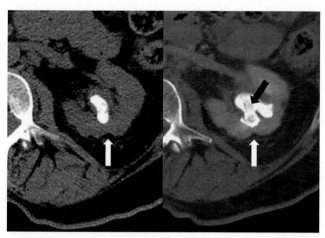

FIGURE 7.15. A calyceal stone is visible in a noncontrast CT **(left)**. Parenchymal scars (*white arrows*) are seen without contrast and in a CT urogram **(right)**. The urogram shows the stone as a filling defect (*black arrow*) in the opacified collecting system; the calyces are blunted.

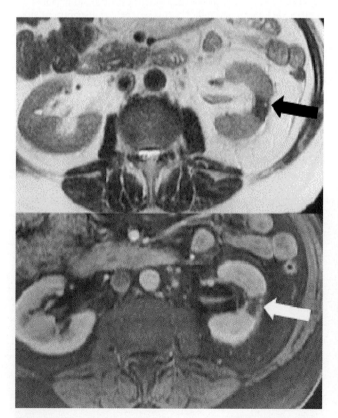

FIGURE 7.14. Chronic atrophic pyelonephritis. T2-weighted image **(top)** and T1-weighted gadolinium-enhanced fat-saturated image **(bottom)** reveal focal region of parenchymal thinning (*arrows*) representing a fibrotic scar.

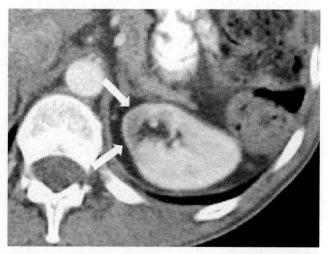

FIGURE 7.16. Radiation-induced scar. The medial aspect of the kidney (*arrows*) was included in a radiation therapy field several years earlier and is now atrophic and has diminished opacification.

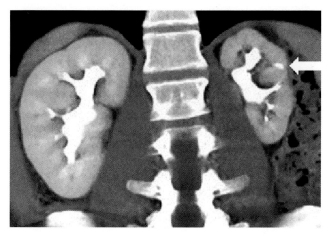

FIGURE 7.17. Chronic focal atrophic pyelonephritis due to childhood reflux. The left kidney is small and demonstrates focal parenchymal loss (*arrow*) with a blunted calyx.

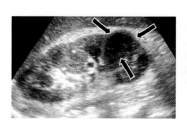
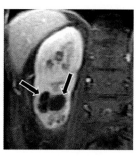

FIGURE 7.18. Renal abscess (*arrows*). The ultrasound **(left)** reveals a moderately thick wall, sparse internal echoes, and enhanced through-transmission. Gadolinium-enhanced MRI **(right)** shows a septum between two compartments of the abscess and an indistinct wall.

Ultrasound changes in patients with chronic atrophic pyelonephritis include focal loss of parenchyma, which can be appreciated on longitudinal or cross-sectional images. Increased echogenicity in the area of the scar may also be demonstrated. The central renal sinus echoes may extend to the periphery of the kidney in the area of abnormality. In contrast to other causes of generalized increased cortical echogenicity, the process appears focal.

Acute Renal Abscess

Renal abscesses form as a result of the coalescence of microabscesses that are often present in acute pyelonephritis. The predominant organisms responsible for abscesses are gram-negative enteric species. Patients with diabetes mellitus, drug abuse, vesicoureteral reflux, or renal calculus disease are most susceptible to abscess formation. Acute abscesses may be solitary or may form simultaneously in multiple locations in the kidney. Multiple lesions are less common and suggest hematogenous dissemination.

The signs and symptoms of an acute renal abscess are difficult to distinguish from those of pyelonephritis, and the diseases often coexist. Fever, leukocytosis, pyuria, and flank pain are common in both. There is frequently a history of prior antibiotic therapy with recrudescence of symptoms on cessation of treatment. Renal abscesses appear as a continuum of conditions. Acute pyelonephritis may progress to a cluster of small abscesses, which may or may not coalesce, so that there may be a single fluid-filled cavity, a multiloculated cavity, or a phlegmonous region in which a network of solid tissue planes separate multiple small abscesses. When fibroblasts migrate into the area of an acute renal abscess and form a barrier between the abscess and the remainder of the kidney, a chronic renal abscess is formed. This may result in a transition zone of inflammatory tissue between the liquid center of the abscess and the normal renal parenchyma.

On sonography, abscesses appear as relatively sonolucent lesions with differing amounts of solid tissue echoes; the pus may contain low-amplitude echoes (Fig. 7.18) and there may be gas bubbles. There is usually enhanced through-transmission of the ultrasound beam. Doppler studies show no flow in the necrotic pus-filled regions; the amount of flow in the wall is variable.

CT is the imaging study of choice for the diagnosis of an acute renal abscess. The lesion is a low-attenuation (10 to 20 HU) rounded or ovoid mass that does not enhance with contrast administration (Fig. 7.19). As a result of the surrounding inflammatory process, the borders of the mass are usually indistinct; the degree

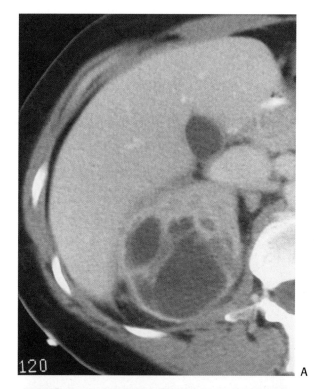

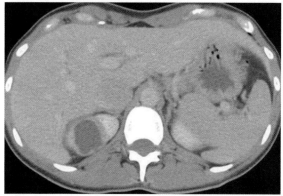

FIGURE 7.19. Two cases of renal abscess. **A:** Acute renal abscess. The cavity is multiloculated. **B:** Chronic renal abscess. There is a zone of inflammatory tissue between the liquid center and the normal renal parenchyma.

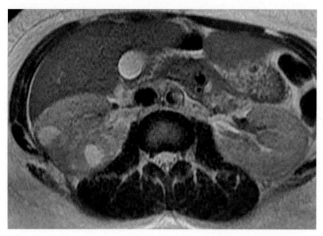

FIGURE 7.20. Renal abscess. In this T2-weighted image, the pus in the two cavities in the right kidney appears bright.

of enhancement of the abscess wall is variable. The presence of gas within a pocket of fluid is virtually pathognomonic of an abscess. There is usually thickening of Gerota fascia, and increased density may be found in the adjacent perinephric and mesenteric fat. The abscess may or may not extend into the perinephric space. MR findings reflect those seen on CT. The center of the abscess has the characteristics of fluid, and the periphery of the lesion, which is of varying thickness, enhances to varying degrees (Figs. 7.19 and 7.20). Radionuclide scanning with technetium-labeled DMSA is occasionally used but has largely been replaced by CT.

Perinephric Abscess

A primary perinephric abscess forms when intrarenal infection breaks through the renal capsule into the perinephric space (Fig. 7.21); a perinephric abscess may also form as a result of obstruction with extravasation of infected urine. Secondary perinephric abscesses may form when infection spreads to the perinephric space hematogenously from an external source or from

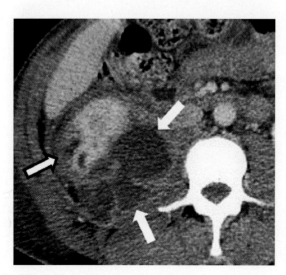

FIGURE 7.21. Multiloculated perinephric abscess (*solid white arrows*). The abscess developed when phlegmonous pyelonephritis (*bordered arrow*) eroded into the perinephric space.

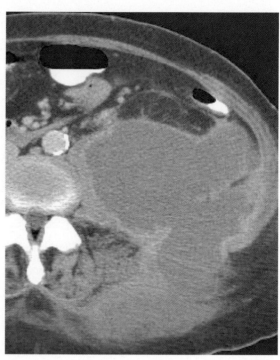

FIGURE 7.22. Left perinephric abscess. The pus-filled cavity involves the psoas muscle and eroded through the posterior abdominal muscular wall.

acute inflammation of an adjacent organ or from perforation of adjacent bowel such as a ruptured appendix or diverticulitis.

The signs and symptoms of a perinephric abscess are nonspecific. In most cases, symptoms of urinary tract infection have been present for periods longer than 2 weeks. Fever is usually intermittent and low grade, and a minority of patients have normal urinalysis. The development of a perinephric abscess as a complication of renal inflammatory disease is more common in patients with large staghorn calculi, pyonephrosis, diabetes mellitus, or a neurogenic bladder. Air secondary to gas-forming organisms is found in a number of large perinephric abscesses. Percutaneous drainage with image guidance is the preferred treatment if the lesion is large; small renal abscesses may be successfully treated by intravenous antibiotics alone.

On ultrasonography, perinephric abscesses appear as masses of variable echogenicity adjacent to the kidney. Any gas within the abscess will demonstrate acoustic shadowing, but when the abscess is anterior to the kidney, gas may be confused with intestinal gas.

The imaging study of choice for the detection of perinephric abscess is CT. The abnormality is usually visible even on unenhanced studies, but abscesses are most easily detected after intravenous contrast administration. The strength of CT is its ability to define precisely the boundaries of the process, so that extension into the psoas muscle (Fig. 7.22), the posterior pararenal space, and the true pelvis may be accurately detected. Like an intrarenal abscess, a perinephric abscess may demonstrate an enhancing rim on CT or MR.

Pyonephrosis

The term *pyonephrosis* refers to a pus-filled obstructed renal collecting system. The clinical seriousness of the condition varies, but when severe, it constitutes a true urologic emergency; if untreated, it may lead to sepsis and death. Most patients with pyonephrosis have clinical evidence of urinary tract infection.

Calculi are the cause of the associated urinary tract obstruction in a majority of cases; metastatic disease, postoperative ureteral strictures, and processes such as retroperitoneal fibrosis account for the remainder.

Plain abdominal radiographs demonstrate obvious urinary tract calculi in approximately one-half of the patients. Sonography may differentiate pyonephrosis from sterile hydronephrosis by demonstrating echoes in the collecting system lumen (Fig. 7.23), which either may diffuse or may appear as dependent layers of debris. In cases of emphysematous infection, echogenic gas bubbles with shadowing may be seen within the pus.

On CT, a grossly dilated collecting system that contains a urine–debris level or an air–fluid level suggests the diagnosis (Fig. 7.24). CT usually shows evidence of hydronephrosis (Fig. 7.25) and generally demonstrates the cause and level of the associated obstruction.

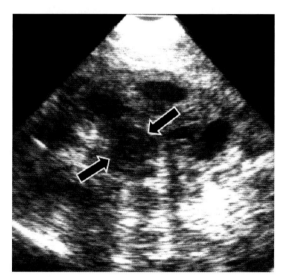

FIGURE 7.23. Obstructive pyonephrosis. The calyces are dilated, and the renal pelvis (*bordered arrows*) contains faint echoes produced by purulent debris.

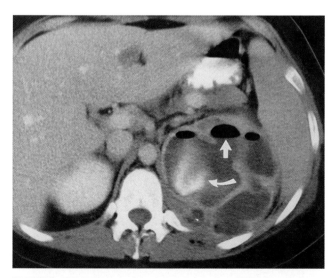

FIGURE 7.24. Pyonephrosis. A grossly dilated collecting system with some contrast medium excretion (*curved arrow*) and an air–fluid level (*arrow*) are present.

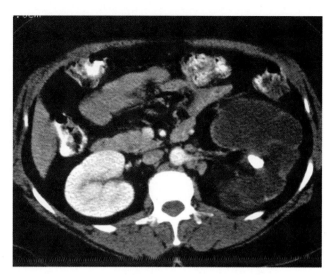

FIGURE 7.25. Pyonephrosis. Severely hydronephrotic left kidney secondary to a calculus obstructing the renal pelvis.

Although rare, layering of contrast medium above purulent material in the collecting system allows a specific diagnosis of pyonephrosis. Percutaneous aspiration of infected urine using radiologic guidance is the definitive diagnostic study in suspected pyonephrosis. Treatment requires drainage by nephrostomy or ureteral stenting along with antibiotics. If percutaneous nephrostomy is performed, care should be taken not to distend the collecting system by injecting contrast because patients may develop serious complications from the procedure including frank sepsis and septic shock.

Gas-Forming Renal Infections

Emphysematous pyelonephritis is an unusual, often severe, variant of upper urinary tract infection in which gas formed by the infecting bacteria appears in the renal parenchyma, adjacent tissues, or collecting system. Patients usually have poorly controlled diabetes mellitus and hyperglycemia. They may also have ureteral obstruction, as emphysematous pyelonephritis may be a complication of pyonephrosis. Patients are usually severely and acutely ill and may have shock and uremia; women are more often affected than men. The pathogen is usually a gram-negative bacterium; *E. coli* is most common, followed by *Klebsiella*, *Aerobacter*, and *Proteus*.

The classic therapy has involved urgent nephrectomy; it was felt that surgery was necessary to prevent a very high mortality from the disease. More recently, it has become apparent that some patients can be treated with antibiotics and drainage of any closed, pus-containing cavity. For cases with ureteral obstruction, percutaneous nephrostomy should be performed (although some urologists will prefer to place ureteral stents), and any abscess should be drained percutaneously. This regimen permits many affected patients to have their infection successfully treated, retain their kidneys, and regain renal function.

The gas may be demonstrated by radiography, CT, or ultrasound; since CT can best delineate the anatomic distribution of the gas, the other signs of infection, and the site and etiology of any ureteral obstruction, it is the best modality for this condition. The gas may appear in a variety of amounts and distribution. It may be present within the collecting system, where it is termed *emphysematous pyelitis* and is usually an indication of less severe disease (Fig. 7.26), or in the perirenal and pararenal spaces, and may occasionally dissect a considerable distance from the kidney (Fig. 7.27). In the parenchyma, it may appear bubbly or in a striated pattern (Fig. 7.28). Any combination of these patterns may appear; rarely, the condition is bilateral. Gas may dissect within the wall

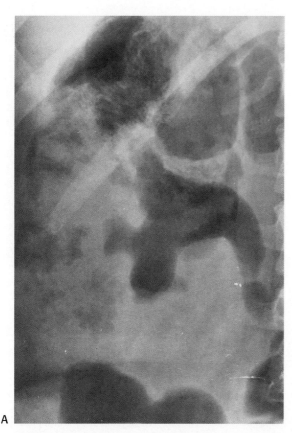

A

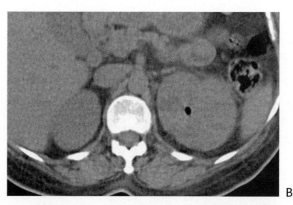

B

FIGURE 7.26. Two cases of emphysematous pyelitis. **A:** Radiograph showing air within renal collecting system and proximal ureter; there is also bubbly air in the renal parenchyma. (Courtesy of David S. Hartman, M.D. and the Armed Forces Institute of Pathology.) **B:** CT with a calyceal air bubble.

of the collecting system and may be present in renal and perirenal abscesses. Although some investigators have found that the anatomic extent of the gas correlates with the severity of the clinical outcome, others have found that the clinical condition is a better predictor of outcome than the amount or distribution of gas.

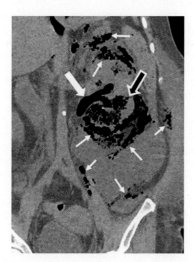

FIGURE 7.27. Emphysematous pyelonephritis with widespread dissection of infection. Noncontrast CT shows air in the parenchyma (*bordered arrow*) and the collecting system (*large white arrow*) widely distributed in the retroperitoneum (*small arrows*).

Renal Fistula

Air or gas in the ureter and collecting system is uncommon. In addition to the emphysematous infections described above, surgery and intubation may introduce air, as may trauma and fistulae to the intestinal tract. Renal fistulae to the alimentary tract are rare. They may result from Crohn disease, from tumors in the kidney or the

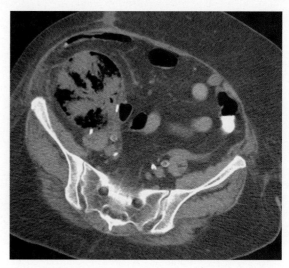

FIGURE 7.28. Severe emphysematous pyelonephritis in a transplanted kidney. There is air throughout the parenchyma.

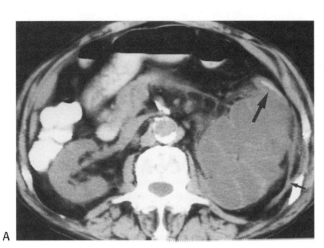 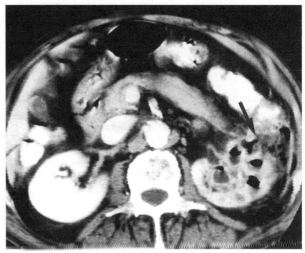

FIGURE 7.29. Renocolic fistula. **A:** Initial CT demonstrates a large hydronephrotic left kidney that displaces and compresses the left colon (*large arrow*). Thickening of Gerota's fascia (*small arrow*) is also present. **B:** Repeat CT demonstrates decompression of the hydronephrosis with air in the collecting system as a result of fistulization to the left colon (*arrow*). (From Parvey HR, Cochran ST, Payan J, et al. Renocolic fistulas: complementary roles of CT and direct pyelography. *Abdom Imaging.* 1997;22:96–99, with permission).

gastrointestinal tract, or from severe renal trauma. Most commonly, however, renal fistulae occur as a result of renal inflammatory disease. Usually, fistulae develop between the kidney and the colon (Fig. 7.29), but the duodenum, stomach, and distal small bowel may also be involved. The site of the fistula is principally determined by the anatomic proximity of the organ to the kidney. Renal fistulae to the skin, pleura, and lung have also been described.

Renal fistulae occur in the setting of renal or perinephric abscesses or pyonephrosis, often complicated by calculi. In the older literature, renal tuberculosis was described as the causative factor in 25% of the cases; it may still be a relatively common factor in undeveloped parts of the world. Although CT will generally be the first study obtained in such patients, it will rarely demonstrate the fistula directly. Indirect signs, such as gas within the collecting system, may be found, but the diagnosis of renal fistula often requires retrograde or antegrade pyelography because the severe inflammatory disease requisite for the development of the fistula will preclude sufficient contrast material excretion for visualization on CTU.

Xanthogranulomatous Pyelonephritis

Xanthogranulomatous pyelonephritis (XGP) is a relatively uncommon form of renal inflammatory disease. It is characterized histologically by the presence of lipid-laden macrophages (xanthoma cells), as well as by other inflammatory cells including plasma cells, leukocytes, and histiocytes. The signs and symptoms of the disease are nonspecific and usually long-standing; fever, malaise, flank pain or tenderness, weight loss, and leukocytosis are the most common presenting complaints. Lower urinary tract symptoms (frequency, dysuria) are present in only one half of patients. Anemia is present in 70% of patients; approximately 25% of patients demonstrate abnormalities in liver function tests; and about 10% of patients have underlying diabetes mellitus. Rarely, XGP may present as a fulminant illness and may be accompanied by an acute renal abscess. Total or partial nephrectomy is the usual treatment. Some series report a female preponderance in XGP as high as 4:1. Although most patients range from 45 to 65 years of age, patients as young as 5 years have been reported. Active urinary tract infection with *E. coli, P. mirabilis, Klebsiella,* or *P. aeruginosa* alone or in combination is present in virtually every case.

XGP probably represents an uncommon reaction by the kidney to a long-standing purulent infection. This is most commonly chronic obstructive pyonephrosis, which is often due to a calculus, but less commonly may be secondary to a congenital ureteropelvic junction obstruction or a ureteral tumor. It may also be seen in patients with long-standing renal abscesses.

The classically described triad of findings includes (1) a staghorn calculus, (2) absent or diminished excretion of contrast medium, and (3) a poorly defined renal mass. Radiography often demonstrates the calculus. Retrograde pyelography may be performed to demonstrate the point of obstruction (Fig. 7.30). The calyces may be grossly irregular, with evidence of superimposed papillary necrosis.

Sonography usually demonstrates diffuse renal enlargement with a central echogenic focus representing the stone. The renal parenchyma demonstrates a diffuse hypoechoic pattern that corresponds to the areas of inflammatory reaction or abscess. In some cases, however, the infected parenchyma may produce an echo pattern similar to that produced by normal renal parenchyma and is a source of potential confusion. The calyces may be seen as multiple fluid-filled regions with echo-producing debris, indistinguishable from pyonephrosis.

Although the CT findings in XGP are not specific for the disease, they usually strongly suggest the correct diagnosis (Fig. 7.31). The kidney is usually enlarged but retains its reniform shape. The renal pelvis is characteristically poorly defined or normal in size, unless there is concomitant ureteropelvic junction obstruction. One or more calculi are generally present, and there may be small flecks of parenchymal calcification. There are often low-density areas at the periphery of the kidney representing atrophic parenchyma; cortical columns of Bertin may separate low-attenuation central areas representing dilated calyces filled with pus and necrotic material. Contrast-enhanced scans demonstrate hyperemia at the periphery of the kidney, around the calyces, and in the renal fascia. Extension to the perinephric space, the posterior pararenal space, the psoas muscles, or the muscles of the back is well demonstrated by CT.

The most common form of XGP results in diffuse involvement of the affected kidney. In an unusual form of XGP, the inflammatory process is limited to a portion of the kidney. This is sometimes referred to as the "tumefactive" form of XGP, and the findings can be confused with those of a poorly enhancing renal tumor (Fig. 7.32). The majority of cases of both forms of XGP demonstrate extensive perinephric inflammation.

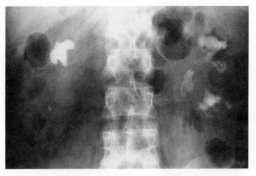

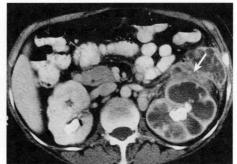

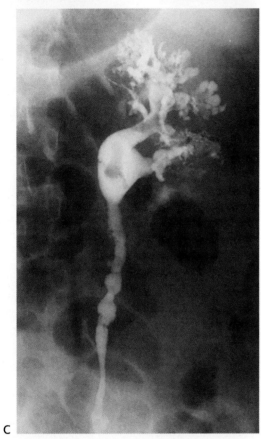

FIGURE 7.30. Xanthogranulomatous pyelonephritis. **A:** Radiography demonstrates bilateral staghorn calculi. **B:** CT demonstrates hydronephrosis and stones with extension of the inflammatory process to the perinephric space (*arrow*). **C:** Retrograde pyelogram demonstrates filling defects in the renal pelvis and calyces from the calculi and gross papillary necrosis.

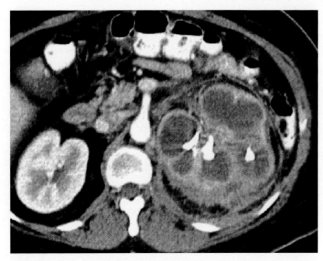

FIGURE 7.31. Xanthogranulomatous pyelonephritis. The left kidney is hydronephrotic, contains several stones, and is surrounded by perinephric inflammation.

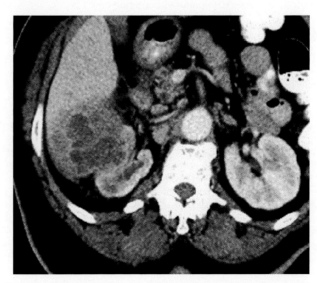

FIGURE 7.32. Tumefactive XGP. The heterogeneous masslike lesion arising from the right kidney was found on resection to be inflammatory and to have the characteristic lipid-laden macrophages of XGP.

RENAL TUBERCULOSIS

Although there has been a decline in the incidence of pulmonary tuberculosis in nonimmunosuppressed patients, the incidence of extrapulmonary tuberculosis has remained unchanged. New cases continue to be diagnosed in the United States, particularly among immigrant populations. A history of tuberculosis in another site—often the thorax—is usually present, but that site may be inactive at the time of presentation with renal involvement.

Renal tuberculosis results from hematogenous dissemination of *Mycobacterium tuberculosis* from a distant site. Bacilli lodge in the corticomedullary junction of the kidney; the resultant small lesions usually heal without sequela. Although these initial lesions are bilateral in nearly all cases, radiologically visible lesions form in only one kidney. Small caseating granulomas may form and then coalesce into larger cavities. They may or may not be accompanied by calcification. The lesions then progress along the nephron to the papillae; sloughing of caseated tissue then produces papillary necrosis. As the bacteria enter the collecting system, they infect the transitional epithelium, first causing it to become thick and inflamed and then causing it to become scarred and contracted. The same process may then progress to the bladder, which first develops a tuberculous cystitis and then forms scars; these scars may markedly reduce bladder capacity and cause sufficient elevation of bladder pressure or ureterovesical junction strictures that obstruction and hydronephrosis of the previously noninvolved side may appear.

The renal lesions progress slowly, often producing few symptoms until the entire urinary tract is affected, so lower urinary tract symptoms like frequency, dysuria, and nocturia are common presenting complaints; some patients have gross hematuria. Patients often have the classic laboratory finding of sterile pyuria—the presence of white blood cells in the urine with subsequently sterile cultures on conventional culture media.

The radiologic findings in renal tuberculosis depend on the extent of the disease process. In the earliest stages of renal tuberculosis, the tips of the papilla demonstrate a moth-eaten, irregular appearance at urography. As the disease progresses, extensive papillary necrosis may be present with the formation of frank cavities (Fig. 7.33), which may communicate with each other as a result of caseous necrosis within the renal parenchyma. Parenchymal scarring may be present, which may be localized to a single area of the kidney (Fig. 7.34) or may involve the entire kidney. The scars are generally associated with underlying calyceal abnormalities and parenchymal calcifications. Advanced renal tuberculosis presents with a nonfunctioning kidney—the "autonephrectomy" (Figs. 7.35 and 7.36) Extensive parenchymal calcification is typically present in such cases, and there may be regional lymphadenopathy (Fig. 7.34).

A hallmark of renal tuberculosis is the development of multiple, irregular infundibular stenoses or strictures with subsequent hydrocalycosis (Figs. 7.37 and 7.38). These stenoses are the result of fibrosis that accompanies the healing process. When the strictures produce complete occlusion, the entire calyx may be excluded

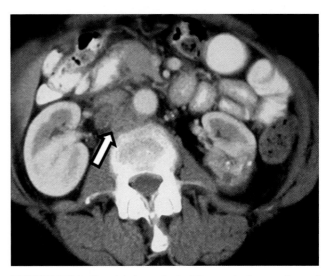

FIGURE 7.34. Renal tuberculosis. The posterior portion of the left kidney is inhomogeneously scarred and has punctate calcifications. There is retrocaval tuberculous lymphadenopathy (*arrow*).

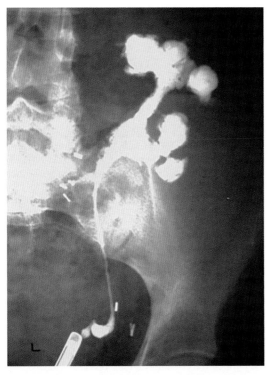

FIGURE 7.33. Renal tuberculosis in a transplanted kidney. Retrograde pyelogram shows papillary necrosis with ragged pyelocalyceal margins. There is also ureteral stenosis.

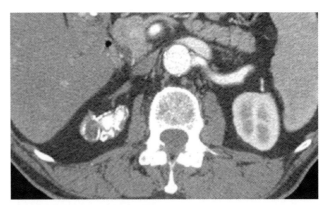

FIGURE 7.35. Tuberculous autonephrectomy. The right kidney is severely shrunken, has extensive amorphous calcification, and does not function.

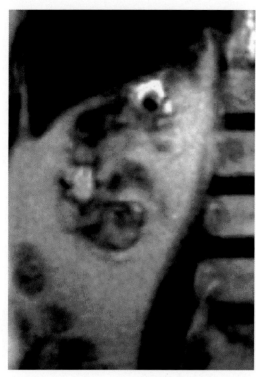

FIGURE 7.36. Tuberculous autonephrectomy. T2-weighted MRI. The kidney is atrophic; the dark areas within it are calcified.

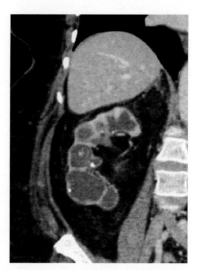

FIGURE 7.38. Tuberculous stricture. The renal pelvis and major infundibuli have been virtually obliterated by strictures; only dilated calyces remain. The renal parenchyma is thinned and there are scattered calcifications.

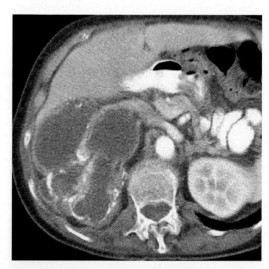

FIGURE 7.39. Renal tuberculosis. A stricture at the right ureteropelvic junction formed while the kidney was still producing urine, leading to severe hydronephrosis. The kidney no longer functions, and there are scattered parenchymal calcifications.

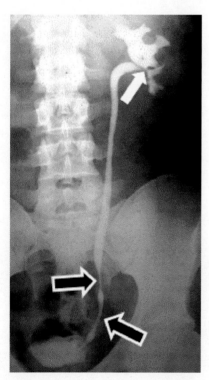

FIGURE 7.37. Tuberculous strictures revealed by retrograde pyelogram. There is a tight renal pelvic stricture (*white arrow*) and less severe distal ureteral strictures (*bordered arrows*).

from the remainder of the collecting system. Similar strictures may involve the renal pelvis and ureter. In end-stage disease, the renal size depends upon the rates of progression of parenchymal destruction and stricture formation; if the former is predominant, a small nonfunctioning kidney may appear (Figs. 7.35 and 7.36), but if renal pelvic or ureteral stenosis progresses while the kidney is still functioning, hydronephrosis may enlarge all or part of the organ (Fig. 7.39).

Descending infection may involve the bladder wall, which first becomes thickened from inflammation; fibrosis may ensue, which diminishes bladder distensibility, sometimes severely (Fig. 7.40). Although upper tract manifestations of tuberculosis are almost always unilateral, this bladder abnormality may cause contralateral ureterovesical junction obstruction.

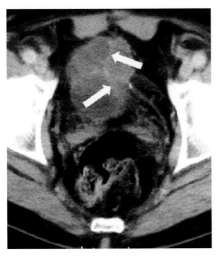

FIGURE 7.40. Tuberculous cystitis. The bladder has been reduced in volume by multiple fibrous bands (*arrows*) due to chronic tuberculosis.

The multiplicity of these findings, and the numerous combinations of them that appear, may make the diagnosis of urinary tract tuberculosis difficult, but there are principles that may aid in differential diagnosis. Papillary necrosis can be caused by a number of entities, but papillary necrosis is not likely to indicate tuberculosis if it appears bilaterally, is not accompanied by caseating cavities or calcification, or creates retained sloughed papillae in the calyces. Renal calcification, which is bilateral or is not accompanied by renal morphologic abnormalities, usually represents stones or nephrocalcinosis, not tuberculosis. "Purse-string" strictures in the renal pelvis, with peripheral calyceal dilatation, are characteristic of tuberculosis. Schistosomiasis may produce bladder and ureteral calcification and ureteral strictures but can usually be distinguished from tuberculosis, as schistosomiasis tends to produce bilaterally symmetrical disease, whereas tuberculosis is usually unilateral, and schistosomiasis abnormalities are usually more severe in the lower ureters and bladder, whereas tuberculosis usually produces abnormalities most severe in the kidneys and collecting systems. Finally, several diseases may produce a unilateral calcified nonfunctioning kidney. A multicystic dysplastic kidney in an adult usually produces a cluster of thin ringlike calcifications in the renal fossa, whereas calcifications from tuberculosis are more amorphous. A calcified renal pelvic stone may be accompanied by a nonfunctioning kidney in cases of severe obstructive atrophy, obstructive pyonephrosis, or XGP, but a calcified stone has a different appearance from the parenchymal and collecting system calcifications of tuberculosis.

UNCOMMON RENAL INFECTIONS

Fungal Infections

Fungal diseases of the kidney develop as opportunistic infections occurring principally in the setting of altered host resistance from conditions such as diabetes mellitus, lengthy use of systemic antibiotics, administration of immunosuppressive and chemotherapeutic agents, acquired immunodeficiency disease, renal transplantation, and chronic catheterization. Renal involvement most commonly occurs with infections secondary to *Candida albicans* or other *Candida* spp. but has been reported in association with *Coccidioidomycosis immitis*, *Cryptococcus neoformans*, *Torulopsis glabrata*, and *Aspergillus fumigatus*. Fungal infections may also complicate conventional gram-negative urinary tract infections.

Candidiasis

Candida is a ubiquitous organism normally found in the pharynx, the gastrointestinal tract, or the vagina. Renal candidiasis is not common and tends to occur in infants and patients with severe immune compromise. Most patients with *Candida* pyelonephritis are diabetic and severely ill with systemic candidiasis. These patients usually have bilateral disease, although occasionally less severe unilateral disease occurs.

The disease produces parenchymal inflammation and multiple abscesses; inflammation of the deep medulla may cause papillary necrosis. Hyphae may proliferate in the collecting systems and form fungus balls, which in turn may obstruct urine outflow and destroy renal function.

Ultrasound typically shows renal enlargement, a general increase and inhomogeneity of parenchymal echogenicity and focal regions of diminished echoes where abscesses have formed. Mycetomas are echogenic but nonshadowing and may form discrete fungus balls (Fig. 7.41) or fill the collecting system as echogenic casts, often with hydronephrosis; occasionally, hyphae in the collecting systems may mimic echogenic debris in the urine. CT also shows the affected kidneys to be enlarged and to have diminished and inhomogeneous parenchymal nephrograms; discrete abscesses may appear as poorly marginated fluid-filled regions (Fig. 7.42). Pyelography may demonstrate hydronephrosis; fungus balls present as lucent filling defects (Fig. 7.43); occasionally, cystography may reveal fungus balls in the bladder. Scalloping of the ureters related to submucosal edema, analogous to the changes in the esophagus produced by oral thrush, has also been reported.

Coccidioidomycosis

Infection with coccidioidomycosis occurs as a result of an active focus of infection elsewhere, usually in the lungs. Renal manifestations including papillary necrosis, cavitation, and parenchymal calcification have all been reported. *Cryptococcus* infection may produce cavitation, papillary necrosis, and multiple parenchymal abscesses.

Brucellosis

Brucellosis of the kidney occurs primarily in meat packers or from the ingestion of unpasteurized milk. The renal infection occurs as

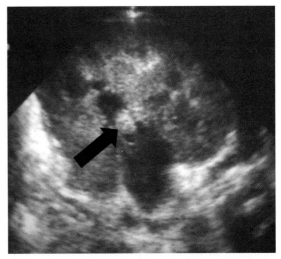

FIGURE 7.41. Renal candidiasis. Ultrasound shows a fungus ball (*arrow*) in the collecting system. The parenchymal echo pattern is heterogeneous, reflecting widespread inflammation and small abscesses.

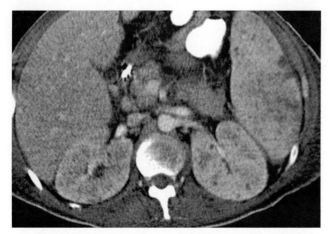

FIGURE 7.42. Extensive renal and splenic candidiasis. Both kidneys and the spleen enhance inhomogeneously; the small lucent portions represent innumerable abscesses.

a result of hematogenous dissemination of the organism. The renal involvement is radiologically similar to that produced by tuberculosis with extensive calcification, cavitation, and infundibular strictures.

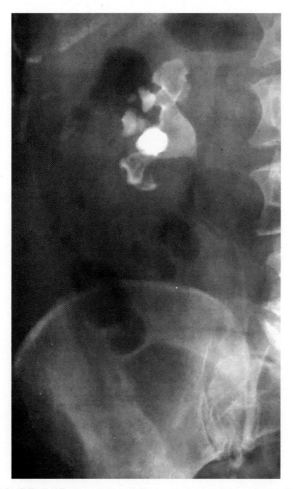

FIGURE 7.43. Renal candidiasis. Retrograde pyelography shows collecting system mycetoma that appears as a lucent filling defect occupying nearly the entire collecting system.

Aspergillosis

Clinical infection with *A. fumigatus* is rare. The fungus may produce renal parenchymal inflammation with large or small abscesses (Fig. 7.44), papillary necrosis, and fungus balls.

Actinomycosis

Actinomycosis of the kidney usually occurs as a result of infection of the gastrointestinal tract that spreads to the kidney through a renoalimentary fistula or by fistulization through the diaphragm from the lung. The causative organism, *Actinomycosis israelii*, although producing mycelial colonies similar to fungi, is actually a bacterium. Infection may result in acute pyelonephritis, pyonephrosis, or a granulomatous renal abscess.

Hydatid Disease

Renal hydatid disease is caused by infestation by a tapeworm, usually *Echinococcus granulosus*. Dogs or other canines constitute the primary host for the disease. The eggs of the worm are swallowed, hatch in the gastrointestinal tract, and then enter the portal circulation, where the oncospheres lodge in multiple organs, mainly the liver and lungs. Renal involvement occurs in only approximately 2% to 3% of patients and may be primary or secondary. Within the kidney, the worms form a characteristic three-layered hydatid cyst that may grow rapidly and destroy the kidney or may progress very slowly, producing minimal clinical symptoms. One or more daughter cysts may form within the mother cyst. Symptoms of renal involvement are nonspecific but include flank pain, renal colic, and eosinophilia. At the time of presentation, the average hydatid cyst is approximately 8 cm in diameter.

All imaging modalities show the lesions to be cystic; they may have curvilinear mural calcification. Ultrasound, CT, and MRI reveal the walls of the daughter cysts; these tend to be within, but at the periphery of, the main (mother) cyst; occasionally, they fill the entirety of the volume of the main cyst. Cyst walls are of various thicknesses and may enhance slightly. Ultrasound may demonstrate internal debris and occasionally shows an inner layer of the wall, which has separated from the wall to form an undulating surface nearer to the center of the cyst. Retrograde urography or CTU may show that the cyst distorts the pyelocalyceal system as any adjacent space-occupying lesion would. Rarely, the cysts rupture into the collecting system; pyelography may reveal the connection. Extensive renal destruction may result in a nonfunctioning kidney. In most cases of renal echinococcosis, hydatid cysts are also seen in the liver.

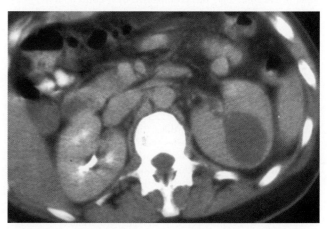

FIGURE 7.44. Renal abscess due to aspergillosis. There is no prominent enhancing ring, but the diminished nephrogram in the left kidney reveals that the organ is diffusely involved.

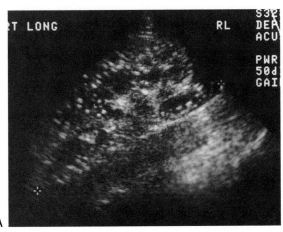 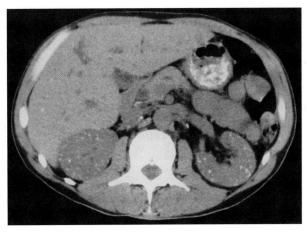

FIGURE 7.45. *Pneumocystis carinii* infection. **A:** Longitudinal ultrasound of the right kidney shows multiple focal areas of increased echogenicity. **B:** Punctate bilateral renal calcification is confirmed by CT. (Courtesy of Alec J. Megibow, M.D.)

The advisability of diagnostic cyst puncture in hydatid disease has been debated for many years. The concern that the puncture will cause spread of the disease to uninfected areas has been raised, and venous intravasation of the cystic fluid has been reported to cause acute anaphylaxis. Yet series have also been published in which aspiration and treatment by sclerosing agents via needle puncture have been successful and safely performed.

SARCOIDOSIS

Sarcoidosis is a systemic inflammatory disease characterized pathologically by noncaseating granulomas. Although most commonly appearing in the thorax, it can involve any organ system. A variety of renal manifestations have been reported including renal masses that mimic lymphoma in appearance. Increased intestinal absorption of calcium, and the resulting hypercalcemia and hypercalcinuria, may lead to nephrolithiasis.

RENAL MANIFESTATIONS OF AIDS

A wide variety of inflammatory abnormalities may be found in the kidneys of patients with acquired immune deficiency syndrome (AIDS). HIV-associated nephropathy appears in about half of patients with advanced disease and pathologically involves focal glomerular sclerosis. The ultrasound findings have predominated in the imaging literature; the kidneys are often enlarged and may be globular in shape, the renal sinus fat is diminished, and the parenchymal echogenicity is increased, sometimes markedly so. The corticomedullary distinction may be increased, decreased, or completely absent. If the condition is long standing, the kidneys may shrink and share the small echogenic kidney appearance of a number of chronic renal parenchymal or small vessel diseases. Patients with HIV have a higher incidence of fungal and bacterial renal infections as well.

Opportunistic Infections

The depletion of T-helper lymphocytes in patients with HIV infection increases the susceptibility to both opportunistic and pyogenic renal infections. Among the opportunistic infections, *Pneumocystis carinii*, although usually thought of primarily as a pulmonary disease, is becoming more common in extrapulmonary sites because of the widespread use of pentamidine inhalers for prophylaxis. The disease may spread by hematogenous and lymphatic dissemination

to a variety of organs, including the kidneys. Punctate renal calcifications (Fig. 7.45) are characteristic of renal involvement but have also been reported in patients with *Mycobacterium avium–intracellulare* (MAI) and cytomegalovirus infection. MAI infection is reported in approximately 5.5% of patients with AIDS. The symptoms of MAI are nonspecific and include fever, generalized lymphadenopathy, and anorexia. Focal echogenic lesions in the kidneys on sonography, as well as the development of renal abscesses, are reported. Disseminated candidiasis may result in acute pyelonephritis, parenchymal microabscesses, and the development of fungus balls. Other opportunistic infections in patients with AIDS include tuberculosis, mucormycosis, and cryptococcosis.

SUGGESTED READINGS

General References/Pathophysiology

Browne RFJ, Zwirewich C, Torreggiani WC. Imaging of urinary tract infection in the adult. *Eur Radiol.* 2004;14(suppl 3):E168–E183.

Goel RH, Unnikrishnan R, Remer E. Acute urinary tract disorders. *Radiol Clin North Am.* 2015;53(6):1273–1292.

Kawashima A, Sandler CM, Goldman SM, et al. CT of renal inflammatory disease. *Radiographics.* 1997;17:851–866.

Kawashima A, Sandler CM, Goldman SM. Current roles and controversies in the imaging evaluation of acute renal infection. *World J Urol.* 1998;16:9–17.

Hammond NA, Nikolaidis P, Miller FF. Infectious and inflammatory diseases of the kidney. *Radiol Clin North Am.* 2012;50(2):259–270.

Parsons CL. Pathogenesis of urinary tract infections. Bacterial adherence, bladder defense mechanisms. *Urol Clin North Am.* 1986;13(4):563.

Talner LB, Davidson AJ, Lebowitz RL, et al. Acute pyelonephritis: can we agree on terminology? *Radiology.* 1994;192:297–305.

Webb JA. The role of imaging in adult acute urinary tract infection. *Eur Radiol.* 1997;7(6):837–843.

Acute Pyelonephritis

Cerwinka WH, Grattan-Smith JD, Jones RA, et al. Comparison of magnetic resonance urography to dimercaptosuccinic acid scan for the identification of renal parenchyma defects in children with vesicoureteral reflux. *J Pediatr Urol.* 2014;10(2):344–351.

Craig WD, Wagner BJ, Travis MD. Pyelonephritis: radiologic–pathologic review. *Radiographics.* 2008;28:255–276.

Dalla-Palma L, Pozzi-Mucelli F, Pozzi-Mucelli RS. Delayed CT findings in acute renal infection. *Clin Radiol.* 1995;50:364–370.

Ditchfield MR, De Campo JF, Cook DK, et al. Vesicoureteral reflux: an accurate predictor of acute pyelonephritis in childhood urinary tract infection? *Radiology.* 1994;190(2):413.

Hammond NA, Nikolaidis P, Miller FH. Infectious and inflammatory diseases of the kidney. *Radiol Clin North Am*. 2012;50(2):259–270.

Hardy RD, Austin JC. DMSA renal scans and the top-down approach to urinary tract infection. *Pediatr Infect Dis J*. 2008;27(5):476–477.

Ishikawa I, Saito Y, Onouchi Z, et al. Delayed contrast enhancement in acute focal bacterial nephritis: CT features. *J Comput Assist Tomogr*. 1985;9(5):89.

Lonergan GJ, Pennington DJ, Morrison JC, et al. Childhood pyelonephritis: comparison of gadolinium-enhanced MR imaging and renal cortical scintigraphy for diagnosis. *Radiology*. 1998;207(2):377–384.

Martina MC, Campanino PP, Caraffo F, et al. Magnetic resonance imaging in acute pyelonephritis. *Radiol Med*. 2010;115(2):287–300.

Rathod SB, Kumbhar SS, Nanivadekar A, et al. Role of diffusion-weighted MRI in acute pyelonephritis: a prospective study. *Acta Radiol*. 2015;56(2):244–249.

Saadeh SA, Mattoo TK. Managing urinary tract infections. *Pediatr Nephrol*. 2011;26(11):1967–1976.

Sakarya ME, Arslan H, Erkoc R, et al. The role of power Doppler ultrasonography in the diagnosis of acute pyelonephritis. *Br J Urol*. 1998;81(3):360–363.

Stunell H, Buckley O, Feeney J, et al. Imaging of acute pyelonephritis in the adult. *Eur Radiol*. 2007;17(7):1820–1828.

Tsugaya M, Hirao N, Sakagami H, et al. Renal cortical scarring in acute pyelonephritis. *Br J Urol*. 1992;69(3):245.

Vivier PH, Sallem A, Beurdeley M, et al. MRI and suspected acute pyelonephritis in children: comparison of diffusion-weighted imaging with gadolinium-enhanced T1-weighted imaging. *Eur Radiol*. 2014;24(1):19–25.

Vourganti S, Agarwal PK, Bodner DR, et al. Ultrasonographic evaluation of renal infections. *Radiol Clin North Am*. 2006;44(6):763–765.

Renal and Perirenal Abscesses

Morgan WR, Nyberg LM Jr. Perinephric and intrarenal abscesses. *Urology*. 1985;26(6):529.

Parvey HR, Cochran ST, Payan J, et al. Renocolic fistulas: complementary roles of computed tomography and direct pyelography. *Abdom Imaging*. 1997;22(1):96–99.

Pyonephrosis

Jeffrey RB, Laing FC, Wing VW, et al. Sensitivity of sonography in pyonephrosis: a reevaluation. *AJR Am J Roentgenol*. 1985;144:71.

Subramanyam BR, Raghavendra BN, Bosniak MA, et al. Sonography of pyonephrosis: a prospective study. *AJR Am J Roentgenol*. 1983;140:991.

Gas-Forming Renal Infections

Roy C, Pfleger DD, Tuchmann CM, et al. Emphysematous pyelitis: findings in five patients. *Radiology*. 2001;218:647–650.

Shokeir AA, El-Azab M, Mohsen T, et al. Emphysematous pyelonephritis: a 15-year experience with 20 cases. *Urology*. 1997;49(3):343–346.

Wan YL, Lee TY, Tsai CC, et al. Acute gas-producing bacterial renal infections: correlation between imaging findings and clinical outcome. *Radiology*. 1996;198:433–438.

Xanthogranulomatous Pyelonephritis

Goldman SM, Hartman DS, Fishman EK, et al. CT of xanthogranulomatous pyelonephritis: radiologic–pathologic correlation. *AJR Am J Roentgenol*. 1984;141:963.

Hayes WS, Hartman DS, Sesterbenn IA. From the Archives of the AFIP: xanthogranulomatous pyelonephritis. *Radiographics*. 1991;11(3):485.

Chronic Pyelonephritis

Cerwinka WH, Grattan-Smith JD, Jones RA, et al. Comparison of magnetic resonance urography to dimercaptosuccinic acid scan for the identification of renal parenchyma defects in children with vesicoureteral reflux. *J Pediatr Urol*. 2014;10(2):344–351.

Oh MM, Jin MH, Bae JH, et al. The role of vesicoureteral reflux in acute renal cortical scintigraphic lesion and ultimate scar formation. *J Urol*. 2008;180(5):2167–2170.

Peters C, Rushton HG. Vesicoureteral reflux associated renal damage: congenital reflux nephropathy and acquired renal scarring. *J Urol*. 2010;184(1):265–273.

Renal Tuberculosis

Gibson MS, Puckett ML, Shelly ME. Renal tuberculosis. *Radiographics*. 2004;24:251–256.

Jung YY, Kim JK, Cho KS. Genitourinary tuberculosis: comprehensive cross-sectional imaging. *AJR Am J Roentgenol*. 2005;184:143–150.

Kollins SA, Hartman GW, Carr DT, et al. Roentgenographic findings in urinary tract tuberculosis. A 10 year review. *AJR Am J Roentgenol*. 1974;121(3):487.

Rui X, Li XD, Cai S, et al. Ultrasonographic diagnosis and typing of renal tuberculosis. *Int J Urol*. 2008;15(2):135–139.

Sallami S, Ghariani R, Hichri A, et al. Imaging findings of urinary tuberculosis on computerized tomography versus excretory urography: through 46 confirmed cases. *Tunis Med*. 2014;92(2):743–747.

Wang Y, Wu JP, Qin GC, et al. Computerised tomography and intravenous pyelography in urinary tuberculosis: a retrospective descriptive study. *Int J Tuberc Lung Dis*. 2015;19(12):1441–1447.

Fungal Infections

Hitchcock RJ, Pallett A, Hall MA, et al. Urinary tract candidiasis in neonates and infants. *Br J Urol*. 1995;76:252–256.

Irby PB, Stoller ML, McAninch JW. Fungal bezoars of the upper urinary tract. *J Urol*. 1990;143:447.

Sadegi BJ, Patel BK, Wilbur AC, et al. Primary renal candidiasis: importance of imaging and clinical history in diagnosis and management. *J Ultrasound Med*. 2009;28(4):507–514.

Wise GJ, Silver DA. Fungal infections of the genitourinary system. *J Urol*. 1993;149:1377–1388.

Zirinsky K, Auh YH, Hartman BJ, et al. Computed tomography of renal aspergillosis. *J Comput Assist Tomogr*. 1987;11:177.

Hydatid Disease

Ishimitsu DN, Saouaf R, Kallman C, et al. Renal hydatid disease. *Radiographics*. 2010;30:334–337.

Pedrosa I, Saiz A, Arrazola J, et al. Hydatid disease: radiologic and pathologic features and complications. *Radiographics*. 2000;20(3):795–817.

Turgut AT, Odev K, Kabaalioglu A, et al. Multitechnique evaluation of renal hydatid disease. *AJR Am J Roentgenol*. 2009;192(2):462–467.

Sarcoidosis

Warshauer DM, Lee JKT. Imaging manifestations of abdominal sarcoidosis. *AJR Am J Roentgenol*. 2004;182:15–28.

Renal Manifestations of AIDS

Di Fiore JL, Rodriguez D, Kaptein EM, et al. Diagnostic sonography of HIV-associated nephropathy: new observations and clinical correlation. *AJR Am J Roentgenol*. 1998;171(3):713–716.

Kay CJ. Renal diseases in patients with AIDS: sonographic findings. *AJR Am J Roentgenol*. 1992;159:551.

Kuhlman JE, Browne D, Shermak M, et al. Retroperitoneal and pelvic CT of patients with AIDS: primary and secondary involvement of the genitourinary tract. *Radiographics*. 1993;11(3):473.

Miller FH, Parikh S, Gore RM, et al. Renal manifestations of AIDS. *Radiographics*. 1993;13:587.

Redvanly RD, Silverstein JE. Intra-abdominal manifestation of AIDS. *Radiol Clin North Am*. 1997;35(5):1083–1125.

Symeonidou C, Standish R, Sahdev A, et al. Imaging and histopathologic features of HIV-related renal disease. *Radiographics*. 2008;28(5):1339.

Renal Failure

RENAL FAILURE

There is no clearly defined set of biochemical or clinical criteria that characterize *renal failure*. Most authors use this term to describe a patient whose renal function is insufficient to maintain homeostasis. The term *renal insufficiency* characterizes a condition in which renal function is abnormal but capable of sustaining essential bodily functions. Uremia, the clinical syndrome that results from renal dysfunction, may be present in untreated patients with both renal insufficiency and renal failure. Uremia may result in symptoms related to a number of different organ systems including the gastrointestinal tract (nausea, vomiting), the cardiovascular system (hypertension, cardiac arrhythmias, pericarditis), the nervous system (personality changes, seizures, somnolence), and the hematopoietic system (anemia, bleeding diathesis). The term *end-stage renal disease* is often used to describe a condition in which chronic renal failure whose renal deterioration is irreversible and requires dialysis or renal transplantation to sustain life.

There are a number of parameters that can be assessed to quantitate particular aspects of renal function. The most frequent with which radiologists deal is the glomerular filtration rate (GFR). This is usually expressed in milliliters per minute (volume of glomerular filtrate created per minute); the normal rate for an average-size adult is about 120 mL/min. The rate varies directly with body size and diminishes normally with age. The most commonly used measure of glomerular filtration is a single determination of serum creatinine (creatinine is freely filtered, but neither secreted nor absorbed by renal tubules). This assessment is not ideal, since glomerular filtration may diminish as much as 50% below normal before serum creatinine rises, and glomerular filtration may change more rapidly than serum creatinine. Normal ranges for serum creatinine differ depending on body size, race, and sex. Determination of actual creatinine clearance rates is difficult, since it requires timed complete urine collections along with urine and serum creatinine levels; certain iodinated contrast agents and radiolabeled compounds can be used for the same purpose; an estimated glomerular filtration rate (eGFR) is sometimes approximated by formulae, such as the Cockroft–Gault method.

The RIFLE criteria divide degrees of renal failure into five clinical categories of increasing severity: **risk** (Cr 1.5X normal, GFR loss >25%, or urine output <0.5 mL/kg/hour × 6 hours), **injury** (Cr 2X normal, GFR loss >50%, or urine output <0.5 mL/kg/hour × 12 hours), **failure** (Cr 3X normal, GFR loss >75%, or urine output <0.3 mL/kg/hour × 24 hours or anuria × 12 hours), **loss** (persistent acute renal failure [ARF] >4 weeks), and **end-stage kidney disease** (complete renal functional loss <3 months).

Acute Renal Failure

ARF is the rapid deterioration in renal function. Classically, the causes of ARF are divided into three broad categories: (1) prerenal, (2) renal, and (3) postrenal.

Prerenal causes are generally associated with volume depletion or renal hypoperfusion and are the most common causes of ARF. Such conditions include shock from sepsis, dehydration, burns, or hemorrhage; congestive heart failure; cirrhosis with ascites; diuretic use; and diabetic ketoacidosis. Acute renal arterial insufficiency or renal vein occlusion may also be responsible.

Renal causes of ARF include damage to any portion of the kidney, including the tubules, the glomeruli, the interstitium, or the small vessels. Acute tubular necrosis (ATN) is among the most common of these causes. Interstitial causes for ARF include acute urate nephropathy, multiple myeloma, and acute interstitial nephritis. Glomerular damage may cause ARF as a result of acute glomerulonephritis, drug toxicity, Goodpasture syndrome, systemic lupus erythematosus, and other causes.

Postrenal ARF refers to the onset of renal failure secondary to acute ureteral or bladder outlet obstruction. Although postrenal causes of ARF account for only about 15% of the cases, this entity is the cause for ARF most frequently sought radiologically, both because acute obstruction represents an easily reversed cause of acute renal dysfunction and because imaging is better able to diagnose obstruction than causes of renal or prerenal failure.

Chronic Renal Failure

The gradual progressive loss of renal function characterizes chronic renal failure. The renal dysfunction is attributable to the loss of functioning renal parenchyma and is usually irreversible. The causes of chronic renal failure are protean, but they may be related to vascular disease (e.g., generalized arteriosclerosis and arterial infarction), intrinsic renal disease (e.g., chronic glomerulonephritis, autosomal dominant polycystic kidney disease, and interstitial nephritis), and systemic disease (e.g., diabetes mellitus and hypertension) or may be the result of long-standing obstruction (e.g., prostate hypertrophy, neurogenic bladder disease, and posterior urethral valves). Severe chronic renal failure often requires dialysis or renal transplantation.

Chronic renal failure, with or without dialysis, is often accompanied by renal osteodystrophy. The imaging findings include osteopenia, bone cysts, subperiosteal bone resorption, and multifocal regions of increased uptake on radionuclide bone scans. There may also be calcification in the soft tissues and in the medium-size arteries more severe than that usually seen in atherosclerosis. The arterial calcification is correlated with an increased risk of the generalized cardiovascular disease, which chronic renal failure confers.

Quantitation of renal size is particularly important in evaluating patients with renal failure. In the absence of renal disease, overall renal volume increases throughout childhood, plateaus in early adult life, diminishes slightly in middle age, and shrinks more rapidly in the elderly. In morphologic examinations, renal volume may be approximated simply by measuring pole-to-pole length. Clearly, direct measurement of renal parenchymal volume by three-dimensional ultrasound, computed tomography (CT), or magnetic resonance imaging (MRI) more accurately assesses functional renal mass and becomes even more accurate if the contents of the renal sinus and the volume of any dilated portions of the collecting system are excluded. Loss of parenchymal mass from any disease is irreversible, and since parenchymal volume is closely related to GFR, quantitation of parenchymal volume is important for prognosis. In some circumstances, renal mass is inversely related to function and prognosis, including the parenchymal hypertrophy that accompanies early diabetic nephropathy, and the progressive increase in renal volume seen in patients with autosomal dominant polycystic disease.

IMAGING STUDIES IN RENAL FAILURE

Plain Radiography

Radiographs can be used to detect obstructing stones (Fig. 8.1), parenchymal calcifications, and renal vascular calcifications and may permit assessment of renal size. They may reveal abnormal gas collections in the patient with urosepsis and allow assessment of the bony pelvis for renal osteodystrophy or metastatic disease.

The Nephrogram

Renal parenchymal opacification (the nephrogram) is almost always reduced during contrast-enhanced CT (much of the investigation of the renal parenchymal enhancement patterns seen in renal failure was originally performed with excretory urography). In both acute and chronic renal failure, the initial opacification of the renal cortex is slowed and diminished as compared with normal, and the washout, or deopacification, occurs at a slower rate than normal. In patients with chronic renal failure, the densest opacification of the cortical or medullary tissue is never as high as that seen in normal patients given the same contrast dose; this is probably due to a diminished GFR and diminished concentrating capacity of the remaining tubules. Patients with ARF share the slowed rate of opacification (Fig. 8.2) and deopacification of renal parenchyma seen with chronic renal failure, but the densest opacification reached is much more variable. In some patients, the

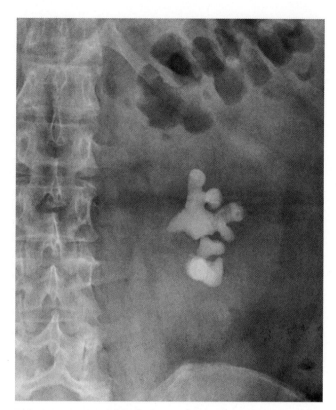

FIGURE 8.1. Staghorn calculus. Plain radiography demonstrates a staghorn calculus.

parenchyma ultimately becomes very densely opacified and, in a few minutes or hours, may become even denser than the maximum normal renal opacification. This nephrogram may involve the cortex only (Fig. 8.3) or both the cortex and the medulla (Fig. 8.4) and is occasionally striated (Fig. 8.5). The mechanism of this dense prolonged nephrogram is not known with certainty. Diminished flow rate of intratubular fluid resulting in abnormally high degrees of absorption of water leading to elevated intratubular contrast concentrations, leak of contrast-containing tubular fluid into the interstitium, and (in cases of acute obstruction) dilatation of the lumina of contrast-containing tubules have all been postulated.

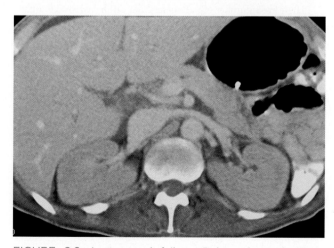

FIGURE 8.2. Acute renal failure. Bolus-enhanced CT in the portal venous phase reveals less than normal cortical enhancement.

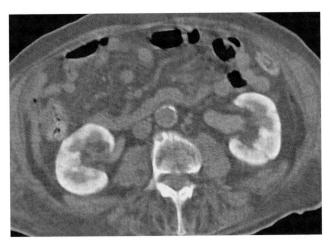

FIGURE 8.3. Acute renal failure. A day after cardiac angiography; the renal cortices remain densely opacified.

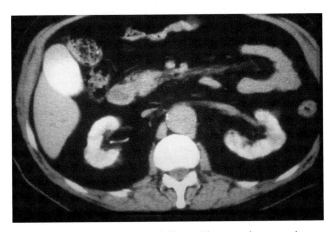

FIGURE 8.4. Acute renal failure. The renal parenchyma remains opacified, and there is vicariously excreted contrast in the gallbladder.

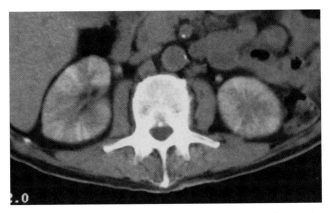

FIGURE 8.5. Acute renal failure. The nephrogram is persistent and striated.

The prolonged dense nephrogram of ARF may be encountered in prerenal, renal, or postrenal failure and is often accompanied by some degree of oliguria. If it is bilaterally symmetrical, it is usually due to shock or ATN. A unilateral prolonged dense nephrogram is usually caused by acute ureteral obstruction—this nephrogram pattern is often called the *obstructive* nephrogram—but occasionally

acute unilateral renal vascular insufficiency, due to conditions such as renal arterial embolization or dissection, or renal vein thrombosis, in which renal blood flow is diminished but not absent, may be causative. A dense prolonged nephrogram is never encountered in patients with chronic renal failure unless there is coexisting ARF.

A bilaterally symmetrical, dense, prolonged nephrogram in a radiograph or CT for which contrast has not been administered has been called a sentinel sign of ARF due to contrast administered for a prior recent examination, such as cardiac angiography. The delayed nephrogram of ARF is not always dense; it may be quite faint and never reach the density of the parenchymal opacification in normal kidneys.

Ultrasound

Ultrasound is the best initial imaging study for the patient with renal failure. In a patient with renal failure, sonography can easily distinguish a patient with normal-size kidneys, who usually has ARF, from one with small kidneys, which generally indicates chronic renal failure (Fig. 8.6). Resistive indices (RIs) are usually elevated in acute and chronic renal failure but are usually normal in patients with prerenal failure. Sonography can also readily identify patients with autosomal dominant polycystic kidney disease and can accurately depict renal calculi as a cause of, or in association with, renal failure.

Ultrasound is effective in screening patients for urinary tract obstruction as the cause of renal failure. Obstructive renal failure is usually chronic in nature and is associated with hydronephrosis and is readily detectable by ultrasound (Fig. 8.7). In patients without known risk factors for urinary obstruction, the incidence of obstructive renal failure is relatively low. The accuracy of ultrasound in screening for chronic renal obstruction is discussed in Chapter 12.

Ultrasound may also provide limited information regarding the nature of the underlying renal disease. Most chronic renal parenchymal diseases result in increased cortical echogenicity (Fig. 8.8). Although such a finding has a high specificity, it has a relatively low sensitivity for detecting renal disease on screening sonography. Increased diffuse renal echogenicity, like diminished parenchymal volume, carries a poor prognosis for recovery of renal function.

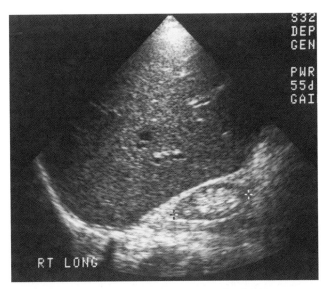

FIGURE 8.6. Chronic renal failure. Longitudinal sonogram of the right upper quadrant demonstrates a small echogenic kidney.

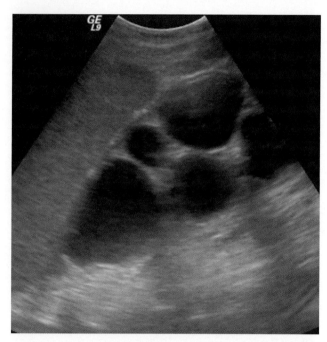

FIGURE 8.7. Hydronephrosis and obstructive atrophy. Longitudinal sonogram of the right kidney shows dilated calyces and thinned renal parenchyma.

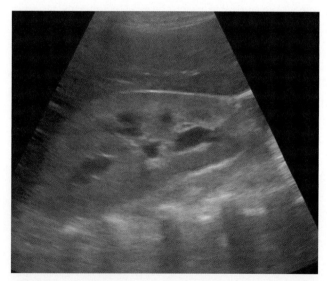

FIGURE 8.8. Chronic renal parenchymal disease. Longitudinal sonogram of the right kidney. The increased echogenicity is specific for identifying abnormal kidneys, but does not permit the diagnosis of the particular disease.

A small number of renal diseases including lymphoma, acute pyelonephritis, and renal vein thrombosis may cause decreased cortical echoes. Gouty nephropathy, medullary nephrocalcinosis, renal tubular acidosis, and medullary sponge kidney may result in increased medullary echogenicity.

Computed Tomography

CT is often used in patients with renal failure when ultrasonography is inconclusive. Even without intravenous contrast administration,

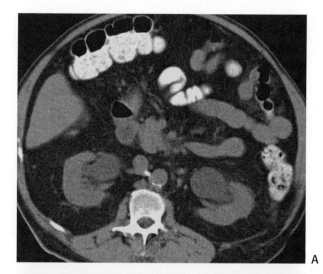

A

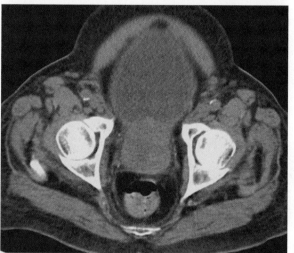

B

FIGURE 8.9. Mild chronic renal failure due to benign prostatic hypertrophy. **A:** Unenhanced CT reveals mild bilateral chronic hydronephrosis. **B:** The prostate is enlarged and the bladder is distended.

CT can detect hydronephrosis and can be useful in delineating the point and nature of an obstruction (Fig. 8.9). CT provides an accurate assessment of renal size and the degree of any cortical atrophy (Fig. 8.10). The degree of cortical atrophy is a good indicator of the amount of irreversible renal functional loss. If contrast is administered despite renal failure, the nephrogram will be faint (Fig. 8.11). Cortical nephrocalcinosis indicates diseases such as Alport syndrome, chronic glomerulonephritis, and oxalosis (Fig. 8.12), which produce renal failure. In some forms of renal cystic disease, CT is the imaging study of choice to detect a complication of the disease process (e.g., hemorrhage complicating adult polycystic disease or the development of a solid renal tumor in patients with acquired cystic disease). Finally, CT is highly sensitive for the detection of renal calculi.

Radionuclide Studies

Because the excretion of radiopharmaceuticals depends on renal function, they cannot be used to evaluate all patients with renal failure. This is particularly the case with technetium-99m diethylenetriaminepentaacetic acid (^{99m}Tc-DTPA), since it is excreted primarily by glomerular filtration. Technetium-99m

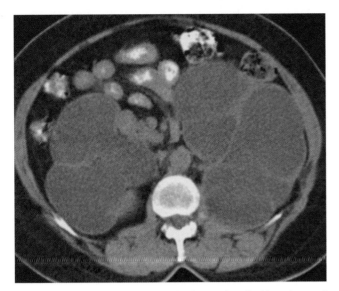

FIGURE 8.10. Severe bilateral hydronephrosis. Unenhanced CT reveals nearly complete loss of renal parenchyma from obstructive atrophy.

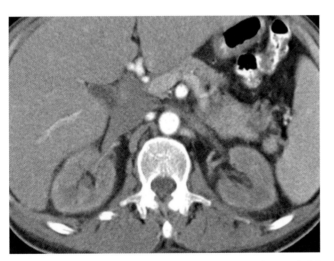

FIGURE 8.11. Chronic renal failure. Contrast-enhanced CT shows only faint enhancement of renal parenchyma.

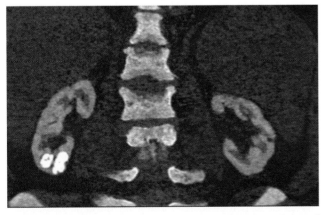

FIGURE 8.12. Oxalosis. Coronal reconstruction of unenhanced CT reveals diffuse renal cortical nephrocalcinosis and right lower pole oxalate stones. (Courtesy of Michael Morris, M.D.)

mercaptoacetyltriglycine (^{99m}Tc-MAG$_3$), however, is excreted by tubular secretion and thus may demonstrate the kidneys even when renal dysfunction is relatively advanced. ^{99m}Tc-MAG$_3$ uptake can be used to estimate function and is useful in predicting how much renal function will remain after a unilateral nephrectomy. ^{99m}Tc-DMSA scans yield similar information. If obstruction is present, a percutaneous nephrostomy tube or ureteral stent should be placed and the kidney allowed sufficient time to recover maximal function before performing a radionuclide scan to estimate residual renal function.

Scintigraphy cannot always identify specific causes of renal failure because many abnormalities of perfusion, parenchymal uptake, and excretion are shared by many diseases. Moderate and severe parenchymal loss can be identified; bilaterally symmetrical parenchymal loss can distinguish small vessel, glomerular, and tubulointerstitial diseases from unilateral disease caused by large vessel diseases, ureteral obstruction, or scarring from stones or reflux. Unilateral persistent intense isotope uptake identifies disease caused by acute ureteral or large vessel obstruction. When bilaterally symmetrical, it is due to shock or acute renal or prerenal failure. Dilated pyeloureteral systems may be visible and indicate ureteral obstruction or severe reflux. Radionuclide determination of the GFR may also be of value.

Magnetic Resonance Imaging

MRI provides useful information in some patients with chronic renal failure. The distinction between the cortex and the less intense medullary pyramids usually seen in T1-weighted images of normal patients often disappears in patients with chronic renal failure, although the loss of the corticomedullary distinction may also occur in normal patients who are well hydrated. Gadolinium enhancement of the parenchyma is reduced in patients with chronic renal failure (Fig. 8.13). The superb anatomic detail afforded by MRI permits assessment of parenchymal volume (Fig. 8.14). Diseases that involve chronic hemolysis, such as hemoglobinopathies, prosthetic heart valves, and paroxysmal nocturnal hemoglobinuria (Fig. 8.15), may cause iron to be deposited in the renal cortex and produce low cortical signal intensity, especially with gradient-echo imaging. Hemochromatosis may produce similar signal loss in the medulla as well as in the cortex.

Angiography

The role of angiography is extremely limited in the diagnostic evaluation of patients with renal failure. Occasionally, the angiographic features of end-stage renal disease will be encountered in patients being evaluated for another purpose. Such features include

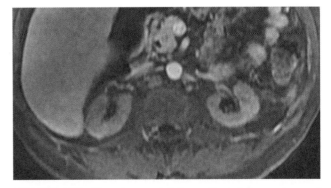

FIGURE 8.13. Chronic renal failure. Gadolinium-enhanced T1-weighted MR image shows markedly diminished cortical enhancement.

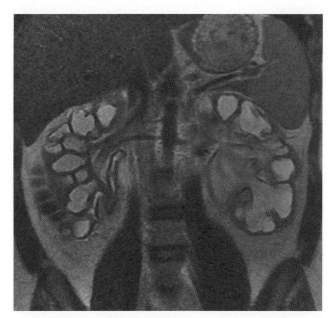

FIGURE 8.14. Reflux nephropathy. T2-weighted MRI shows marked bilateral parenchymal loss from severe vesicoureteral reflux.

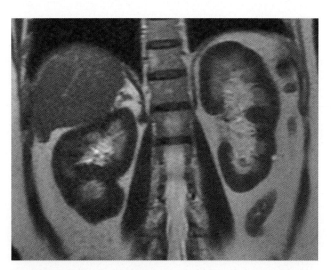

FIGURE 8.15. Paroxysmal nocturnal hemoglobinuria. T2-weighted spin-echo MRI reveals abnormally dark renal cortices because of deposited iron.

a pruned, tortuous appearance of the intrarenal vessels, thinning of the renal cortex, and a slowing of arterial flow within the kidneys. The angiographic nephrogram may have a mottled or lucent appearance. A number of systemic diseases associated with renal failure may demonstrate multiple microaneurysms, including Wegener granulomatosis, polyarteritis nodosa, and systemic lupus erythematosus (see Chapter 10). Renal venography may be used to confirm the diagnosis of renal vein thrombosis if findings on CT or MRI are not definitive.

Pyelography

Antegrade and retrograde pyelography may be useful in establishing the diagnosis of ureteral obstruction as a cause for renal failure (see Chapter 12).

MEDICAL RENAL DISEASE

Diseases of the main renal vessels, and conditions that produce ureteral obstruction or reflux, are causes of renal failure that are dealt with in other parts of this text. Diseases of the renal parenchyma or small vessels may or may not be amenable to differential diagnosis by radiologic examinations. When a specific diagnosis is not possible, they are often referred to as *medical renal disease*. This phrase is frequently used in ultrasound practice for the conditions that produce small kidneys with uniform increased echogenicity, and it is sometimes applied to the conditions that produce uniformly shrunken kidneys seen on CT or magnetic resonance (MR) examinations. These diseases are not amenable to surgical cure and are managed with drugs and diet, but radiologists should be aware that the term *medical renal disease* is not widely used among clinicians to denote any particular group of conditions.

Acute Tubular Necrosis

ATN is the most common form of reversible ARF. It has a wide range of causes including hemolysis, dehydration, hypotension, drugs (such as cisplatin, aminoglycosides, and other antibiotics), heavy metals, and solvent exposure. Despite the long-standing conviction that contrast nephropathy is common, and may lead to chronic renal failure, prolonged hospitalization, and even death, recent investigations have demonstrated that intravenous contrast only rarely leads to nephropathy. ATN is commonly seen after cadaveric renal transplantation. The exact pathogenesis of ATN is poorly understood, but some authorities believe that direct tubular damage is the initiating event and results in filling of the tubular lumen with cellular debris. Others, however, believe that ATN is related to a global decrease in renal blood flow, possibly due to abnormalities of the renin–angiotensin system. Proponents of this theory prefer the term *acute vasomotor nephropathy* because they believe that there is little primary tubular damage and that the renal failure occurs as a result of a redistribution of blood flow within the kidney. Intratubular obstruction is sometimes invoked as a cause of ATN. ARF is a commonly used synonym.

The renal failure may be oliguric or nonoliguric. During the acute phase, azotemia is present, with blood urea nitrogen and creatinine levels peaking in a few days to a few weeks. The return of renal function is typically heralded by the onset of a diuresis.

The kidneys in patients with ATN are often enlarged bilaterally. If contrast is administered, an increasingly dense, persistent nephrogram, as discussed earlier (Figs. 8.3 to 8.5), may appear. The nephrogram may persist for hours or even days after contrast administration. There is typically no opacification of the collecting system, and if a pyelogram does appear, it is usually faint. ARF following strenuous exercise may produce wedge-shaped regions of diminished parenchymal opacification.

A variety of sonographic appearances of ATN have been reported. Some authors have reported an increase in cortical echogenicity with preservation of the corticomedullary definition; others have noted an increase in the echogenicity of the pyramids with a normal cortical appearance, whereas the opposite appearance (i.e., a decrease in the echogenicity and swelling of the pyramids) has been observed by still others. Several studies have suggested that an elevated RI on duplex Doppler imaging is present in a majority of patients with renal failure secondary to ATN and may even precede a rise in creatinine. An elevated RI is less common in patients with prerenal causes.

MRI sometimes demonstrates loss of the normal corticomedullary differentiation often seen in normal kidneys on T1-weighted images. Initial enthusiastic reports that MRI would be helpful in differentiating renal transplant rejection from ATN have not been borne out.

Acute Cortical Necrosis

Acute cortical necrosis is a distinct form of ARF that results in ischemic necrosis of the renal cortex, including the columns of Bertin, whereas the medullary portions of the kidney are relatively spared. The process may occur diffusely throughout both kidneys and may result in complete absence of renal function or may occur in a patchy distribution, resulting in renal insufficiency. In both instances, there is a characteristic sparing of a thin rim of cortical tissue on the outer surface of the kidney because of preservation of the capsular blood supply. A large number of conditions are reported in association with cortical necrosis including burns, sepsis, snake bites, toxins, transfusion of incompatible blood, dehydration, and peritonitis. More than two-thirds of the cases, however, are reported to be associated with pregnancy, especially those complicated by placental abruption, septic abortion, or placenta previa. The precise mechanism by which cortical necrosis occurs remains obscure; a transient episode of intrarenal vasospasm leading to cortical ischemia is a possible mechanism. Other possible explanations include intravascular thrombosis and damage to the glomerular capillary endothelium.

The radiographic findings depend on the stage of the illness. In the early stages of the disease, the kidneys are diffusely enlarged. On contrast-enhanced CT scans, a zone of absent contrast enhancement at the periphery of the kidneys is characteristic (Fig. 8.16), and arteriography will reveal absent cortical perfusion. Over the course of several months, there will be smooth renal shrinking. Characteristically, this will be accompanied by a distinctive form of calcification at the margins of the cortex, including the septal cortex. The appearance of this calcification has been reported as early as 24 days after the onset of the illness, but more characteristically, it is found after several months. On ultrasonography, the outer cortex is hypoechoic before calcification has occurred, a finding that has been reported soon after the onset of the disease.

Acute Interstitial Nephritis

Acute interstitial nephritis may result in renal insufficiency or frank renal failure. Three forms have been described, including that associated with a variety of drugs, nephritis associated with a number of

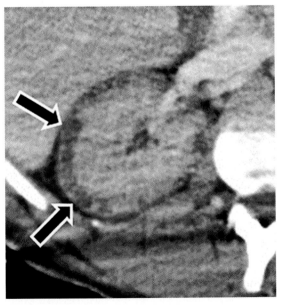

FIGURE 8.16. Acute cortical necrosis. In this contrast-enhanced CT, the medullary regions are enhanced, but there is virtually no enhancement of the renal cortex (*arrows*).

nonrenal infectious processes (e.g., infectious mononucleosis), and idiopathic nephritis. Drug-induced interstitial nephritis is the most common of these. More than 40 compounds, including penicillin, particularly methicillin, rifampin, sulfonamide derivatives, nonsteroidal anti-inflammatory drugs (NSAIDs), cimetidine, furosemide, and thiazide diuretics, have been associated with acute interstitial nephritis. Typically, there is recovery from the renal failure on withdrawal of the drug.

Bilateral nephromegaly with diminished contrast enhancement of the collecting system has been reported. On ultrasound, increased cortical echogenicity and renal enlargement may be found. Increased accumulation of gallium-67 (^{67}Ga) citrate in the kidneys has also been reported.

Hematologic Disorders

Sickle Cell Anemia

A variety of morphologic abnormalities, including bilateral renal enlargement, lobar infarction, and papillary necrosis (Fig. 8.17), have been described in patients with heterozygous and homozygous sickle cell disease. In addition to these structural defects, a number of functional abnormalities including hyposthenuria, hematuria, renal tubular acidosis, and progressive renal insufficiency appear. This constellation of functional abnormalities is known as sickle cell nephropathy.

Papillary necrosis is present in approximately 25% to 40% of patients with homozygous sickle cell disease. The appearance of the radiologic abnormalities, however, does not necessarily correlate with the presence of renal functional abnormalities. Papillary necrosis is thought to occur as a result of low oxygen tension in the renal papilla that promotes sickling of the abnormal red blood cells. This, in turn, results in necrosis and ischemia of the papillary tips. Doppler ultrasound reveals elevated resistive and pulsatility indices in many patients with sickle cell disease or trait. Patients with sickle cell disease occasionally display iron deposition in the renal cortex. Ordinarily, sickle cell disease, thalassemia, and other hemoglobinopathies produce abnormal red blood cells that are sequestered and undergo lysis in reticuloendothelial tissue, so that the deposited iron is seen in the spleen, liver, and lymph nodes; therefore, renal iron deposition more often suggests conditions producing intravascular hemolysis, such as paroxysmal nocturnal hemoglobinuria and certain prosthetic heart valves, or abnormalities of iron metabolism such as primary hemochromatosis. Nevertheless, chronic hemolysis and multiple transfusions may deposit iron in the kidneys in patients with hemoglobinopathies as well.

Hemophilia

A variety of abnormalities including bilateral renal enlargement, retroperitoneal hemorrhage, and obstructive uropathy secondary to blood clots within the collecting system or ureter have been described in patients with hemophilia. Intramural renal pelvic or ureteral hemorrhage may occur, but are rare. The most striking feature, bilateral nephromegaly, is of uncertain etiology. Papillary necrosis, thought to be related to concomitant analgesic ingestion, has also been described.

Acute Leukemia

Leukemia is the most common malignant cause of bilateral nephromegaly in children (Fig. 8.18). The renal enlargement is commonly attributed to infiltration of the kidneys by leukemic cells; however, intrarenal hemorrhage and edema also contribute to this appearance. The degree of renal enlargement may be striking, simulating the appearance of polycystic kidney disease. In some cases, the renal enlargement may be asymmetric, and rarely, it may occur as a focal intrarenal mass (chloroma). The collecting system

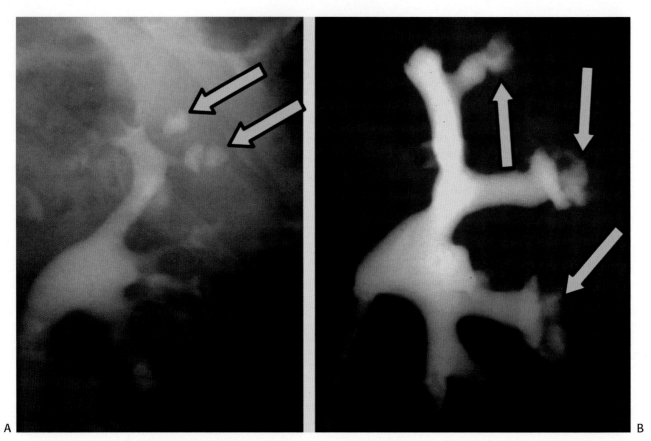

FIGURE 8.17. Two cases of papillary necrosis. Excretory urography **(A)** and retrograde pyelography **(B)** reveal collections of contrast material *(arrows)* in the space left by the sloughed papillary tips.

is generally attenuated, and there may be filling defects in the renal pelvis or calyces secondary to blood clots or uric acid stones.

Multiple Myeloma

Multiple myeloma is one of a group of plasma cell dyscrasias that include Waldenström macroglobulinemia, heavy- and light chain

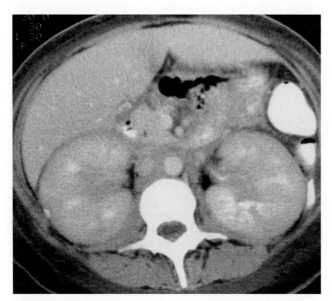

FIGURE 8.18. Leukemic infiltration. Marked nephromegaly is present in this child with leukemic infiltration of the kidneys.

disease, and benign monoclonal gammopathy. The disease results in excess production of immunoglobulins and is characterized by Bence Jones proteins in the urine. Renal failure occurs in 30% to 50% of such patients and has been attributed to the abnormal precipitation of myeloma proteins within the renal tubules, dehydration, or superimposed renal infection. Hypercalcemia, as a result of the bone destruction that accompanies the myelomatous lesions in bone, may result in nephrocalcinosis. Because there is excess uric acid production, uric acid calculi may also be found. Amyloidosis develops in approximately 10% of the patients.

Radiologically, the kidneys are enlarged, and there may be attenuation of the collecting system as the result of interstitial edema. After contrast administration, the density of the nephrogram and excreted urine is diminished. On ultrasonography, the kidneys are enlarged with decreased echogenicity.

The administration of intravenous contrast media to patients with multiple myeloma was thought to be contraindicated because of reports that contrast media caused precipitation of the myeloma proteins within the renal tubules, thereby hastening the onset of renal failure. More recent literature, however, suggests that the risks associated with contrast administration in patients with myeloma are more closely correlated with the status of renal function and can be minimized by hydration.

Amyloidosis

Amyloidosis is characterized by the extracellular deposition of an insoluble fibrillar proteinaceous material often referred to as amyloid fibrils. Although the disease may be localized to one organ, a systemic, multiorgan form of involvement is present in more than 85% of the cases. The disease is known to occur as an idiopathic systemic process (primary amyloidosis); in association with a variety of other chronic diseases including rheumatoid arthritis, tuberculosis, leprosy, chronic osteomyelitis, and some malignancies (secondary amyloidosis); as a familial form including that associated with familial Mediterranean fever; in a senile form; or in association with endocrine disorders, including medullary carcinoma of the thyroid and diabetes mellitus. A specific form of amyloidosis has been recognized that results in a multiarticular arthropathy in patients on long-term hemodialysis.

Virtually every organ in the body may be involved with amyloidosis; men are affected more commonly than women. The usual age of onset is 55 to 60 years. Most patients experience nonspecific symptoms including weight loss, weakness, and fatigue. Renal involvement occurs more frequently in patients with secondary amyloidosis than in those with the primary disease. Fifty percent of patients with secondary amyloidosis die of renal failure. Although the kidneys are the most commonly involved organ in the urinary tract, isolated involvement of the renal pelvis, ureter, bladder, urethra, prostate, retroperitoneum, and seminal vesicles has been described. Amyloidosis of the renal pelvis, without renal parenchymal involvement, may be associated with a characteristic pattern of submucosal calcification. Renal vein thrombosis is a well-described complication of renal amyloidosis and may affect only the segmental or interlobar veins as a unique feature. The sudden onset of the nephrotic syndrome in a patient with amyloidosis should suggest the development of this complication.

The radiologic findings in renal amyloidosis are nonspecific. Although some patients have normal-size kidneys, the most consistently described feature is smooth bilateral renal enlargement. As the disease progresses and renal failure ensues, the kidneys decrease in size while retaining their smooth contour. After contrast administration, the nephrogram is typically diminished, and there may be attenuation of the collecting system. On sonography, there is renal enlargement in the acute phase with an increase in cortical echogenicity (Fig. 8.19), presumably related to the abnormal protein deposition. Angiographic features include tortuosity and irregularity of the interlobar arteries, which may be localized to one portion of the kidney. An abnormal accumulation of ^{67}Ga citrate in the kidneys 48 to 72 hours after injection has been described on radionuclide examination.

Rhabdomyolysis and Myoglobinuria

Rhabdomyolysis, an acute disruption of the structural integrity of skeletal muscle cells, is a frequent complication of trauma. Other causes include thermal or ischemic muscle necrosis, drugs (including heroin, amphetamines, and alcohol), and polymyositis. Such injuries result in an increase in the serum concentration of creatine phosphokinase (CPK) and the excretion of an excessive quantity of myoglobin in the urine. Although myoglobin is considered to

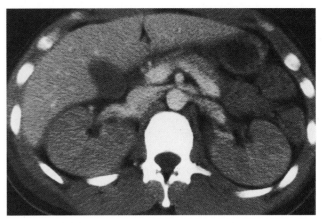

FIGURE 8.20. ARF secondary to rhabdomyolysis. The nephrogram is virtually absent despite excellent enhancement of the renal veins, inferior vena cava, and aorta. (Courtesy of Akira Kawashima, M.S.)

be nephrotoxic, there is a poor correlation between urine myoglobin levels and degree of renal failure. In most instances, the renal failure is transient with the eventual return of normal renal function.

Imaging findings have been reported in a few cases. Nephromegaly with an increasingly dense or striated nephrogram may be found on CT. With more advanced renal failure, severe impairment of contrast excretion may be present (Fig. 8.20).

Acute Urate Nephropathy

Increased nucleoprotein catabolism may occur as a complication of chemotherapy or radiation therapy in patients with leukemia, lymphoma, and other neoplastic disorders. As a consequence, there is a marked increase in plasma uric acid concentration, increased renal tubular secretion, and possibly decreased resorption of the filtered urate load. In such cases, precipitation of urate crystals within the tubules resulting in oliguric renal failure may occur. This form of ARF is termed *urate nephropathy*.

An increasingly dense nephrogram with enlarged kidneys and an absent or markedly diminished pyelogram have been reported (Fig. 8.21). As contrast medium is a known uricosuric agent, precipitation of acute urate nephropathy in patients with high plasma uric acid concentrations may also occur after contrast administration.

Increased medullary echogenicity on ultrasonography has been reported in patients with hyperuricemia and clinical evidence of gout.

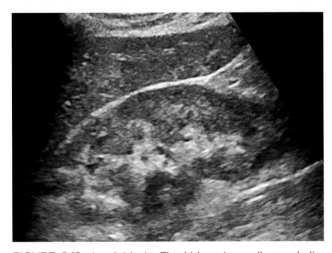

FIGURE 8.19. Amyloidosis. The kidney is swollen and displays increased echogenicity.

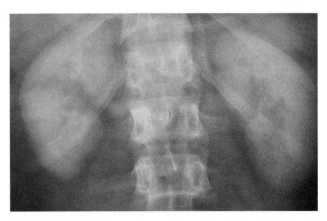

FIGURE 8.21. Acute urate nephropathy. A prolonged and dense nephrogram is seen in this patient with acute urate nephropathy.

Diabetic Nephropathy

Diabetic nephropathy is the most common cause of chronic renal failure in the United States. It is believed to occur as a result of glomerular hyperperfusion that results in glomerular hypertension. This results in an increase in transcapillary pressure and protein leakage into the mesangium, which leads to microalbuminuria and glomerular sclerosis.

The occurrence of diabetic nephropathy is highly correlated with insulin dependence and has recently been correlated with poor glycemic control. The incidence of diabetic nephropathy has declined, as the importance of glucose control has been recognized. The fully developed nephrotic syndrome generally occurs after 15 to 20 years of insulin dependence, with a resultant decrease in GFR heralding the onset of overt renal failure.

Early in the course of diabetes, imaging studies frequently show generalized nephromegaly. In some cases, the nephromegaly may be found before overt glycosuria develops. Although the exact etiology of the renal enlargement is not known, nephron hypertrophy is a possible explanation. Later in the disease process, there is a progressive reduction in renal size and an increase in echogenicity of the renal cortex with preservation of the corticomedullary junction on ultrasonography. With overt renal failure, the kidneys become small, with the echogenicity of the medulla equal to that of the cortex. An elevated RI may be seen in patients with diabetic nephropathy and is a poor prognostic sign.

Human Immunodeficiency Virus Nephropathy

Azotemia, with moderate to severe proteinuria, may occur in patients with human immunodeficiency virus (HIV) infection. A variety of glomerular lesions, including focal and segmental glomerulosclerosis with mesangial deposits of complement C3, immunoglobulin M (IgM), or IgG, as well as tubular atrophy, have been found on histologic examination. Other forms of glomerulopathy have also been described. The combination of renal insufficiency, nephrotic syndrome, and glomerular changes has been called *HIV nephropathy*. Because renal insufficiency may be the first manifestation of HIV infection, the disorder is properly termed *HIV-associated nephropathy* rather than acquired immunodeficiency syndrome (AIDS) associated nephropathy. There is a striking predominance of male African American patients. Modern retroviral therapy has significantly reduced the incidence of this condition.

Ultrasound examinations are normal in approximately 50% of the patients with abnormal renal function, whereas the remainder show increased cortical echogenicity (Fig. 8.22) with normal-size or enlarged kidneys. A decrease in renal sinus fat has also been described.

On CT, global renal enlargement with or without hydronephrosis and cortical scarring has been described (Fig. 8.23). On MRI, nephromegaly with loss of corticomedullary distinction on T1-weighted images has been found, but is a nonspecific finding.

Glomerulonephritis

The various types of glomerulonephritis are important clinically, but cannot be reliably distinguished by imaging. In acute severe glomerulonephritis, the kidneys may be enlarged; the enlargement is symmetrical and smooth. Little has been published about CT in this condition, though based on information from excretory urography, the concentration of contrast in excreted urine may be diminished. There is sometimes an increase in cortical echogenicity on ultrasound. In chronic glomerulonephritis, the kidneys often shrink smoothly and symmetrically, and the parenchyma remains

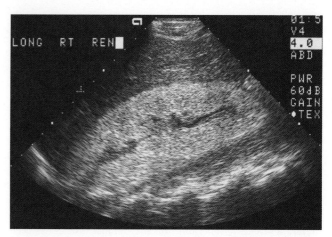

FIGURE 8.22. HIV nephropathy. Ultrasound shows a diffusely echogenic right kidney.

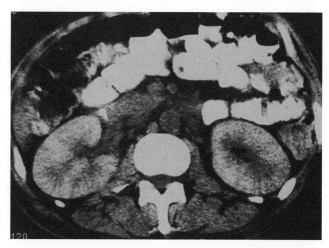

FIGURE 8.23. HIV nephropathy with ARF. CT demonstrates bilateral nephromegaly and a striated persistent nephrogram. Contrast had been administered a day earlier.

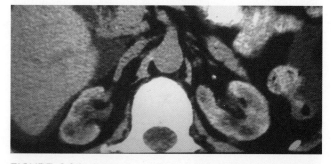

FIGURE 8.24. Cortical nephrocalcinosis from chronic glomerulonephritis. Unenhanced CT demonstrates dense renal parenchyma.

abnormally hyperechogenic. The concentration of excreted contrast and excreted radionuclides is diminished. The small, smooth kidneys of chronic glomerulonephritis cannot be distinguished from the small, smooth kidneys that are the end stage of a number of other generalized renal diseases such as diabetic or hypertensive nephropathy. Some cases progress to cortical nephrocalcinosis (Fig. 8.24).

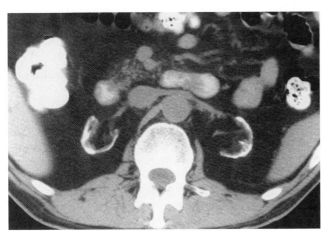

FIGURE 8.25. Alport syndrome. An unenhanced CT demonstrates small kidneys with atrophied and calcified renal cortices.

Alport Syndrome

The association of chronic hereditary renal disease, deafness, and ocular abnormalities is known as *Alport syndrome*. Although both sexes are affected equally, male patients have a much worse prognosis and usually die of renal failure at an earlier age than do female patients. Symptoms begin in early childhood and include episodic hematuria, progressive renal failure, and progressive, high-frequency nerve deafness. Ocular abnormalities include congenital cataracts, nystagmus, and myopia. Although there is typically a strong familial history of renal failure, the precise mode of transmission has not been established. On pathologic examination, the kidneys are small but smooth and exhibit a variety of histologic abnormalities including interstitial fibrosis with patchy glomerular involvement.

Small, smooth kidneys with impaired excretion of contrast medium are found on radiologic examination. Pruning of the interlobar arteries with an indistinct corticomedullary junction has been reported on angiography. Cortical nephrocalcinosis may develop (Fig. 8.25).

Balkan Nephropathy

Balkan endemic nephropathy is a clinical entity resulting in chronic renal failure as a result of interstitial nephritis with a long latency period, which occurs in the localized area of Bulgaria, Romania, and the former Republic of Yugoslavia. Although the precise etiology is unknown, a familial or environmental etiology, or a combination of these two factors, has been suggested. In addition to chronic renal failure, there is a striking increased incidence of renal cell carcinoma and urothelial neoplasms including carcinomas of the renal pelvis or urinary bladder. On ultrasound, small kidneys may be found bilaterally.

Miscellaneous Conditions

Nephromegaly has been reported in a variety of other medical conditions including hepatic cirrhosis, diabetes mellitus, infectious mononucleosis, hyperalimentation, paroxysmal nocturnal hemoglobinuria, acute glomerulonephritis, heroin abuse, and Fabry disease.

SUGGESTED READINGS

General References and Imaging Studies in Renal Failure

Beland MD, Walle NL, Machan JT, et al. Renal cortical thickness measured at ultrasound: is it better than renal length as an indicator of renal function in chronic kidney disease? *AJR Am J Roentgenol.* 2010;195(2):W146–W149.

Cansu A, Kupeli A, Kul S, et al. Evaluation of the relationship between renal function and renal volume-vascular indices using 3D power Doppler ultrasound. *Eur J Radiol.* 2014;83(7):1080–1085.

DiSalvo DN, Park J, Laing FC. Lithium nephropathy: unique sonographic findings. *J Ultrasound Med.* 2012;31(4):637–644.

Dyer RB, Munitz HA, Bechtold R, et al. The abnormal nephrogram. *Radiographics.* 1986;6(6):1039.

Faubel S, Patel NY, Lockhart ME, et al. Renal relevant radiology: use of ultrasonography in patients with AKI. *Clin J Am Soc Nephrol.* 2014;9(2):382–394.

Gupta S, Singh AH, Shabbir A, et al. Assessing renal parenchymal volume on unenhanced CT as a marker for predicting renal function in patients with chronic kidney disease. *Acad Radiol.* 2012;19(6):654–660.

Haufe SE, Riedmuller K, Haberkorn U. Nuclear medicine procedures for the diagnosis of acute and chronic renal failure. *Nephron.* 2006;103(2):c77.

Heine GH, Reichart B, Ulrich C, et al. Do ultrasound renal resistance indices reflect systemic rather than renal vascular damage in chronic kidney disease? *Nephrol Dial Transplant.* 2007;22(1):163–170.

Karivanna SS, Light RP, Agarwal R. A longitudinal study of kidney structure and function in adults. *Nephrol Dial Transplant.* 2010;25(4):1120–1126.

Khati NJ, Hill MC, Kimmel PL. The role of ultrasound in renal insufficiency: the essentials. *Ultrasound Q.* 2005;21:227.

Kim HC, Yang DM, Jin W, et al. Relation between total renal volume and renal function: usefulness of 3D sonographic measurements with a matrix array transducer. *AJR Am J Roentgenol.* 2010;194(2):W186–W192.

Mucelli RP, Bertolotto M. Imaging techniques in acute renal failure. *Kidney Int Suppl.* 1998;66:S102–S105.

Mullerad M, Dastin A, Issaq E, et al. The value of quantitative 99M technetium dimercaptosuccinic acid renal scintigraphy for predicting postoperative renal insufficiency in patients undergoing nephrectomy. *J Urol.* 2003;169:24.

O'Neill WC. B-mode sonography in acute renal failure. *Nephron.* 2006;103:19.

Page JE, Morgan SH, Eastwood JB, et al. Ultrasound findings in renal parenchymal disease: comparison with histological appearances. *Clin Radiol.* 1994;49(12):867–870.

Platt JF, Rubin JM, Bowerman RA, et al. The inability to detect kidney disease on the basis of echogenicity. *AJR Am J Roentgenol.* 1988;151:317.

Rimola J, Martin J, Puig J, et al. The kidney in paroxysmal nocturnal haemoglobinuria: MRI findings. *Br J Radiol.* 2004;77:953.

Ritchie WW, Vick CW, Glocheski SK, et al. Evaluation of azotemic patients: diagnostic yield of initial US examination. *Radiology.* 1988;167:245.

Schein A, Enriquez C, Coates TD, et al. Magnetic resonance detection of kidney iron deposition in sickle cell disease: a marker of chronic hemolysis. *J Mag Reson Imaging.* 2008;28(3):698–704.

Suzukawa K, Ninomiya H, Mitsuhashi S, et al. Demonstration of the deposition of hemosiderin in the kidneys of patients with paroxysmal nocturnal hemoglobinuria by magnetic resonance imaging. *Internal Med.* 1993;32(9):686–690.

Acute Tubular Necrosis

Bahser N, Godehardt E, Hess AP, et al. Examination of intrarenal resistance indices indicate the involvement of renal pathology as a significant diagnostic classifier of preeclampsia. *Am J Hypertens.* 2014;27(5):742–749.

Giustiniano E, Meco M, Morenghi E, et al. May renal resistive index be an early predictive tool of postoperative complications in major surgery? Preliminary results. *BioMed Res Int.* 2014;201:917–985.

Ishikawa I. Acute renal failure with severe loin pain and patchy renal ischemia after anaerobic exercise in patients with or without renal hypouricemia. *Nephron.* 2002;91:559.

Marty P, Szatjnic S, Ferre F, et al. Doppler renal resistive index for early detection of acute kidney injury after major orthopedic surgery: a prospective observational study. *Eur J Anaesthesiol.* 2013;32(1):37–43.

Platt JH, Rubin JH, Ellis JH. Acute renal failure: possible role of duplex Doppler US in distinction between acute prerenal failure and acute tubular necrosis. *Radiology.* 1991;179(2):419.

Acute Cortical Necrosis

Goergen TG, Lindstrom RR, Tan H, et al. CT appearance of acute renal cortical necrosis. *AJR Am J Roentgenol.* 1981;137:176.

Sefczek RJ, Beckman I, Lupetin AR, et al. Sonography of acute renal cortical necrosis. *AJR Am J Roentgenol.* 1984;142:553.

Acute Interstitial Nephritis

Ten RM, Torres VE, Milliner DS, et al. Acute interstitial nephritis: immunologic and clinical aspects. *Mayo Clin Proc.* 1988;63:921.

Hematologic Disorders

Davidson AJ, Choyke PL, Hartman DS, et al. Renal medullary carcinoma associated with sickle cell trait: radiologic findings. *Radiology.* 1995;195(1):83.

Kawashima A, Alleman WG, Takahashi N, et al. Imaging evaluation of amyloidosis of the urinary tract and retroperitoneum. *Radiographics.* 2011;31:1569.

Lande IM, Glazer GM, Sarnaik S, et al. Sickle-cell nephropathy: MR imaging. *Radiology.* 1986;158:379.

Mangano FA, Zaontz M, Pahira JJ, et al. Computed tomography of acute renal failure secondary to rhabdomyolysis. *J Comput Assist Tomogr.* 1985;9(4):777.

Purysko AS, Westphalen AC, Remer EM, et al. Imaging manifestations of hematologic diseases with renal and perinephric involvement. *Radiographics.* 2016;36:1038.

Scott PP, Scott WW Jr, Siegelman SS. Amyloidosis: an overview. *Semin Roentgenol.* 1986;21(2):103.

Taori KB, Chaudhary RS, Attarde V, et al. Renal Doppler indices in sickle cell disease: early radiologic predictors of renovascular changes. *AJR Am J Roentgenol.* 2008;191(1):239–242.

Wheeler DC, Feehally J, Burton P, et al. The kidney in myeloma. *Br Med J.* 1986;292:339.

Acute Urate Nephropathy

Martin DJ, Jaffe N. Prolonged nephrogram due to hyperuricaemia. *Br J Radiol.* 1971;44:806.

Diabetic Nephropathy

Brkljacic B, Mrzljak V, Drinkovic I, et al. Renal vascular resistance in diabetic nephropathy: duplex Doppler US evaluation. *Radiology.* 1994;192(2):549–554.

Buturovic-Ponikvar J, Visnar-Perovic A. Ultrasonography in chronic renal failure. *Eur J Radiol.* 2003;46:115.

Mancini M, Masulli M, Liuzzi R, et al. Renal duplex sonographic evaluation of type 2 diabetic patients. *J Ultrasound Med.* 2013;32(6):1033–1040.

Nosadini R, Velussi M, Brocco E, et al. Increased renal arterial resistance predicts the course of renal function in type 2 diabetes with microalbuminuria. *Diabetes.* 2006;55:234.

Ohta Y, Fujii D, Arima H, et al. Increased renal resistive index in atherosclerosis and diabetic nephropathy assessed by Doppler sonography. *J Hypertens.* 2005;23:1905.

Rodriguez-de-Velascuez A, Yoder IC, Velasquez RA, et al. Imaging the effects of diabetes on the genitourinary system. *Radiographics.* 1995;15:1501.

HIV Nephropathy

Bourgoignie JJ, Pardo V. HIV-associated nephropathies. *N Engl J Med.* 1992;327(10):729.

Coleburn NH, Scholes JV, Lowe FC. Renal failure in patients with AIDS-related complex. *Urology.* 1991;37(6):523.

DiFiori JL, Rodriguez D, Kaptein EM, et al. Diagnostic sonography of HIV-associated nephropathy: new observations and clinical correlation. *AJR Am J Roentgenol.* 1998;171(3):713–716.

Gore RM, Miller FH, Taghmai V. Acquired immunodeficiency syndrome (AIDS) of the abdominal organs: imaging features. *Semin Ultrasound CT MR.* 1998;19(2):175–189.

Hamper UM, Goldblum LE, Hutchins GM, et al. Renal involvement in AIDS: sonographic-pathologic correlation. *AJR Am J Roentgenol.* 1988;150:1321.

Redvanly RD, Silverstein JE. Intra-abdominal manifestations of AIDS. *Radiol Clin North Am.* 1997;35(5):1083–1125.

Alport Syndrome

Chuang VP, Reuter SR. Angiographic features of Alport's syndrome. *AJR Am J Roentgenol.* 1974;121(3):539.

Renal Transplantation

The incidence of end-stage renal disease is rising, and renal transplantation is the most desirable treatment for many of these patients, as it permits homeostasis and a quality of life superior to that achievable by dialysis. More than half of the almost 30,000 organ transplants performed in the United States in 2014 were renal. The two sources of donor kidneys are cadavers and living donors. The shortage of deceased donor kidneys has increased the need for living donors.

The results of renal transplantation are quite good. Currently, 90% to 95% of transplant recipients survive the first year after surgery, and at least 80% of those transplanted kidneys are functioning at that time. Short-term and long-term survival rates of functioning transplanted kidneys correlate positively with meticulous immunosuppression, careful human leukocyte antigen (HLA) matching, the experience of the transplant team, and an ideal recipient age (5 to 50 years). However, even among elderly patients (>70 years), transplantation offers significantly lower mortality than dialysis. The duration of a successful transplant is limited. Despite careful selection and management of patients, only a minority of transplanted kidneys retain useful function longer than 10 years. Patients may receive subsequent grafts after a first one has failed, and the duration of function of the first graft is a useful predictor of the longevity of the next transplantation.

A variety of radiologic procedures are used in the selection of donors and recipients, as well as in the management and detection of posttransplant complications.

PRETRANSPLANT EVALUATION

Living Donor Evaluation

About 20% of transplanted kidneys are obtained from living donors, and most donors are related to the recipients. After appropriate HLA matching is performed, the donor undergoes radiologic evaluation to be sure that the kidney considered for donation does not have a morphologic or vascular abnormality that would contraindicate surgery. The remaining kidney must be sufficiently normal that the donor is not at risk for subsequent renal insufficiency.

Laparoscopic nephrectomy has become the preferred method of harvesting the donor kidney. Since the exposure is limited, it is important to provide an imaging evaluation to guide the procedure. Computed tomography (CT) is the preferred modality due to its high spatial resolution and sensitivity to vascular calcification and renal stones.

Both computed tomography angiography (CTA; Fig. 9.1) and magnetic resonance angiography (MRA; Fig. 9.2) have proven to be accurate in distinguishing whether each kidney has one or two

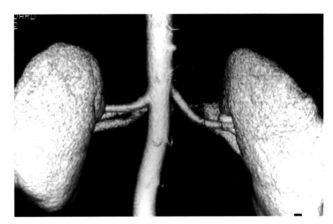

FIGURE 9.1. CTA. Single renal arteries are seen on this volume-rendered image. Portions of the renal veins are also visible.

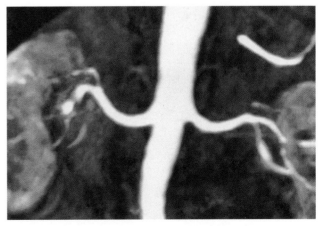

FIGURE 9.2. MRA. Single renal arteries are seen on this T1-weighted three-dimensional spoiled gradient-echo image.

main renal arteries. CT is used more commonly than MR to evaluate prospective renal donors, and images are routinely reformatted to display the anatomy of the artery and to identify the point at which the first branch occurs (Fig. 9.3). These CT-reformatted images are also used to depict renal venous anatomy (Figs. 9.4 to 9.6). MRA has the disadvantage of low sensitivity for small renal stones and is more likely than CTA to miss tiny polar accessory arteries, further supporting CT as the primary imaging modality for evaluating prospective renal donors.

Several techniques are available to reduce the radiation dose of the donor CT examination. Unenhanced views of the kidneys are necessary to find small stones and are helpful in detecting vascular calcification. Arterial phase images are obtained to assess the vascular supply, and delayed images are useful to evaluate the collecting system. The scout view from a CT urogram depicts the renal collecting systems, bladder, and ureter (Fig. 9.7). Axial images collimated to 1.5 mm as well as coronal, sagittal, and 3D-reconstructed images should be available for review at the workstation.

Evaluation of the kidneys should include an assessment of renal volume, as this parameter closely predicts renal function. Large kidneys are preferable; donors with large remaining kidneys achieve better renal function than those with small ones; large donated kidneys have fewer complications in recipients; and small transplanted kidneys may have insufficient function to serve a large recipient. Simple cysts and small nonobstructing stones may not absolutely disqualify a donor candidate, but tumors, postinflammatory fibrosis, hydronephrosis, and other conditions can jeopardize the health of the donor and/or recipient and usually prohibit transplantation.

Renal vascular assessment is crucial. Arterial conditions such as atherosclerosis or fibromuscular disease (Fig. 9.8) are contraindications to donor nephrectomy. Accessory renal arteries are important to demonstrate (Fig. 9.9). Duplicated renal arteries are not an absolute contraindication, but arterial luminal diameters should be measured because arteries smaller than 3 mm are difficult to anastomose to recipient vessels. Triplicated renal arteries usually preclude donor nephrectomy. Very small polar arteries can often be sacrificed, but since small lower pole arteries may give branches to the renal pelvis and proximal ureter, postoperative ureteral complications are more likely if these vessels are occluded. The distances between the origin from the aorta and first bifurcation of all major renal arteries should be measured; if these segments are short, surgery becomes more difficult.

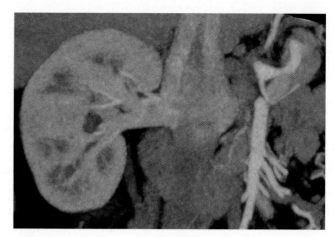

FIGURE 9.4. CTA. A single right renal vein is clearly demonstrated.

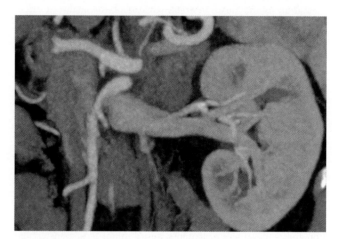

FIGURE 9.5. CTA. A single left renal vein is clearly demonstrated.

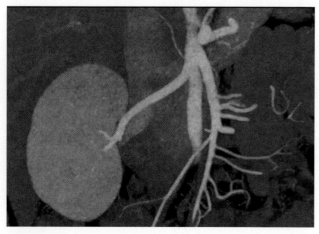

FIGURE 9.3. CTA. A single right renal artery is reformatted to clearly display the first branching vessel.

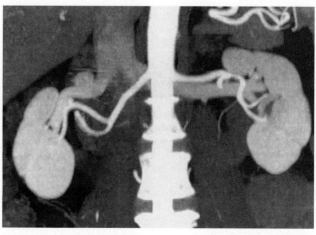

FIGURE 9.6. CT angiogram reveals a single artery and vein supplying each kidney.

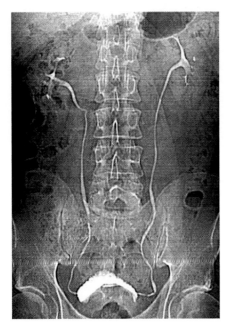

FIGURE 9.7. CT urography. A scout view demonstrates a single ureter bilaterally. The prostate is enlarged, there is a TURP defect, and the bladder is trabeculated.

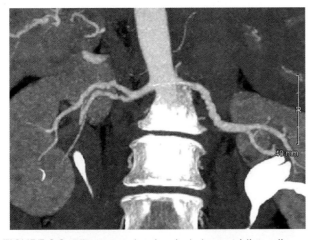

FIGURE 9.8. Fibromuscular dysplasia is seen bilaterally.

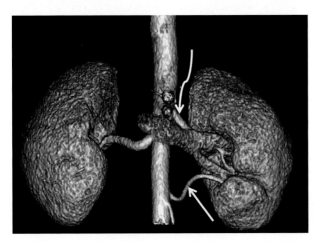

FIGURE 9.9. Accessory renal artery. Volume-rendered image from CTA demonstrates two left renal arteries (*arrows*).

Renal venous anatomy must also be analyzed. Retroaortic or circumaortic left renal veins are found in approximately 5% of potential donors and are important to recognize, as are duplicated right renal veins, found in almost 15% of donor evaluations. The distance between the junction of the vein with the inferior vena cava and the first bifurcation should be measured. Finally, renal venous tributaries, such as adrenal, lumbar, and gonadal veins, should be described.

The left kidney is preferred for donation, as the left renal vein is longer and surgical resection is often easier (Fig. 9.5). Single renal arteries are preferred, though small accessory arteries may sometimes be ignored. Potential donors with accessory arteries at the lower pole may have branches supplying the renal pelvis or ureter and are usually avoided.

Perirenal fat is removed from the donor kidney before transplantation. Thus, an assessment of the amount of fat in the perirenal space is useful. Simple renal cysts are seldom a problem as they are easily excised. Indeterminant lesions should be carefully evaluated before surgery. Ureteral duplication, found in 1% of the population, presents a technical challenge, but is not an absolute contraindication for transplantation.

Chu et al. found renal or extrarenal abnormalities in more than 40% of potential renal donors, though most were incidental findings that did not prevent organ donation. Renal abnormalities, which are absolute contraindications to transplantation including solitary kidney, horseshoe kidney, or polycystic kidney disease, were found in <1% of potential donors.

Recipient Evaluation

Due to the success of heterotopic renal transplantation, orthotopic transplantation is rarely performed. With heterotopic transplantation, the donor kidney is placed in an extraperitoneal location in the iliac fossa. CT is helpful in confirming that there is space within the fossa for the transplanted kidney. The renal artery and vein are anastomosed to the external iliac vessels. There are many techniques for reconstructing the urinary tract, but an antirefluxing ureteroneocystostomy is commonly created.

Virtually all recipients have their kidneys imaged in the course of treatment for renal failure, often a combination of ultrasound, CT, MRI, and radionuclide studies. Sometimes, specific imaging of the recipient's native kidneys will be necessary during the pretransplant workup. Evaluation for acquired renal cystic disease and the neoplasms that such kidneys develop is best performed by CT. Patients with autosomal dominant polycystic kidney disease may also benefit from a CT examination prior to transplantation if extreme enlargement or persistent bleeding makes them candidates for nephrectomy. Patients with severe vesicoureteral reflux may require surgical therapy, so voiding cystourethrography may be necessary in patients with recurrent urinary tract infections. Voiding cystourethrography may also be indicated in patients who have been anuric so long that their ability to void normally after transplantation is questioned. Bladders in such patients may have only a small capacity and, when studied by cystography, may demonstrate benign extravasation. This finding does not indicate gross perforation of the bladder and is not a contraindication to transplantation.

Evaluation of the vessels to which the transplanted kidney's artery and vein will be anastomosed is important. An unenhanced CT permits assessment of the degree of recipient vascular calcification; the severity of calcification is directly proportional to the degree of difficulty in performing the anastomosis. Some centers perform CTA of the common and external iliac arteries as well to evaluate them for stenosis or occlusion.

Patients with end-stage renal disease often have undergone one or more biopsies. These may lead to an arteriovenous fistula or pseudoaneurysm. While most of these are asymptomatic, some may lead to hematuria or hypertension and should be treated prior to transplantation.

COMPLICATIONS OF RENAL TRANSPLANTATION

Since it requires no intravascular contrast administration and has no ionizing radiation, ultrasound is usually the imaging modality chosen to evaluate patients after renal transplantation. Imaging of the recipient (Fig. 9.10) may show no abnormalities.

Complications of renal transplantation may be divided into those that affect the renal parenchyma and its small vessels, those that involve primarily the large vessels and their surgery, those that involve the transplanted ureter and its anastomosis, and those that appear as fluid collections in the surgical bed of the recipient. Long-term complications of renal transplantation consist primarily of neoplasms for which recipients are at increased risk due to immunosuppression.

Renal Complications

Table 9.1 reveals the times during or after transplantation that these complications are most likely to appear. These times, and some of the clinical and radiologic data that can be acquired, frequently permit a confident diagnosis of the specific complication. However, it is often difficult to establish a specific diagnosis without biopsy of the renal cortex for histologic examination.

Acute Tubular Necrosis

Acute tubular necrosis (ATN) usually occurs in the period immediately after transplantation and is related to ischemia of the transplanted kidney before vascular anastomosis. Such ischemia may occur in cadaveric donors during the agonal period of the donor and in any donor kidney during the delay between the harvesting of the kidney and the completion of vascular anastomoses in the recipient. The duration of the ischemia is directly related to the likelihood of ATN. Most episodes of ATN resolve sponta-

TABLE 9.1	
Temporal Sequence of Causes of Parenchymal Complications of Renal Transplants	
ATN	During or immediately after surgery
Hyperacute rejection	During surgery to a few hours afterward
Accelerated acute rejection	First week after surgery
Acute rejection	1–4 wk after surgery
Chronic rejection	Months to years after surgery
Cyclosporine toxicity	1–3 mo after surgery

neously and appear to have little adverse effect on ultimate graft survival.

ATN may manifest as anuria, rising creatinine, and mild enlargement and tenderness of the graft. Graft tenderness and fever are less likely to be prominent signs of ATN than of cases of acute rejection, but the clinical picture seldom allows confident differentiation between the two conditions. ATN usually appears within 1 or 2 days after transplantation and usually resolves within a few days to a few weeks of initial onset; however, some cases may persist for several weeks before recovery. Patients who experience ATN after transplantation may require dialysis for a week until renal function returns. ATN is much more common in cadaveric transplants than living related donors.

Cyclosporine Nephrotoxicity

Cyclosporine, together with prednisone, has been the mainstay of immunosuppressive therapy. It is, however, both nephrotoxic and hepatotoxic. Newer drugs, including sirolimus, tacrolimus, and mycophenolate mofetil, permit reduction in doses of cyclosporine and diminished nephrotoxicity, albeit at the cost of increased risk of hyperlipidemia and diabetes. Cyclosporine nephrotoxicity may be acute, subacute, or chronic. Both acute and subacute

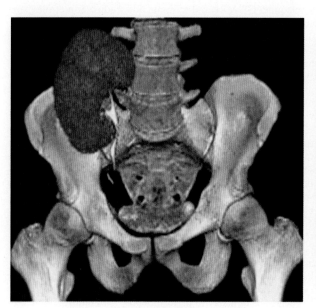
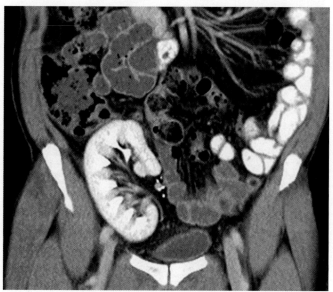

FIGURE 9.10. CT urography of two patients with kidneys transplanted into their right iliac fossae. **Left:** Volume-rendered image. **Right:** Coronal reformat.

nephrotoxicity may be treated by lowering the dose of cyclosporine; chronic nephrotoxicity is seldom reversible. Acute toxicity appears to potentiate initial graft dysfunction related to ischemia and may also prolong it. Because measurement of blood cyclosporine levels does not always permit distinction of cyclosporine nephrotoxicity from other causes of transplant dysfunction, imaging data may be critical in the differential diagnosis of a failing transplant.

Rejection

Graft rejection continues to represent a significant source of morbidity in the transplant patient. Rejection is classified into four categories: (1) hyperacute rejection, (2) accelerated acute rejection, (3) acute rejection, and (4) chronic rejection. Virtually every patient experiences some form of rejection after transplantation. Differentiation of graft rejection from other causes of intrinsic renal dysfunction is crucial because rejection may require increasing the dose of immunosuppressive therapy, whereas cyclosporine nephrotoxicity should be treated in the opposite way.

Hyperacute rejection is mediated by hormonal antibodies and is often manifested during surgery; the antigen–antibody reaction causes complement activation, which in turn damages the vascular endothelium, particularly in small vessels. These vessels become filled with fibrin thrombi, thereby making extensive cortical necrosis inevitable. A graft exhibiting hyperacute rejection is seldom salvageable, and transplant nephrectomy is performed immediately.

Some authors believe that accelerated acute rejection is an antibody-mediated form of rejection identical to hyperacute rejection, but with an onset delayed until 2 or 3 days after surgery. Others believe it is a manifestation of cell-mediated immunity. Diagnosis of an accelerated acute rejection usually occurs when a rejection episode occurs in the first week of transplantation. It is frequently, but not always, successfully treated with immunosuppression.

Acute rejection constitutes functional and pathologic changes characterized by a relatively rapid increase in serum creatinine (a rise of 25% or more above the baseline level occurring within 24 to 48 hours), graft swelling and tenderness, and fever. There is usually oliguria. Acute rejection is thought to occur because of a proliferation of C-lymphocytes and to represent a cell-mediated form of immunity. Histologically, acute rejection is characterized by a proliferation of mononuclear cells, eosinophils, and plasma cells that infiltrate the interstitium of the kidney. A vascular component may also be present. Biopsy specimens in acute rejection sometimes are classified as showing primarily interstitial rejection or both interstitial and vascular abnormalities. A vascular component connotes a poorer prognosis. Acute rejection may occur at any time after transplantation, but is most often encountered during the first 10 weeks after surgery.

Chronic rejection may appear months to years after surgery and usually has a more insidious onset than acute rejection. Graft swelling and tenderness and fever are less prominent features of chronic rejection than acute rejection. Pathologic examination may reveal endothelial swelling, smooth muscle proliferation in small vessels, and glomerular changes, as well as tubular atrophy, segmental fibrosis, and diffuse infiltration with inflammatory cells. In general, the changes of chronic rejection are irreversible and lead to progressive azotemia and hypertension. Chronic allograft nephropathy is often due to a combination of chronic rejection, antirejection drug nephrotoxicity, and a vasculopathy due to more protean risk factors such as hypertension, hyperlipidemia, diabetes, and smoking. Decline in renal function may be slowed by careful management of drugs, but is rarely, if ever, halted completely.

Imaging

Imaging of patients with functional abnormalities of transplanted kidneys is a critical step in the differential diagnosis of the cause of the transplant dysfunction, but imaging findings, considered alone, do not always allow an accurate and specific diagnosis. Sometimes, the abnormality is clear, but frequently, the clinical or laboratory data must be considered along with the radiologic findings to reach a firm diagnosis. Although nuclear medicine and Doppler ultrasound findings have been the subjects of considerable investigation, findings that permit accurate distinction among rejection, cyclosporine nephrotoxicity, and ATN in the absence of clinical information have been elusive, and biopsy is frequently necessary. Scintigraphy provides quantifiable assessment of the transplant's handling of specific compounds, but the ability of gray-scale, Doppler, and color Doppler ultrasound to evaluate vessels, flow dynamics, anatomy, and peritransplant structures has led to its usual choice as the first imaging technique.

Hyperacute rejection infrequently leads to an imaging evaluation because it usually occurs in the operating room. Because renal cortical perfusion is markedly diminished or completely absent, Doppler ultrasound will reveal little or no cortical blood flow, radionuclide examinations will show almost complete absence of perfusion or tubular accumulation (Fig. 9.11), and angiography will reveal total or near-total lack of filling of small vessels.

Accelerated acute rejection demonstrates imaging findings consistent with acute rejection, but occurs within the first week after transplantation. Rare cases of cortical nephrocalcinosis (Fig. 9.12) have been described in patients whose transplants underwent severe immediate rejection but were left in situ for several years.

Gray-scale images (Fig. 9.13) of patients with acute transplant rejection may show an increase in the volume of the kidney,

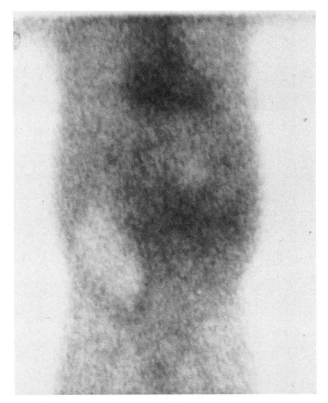

FIGURE 9.11. Hyperacute rejection. Scintigram obtained a day after transplantation shows nearly complete absence of activity in transplanted kidney. (Courtesy of Rashid Fawwaz, M.D.)

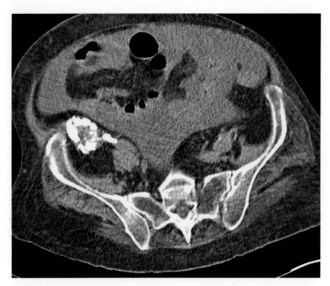

FIGURE 9.12. Cortical nephrocalcinosis from acute severe rejection. Small, calcified renal allograft is in right lower quadrant.

swelling, and altered echogenicity of the renal pyramids and the cortex. The high echogenicity of the sinus of a normal kidney may be diminished. These findings are thought to reflect edema of the parenchyma and of the renal sinus fat. Edema of the collecting system walls may make them appear thickened. The sensitivity of these findings to diagnose rejection, however, and the ability to distinguish rejection from cyclosporine nephrotoxicity and ATN when the findings are not clearly present are poor.

There is diminution of renal blood flow in rejection, cyclosporine nephrotoxicity, and ATN. Although there are variations in the severity of oligemia among cases of each condition, attempts have been made to use Doppler flow studies to distinguish acute rejection from ATN and cyclosporine nephrotoxicity by analyzing signals from the main renal artery and from intrarenal branches. In patients with acute rejection—especially those in whom vascular changes predominate in biopsy specimens, as opposed to those in whom the histologic changes are primarily interstitial where the resistive index (RI) is often elevated (Fig. 9.13). When the RI is 0.90 or higher, acute rejection is likely, although occasionally elevated RIs may be caused by arterial stenosis, renal vein thrombosis, acute severe ureteral obstruction, severe ATN, acute cyclosporine nephrotoxicity, pyelonephritis, and compression of the kidney by a perirenal fluid collection. With lower RIs, primarily interstitial acute

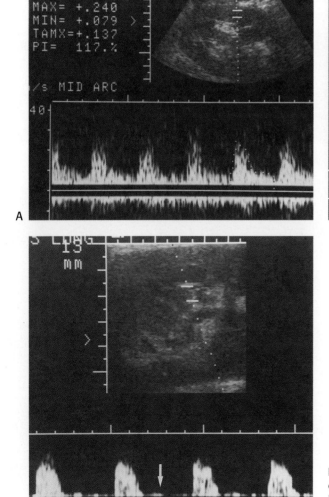

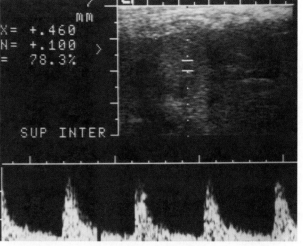

FIGURE 9.13. Duplex Doppler ultrasonograms. **A:** Normal duplex study with a PI of 1.17. **B:** Mild rejection; RI = 0.78, PI = 1.7. **C:** Severe rejection with virtually complete absence of diastolic flow (*arrow*).

rejection, cyclosporine nephrotoxicity, and ATN are possible etiologies. Because rejection and ATN may not affect the entire kidney uniformly and because RIs may vary from observer to observer, the accuracy of this method of differential diagnosis is far from ideal and many authors feel that RI measurements are not useful. In some centers, the pulsatility index (PI) ([peak systolic frequency shift–diastolic frequency shift]/the mean frequency shift) is used as an alternative to measurement of the RI. A PI of 1.5 or greater is generally considered indicative of rejection. In patients with ATN, higher RI and PI values are associated with longer periods of recovery of function. Power Doppler findings have not improved upon the differentiation between acute rejection and other causes of graft failure.

RI and PI values may have prognostic significance as well. If they remain elevated in the first transplant month, even in patients with stable renal function, the kidneys are at increased risk to develop chronic allograft nephropathy, and the risk is worse if there are progressive rises in these indices. An elevated RI in the graft vessels also indicates an increased risk for the subsequent development or worsening of general cardiovascular disease, possibly because this parameter not only reflects abnormal vessels in the graft but also indicates decreased compliance of the systemic arteries in the rest of the body.

Although experimental evidence shows that renal blood flow is lower than normal in cases of ATN, Doppler and radionuclide examinations do not always suggest ischemia. The early phase in a technetium-99m-diethylenetriaminepentaacetic acid (^{99m}Tc-DTPA) renogram (the "perfusion" phase) is relatively well maintained (Fig. 9.14), even though the later phases and the technetium-99m-mercaptoacetyltriglycine (^{99m}Tc-MAG3) curves fail to show rapid parenchymal washout and even show persistent accumulation of the isotope. Sonography, including Doppler, may be normal, or the RI may be increased (Fig. 9.13).

Like Doppler ultrasound, scintigraphy interpreted in the absence of other data can seldom accurately distinguish among the several causes of renal parenchymal dysfunction in transplant patients, but it may be of value when considered with all available information. In acute rejection associated primarily with vascular changes (Fig. 9.15), the rapid increase in activity seen normally is attenuated; the maximum intensity of activity seen in early images is diminished, and the delay between the time of peak activity in the aorta and peak activity in the kidney is prolonged. These findings may also occur in rejection that is primarily of the cellular type, as well as in ATN and cyclosporine nephrotoxicity, but are less severe in those conditions. The findings may precede clinical evidence of rejection. All parenchymal causes of graft dysfunction exhibit deteriorating tubular function manifested by diminished activity in the later parts of the examination. Once established, ATN and acute rejection may produce scintigraphic findings that are difficult to distinguish. But if the first scans after surgery are abnormal, ATN is likely to be present, whereas if the scans were initially normal, but subsequently became abnormal, acute rejection is more likely to be the diagnosis. ATN followed by acute rejection is difficult to distinguish from ATN without recovery, although the usual course of ATN is a spontaneous return toward normal within 1 or 2 weeks of onset. Severe diminution of activity in the kidney, or complete failure of the kidney to accumulate isotope, is a poor prognostic sign.

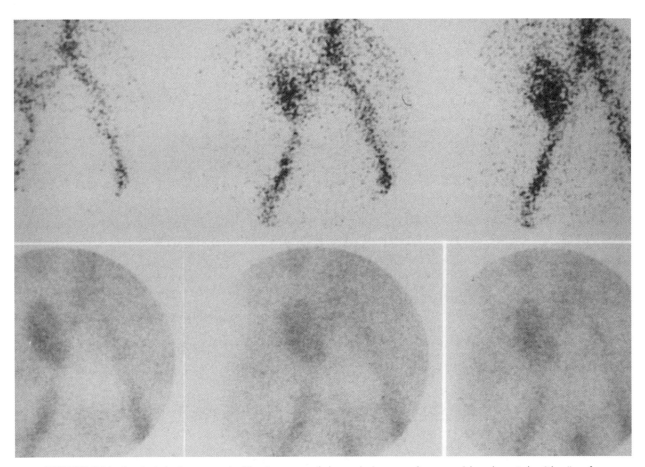

FIGURE 9.14. Acute tubular necrosis. The top row of dynamic images shows rapid early uptake (the "perfusion" phase). The lower row of images, obtained 1, 10, and 20 minutes after administration of isotope, reveals persistence of activity and little excretion into the bladder. (Courtesy of Rashid Fawwaz, M.D.)

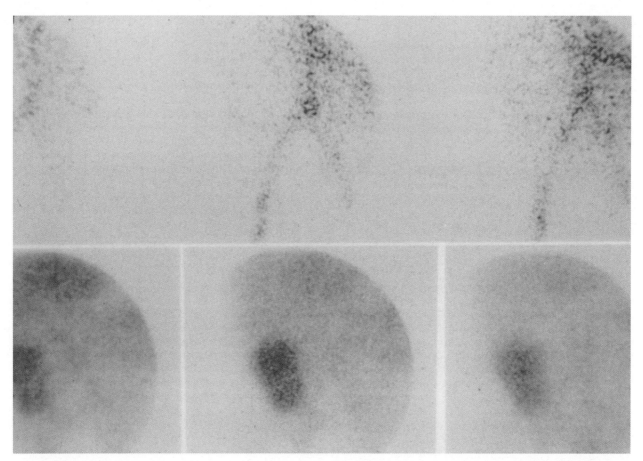

FIGURE 9.15. Acute vascular rejection. The upper row of scintigrams consists of dynamic images and reveals diminished renal perfusion as the isotope traverses the iliac arteries. The lower images were obtained 1, 10, and 20 minutes after isotope administration and reveal persistence of activity in the parenchyma.

Gadolinium-enhanced MRI is able to assess local transplant parenchymal perfusion abnormalities. T1-weighted unenhanced images of transplanted kidneys may reveal loss of the normal corticomedullary differentiation, but this feature is not specific for any particular cause of transplant dysfunction.

Catheter angiography is not performed to diagnose rejection, but may be indicated for other reasons in transplant patients. With acute rejection, there is often a prolonged arterial phase with poor washout. The nephrogram is diminished, demonstrates patchy opacification, and reveals poor definition of the corticomedullary junction. Arteriovenous shunting may be present. Angiographic findings of acute rejection may be focal.

Chronic rejection produces imaging findings that vary in severity and tend to differ from those of acute processes. For example, ^{99m}Tc-DTPA scans may display a diminution in perfusion, which precedes the diminution in uptake, but the findings may not permit differentiation of rejection from other chronic conditions affecting a transplanted kidney, such as chronic cyclosporine nephrotoxicity, or the superimposition of diseases, such as hypertension or diabetic nephropathy.

In patients with chronic rejection, the kidneys are often small. Ultrasound may show thinning and increased echogenicity of the cortex (Fig. 9.16); in the rare cases in which mild cortical nephrocalcinosis occurs, cortical echoes may be very strong. The RI value may be normal or elevated (Fig. 9.17). A radionuclide scan tends to show relatively rapid uptake and washout; the pattern of poor initial uptake but gradually increasing activity seen with some acute processes is not a feature of chronic rejection (although a bout of

acute rejection may be superimposed on a kidney that has been chronically rejecting). Although angiography is not indicated in the diagnosis of chronic rejection, it may be performed on chronically rejecting kidneys when renal artery stenosis is a possibility. The

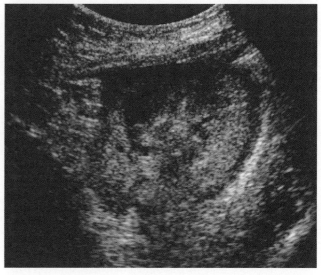

FIGURE 9.16. Chronic rejection. Ultrasound reveals very echogenic cortex.

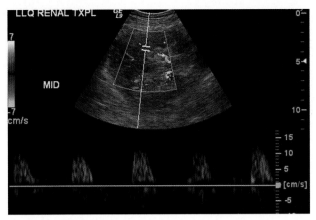

FIGURE 9.17. Chronic rejection. Doppler ultrasound shows negligible diastolic flow.

rejection may be manifested as a thinned cortex with a diminished nephrogram; the small vessels are sparse, diminutive, and pruned. T1-weighted spin-echo MRI may reveal the absence of corticomedullary distinction seen in a number of chronic renal parenchymal diseases.

Sonographic findings in cyclosporine nephrotoxicity are similar to those in rejection and ATN; the resistive and pulsatility indices tend to be elevated. In the chronic phase, the transplanted kidney may be small and/or echogenic. There may be a dissociation between the perfusion phase of a ^{99m}Tc-DTPA study (Fig. 9.18), which tends to remain relatively intact, and the clearance phase of a hippuran or ^{99m}TC-MAG3 study, which often reveals a prolonged rate of clearance. This is particularly the case in patients with subacute nephrotoxicity. The scintigraphic findings in cyclosporine toxicity are similar to the abnormalities produced by ATN or rejection. The diagnosis is often based on measurements of cyclosporine in the blood and on monitoring the effect of dose adjustments.

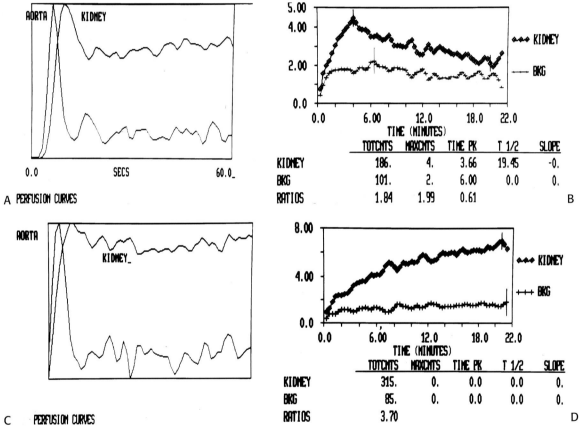

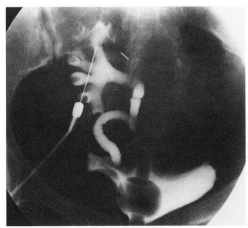

FIGURE 9.18. Cyclosporine nephrotoxicity. Immediate post-transplant ^{99m}Tc-DTPA perfusion **(A)** and ^{131}I-hippuran renogram **(B)** curves in a patient who received a living related kidney show good perfusion and excretion. Three days later, the perfusion curve **(C)** remains relatively intact; however, the hippuran curve **(D)** now demonstrates an ascending slope. An antegrade pyelogram **(E)** shows no evidence of obstruction, confirming that the cause of the transplant dysfunction is cyclosporine nephrotoxicity.

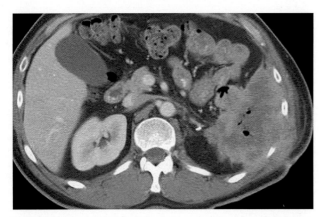

FIGURE 9.19. An abscess is seen in the renal bed after nephrectomy.

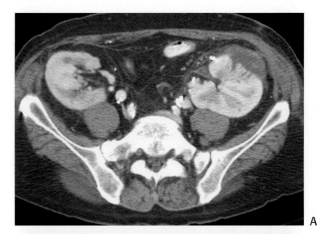

A

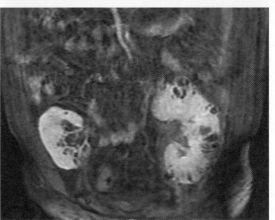

B

FIGURE 9.20. **A:** Graft infection in a patient with two transplanted kidneys. **B:** CT reveals focal diminution and striation in the nephrogram adjacent to a small perinephric collection. T1-weighted gadolinium-enhanced MRI performed a week later shows multiple bilateral abscesses.

Graft Infection

Infection may occur in the renal donor (Fig. 9.19), but is more common in the graft recipient due to the immunosuppression therapy. Many patients receiving renal allografts require treatment for urinary tract infection within the first 4 months after surgery, and some may develop frank sepsis. The incidence and severity of the infection depend on the dose of immunosuppressive therapy, the presence and degree of control of diabetes mellitus, and the coexistence of graft dysfunction. The organisms responsible are the same gram-negative pathogens commonly found in other patients with urinary tract infection. Graft recipients may also be infected with cytomegalovirus or herpes simplex virus. Symptoms may not be as obvious in suggesting pyelonephritis in transplanted kidneys as they are in patients with normal kidneys.

The imaging findings of pyelonephritis of transplanted kidneys are similar to those encountered in infected native kidneys (Fig. 9.20). Ultrasound may reveal parenchymal swelling and an elevated RI. Focal inflammation may cause focal diminution of perfusion; if contrast-enhanced ultrasound is available, these regions may more easily be seen. Both DTPA and MAG3 scans may show diminished activity in infected regions.

Several cases of emphysematous pyelonephritis have been reported in transplant patients; the diagnosis may be established by demonstrating gas within the renal parenchyma by CT (Fig. 9.21) or ultrasound.

There is a relationship between reflux into the transplanted ureter and infection. If a graft recipient suffers multiple infections and if ureteroneocystostomy would be considered if severe reflux were present, voiding cystography should be performed (Fig. 9.22).

Renal Transplant Rupture

This is a dramatic but unusual complication that usually occurs within the first 2 weeks of the transplant surgery. The etiology of rupture is not known, but it has been speculated that acute rejection, ATN, and vascular occlusion may be predisposing causes. Trauma caused by biopsies may also be contributory.

The imaging findings include renal parenchymal laceration, intrarenal hematoma, and perirenal hematoma. Ultrasound may reveal a hypoechoic fluid collection representing a hematoma within the laceration and/or perinephric space; in the acute phase, CT will demonstrate dense clot within the laceration or perinephric space (Fig. 9.23); and radionuclide scans may reveal a focal photopenic region at the site of the laceration.

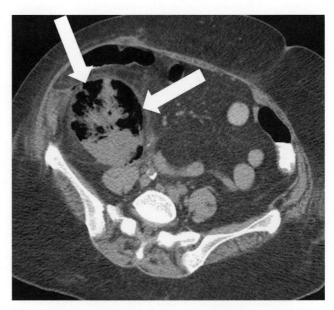

FIGURE 9.21. Emphysematous pyelonephritis in a diabetic patient. Gas (*arrows*) infiltrates the renal parenchyma.

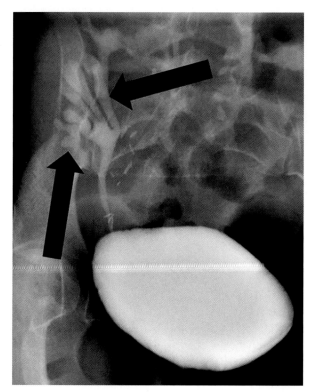

FIGURE 9.22. Vesicoureteral reflux into a transplanted kidney. A cystogram shows reflux into the collecting system (*arrows*).

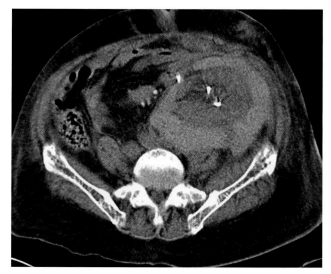

FIGURE 9.23. Perirenal hematoma. High-density fluid is seen surrounding the renal allograft on this unenhanced CT. The kidney has a stent within the collecting system, and there is a surgical clip adjacent to the anterior surface of its cortex.

Vascular Complications

Thrombosis

Thrombosis of the renal artery may occur in the immediate postoperative period; it may be caused by complete or partial occlusion at the anastomotic site or may form as a result of an intimal flap. Renal arterial thrombosis is more common in kidneys that have more than one renal artery and in association

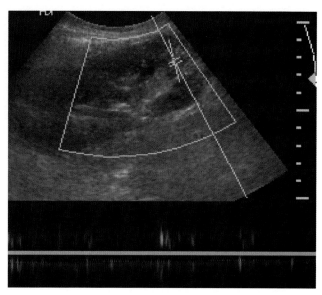

FIGURE 9.24. Renal artery occlusion. Color Doppler image and waveform show very little flow.

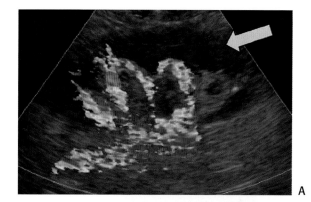

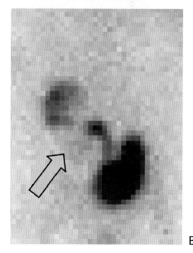

FIGURE 9.25. **A:** Color Doppler image shows no flow in inferior portion of transplanted kidney (*arrow*). **B:** The scintigram shows very little isotope in the same region (*arrow*).

with hyperacute rejection. If diminution in renal blood flow is severe or complete, Doppler ultrasound will reveal no evidence of flow within the kidney (Fig. 9.24), radionuclide scintigrams will show no perfusion (Fig. 9.25), and contrast-enhanced MR

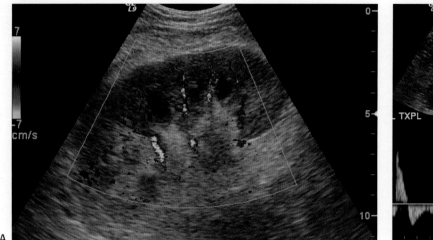
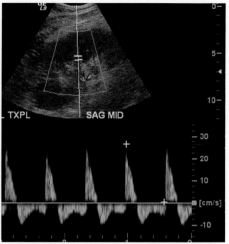

FIGURE 9.26. Renal vein thrombosis. Color Doppler image **(A)** shows very little flow and waveform **(B)** shows reversal of diastolic flow.

or CT will reveal an absent nephrogram. An infarcted kidney, or infarcted portion of kidney, will appear swollen and relatively hypoechoic on gray-scale ultrasound; a hemorrhagic infarct may appear more echogenic.

Renal vein thrombosis in transplanted kidneys is quite rare. It presents with graft tenderness and swelling, usually in the first week after transplantation. The imaging findings are the same as those associated with renal vein thrombosis in native kidneys (Fig. 9.26), including echogenic material and absence of flow in the renal vein, markedly elevated RIs, or reversal of diastolic flow and parenchymal swelling.

Renal Artery Stenosis

Renal artery stenosis is the most common vascular complication of transplantation and is reported to occur in up to 10% of renal transplant recipients. The real incidence may be higher because asymptomatic patients are not evaluated. Renal artery stenosis may cause diminution in renal function, hypertension, and a bruit. Evidence of mild anastomotic narrowing in the period immediately after transplantation may reflect transient edema, which usually resolves.

Stenoses in the host artery proximal to the anastomosis may be related to general atherosclerosis, especially in patients with diabetes, or may be related to trauma suffered at the time of surgery. Stenoses at the anastomotic site may be related to the surgical technique, the suture material, or perfusion injury of the vessels themselves. Postanastomotic stenosis may be related to rejection, abnormal local hemodynamics, or extrinsic compression. Stenoses involving the recipient's arteries are rare.

Posttransplant renal artery stenosis requires arterial imaging for accurate evaluation (Fig. 9.27). Either hypertension or declining graft function may prompt a search for arterial stenosis. Doppler ultrasound (Fig. 9.28) often reveals elevated flow rates within the

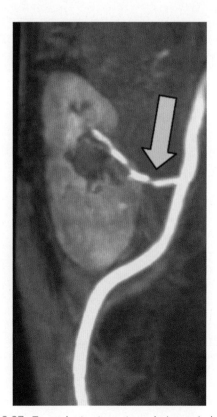

FIGURE 9.27. Transplant artery stenosis (*arrow*) shown with MRA.

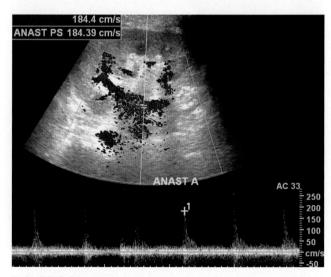

FIGURE 9.28. Transplant artery stenosis. Doppler waveform shows high-velocity systolic flow and turbulence.

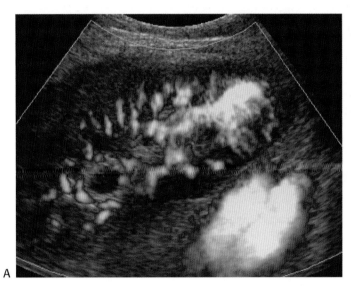
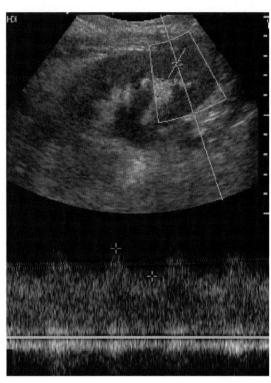

FIGURE 9.29. Arteriovenous fistula in transplant after biopsy **(A)**. Power Doppler reveals region of increased flow **(B)**; Doppler waveform shows severe turbulence.

stenotic area and spectral broadening within and immediately distal to the stenosis; care must be taken not to ascribe the elevated peak velocities sometimes produced by severe changes in flow direction at arterial anastomoses to stenosis. Peak velocities may also be elevated in the immediate posttransplant period without stenosis. Both MRA and CTA have been found to be accurate in diagnosing or excluding renal artery stenosis.

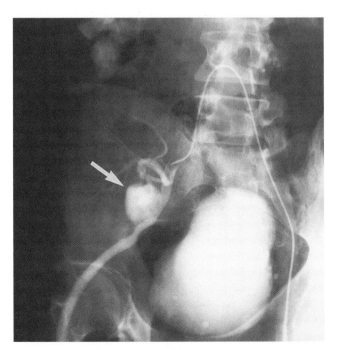

FIGURE 9.30. A pseudoaneurysm (*arrow*) in the external iliac artery adjacent to the transplant anastomosis is present.

Percutaneous transluminal angioplasty has become the preferred method by which such stenoses are treated; a large majority of patients have successful outcomes, at least in the short term. The success rates are higher with end-to-side anastomoses than with end-to-end anastomoses. The technique and potential complications are similar to those encountered during percutaneous transluminal angioplasty in native renal arteries.

Renal Arteriovenous Fistula

Because transplanted kidneys frequently undergo biopsy, small arteriovenous fistulae and pseudoaneurysms are common. They usually close quickly and spontaneously, but persist in 1% or 2% of patients, and may cause transplant dysfunction or significant arteriovenous shunting. Rupture may result in hematuria or a perirenal hematoma. Doppler ultrasound (Fig. 9.29) may reveal low-impedance, high-velocity flow through the afferent artery; the draining vein may reveal pulsatile, high-velocity flow, and the draining veins may demonstrate an arterial-type pulsatile waveform. Pseudoaneurysms (Fig. 9.30) are seen on ultrasound studies as cystic or complex lesions with Doppler evidence of disorganized flow or alternative patterns of flow toward and away from the transducer.

Angiographic findings are the same as those encountered in small arteriovenous fistulae or pseudoaneurysms in native kidneys. If they require therapy, they may be amenable to transarterial embolization with coils (Fig. 9.31) or Gelfoam (Upjohn, Kalamazoo, Michigan).

Urologic Complications

Urinary Leak

Urinary leak (Fig. 9.32) most often occurs in the first 3 months after transplantation and is usually discovered within the first few postoperative weeks. Urine may leak from the ureterovesical anastomosis, from a vesicostomy site, or even from injury to the transplanted

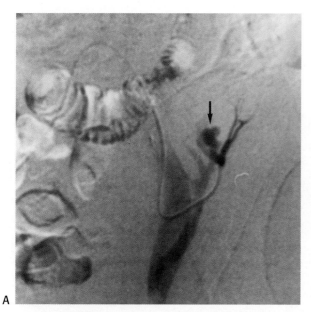
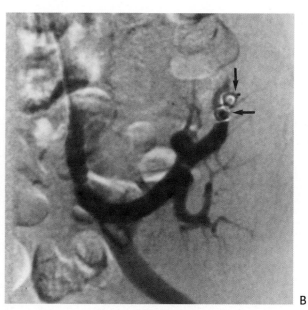

A

B

FIGURE 9.31. A: Subselective renal angiogram shows a large arteriovenous fistula (*arrow*). **B:** After embolization with Gianturco coils (*arrows*), a repeat arteriogram shows closure of the fistula.

renal pelvis. If the leak is small and transient, the urine is usually resorbed; if it persists, a urinoma frequently forms.

Ultrasound, CT, and MRI may all demonstrate leaks as small irregularly margined fluid collections, which may become encapsulated if they persist as chronic urinomas. The fluid may be difficult to distinguish from a seroma or lymphocele, but CT urography or scintigraphy may diagnose an acute urine leak by demonstrating that contrast or isotope reaches the collections.

Ureteral Necrosis

Necrosis and sloughing of the distal ureter (Fig. 9.33) are common urologic complications and often cause a urinary leak. It may occur in up to 4% of patients, usually before the sixth postoperative month. It is thought to be caused by ischemia of the distal ureter from interruption of the arterial blood supply to the ureter or from a tight submucosal tunnel in the bladder; it may also appear because of rejection.

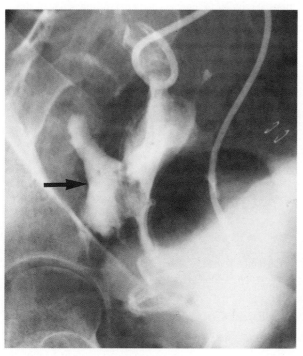
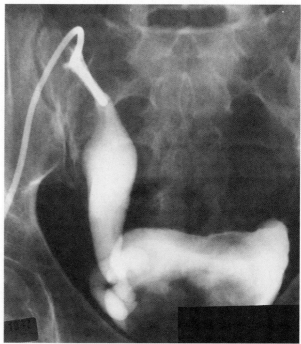

A

B

FIGURE 9.32. A: Nephrostogram demonstrates extravasation from the tear of the renal pelvis (*arrow*). **B:** After removal of the ureteral stent and several weeks of nephrostomy drainage, the leak has healed completely.

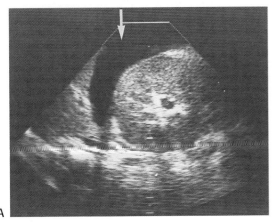
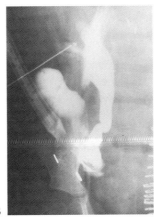
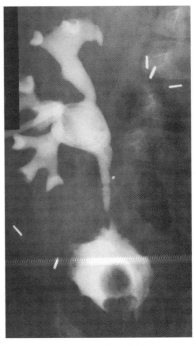

A B C

FIGURE 9.33. Ureteral necrosis. **A:** An ultrasound examination demonstrates fluid around the transplant kidney (*arrow*). **B:** Antegrade pyelogram shows extravasation from the distal ureter as a result of ureteral necrosis. **C:** After percutaneous nephrostomy and stent placement, a nephrostogram shows complete healing.

Ureteral Obstruction

Transient obstruction at the site of the ureteral implantation is common in the immediate postoperative period; it is usually caused by edema and subsides quickly. Ureteral obstruction that appears months to years after transplantation is more likely due to ureteral strictures caused by ischemia. Rarely, acute obstruction is caused by blood clots, calculi, fungus balls, or sloughed papillae. Stones are reported to occur in approximately 1% of patients with renal allografts; most stone formers are thought to have underlying predisposing conditions. Occasionally, undetected calculi in donor kidneys may cause complications in recipients. Acute ureteral obstruction from a stone may produce pain and graft swelling that simulates acute rejection. Patients may suddenly become oliguric or anuric. A suture at the site of ureteral implantation or vesicostomy may act as a nidus for the formation of a bladder stone. Any fluid collection may compress the ureter and cause obstruction. The imaging signs of obstruction in a transplanted kidney are the same as those of ureteral obstruction in a native kidney (Fig. 9.34).

Torsion

Torsion of a renal transplant is a very rare complication. The kidney rotates around its vascular pedicle, causing vascular occlusion and infarction. Torsion is more likely to occur when the transplant

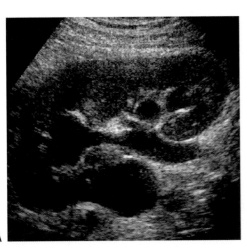
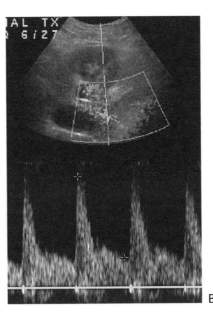

A B

FIGURE 9.34. Ureteral obstruction in transplanted kidney. **A:** Ultrasound reveals moderate hydronephrosis. **B:** Doppler waveform shows elevated RI.

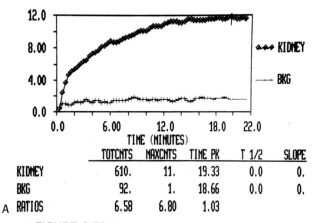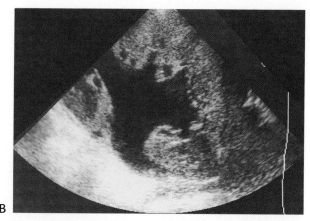

FIGURE 9.35. Transplant obstruction. **A:** A renogram curve demonstrates an ascending slope compatible with obstruction. **B:** Ultrasound examination confirms that transplant hydronephrosis is present.

kidney is placed in the peritoneal cavity. Imaging studies demonstrate a change in the renal axis. If vascular compromise occurs, there may be parenchymal swelling or diminished enhancement.

Imaging

A variety of radiologic examinations may be helpful in investigating urologic complications. Plain films may show large urinomas or other fluid collections and may also demonstrate stones. However, because the transplanted kidney and collecting system frequently overlie the iliac bone and sacrum, small or faintly calcified stones may be hard to find. An unenhanced CT examination is more sensitive and specific than plain films in evaluating transplant patients for stone disease.

Ultrasound studies are extremely useful for investigating urologic complications. Ultrasound may show hydronephrosis (Fig. 9.34), and the degree to which this represents ongoing obstruction may be made clearer by searching for abnormal RIs and absent ureteral jets with Doppler. It may detect renal or ureteral calculi and peritransplant fluid collections. Hydronephrosis is found frequently in patients with ureteral sloughing and urinary extravasation.

Retrograde pyelography is sometimes difficult to perform on transplanted kidneys and ureters because it is difficult to catheterize a ureter through a ureteroneocystostomy, but contrast may reflux into the transplant ureter during cystography. Cystography may demonstrate a urinary leak with the source in the wall of the bladder, but may give false-negative results in patients in whom the leak arises from the distal ureter.

Radionuclide examinations are often used to investigate transplant dysfunction. Patients with urinomas may, in early images, demonstrate a photopenic region corresponding to the urinoma; the region gradually will accumulate activity in the delayed images if urine is actively excreted into the collection. Ureteral obstruction can also be identified on radionuclide studies. The perfusion phase in a ^{99m}Tc-DTPA examination may be relatively well preserved, and with a ^{99m}Tc-MAG3 examination, there is relatively prompt uptake of the radiopharmaceutical by the transplant kidney. The excretory portion of the study is prolonged, and the renogram curve may have an ascending slope (Fig. 9.35). These findings are similar to those accompanying ATN and acute cyclosporine nephrotoxicity. Sometimes, direct demonstration of hydronephrosis and hydroureter by scintigraphy, or by other imaging modalities (Fig. 9.34), makes the diagnosis more specific.

CT may reveal urinomas or other fluid collections (Fig. 9.36), which can be characterized further with percutaneous aspiration.

Fine-needle antegrade pyelography is sometimes useful in diagnosing and locating transplant ureteral obstruction and in detecting and outlining ureteral fistulas. Although it is an invasive technique and is associated with the risk of hemorrhage and infection, the actual complication rate is quite low.

Interventional procedures may be used to treat most urologic complications. Percutaneous nephrostomy provides relief of obstruction, and once inserted, a percutaneous nephrostomy tube may be used for other procedures or to treat stones and urinary leaks. Urinary tract calculi can be extracted using techniques similar to those employed in the native kidneys. Ureteral or anastomotic leaks may be managed successfully with percutaneous diversion and stent placement. Some ureteral strictures may be treated successfully with percutaneous balloon dilatation or ureteral stent placement. Although there is a significant rate of short-term failure and long-term restenosis of transplant ureters after balloon dilatation, the technique may provide transient or even permanent relief of obstruction in some patients.

Fluid Collections

A fluid collection around the transplanted kidney may represent a hematoma, urinoma, lymphocele, or abscess.

Hematomas

Hematomas usually form in the immediate postoperative period. Ultrasound reveals them as fluid collections, but clots or red

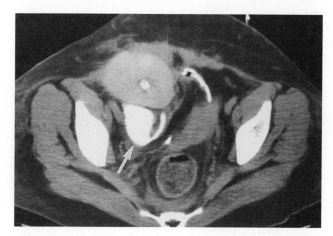

FIGURE 9.36. Urinoma. CT demonstrates a collection of extravasated contrast (*arrow*) behind the transplanted kidney.

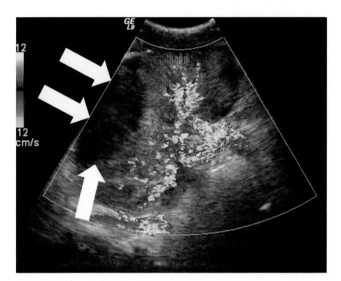

FIGURE 9.37. Subcapsular hematoma. The collection of blood (*arrows*) adjacent to the transplanted kidney contains echoes and indents the cortex.

cell debris may produce regions of echogenicity within them (Fig. 9.37). Hematomas may be resorbed. If not, the red cells lyse, forming seromas. If subcapsular in location, either a hematoma or seroma may sufficiently compress the renal parenchyma to cause renin-mediated hypertension, which is often referred to as a *Page kidney* (Fig. 9.38). Fluid collections in the perirenal space, outside the renal capsule, do not compress the renal parenchyma. Clots or layers of debris may appear on unenhanced CT images as regions denser than adjacent solid tissues (Fig. 9.23). Hematomas appear photopenic on the early phases of a radionuclide studies, and MRI reveals the same features of hematomas as are seen with extracranial hematomas arising elsewhere.

Urinomas

Urinomas also form relatively early after transplantation because they are usually caused by acute leaks from the ureteral anastomosis. The fluid in urinomas appears echo-free on ultrasound, has a density near water on CT, and demonstrates the features of protein-free fluid (dark on T1-weighted images and bright on T2-weighted images) on MRI. If urine is actively flowing into the urinoma at the time of a radionuclide examination, the urinoma may become quite active if any renal-excreted compound is used. Eventually, leaking may cease, and an encapsulated urinoma may no longer accumulate excreted radionuclide or excreted contrast media.

Lymphoceles

Lymphoceles are the most common peritransplant fluid collection; they occur in 1% to 15% of all transplant recipients. They usually appear 4 to 6 weeks after transplantation and are frequently associated with previous episodes of rejection. They are believed to be caused by disruption of the recipient's lymphatics at the time of surgery, but there may be a contribution from the transplanted kidney as well.

Lymphoceles are frequently asymptomatic, but when large, they may compress the collecting system or the ureter and even produce obstruction and impairment of function. They may be palpable and may be associated with pain and ipsilateral leg edema.

Lymphoceles may be detected by a variety of imaging modalities. Ultrasound demonstrates fluid-filled structures that often contain fine septations that may be difficult to distinguish from urinomas. They are usually seen at the inferior margin of the renal allograft between the kidney and the bladder. On CT, lymphoceles are demonstrated as round or oval collections with sharp borders and CT values ranging from 0 to 20 Hounsfield units. Without contrast, they may be difficult to distinguish from urinomas. After intravenous contrast injection, many but not all urinomas opacify, whereas lymphoceles do not. On radionuclide examinations, they are seen as photopenic areas near the transplanted kidney or the bladder that do not accumulate activity on delayed views. Lymphoceles have a low signal intensity on T1-weighted MR images and are bright on T2-weighted sequences (Fig. 9.39).

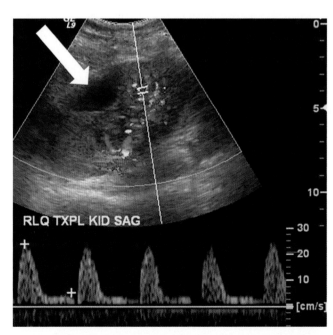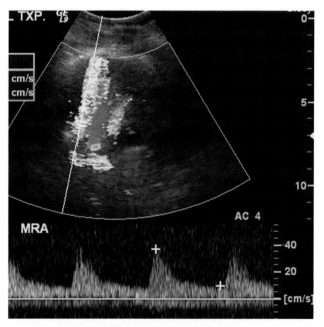

FIGURE 9.38. Seroma after perinephric hematoma producing a Page kidney and hypertension. **Left:** The fluid collection (*arrow*) compresses the kidney, causing an elevated RI. **Right:** After percutaneous drainage, the Doppler spectrum has returned to normal; the hypertension resolved.

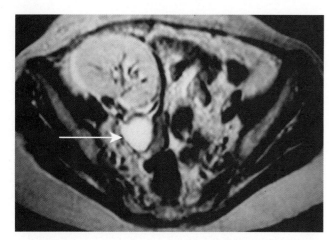

FIGURE 9.39. Lymphocele. T2-weighted MRI reveals a small fluid collection (*arrow*) posterior to the transplanted kidney.

The role of percutaneous drainage of lymphoceles is controversial. Although they may be drained and cured, they recur with sufficient frequency that instillation of a sclerosing agent or surgical therapy is often needed.

Abscess

The incidence of peritransplant abscess is difficult to estimate from the reported series. Most occur as a complication of pyelonephritis, although abscess as a direct complication of surgery may also occur. Peritransplant fluid collections such as urinomas, hematomas, or lymphoceles may become infected secondarily.

CT and ultrasound are the most helpful imaging modalities in detecting abscesses, but they are often indistinguishable from sterile collections by imaging techniques alone. The diagnosis of abscess depends on the combination of clinical evidence and imaging findings. Needle aspiration is relatively easy to perform to detect abscesses, and the abscesses usually respond to antibiotics and percutaneous catheter drainage.

Neoplasms

There is an increased incidence of malignancy in patients treated with immunosuppressive drugs over a long period of time. There is a positive correlation between the dose of the immunosuppressive drug and the duration in which it is given with the incidence of secondary malignancies. There is also an increased risk of viral derived malignancies among organ transplant recipients.

Patients receiving renal transplants are prone to developing lymphoproliferative disorders (PTLD) and the incidence increases with the level and duration of immunosuppression. Patients infected with the Epstein–Barr virus are also at increased risk. The majority of these PTLD cases occur in the abdomen, and they may develop in the renal allograft.

The risk of developing a renal cell carcinoma (RCC) after renal transplantation is estimated to be 2%, with the RCC developing in either the native or transplant kidney. RCCs develop in the native kidneys, especially those with acquired cystic kidney disease, 100 times more frequently than in the general population. The most common cell type is papillary carcinoma.

Frick and colleagues have reported the CT appearance of abdominal lymphoma that develops after renal transplantation. The incidence in their series was 1.3% of the transplant population. The lymphomas differed from the usual ones in that they frequently involved extranodal sites, especially in the central nervous system.

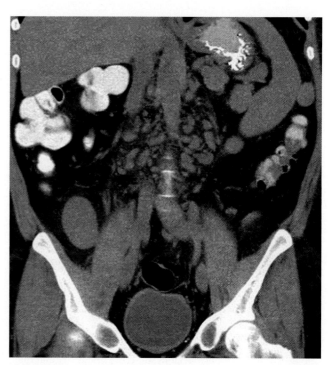

FIGURE 9.40. Posttransplant lymphoma. Multiple enlarged mesenteric lymph nodes are demonstrated on this coronal CT.

CT of posttransplant lymphomas in the abdomen usually reveals bulky masses with inhomogeneous attenuation or diffuse lymphadenopathy (Fig. 9.40).

SUGGESTED READINGS

General

Akbar SA, Jafri SZ, Amendola MA, et al. Complications of renal transplantation. *Radiographics.* 2005;25:1335–1356.

Brown ED, Chen MY, Wolfman NT, et al. Complications of renal transplantation: evaluation with US and radionuclide imaging. *Radiographics.* 2000;20(3):607.

Catala V, Marti T, Diaz JM, et al. Use of Multidetector CT in presurgical evaluation of potential kidney transplant recipients. *Radiographics.* 2010;30:517–531.

Fananapazir G, Troppmann C, Corwin MT, et al. Incidences of acute kidney injury, dialysis and graft loss following intravenous administration of low-osmolality iodinated contrast in patients with kidney transplants. *Abdom Radiol.* 2016;41:2182–2186.

Nankivell BJ, Alexander SI. Rejection of the kidney allograft. *N Engl J Med.* 2010;363(15):1451–1462.

O'Neill WC, Baumgarten DA. Ultrasonography in renal transplantation. *Am J Kidney Dis.* 2002;39(4):663.

Rajiah P, Lim YY, Taylor P. Renal transplant imaging and complications. *Abdom Imaging.* 2006;31(6):735–746.

Rao PS, Merion RSM, Ashley VB, et al. Renal transplantation in elderly patients older than 70 years of age: results from the Scientific Registry of Transplant Recipients. *Transplantation.* 2007;83:1069—1074.

Shapiro R, Sarwal MM. Pediatric kidney transplantation. *Pediatr Clin North Am.* 2010;57(2):393–400.

Sharfuddin A. Renal relevant radiology: imaging in kidney transplantation. *Clin J Am Soc Nephrol.* 2014;9:416–429.

Singh AK, Sahani DV. Imaging of the renal donor and transplant recipient. *Radiol Clin North Am.* 2008;46(1):79–93.

Living Donor Evaluation

Catala V, Marti T, Diaz JM, et al. Use of multidetector CT in presurgical evaluation of potential kidney transplant recipients. *Radiographics.* 2010;30(2):517–531.

Feifer AH, Fong BC, Feldman L, et al. Preoperative evaluation of laparoscopic living renal donors with computerized tomography and its effect on donor morbidity and graft function. *Can J Urol.* 2005;12(3):2713–2721.

Hanninen EL, Denecke T, Stelter L, et al. Preoperative evaluation of living kidney donors using multirow detector computed tomography: comparison with digital subtraction angiography and intraoperative findings. *Transpl Int.* 2005;18(10):1134.

Rossi C, Boss A, Artunc F, et al. Comprehensive assessment of renal function and vessel morphology in potential living kidney donors: an MRI-based approach. *Invest Radiol.* 2009;44(11):705–711.

Sebastia C, Peri L, Salvador R, et al. Multidetector CT of living renal donors: lessons learned from surgeons. *Radiographics.* 2010;30(7):1875–1890.

Su C, Yan C, Guo Y, et al. Multi-detector row CT as a "one-stop" examination in the preoperative evaluation of the morphology and function of living renal donors: preliminary study. *Abdom Imaging.* 2011;36:86–90.

Zamboni GA, Romero JY, Raptopoulos VD. Combined vascular-excretory phase MDCT angiography in the preoperative evaluation of renal donors. *AJR Am J Roentgenol.* 2010;194(1):145–150.

Infection

Al-Geizawi SM, Farney AC, Rogers J, et al. Renal allograft failure due to emphysematous pyelonephritis: successful non operative management and proposed new classification scheme based on literature review. *Transpl Infect Dis.* 2010;12(6):543–550.

Radionuclide Studies

Aktas A, Aras M, Colak T, et al. Indicators of acute rejection on Tc-99m DTPA renal scintigraphy. *Transpl Proc.* 2006;38(2):443–448.

Dubovsky EV, Russell CD, Erbas B. Radionuclide evaluation of renal transplants. *Semin Nucl Med.* 1995;25(1):49.

Guignard R, Mourad G, Mariano-Goulart D. Utility of postsurgical renal scintigraphy to predict one-year outcome of renal transplants in patients with delayed graft function. *Nucl Med Commun.* 2011;32(4):314–319.

Shah AN. Radionuclide imaging in organ transplantation. *Radiol Clin North Am.* 1995;33(3):447.

Acute Rejection: Ultrasound Studies

Chudek J, Kolonko A, Krol R, et al. The intrarenal vascular resistance parameters measured by duplex Doppler ultrasound shortly after kidney transplantation in patients with immediate, slow and delayed graft function. *Transpl Proc.* 2006;38(1):42.

Cosgrove DO, Chan KE. Renal transplants: what ultrasound can and cannot do. *Ultrasound Q.* 2008;24(2):77–87.

Gao J, Rubin JM, Xiang DY, et al. Doppler parameters in renal transplant dysfunction: correlations with histopathologic changes. *J Ultrasound Med.* 2011;30(2):169–175.

Irshad A, Ackerman S, Sosnouski D, et al. A review of sonographic evaluation of renal transplant complications. *Curr Probl Diagn Radiol.* 2008;37(2):67–79.

Krejci K, Zadrazil J, Tichy T, et al. Sonographic findings in borderline changes and subclinical acute renal allograft rejection. *Eur J Radiol.* 2009;71(2):288–295.

Loock MT, Bamoulid J, Courivaud C, et al. Significant increase in 1-year posttransplant renal arterial index predicts graft loss. *Clin J Am Soc Nephrol.* 2010;5(10):1867–1872.

McArthur C, Geddes CC, Baxter GM. Early measurement of pulsatility and resistive indexes: correlation with long-term renal transplant function. *Radiology.* 2011;259(1):278–285.

O'Neill WC, Baumgarten DA. Ultrasonography in renal transplantation. *Am J Kidney Dis.* 2002;39(4):663–678.

Park SB, Kim JK, Cho KS. Complications of renal transplantation: ultrasonographic evaluation. *J Ultrasound Med.* 2007;26(5):615–633.

Magnetic Resonance Imaging

Baumgartner RB, Nelson RC, Ball TI, et al. MR imaging of renal transplants. *AJR Am J Roentgenol.* 1986;147:949.

Klehr HU, Spannbrucker N, Molitor D, et al. Magnetic resonance imaging in renal transplants. *Transpl Proc.* 1987;19(5):3716.

Pereira RS, Gonul II, McLaughlin K, et al. Assessment of chronic renal allograft nephropathy using contrast-enhanced MRI: a pilot study. *AJR Am J Roentgenol.* 2010;194(5):W407–W413.

Steinberg HV, Nelson RC, Murphy FB, et al. Renal allograft rejection evaluation by Doppler US and MR imaging. *Radiology.* 1987;163:337.

Transplant Rupture

Ostrovsky PD, Cart L, Goodman JC, et al. Ultrasound findings in renal transplant rupture. *J Clin Ultrasound.* 1985;13:132.

Computed Tomography

Chu LC, Sheth S, Segev DL, et al. Role of MDCT angiography in selection and presurgical planning of potential renal donors. *AJR Am J Roentgenol.* 2012;199:1035–1041.

Gayer G, Apter S, Katz R, et al. CT findings in ten patients with failed renal allografts; comparison with findings in functional grafts. *Eur J Radiol.* 2000;36(3):133.

Yano M, Lin MF, Hoffman KA, et al. Renal measurements on CT angiograms: correlation with graft function at living donor renal transplantation. *Radiology.* 2012;285:151–157.

Vascular Complications

Al-Katib S, Shetty M, Jafri SMA, et al. Radiologic assessment of native renal vasculature: a multimodality review. *Radiographics.* 2017;37:136–156.

Ghazanfar A, Tavakoli A, Augustine T, et al. Management of transplant renal artery stenosis and its impact on long-term allograft survival: a single-centre experience. *Nephrol Dial Transplant.* 2011;26(1):336–343.

Loubeyre P, Cahen R, Grozel F, et al. Transplant renal artery stenosis. Evaluation of diagnosis with magnetic resonance angiography compared with color duplex sonography and arteriography. *Transplantation.* 1996;62(4):446–450.

Urologic Complications

Gottlieb RH, Voci SL, Cholewinski SP, et al. Urine leaks in renal transplant patients. Diagnostic usefulness of sonography and renography. *Clin Imaging.* 1999;23(1):35–39.

Sciascia N, Zompatori M, Di Scioscio V, et al. Multidetector CT-urography in the study of urological complications in renal transplant. *Radiol Med.* 2002;103(5–6):501–510.

Sutherland T, Temple F, Chang S, et al. Sonographic evaluation of renal transplant complications. *J Med Imaging Radiat Oncol.* 2010;54(3):211–218.

Wong-You-Cheong JJ, Grumbach K, Krebs TL, et al. Torsion of intraperitoneal renal transplants: imaging appearances. *AJR Am J Roentgenol.* 1998;171:1355.

Long-Term Complications of Renal Transplantation

Frick MP, Salomonwitz E, Hanto DW, et al. CT of abdominal lymphoma after renal transplantation. *AJR Am J Roentgol.* 1984;142:97.

Katabathina VS, Menias CO, Tammisetti VS, et al. Malignancy after solid organ transplantation: comprehensive imaging review. *Radiographics.* 2016;36:1390–1407.

Miller WT Jr, Siegel SG, Montone KT. Posttransplantation lymphoproliferative disorder: changing manifestations of disease in a renal transplant population. *Crit Rev Diagn Imaging.* 1997;38(6):569–585.

10

Vascular Diseases

ANATOMY

Arterial

The renal arteries branch from the aorta near the level of the L-1 to L-2 interspace. The right renal artery usually arises from the lateral or anterolateral aspect of the aorta and is slightly lower than the left renal artery, which arises from the lateral or posterolateral aspect of the aorta. Although this is usually readily apparent on CT or MR examinations, catheter aortography should be performed in the anteroposterior or slight right posterior oblique projections to demonstrate the origin of the renal arteries to best advantage.

In as many as 40% of patients, one or both kidneys are supplied by more than one renal artery. Accessory renal arteries arise from the aorta and are usually inferior to the main renal artery. Occasionally, an accessory renal artery supplies the upper pole of the kidney; rarely, an accessory renal artery may arise from the celiac, hepatic, or mesenteric arteries. Anomalous kidneys, such as a horseshoe or pelvic kidney, almost always have multiple renal arteries that arise from the aorta or iliac arteries near the kidneys. Accessory renal arteries are regularly seen on computed tomography angiography (CTA) (Fig. 10.1) or magnetic resonance angiography (MRA) and are often found on routine abdominal CT examinations (Fig. 10.2).

The inferior adrenal artery and arteries supplying the renal capsule, renal pelvis, and ureter arise from the main renal artery. Occasionally, the gonadal, middle adrenal, or inferior phrenic arteries may also arise from the renal artery.

The main renal artery divides into dorsal and ventral rami that run posterior and anterior to the renal pelvis. The larger ventral division supplies the anterior and superior aspects of the kidney, whereas the dorsal division supplies the posterior and inferior portions of the kidney. The junction of these ventral and dorsal divisions creates a relatively avascular plane (Brodel's line), which is the preferred track for placing percutaneous nephrostomies.

Segmental branches arise from the dorsal and ventral rami and run along the infundibula before dividing into interlobar arteries. These interlobar arteries course between the pyramids and the cortical columns parallel to the outer surface of the kidneys before branching into arcuate arteries, which run along the bases of the medullary pyramids.

Collateral pathways that provide arterial supply to the kidney when the main renal artery is compromised include the inferior adrenal, capsular, ureteric, gonadal, intercostal, lumbar, and pelvic arteries. The upper three lumbar arteries allow blood from the aorta to communicate with pelvic, ureteral, or capsular arteries, which anastomose with renal branch arteries. When the ureteral artery serves as a major collateral artery, the dilation and tortuosity resulting from increased blood flow may cause the artery to impinge on the ureter, causing notching.

Venous

In general, the venous anatomy parallels the arterial circulation. Accessory renal veins are less frequent than accessory arteries and occur more commonly on the right side. The left renal vein may bifurcate to encircle the aorta and become a circumaortic renal vein. This anomaly is caused by the persistence of the posteriorly located left supracardinal vein and by a midline supracardinal anastomosis between right and left vessels. It is a relatively common anomaly, reported in 2% to 16% of patients, according to anatomic and angiographic studies. Using CT, Reed et al. (1982) found a circumaortic left renal vein in 19 (4.4%) of 433 patients (Fig. 10.3). The posterior portion of this venous collar typically runs inferiorly before crossing behind the aorta to reach the inferior vena

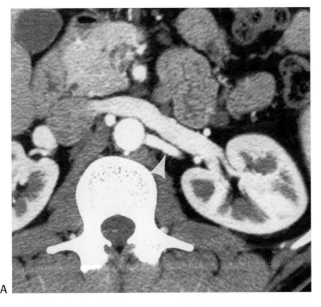

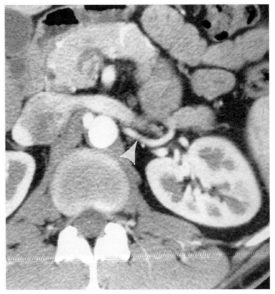

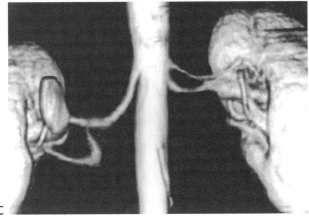

FIGURE 10.1. Accessory renal artery. **A:** The main renal artery (*arrowhead*) is seen arising from the aorta. **B:** An accessory renal artery (*arrowhead*) is identified just cephalad to the main renal artery. **C:** Both left renal arteries are nicely displayed on this shaded surface display.

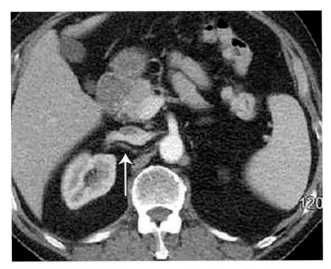

FIGURE 10.2. Accessory renal artery. A small right renal artery (*arrow*) is arising from the aorta.

cava (IVC). The ventral vein usually drains the ventral and inferior portions of the kidney, whereas the dorsal component drains the dorsal and superior segments. Knowledge of this anomaly is important when surgery is contemplated or during collection of renal or adrenal vein samples.

Another common anomaly, the retroaortic left renal vein, is seen less frequently. In the same series of CT examinations reported by Reed et al., 8 (1.8%) of 433 patients had a single retroaortic renal vein (Figs. 10.4 and 10.5). Both of these anomalies can be recognized on CT, and venography is seldom necessary for confirmation. The retroaortic component often extends caudally before passing behind the aorta. It is important not to confuse this with an enlarged lymph node on the axial CT image (Fig. 10.3). Patients are asymptomatic, but recognition is important if surgery involving this region is planned.

The left renal vein receives the inferior phrenic, capsular, ureteric, adrenal, and gonadal veins. In addition, rich collateral vessels usually anastomose with branches of the hemiazygos and ascending lumbar veins. These vessels are particularly important because they may preserve the kidney, should venous thrombosis occur. In patients with a left-sided IVC, the left common iliac vein continues cephalad as the left IVC and drains into the inferior aspect of the left renal vein.

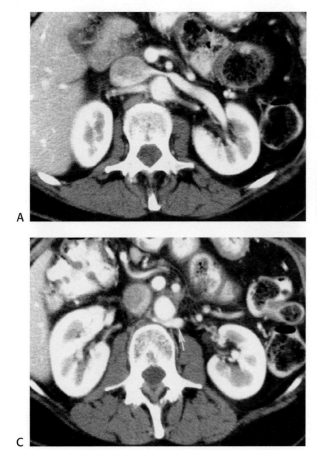

A

B

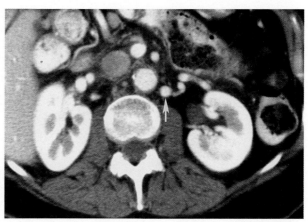

C

FIGURE 10.3. Circumaortic left renal vein. **A:** The anterior portion of a circumaortic left renal vein is in its normal location. **B:** The posterior portion (*arrow*) runs caudally. **C:** The posterior portion (*arrow*) runs behind the aorta.

The right renal vein is shorter than the left and has a more oblique course to the IVC. It receives capsular and ureteric veins as well as some retroperitoneal collateral veins, but the right inferior phrenic and gonadal veins enter directly into the IVC.

Valves may occur in the renal veins. They are infrequently seen on venography, and there is a marked variation in the reported incidence of renal vein valves in anatomic studies, ranging from 28% to 70% on the right and from 4% to 36% on the left. Their significance lies in surgical planning.

Renal vein varices may be idiopathic or may result from renal vein thrombosis or portal hypertension. Like varicoceles, renal vein varices are more common on the left than on the right. Thus, an anatomic etiology is postulated. Compression of the left renal vein between the superior mesenteric artery and the aorta ("nutcracker" phenomenon) may result in left renal vein hypertension, hematuria, and varix formation. Obstruction of the left renal vein by the superior mesenteric artery is more likely to occur in thin patients in whom there is a paucity of retroperitoneal fat. Because a distended

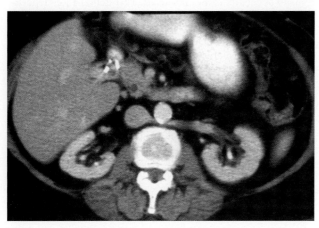

FIGURE 10.4. Retroaortic left renal vein. The left renal vein passes behind the aorta to enter the IVC.

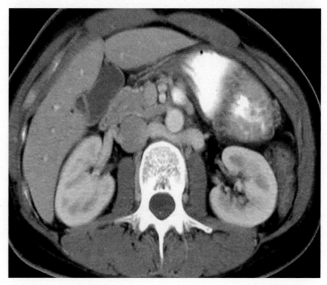

FIGURE 10.5. Retroaortic left renal vein. The vein is seen passing behind the aorta.

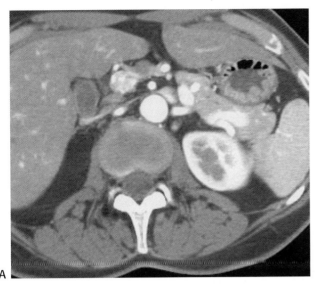
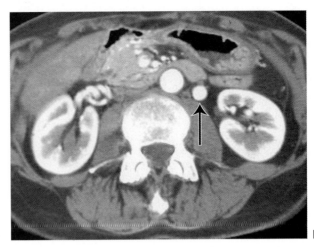

FIGURE 10.6. Nutcracker phenomenon. **A:** The left renal vein is squeezed between the superior mesenteric artery and the aorta. **B:** The left gonadal vein (*arrow*) is enlarged as it is a collateral pathway for renal blood flow.

left renal vein may be seen by CT (Fig. 10.6) or ultrasound in 51% to 72% of the normal population, measurement of a pressure gradient between the IVC and the left renal vein is needed before renal vein compression should be diagnosed. The demonstration of collateral veins using color-flow Doppler provides noninvasive evidence of renal vein compression.

Collateral pathways exist for venous drainage of blood from the kidney in case of occlusion of the main renal vein. Inferior phrenic or adrenal, gonadal, and ureteric veins commonly enter the left renal vein, whereas only the ureteric vein enters the right renal vein. Any of these vessels, as well as a variety of small retroperitoneal veins that enter the renal veins, may function as collateral vessels. The right adrenal, inferior phrenic, and gonadal veins enter directly into the IVC.

In renal vein thrombosis, the clot usually propagates along the entire renal vein, and these collateral vessels are also occluded. A local occlusion, such as surgical ligation, however, may allow these collaterals to take over drainage of the kidney. This occurs much more readily with occlusion of the left renal vein, as it receives more potential collateral vessels than the right renal vein.

Circumcaval (Retrocaval) Ureter

Persistence of the right subcardinal vein traps the ureter behind the IVC. The ureter crosses posterior to the IVC and then passes around the medial border anteriorly to partially encircle the cava. This anomaly, which occurs in approximately 1 in 1,100 patients, has been termed a retrocaval, or circumcaval, ureter. The term *circumcaval ureter* is preferred because it is possible for the ureter to lie behind the vena cava without encircling it. A circumcaval ureter is usually an incidental finding and is more common in men than in women. Most patients are asymptomatic, although right flank pain may be sufficient to bring this anomaly to attention.

The most common complication is obstruction, caused by constriction of the retrocaval segment of the ureter by the IVC. In a few cases, fibrous bands or adhesions of this segment of the ureter have been reported. The hydronephrosis and stasis predispose to stone formation and infection.

Two radiographic patterns of circumcaval ureter have been recognized. The more common form, type I, has an S-shaped deformity of the midureter as it courses around the IVC. The narrowing of the ureter occurs at the lateral border of the psoas muscle, suggesting that the obstruction is not caused by compression by the IVC. The

second type (type II) has less severe hydronephrosis, but the point of obstruction is at the lateral wall of the IVC. However, ureteral obstruction is not necessarily present in a circumcaval ureter.

When the classic (type I) appearance is seen in urography, the diagnosis of circumcaval ureter can be suggested ((Figs. 10.7 and 10.8)). However, an inferior vena cavogram or CT (Fig. 10.8) is needed for confirmation. In the less severe form (type II), medial deviation must be distinguished from other etiologies, such as retroperitoneal fibrosis or a retroperitoneal mass.

Circumcaval ureter can be recognized on CT by following the opacified ureter around the IVC. CT also demonstrates the more lateral location of the cava, which usually lies lateral to the right pedicle of the third lumbar vertebral body.

Lymphatic

There is an extensive lymphatic system within the kidney that provides an accessory drainage route for excess fluid. In normal states, approximately one-fourth of lymphatic flow from the kidney

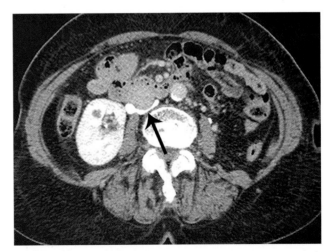

FIGURE 10.7. Circumcaval ureter. Failure of regression of the postcardinal vein traps the ureter (*arrow*) behind the IVC.

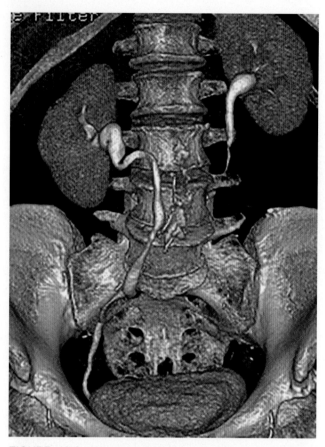

FIGURE 10.8. Circumcaval ureter. Reconstructed images from a CT urogram demonstrate a dilated proximal ureter, which courses behind the IVC.

occurs through small lymphatic vessels that permeate the capsule and communicate with lymph vessels in the perinephric space. The remainder of the renal lymph fluid is drained into large lymph vessels in the renal hilum. The renal lymphatics are not directly imaged, but enlarged vessels may be detected by CT.

DISEASES OF INTRARENAL ARTERIES

A variety of entities affect intrarenal arteries. Although the etiology and clinical course may be different, the radiographic manifestations are similar. Because the disease process is usually generalized, both kidneys are affected and are reduced in size. Small infarcts result in a slightly irregular contour. Renal function may be markedly impaired, but the renal collecting system will be normal. The most characteristic findings of diseases affecting intrarenal arteries are the multiple microaneurysms seen with renal arteriography.

Collagen Vascular Diseases

The vasculitides, which may occur as a primary process or secondary to another disease, are characterized by inflammatory leukocytes, which damage the vessel walls. Although any of the systemic vasculitides may involve the kidneys, this discussion will concentrate on those that do so commonly. They may be classified as large, medium or small vessel arteritis.

Large Vessel Arteritis

Large vessel vasculitides include Takayasu arteritis and giant cell arteritis.

Takayasu disease is a granulomatous arteritis that commonly involves the aorta and its major branches. It has a marked female preponderance and is usually seen in patients younger than 35 years of age. Although primarily seen in Asians, cases are being reported with increasing frequency in western nations. Giant cell or temporal arteritis is histologically similar, but predominantly involves branches of the carotid artery, including the temporal artery; it is typically found in older patients.

Because major branches of the abdominal aorta are often affected, hypertension is a common complication of Takayasu disease. The hypertension may be caused by coarctation of the aorta or main renal artery stenosis (RAS). Symptoms of Takayasu aortitis are nonspecific and are often not recognized until the disease is well advanced.

Takayasu disease is classified into four types. Arteriography demonstrates vascular narrowing of the aortic arch or great vessels arising from the arch (type I); descending thoracic and upper abdominal aorta (type II); aortic arch vessels, abdominal aorta, and major branches (type III); or pulmonary arteries (type IV). Typically, there is a smooth, tapered narrowing of the affected artery. Skip areas may occur, and multiple vessels are commonly involved. The disease may progress to complete occlusion. Treatment is usually surgical, but successful transluminal angioplasty has been reported.

Medium Vessel Arteritis

Polyarteritis nodosa (PAN) and Kawasaki disease are medium vessel vasculitides.

PAN is a panarteritis with foci of fibrinoid necrosis that begin in the media. The subsequent inflammation that spreads to involve the intima and adventitia results in small aneurysms and vascular thrombosis. Although the etiology of PAN is unknown, it is associated with rheumatoid arthritis, Sjögren syndrome, hepatitis B, cryoglobulinemia, and hairy cell leukemia. Renal involvement occurs in 90% of patients with PAN. Patients often present with hematuria, and renin-mediated hypertension is common. The small aneurysms seen in PAN may occasionally rupture and produce an intraparenchymal or perinephric hematoma.

With the exception of arteriography, radiographic imaging studies demonstrate nonspecific findings. Parenchymal scarring may be seen with urography, ultrasound, or CT. Areas of hemorrhage due to aneurysm rupture are best defined by CT but, if large, can also be detected by ultrasonography. The most definitive radiographic examination is arteriography, where small aneurysms occur at the bifurcation of interlobular or arcuate arteries (Fig. 10.9). These aneurysms are not limited to the kidneys, and arteries in the liver, spleen, pancreas, muscle, and gastrointestinal tract are often involved.

Although these small aneurysms are typical of PAN, they are not pathognomonic. Similar aneurysms may be seen in patients with systemic lupus erythematosus, Wegener granulomatosis, and intravenous drug abuse.

Kawasaki disease is an acute febrile illness affecting infants and small children. It is frequently accompanied by a mucocutaneous lymph node syndrome. This vasculitis involves small- and medium-sized arteries with a predilection for the coronary arteries.

Small Vessel Arteritis

Small vessel arteritides include Wegener granulomatosis (granulomatosis with polyangiitis), eosinophilic granulomatosis with polyangiitis (Churg–Strauss), and IgA vasculitis (Henoch–Schönlein purpura).

Patients with Wegener granulomatosis have necrotizing granulomas of the respiratory tract, a focal necrotizing angiitis involving small arteries and veins, and a focal necrotizing glomerulitis that leads to fibrin thrombi and local necrosis of individual glomerular tufts. It occurs most commonly in the fourth and fifth decades and has a slight male preponderance. Symptoms of upper airway involvement dominate the clinical presentation. Although nodular,

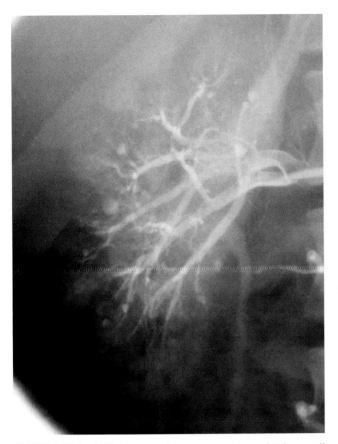

FIGURE 10.9. PAN. An arteriogram reveals multiple small aneurysms of the intrarenal arteries.

infiltrative, or cavitary lung lesions are commonly seen, the pulmonary involvement is generally asymptomatic.

Renal disease may be absent in the limited form of Wegener granulomatosis, but a rapidly progressive glomerulonephritis is life threatening in the full syndrome. The most common manifestations of renal disease are hematuria and proteinuria. The radiographic manifestations in the kidneys are nonspecific but include microaneurysms, renal infarction (Fig. 10.10), parenchymal scarring, and areas of hemorrhage. The findings are indistinguishable

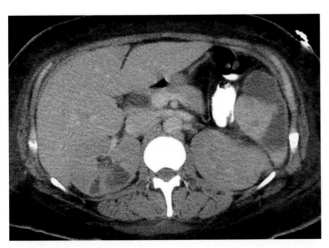

FIGURE 10.10. Wegener granulomatosis. A wedge-shaped area of infarction is seen in the posterior aspect of the right kidney.

from those of PAN. Rarely, a renal mass may be seen as a manifestation of the disease.

Eosinophilic granulomatosis with polyangiitis, or Churg–Strauss vasculitis, is similar to Wegener granulomatosis but rarely involves the kidneys.

Arteritis Affecting any Size Artery

Some vasculitides may affect arteries of any size. Those include systemic lupus erythematosus and Behcet syndrome.

Most patients with systemic lupus erythematosus have renal involvement, and many die of renal failure. The larger renal vessels are usually unaffected, but interlobular arteries may be affected by inflammatory changes and may be narrowed. The predominant renal changes consist of a focal glomerulonephritis with thickening of the basement membrane resulting in the "wire-loop" appearance on histologic preparations.

The radiographic appearance depends on the stage of involvement. Before the onset of renal failure, the kidneys appear normal. Microaneurysms, similar to those seen in PAN, may occasionally be seen on angiography, and renal infarcts are common. Conventional ultrasound examination is often normal, but an elevated resistive index may be predictive of worsening renal function.

Intravenous Drug Abuse

The vasculitis associated with intravenous drug abuse has clinical and pathologic features similar to PAN. Although methamphetamine is a common drug used by patients in whom a vasculitis develops, they are usually exposed to multiple drugs. Circulating hepatitis antigen–antibody complexes or drug contaminants may also be responsible for vascular injury. The radiographic appearance of multiple aneurysms 1 to 5 mm in diameter occurring at bifurcations, vascular stenoses, and complete vascular occlusion with infarction is indistinguishable from other vasculitides.

Scleroderma

Progressive systemic sclerosis is a generalized disorder manifested by vascular and connective tissue fibrosis. Narrowing of the interlobular arteries due to intimal thickening may be present, as may fibrinoid necrosis of the afferent arterioles. It occurs most commonly in the fourth and fifth decades and shows a significant female preponderance. The kidneys may be affected in up to 80% of patients, and renal failure is often the cause of death.

The radiographic manifestations are nonspecific. Before the onset of renal failure, the kidneys may appear normal. Hypertension is common, such that the vascular changes seen on angiography may be due to either nephrosclerosis or scleroderma. However, the microaneurysms seen with the vasculitides are not seen with scleroderma.

Radiation Nephritis

Radiation nephritis is a degenerative process that affects the tubules and glomeruli. It may be acute or chronic, cause hypertension, or result merely in proteinuria. The vascular changes of fibrinoid necrosis occur late in the course and involve primarily arcuate and interlobar arteries. Doses of at least 20 Gy (2,000 rads) within a 5-week period are needed to cause significant renal damage.

Acute radiation nephritis is manifested by proteinuria and hypertension after a latent period of 6 to 12 months. Uremia, malignant hypertension, and congestive heart failure follow. The prognosis of these patients is poor, with a mortality of approximately 50%.

Patients who develop chronic radiation nephritis may or may not have been affected by acute radiation nephritis. Chronic radiation nephritis has an insidious onset of mild proteinuria,

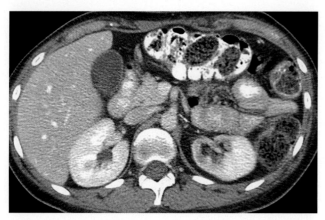

FIGURE 10.11. Radiation nephritis. A thin cortical margin is seen in the upper pole of the left kidney after irradiation of a left adrenal tumor.

anemia, and azotemia, beginning 18 months to several years after radiation exposure. Although the clinical course is more protracted, the mortality of 50% is similar to acute radiation nephritis.

The radiographic appearance of radiation nephritis depends on the radiation dose and the time between the radiation exposure and the imaging study. In the acute phase, diminished renal function may be manifested only by decreased concentration of excreted contrast medium. In the chronic phase, an area of diminished enhancement is seen (Fig. 10.11).

Arteriolar Nephrosclerosis

Systemic hypertension affects the vascular tree of the kidney more consistently and more extensively than any other region of the body. The degree of change is largely a function of the severity and duration of the hypertension.

The clinical symptoms of patients with benign nephrosclerosis are usually limited to those of hypertension. In malignant nephrosclerosis, patients have a diastolic blood pressure >130 mm Hg and have papilledema. Neurologic symptoms and renal failure are common. Elevated plasma renin and aldosterone along with hypokalemia are manifestations of secondary aldosteronism, and proteinuria is common. Untreated malignant hypertension has a poor prognosis, and renal failure is the most common cause of death.

The radiographic findings reflect the degree of involvement of the kidneys. Unless there is a RAS to protect one of the kidneys,

involvement is systemic. The kidneys are normal to small in size. The calyces remain normal, even in areas of marked cortical thinning. Increased tortuosity and more rapid tapering of intrarenal arteries are seen with angiography. More severe changes include filling defects and loss of cortical vessels.

EMBOLISM AND INFARCTION

The most common source of renal artery emboli is a diseased heart. Patients with atrial enlargement secondary to valvular heart disease or a dyskinetic left ventricle after myocardial infarction provide the source of mural thrombi that may dislodge and become renal artery emboli. Smaller emboli may arise from an ectatic or aneurysmal aorta or even from cholesterol plaques in a patient with severe atherosclerosis.

Unlike arterial stenoses that are slowly progressive and may cause atrophy or collateralization, emboli produce acute ischemia that may result in infarction. The typical clinical features include the sudden onset of flank pain, hematuria, proteinuria, fever, and leukocytosis. However, the presentation is variable, and the diagnosis often is missed. Despite documented unilateral involvement, a decrease in renal function is seen in many patients.

The radiographic appearance of renal embolism depends on the size of the embolus and location of the arterial occlusion. There is no enhancement of the affected segment of the kidney, reflecting lack of vascular perfusion. If the main renal artery is occluded, there is no renal function in the affected kidney. A swollen, edematous kidney is seen on ultrasound as an enlarged kidney with decreased echogenicity. Retrograde pyelography reveals a normal collecting system with sharply cupped calyces. If there is much swelling, there may be attenuation of the intrarenal collecting system.

The absence of contrast enhancement in the affected renal tissue is best demonstrated by CT. Smaller infarcts are seen as wedge-shaped, low-density areas within an otherwise normal-appearing kidney (Fig. 10.12). If the entire kidney is affected, the increase in size due to edema can be identified by the large size and more rounded configuration. Even if the entire renal artery is occluded, capsular branches remain patent and enhance the outer rim of the kidney. The preservation of this outer 2 to 4 mm of the cortex is best seen on CT (Figs. 10.10 and 10.12).

Occasionally, high-grade stenosis of an intrarenal artery will diminish opacification, but will not cause frank infarction with scarring. Images obtained after contrast has washed out of the normal renal parenchyma may demonstrate persistent enhancement of this hypoperfused area (Fig. 10.13).

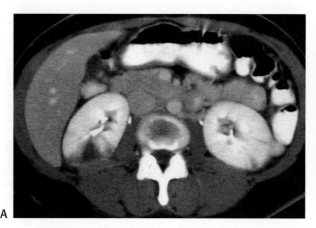
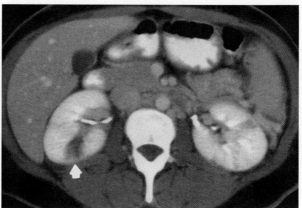

A   B

FIGURE 10.12. Renal infarction. **A:** Several wedge-shaped unenhancing areas indicate infarction because of emboli from subacute bacterial endocarditis. **B:** Capsular vessels preserve a thin peripheral rim (*arrow*).

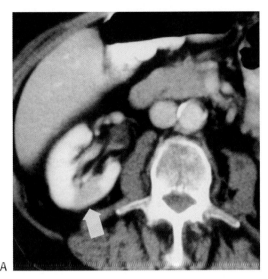 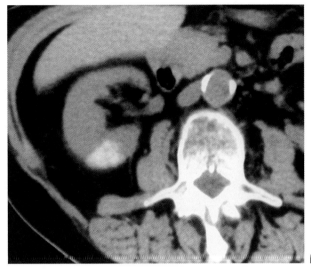

FIGURE 10.13. Localized hypoperfusion. **A:** An area of poor enhancement is seen in the posterior aspect of the right kidney (*arrow*). **B:** An unenhanced examination obtained 2 days later reveals persistent opacification of the hypoperfused area.

Arteriography is no longer needed for a definitive diagnosis of renal infarction, as CT or MR is usually sufficient. If the infarct is due to a renal embolus, arteriography can demonstrate a sharp vessel cutoff when the embolus completely occludes arterial flow. Incompletely occluding emboli appear as a filling defect within a contrast-filled artery (Fig. 10.14).

After the acute phase of renal infarction, atrophy begins. The infarcted tissue contracts, leaving a cortical scar (Fig. 10.15). The parenchymal loss reflects the distribution of the affected artery.

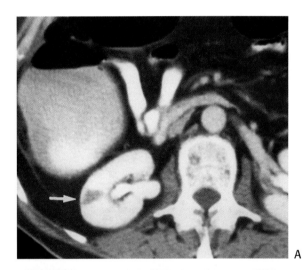

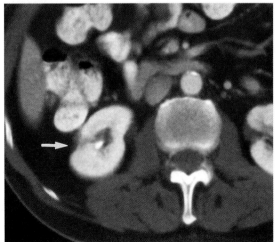

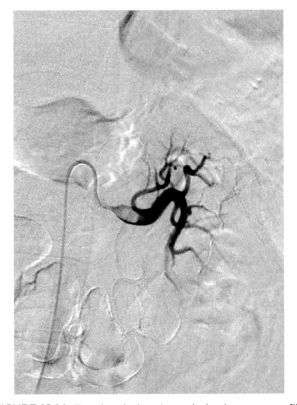

FIGURE 10.14. Renal embolus. An embolus is seen as a filling defect in the left renal artery.

FIGURE 10.15. Chronic infarction. **A:** An acute infarction is seen as a wedge-shaped unenhanced area with preservation of the periphery by capsular vessels (*arrow*). **B:** Six months later, a cortical scar is present (*arrow*).

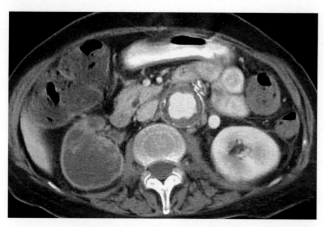

FIGURE 10.16. Renal infarction. An enhanced CT demonstrates preservation of a thin cortical rim supplied by capsular vessels.

If the main renal artery is occluded, the entire kidney will be affected. The kidney will show no enhancement but may demonstrate a viable thin cortical rim supplied by capsular arteries (Fig. 10.16). Later, the kidney atrophies uniformly. There is no appreciable renal function, but renin may be elaborated and may cause hypertension.

Treatment of renal artery embolism depends on the patient's underlying medical condition and the status of the contralateral kidney. Attempts at revascularization can be made with lytic therapy delivered directly into the renal artery through an arterial catheter. Although this is not rewarding as often as lysis of clot that forms behind an arterial stenosis, excellent results have been reported. Many patients are treated with anticoagulant therapy, although surgical revascularization may be attempted in selected cases.

Arterial Thrombosis

Thrombosis of the renal artery occurs most commonly as a complication of severe atherosclerosis and may occasionally be seen on CT (Fig. 10.17). In such cases, atherosclerosis usually involves a variety of other arteries, including coronary and carotid arteries that dominate the clinical picture. This gradual occlusion of the renal

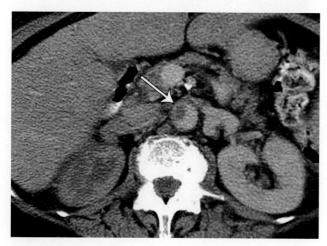

FIGURE 10.17. Renal infarction. Thrombus (arrow) is seen in the aorta at the expected origin of the right renal artery. The right renal cortex shows only minimal enhancement.

artery that finally results in thrombosis is usually clinically silent and results in ipsilateral renal atrophy.

Acute thrombosis of the renal artery may occur after trauma. It usually follows blunt abdominal trauma in which the forces of acceleration or deceleration produce intimal tears, with resulting dissection of the renal artery and thrombosis. Renal artery thrombosis may also result from subintimal dissection of the renal artery during arteriography. This is more likely to occur during an attempted transluminal angioplasty than during a diagnostic renal arteriogram.

With acute renal artery thrombosis, the kidney remains normal in size. Unless extensive renal artery collaterals have developed, there is no renal function, and intravascular contrast medium will not be excreted. Retrograde pyelography demonstrates a normal collecting system.

Color-flow Doppler ultrasound may also be used in the diagnosis of renal artery thrombosis. The most common finding is absence of an intrarenal arterial signal. If there is incomplete occlusion or collateral vessels are present, a severe tardus-parvus abnormality is detected. In some patients, ultrasound may demonstrate a proximal renal artery stump.

CT reveals lack of enhancement, although a thin peripheral rim often remains viable because of collateral circulation through capsular arteries (Fig. 10.16). Because collateral blood flow may also come from ureteric, gonadal, lumbar, or adrenal arteries, additional portions of the kidney, such as the medulla, may also be preserved. Arteriography may be used to confirm the diagnosis of an occluded main renal artery.

With gradual occlusion, the kidney usually diminishes in size over time and a small kidney remains. If collateral vessels are present, there may be a small amount of renal function preserved. The renal contour is smooth, unless small infarcts have already occurred, and the calyces remain normal.

ANEURYSM

Atherosclerotic Aneurysm

Aneurysms of the renal arteries are uncommon. The most common etiology is atherosclerosis, but a dissecting aneurysm may also involve the renal artery. Mycotic aneurysms usually involve the aorta but may occasionally affect the renal artery.

Most patients are asymptomatic, and the aneurysm is often discovered incidentally on imaging studies. Because hypertensive patients often undergo angiography to identify a renovascular etiology, it is not surprising that many patients found to have a renal artery aneurysm are hypertensive. In some patients, surgical resection of the aneurysm results in cure of the hypertension; however, these patients usually have an associated RAS and lateralizing renal vein renin levels.

Renal artery aneurysms often contain clot and may give rise to renal emboli with or without infarction. The risk of rupture is small but is more likely in hypertensive or pregnant patients. Calcified aneurysms rarely rupture.

If calcified, a renal artery aneurysm can be recognized on the plain abdominal radiograph (Fig. 10.18). However, the appearance of a curvilinear calcification could be caused by a tortuous or wandering splenic artery or even a nonvascular etiology.

On ultrasound, an aneurysm is seen as a hypoechoic mass along the course of the renal artery. The Doppler signal arising from the aneurysm depends on the amount of thrombus and the size of the neck of the aneurysm.

Renal artery aneurysms may also be demonstrated by CT. Calcification along the wall of the aneurysm is readily detected on unenhanced images (Fig. 10.19). After contrast administration, variable enhancement is found, depending on the amount of thrombus within the aneurysm.

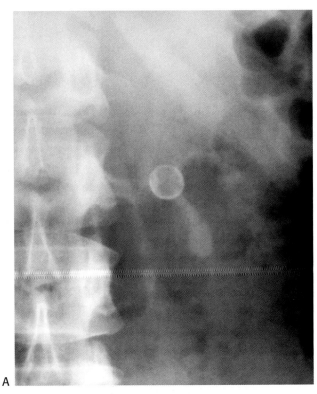
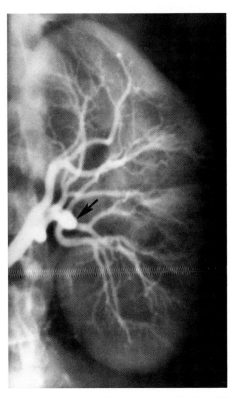

A   B

FIGURE 10.18. Renal artery aneurysm. **A:** A ring of calcium in the region of the left renal artery is identified on an abdominal radiograph. **B:** A selective left renal arteriogram reveals a renal artery aneurysm (*arrow*).

Renal artery aneurysms may be demonstrated on MR using a variety of techniques. Gadolinium-enhanced T1-weighted images using a phased array coil system are commonly employed (Fig. 10.20).

Arteriography may be required for a definitive diagnosis (Fig. 10.18), and even small, noncalcified aneurysms are easily identified unless thrombosed. The aneurysm may be partially or completely filled with thrombus, which prevents its opacification. Thus, thrombosed, uncalcified aneurysms may be missed by arteriography.

Surgical treatment for a renal artery aneurysm is seldom necessary. If renin-dependent hypertension can be demonstrated, resection is indicated. However, the presence of symptoms including flank pain or hematuria may be coincidental with, but not caused by, the aneurysm.

Mycotic Aneurysm

A mycotic aneurysm is one that arises as a result of an infectious process in the arterial wall. They may occur as a result of septic emboli, often from bacterial endocarditis, but also are seen in intravenous drug abusers. Septic emboli tend to lodge at a branch point, a site of rapid

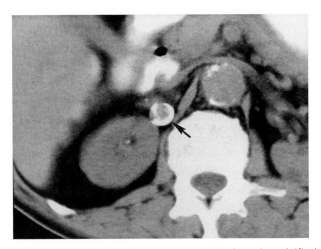

FIGURE 10.19. Renal artery aneurysm. A densely calcified right renal artery aneurysm (*arrow*) is clearly visible on this unenhanced CT examination.

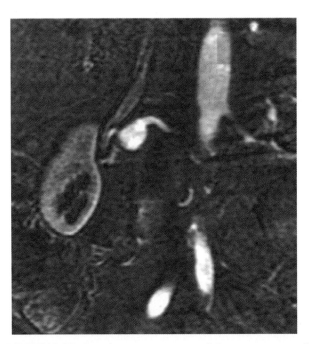

FIGURE 10.20. Renal artery aneurysm. A 3-cm aneurysm of the right renal artery is demonstrated on this gadolinium-enhanced T1-weighted MR image.

vessel tapering, or a sharp bend in the artery. Mycotic aneurysms may also result from direct spread from a contiguous infection or from bacteria lodging in the vasa vasorum or in the diseased intima.

Once established, the infection weakens the arterial wall and has a high incidence of rupture. Identification of a mycotic aneurysm may also be the first clue to an underlying bacterial endocarditis. Because the aneurysm may harbor bacteria despite antibiotic therapy, surgery may be needed to eradicate the site of infection.

ARTERIOVENOUS FISTULA

An arteriovenous fistula is an abnormal communication between the arterial and the venous circulations that bypasses the capillary bed. Congenital fistulae or arteriovenous malformations (AVMs), also known as angiomas or angiodysplasias, are uncommon. Acquired arteriovenous fistulae are usually due to trauma.

Congenital

Congenital AVMs are often asymptomatic and may not be detected in patients until they are well into adult life. They are found more often in women than in men, and hematuria is the most common presenting complaint. If large enough, an AVM may decrease perfusion to the renal parenchyma, resulting in renal ischemia and renin-mediated hypertension.

The findings on imaging studies are dependent on the size and location of the lesions. Large AVMs located near the collecting system may cause extrinsic compression on the renal pelvis. If there is hematuria, blood clots may be seen. Early and delayed phase imaging is important for their detection and characterization on CT. They enhance during the arterial phase and wash out quickly.

Color-flow Doppler ultrasound has become the best non-invasive modality to evaluate AVMs and arteriovenous fistulae. Malformations are seen as focal flow areas with a mixing of Doppler shift frequencies. However, this technique is insensitive to AVMs with minimal flow.

Arteriography may be needed for a definite diagnosis, and many small AVMs can be detected only with selective-magnification renal arteriography. AVMs are often classified as cirsoid or aneurysmal. Cirsoid AVMs have multiple small arteriovenous communications (Fig. 10.21), whereas aneurysmal AVMs have only a solitary communication. The cirsoid variety tends to be located adjacent to the collecting system and often causes hematuria. The aneurysmal AVM is more likely to cause an abdominal bruit and hypertension.

Acquired

Acquired arteriovenous fistulae do not have the female preponderance seen with congenital AVMs. Because trauma due to a penetrating injury or biopsy is the most common etiology, they more often are seen in men.

The physiologic effect of an arteriovenous fistula depends on the size of the fistula and its specific location. The artery supplying the fistula enlarges, and collateral vessels may develop if the fistula is larger than the artery feeding it. In some cases, retrograde flow may occur in the artery distal to the fistula. The draining veins are dilated, and their walls are thickened. This venous arterialization may even be associated with the development of atherosclerotic plaques.

The most common clinical manifestation of renal arteriovenous fistulae is an abdominal bruit. Approximately half of symptomatic patients have cardiomegaly and congestive heart failure. Hematuria is also common. Hypertension, which is usually diastolic, is renin mediated. The renal artery blood pressure and flow distal to the shunt are diminished. This relative renal ischemia stimulates renin secretion.

The most frequent etiology of an acquired arteriovenous fistula (Fig. 10.22) is renal biopsy. Many more acquired arteriovenous

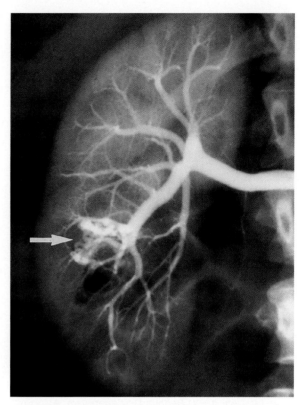

FIGURE 10.21. Congenital AVM. A tangle of vessels is seen in the right kidney (*arrow*).

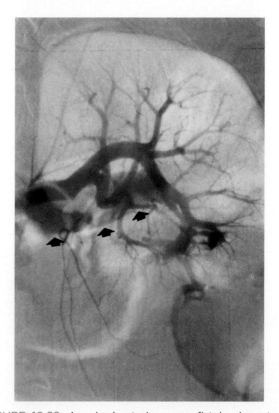

FIGURE 10.22. Acquired arteriovenous fistula. An arteriogram demonstrates rapid filling of the renal vein (*arrows*) after renal biopsy. Both the supplying artery and the draining vein are enlarged.

fistulae occur than are probably diagnosed because imaging is performed only in those patients symptomatic enough to suggest a large fistula. Arteriovenous fistulae may also be seen as a complication of selective renal arteriography, especially during percutaneous transluminal angioplasty (PTA). Acquired arteriovenous fistulae may be easier to detect with ultrasound than congenital AVMs. Increased flow velocity is found in the feeding artery and the draining vein. The flow at the shunt site is highly turbulent. The resistive index in the feeding artery is markedly reduced.

Small arteriovenous fistulae may heal spontaneously. Thus, many patients who develop a fistula after renal biopsy or angiography are not treated unless symptoms develop. Some of these fistulae may enlarge and require treatment.

Significant arteriovenous fistulae may be treated with transcatheter occlusion. It is critical to assess the size of the communication and be sure that any embolic material will be captured in the fistula and not pass through to become a pulmonary embolus. The most common indications for treatment are persistent hematuria or hypertension that can be localized to the kidney containing the fistula. If all the communicating branches can be occluded, percutaneous therapy should be successful. If transcatheter occlusion cannot be performed, surgery may be needed.

Postnephrectomy

Although uncommon, fistulae may develop between the stump of the renal artery and the stump of the renal vein or vena cava after nephrectomy. Postoperative infection or excessive bleeding requiring packing during surgery contributes to their development. These fistulae tend to be large and may be hemodynamically significant.

Idiopathic

Arteriovenous fistulae that appear to be acquired rather than congenital, but do not have an identifiable etiology, are classified as idiopathic. They may arise by erosion of a renal artery aneurysm into the adjacent vein.

RENAL HYPERTENSION

Renal Parenchymal Hypertension

A large number of parenchymal abnormalities have been associated with hypertension including pyelonephritis, glomerulopathies, ureteral obstruction, and renal mass lesions. Although many of these entities are common, they are seldom causally related to hypertension. However, documentation of a causal role has been shown in some cases, with relief of hypertension when the parenchymal abnormality has been alleviated.

Hydronephrosis

Unilateral ureteral obstruction may cause hypertension by activating the renin–angiotensin system. Acute ureteral occlusion has been shown to result in unilateral renin secretion and the development of hypertension in dogs. Human data confirm this increased renin secretion in patients with acute ureteral obstruction, but not in patients with chronic ureteral obstruction. Surgical intervention should cure those patients with lateralizing renin levels.

Renal Cyst

Renal cysts, as well as other masses, may rarely cause renin-mediated hypertension. This may be due to compression of the main renal artery or a branch renal artery causing ischemia. The resultant increased serum renin level leads to hypertension. Decompression of the cyst relieves the pressure on the renal artery and cures the

hypertension. Cyst drainage can be performed percutaneously, but sclerosis may be needed to prevent recurrence.

Chronic Pyelonephritis

Chronic pyelonephritis is another curable etiology of hypertension, although hypertension in most patients with chronic pyelonephritis is idiopathic. Patients more likely to become normotensive after nephrectomy for chronic pyelonephritis are younger, have a more recent onset of hypertension, have a more severely involved ipsilateral kidney, and have a nearly normal contralateral kidney. Lateralizing renal vein renin levels may be used to predict patients likely to respond to surgery.

Renal Carcinoma

Both renal adenocarcinoma and Wilms tumor may cause hypertension in several different ways. The mass may cause extrinsic compression on the renal artery, resulting in ischemia and increased renin secretion. Very vascular tumors may cause hypertension because of arteriovenous shunting. Rarely, a renal carcinoma or Wilms tumor may produce renin. In some patients, hypertension may be the presenting finding, and the renal tumor may be detected during the hypertension workup. Arteriography performed in these patients must include both main renal arteries to exclude a significant RAS and possible renovascular hypertension in the contralateral kidney.

Juxtaglomerular Tumors

A renin-secreting tumor of the juxtaglomerular cells is a rare cause of hypertension. Patients with a juxtaglomerular tumor, or reninoma, range in age from 7 to 58 years but often are younger than 20 years. The tumors are almost twice as common among women than among men. The most frequent symptoms are related to the hypertension and include headache, polydipsia, polyuria, and neuromuscular complaints resulting from hypokalemia. Hypertension in these patients is usually moderate to severe.

The tumor is usually small and confined to the kidney, although a large (6.5 cm) tumor and a reninoma arising in the perinephric space have been reported. Juxtaglomerular tumors are usually sharply marginated and may be separated from the normal renal parenchyma by a pseudocapsule.

Ultrasound is seldom used to detect juxtaglomerular tumors, but when found, they are relatively echogenic because of the numerous interfaces caused by the small vascular channels in the tumor.

CT is quite sensitive in detecting juxtaglomerular tumors (Fig. 10.23), but their appearance is nonspecific. Contrast

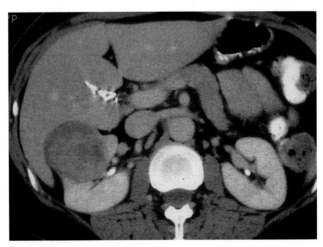

FIGURE 10.23. Juxtaglomerular tumor. A well-defined, soft-tissue mass is seen in the right kidney on this enhanced CT examination.

enhancement is needed, because the tumor may be isodense with normal renal parenchyma on unenhanced scans.

Reninomas may be detected at arteriography during an evaluation for possible renovascular hypertension. The tumor is typically hypovascular, even on selective renal arteriography. Thus, it is important to include the kidneys in the field of view and not focus merely on the aorta and main renal arteries. Juxtaglomerular tumors are detected by displacement of small intrarenal arteries.

Renal vein renin sampling will demonstrate elevated renin levels arising from the tumor; however, selective sampling from branch renal veins may be needed to confirm the abnormal renin secretion.

Although few juxtaglomerular tumors have been reported, they appear to be benign. Thus, simple tumorectomy or partial nephrectomy is curative.

Ask-Upmark Kidney

Segmental hypoplasia has been recognized as a cause of hypertension since Ask-Upmark reported findings regarding six patients in 1929. The affected kidney is small, has few pyramids, and has a deep cortical groove overlying an abnormal calyx. Hyperplasia of juxtaglomerular cells has been reported, and excess renin secretion has been documented in some cases. The process may be unilateral or bilateral.

An Ask-Upmark kidney may be seen in children and adults. Most children with an Ask-Upmark kidney are hypertensive, and often the hypertension is severe. The condition is more common in female patients and is highly associated with vesicoureteral reflux and urinary tract infection.

On CT, the affected kidney is small and contains one or more deep cortical scars. The contralateral kidney often demonstrates compensatory hypertrophy. The calyx underlying the cortical scar is dilated and clubbed. Hypertrophy of adjacent renal tissue may splay the infundibulum, creating a mass effect. Arteriography demonstrates a renal artery proportional to the size of the kidney, which is often small. The size of the orifice of the renal artery is also proportional to the size of the vessel, indicating its congenital etiology.

Trauma

Trauma may cause hypertension by causing injury to the renal artery, or hypertension may be due to the compressive effect of a subcapsular hematoma. Traumatic injury may create an intimal hematoma or partial tear of the renal artery that results in renal ischemia. Selective renal arteriography is needed to detect the arterial lesion, which may affect the main renal artery or a branch vessel. Those patients with partial renal damage may be treated medically because the hypertension may resolve spontaneously. If the kidney is threatened, however, urgent repair is required.

Another mechanism of trauma-induced hypertension is the development of a subcapsular hematoma that compresses the renal parenchyma, creating local ischemia and resulting in increased renin secretion. This is often called a "Page Kidney," named for Irvine Page, who demonstrated this phenomenon in the laboratory. The development of hypertension is not acute, but may take months or even years to develop after the trauma.

A subcapsular hematoma is easily seen on CT (Fig. 10.24). If hypertension develops subsequently, renal vein renin levels should be measured. These will usually lateralize to the affected kidney. Arteriography shows no arterial injury, but the renal distortion by the subcapsular mass is seen. Evacuation of the hematoma should result in cure.

Renovascular Hypertension

Only a small minority of hypertensive patients have a renovascular etiology; the vast majority of patients have essential hypertension.

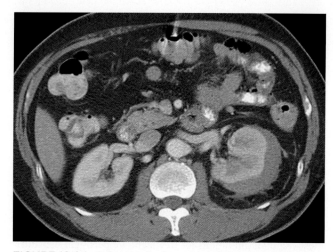

FIGURE 10.24. Subcapsular hematoma. Compression of the renal parenchyma indicates the subcapsular location. The compression creates local ischemia resulting in increased renin secretion.

Estimates vary, but the prevalence of renovascular hypertension among all hypertensive patients is only approximately 1% to 4%. It is difficult to predict on a clinical basis, which patients have renovascular hypertension, but some characteristics make it more likely.

Renovascular hypertension is more common among patients at either age extreme. Patients younger than 20 years or older than 50 years are more likely to have a renovascular etiology, whereas patients with essential hypertension are usually between 30 and 50 years at onset. However, fibromuscular dysplasia (FMD), the second most common cause of renovascular hypertension, typically affects women between 30 and 55 years. Rapid acceleration or severe hypertension is another indication of a renovascular etiology, as is a severe hypertensive retinopathy. A flank bruit found on physical examination also suggests a renovascular etiology; it is especially common in patients with FMD. A family history of hypertension is found more often in patients with essential hypertension. Renovascular hypertension is renin mediated and occurs as a response to renal ischemia. The most important factor governing renin release is the afferent arteriole, which acts as a baroreceptor. The transmural pressure across this arteriole may decrease as a result of a reduction in perfusion pressure or decreased compliance of the arteriole.

Although many different processes may cause stenosis of the main renal artery, the most common are atherosclerosis and FMD.

Atherosclerosis

Atherosclerosis begins as a proliferation of smooth muscle cells in the intima and creates a mound that protrudes into the lumen. Lipid deposition follows with inflammation, necrosis, and formation of atherosclerotic plaque. It accounts for approximately two-thirds of cases of significant narrowing of the main renal artery. The lesions occur usually at the origin of the renal artery or within the first 2 cm (Fig. 10.25). They are often circumferential but may be eccentric. Because atherosclerosis is a generalized process, both renal arteries are frequently affected. If atherosclerosis is present at the renal ostia, it may not be possible to determine whether the plaque is renal or aortic in location.

Atherosclerosis is more common in men than in women and is accelerated by smoking. The age at which patients present with hypertension is considerably older than in those with FMD.

Fibromuscular Dysplasia

FMD accounts for almost one-third of cases of renovascular hypertension. It may involve any layer of the renal artery and is classified

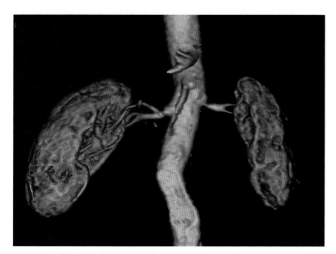

FIGURE 10.25. Renal artery stenosis. High-grade stenosis at the origin of the left renal artery is seen on this volume-rendered MR angiogram.

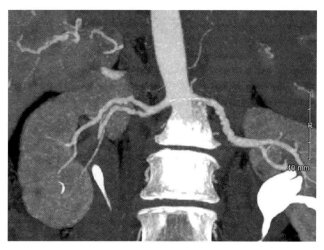

FIGURE 10.27. FMD. The classic string of beads appearance is seen on these reconstructed images from a CTA examination.

as intimal, medial, or adventitial. The medial variety can be subdivided into several more categories.

Intimal fibroplasia consists of a concentric accumulation of collagen beneath the internal elastic membrane. This creates a smooth stenosis, usually in the midportion of the renal artery. It is more common among children and is progressive.

Medial dysplasia is the most common type of FMD and accounts for approximately 90% of cases. The subcategories reflect involvement of the inner or outer media and the presence of collagenous infiltration, smooth muscle hypertrophy, or medial dissection.

Medial fibroplasia is the most common subtype of dysplasia. There is replacement of smooth muscle by collagen that forms thick ridges. These alternate with areas of small aneurysm formation and result in the classic "string of beads" appearance seen with conventional arteriography (Fig. 10.26), CTA (Fig. 10.27), or on reconstructed images (Fig. 10.28). This type of medial dysplasia is most commonly seen in women between 15 and 50 years. Although it is progressive, it is usually responsive to PTA.

Collagen infiltrates the outer layer of the media in perimedial fibroplasia. A beaded appearance similar to that seen in medial fibroplasia is present in the renal arteries but is less dramatic because true aneurysms do not develop.

True medial hyperplasia is an uncommon form of medial dysplasia and consists of hyperplastic smooth muscle and fibrous tissue. Focal stenoses are seen, but aneurysm formation is not present (Fig. 10.29).

Medial dissection is also uncommon and may be histologically indistinguishable from other forms of medial dysplasia. In this form, a new channel is formed in the outer third of the media.

In adventitial dysplasia, a collagenous infiltrate surrounds the adventitia. Either discrete focal or longer tubular stenoses may be produced.

FMD is not limited to the renal arteries, but is also seen in visceral and peripheral arteries. FMD may involve the carotid and vertebral arteries but tends to spare the intracranial vessels. Transient ischemic attacks may be due to involvement of cephalic vessels by FMD. Most patients are asymptomatic when the visceral arteries are affected by FMD, although symptoms of intestinal angina have been reported because of lesions in the superior mesenteric artery.

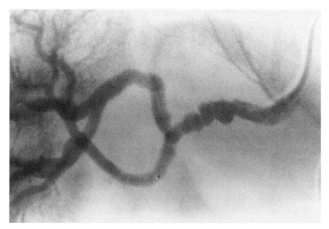

FIGURE 10.26. FMD. Thick ridges of collagen alternate with aneurysms to create a string of beads appearance typical of medial fibroplasia.

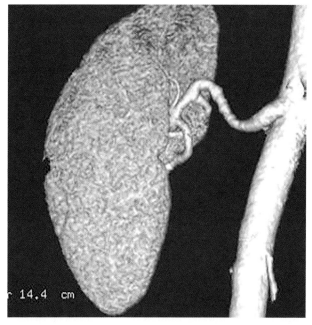

FIGURE 10.28. FMD. Reformatted CT image demonstrates the string of beads appearance.

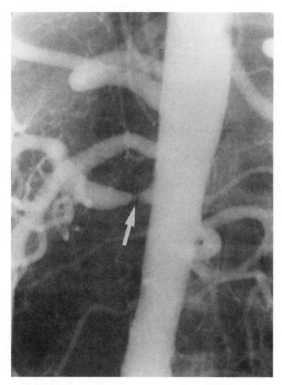

FIGURE 10.29. Focal stenosis. A high-grade stenosis of the proximal renal artery identified on this conventional aortogram (*arrow*) suggests FMD.

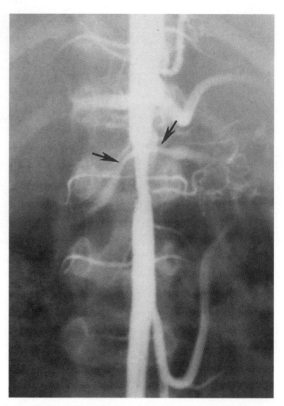

FIGURE 10.30. Middle aortic syndrome. Tubular narrowing of the midaorta has resulted in bilateral RAS (*arrows*).

The hepatic artery may also be involved, but seldom causes symptoms. Peripheral arteries are seldom affected, but reports have confirmed involvement of most medium and large muscular arteries.

Middle Aortic Syndrome

This rare syndrome of diffuse narrowing of the abdominal aorta often affects the visceral and renal arteries. It occurs in young patients, most often in the second decade of life. Hypertension is typically severe. An abdominal bruit and diminished femoral pulses in a young patient may suggest the diagnosis. The prognosis is poor; the patients often die from cerebral hemorrhage, hypertensive encephalopathy, stroke, and congestive heart failure.

The middle aortic syndrome is distinct from aortic coarctation, which is a congenital lesion. Multiple etiologies are responsible for the middle aortic syndrome and include a chronic inflammatory aortitis, atherosclerosis, and cystic medial necrosis. The disease is progressive and does not respond well to transluminal angioplasty. Thus, treatment consists of surgical revascularization. Although surgery is best performed after the patient is fully grown, the severity of disease may mandate an earlier aggressive surgical approach.

The radiographic manifestations depend on the specific vessels involved. Stenosis of a renal artery may result in a small kidney with delayed excretion of contrast medium. Arteriography is required to define the vascular involvement. A smooth tapering of the distal thoracic or abdominal aorta is seen. Narrowing is often severe and is usually most marked in the infrarenal aorta. The renal arteries are commonly affected with long stenoses (Fig. 10.30). Lateral views may demonstrate narrowing of the celiac or superior mesenteric arteries in as many as 90% of patients.

The middle aortic syndrome must be distinguished from Takayasu disease. Patients with Takayasu disease are usually slightly older and have other manifestations of arteritis, such as fever and an elevated sedimentation rate. The great vessels of the chest are often involved in Takayasu disease, but not in the middle aortic syndrome.

Renal Transplantation

Approximately 50% of patients develop hypertension after receiving a renal allograft. In the early period after transplantation, acute rejection is the most common cause of hypertension. High-dose glucocorticoid therapy contributes to hypertension, but this can be reduced by using an alternate-day regimen for long-term therapy. Stenosis of the transplant renal artery is another possible cause of hypertension. This stenosis may be caused by acute angulation or extrinsic compression of the artery, ischemic injury during vascular clamping, or intimal fibrosis due to rejection.

The incidence of hypertension is higher if the native kidneys are left in place than if they are removed. This is most likely due to activation of the renin–angiotensin system because elevated renin levels can be measured in the native renal veins.

Renal Artery Aneurysm

There is an association between renal artery aneurysms and hypertension; however, it is not clear how often the hypertension is caused by the aneurysm (Fig. 10.31). Renin-mediated hypertension may be produced by extrinsic compression of the main renal artery or an intrarenal branch artery by the aneurysm or by thrombus formation and occlusion of a branch artery.

Evaluation and Treatment

Because it is extremely difficult to predict on a clinical basis which patients have renovascular hypertension, a radiographic screening test is needed. However, the prevalence of renovascular hypertension is <5% of all hypertensive patients, so it is impractical to apply these tests to all hypertensive patients. Thus, a group of patients at increased risk for renovascular hypertension is selected to undergo radiographic screening for renovascular hypertension. The following criteria are often used to select patients for radiographic screening:

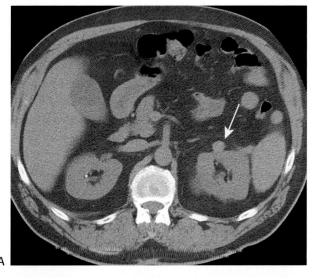

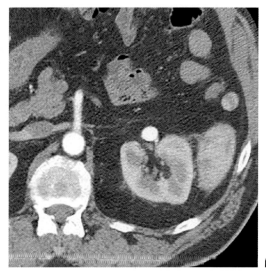

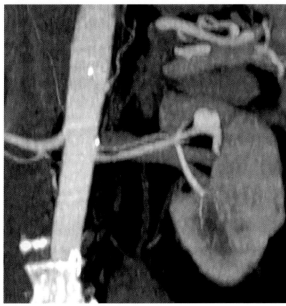

FIGURE 10.31. Renal artery aneurysm. **A:** A small mass lies near the left renal hilum (*arrow*). **B:** It enhances the same as the aorta. **C:** Reconstructed image in the coronal plane demonstrates its connection to the renal artery.

- Age extreme, usually younger than 20 or older than 50 years
- Recent onset of hypertension (<1 year)
- Rapid acceleration of hypertension
- Malignant hypertension
- A flank bruit

A variety of radiographic screening tests have been used, and the choice may reflect equipment available, physician interest or expertise, and the characteristics of the patient population. The goal of these screening examinations is not only to detect RAS but also to predict which patients will respond to revascularization.

Doppler Ultrasound

Doppler ultrasound has become the preferred screening modality for RAS. It is noninvasive, has no ionizing radiation, is relatively inexpensive, and has no contraindications in patients with azotemia or contrast allergy. However, it is operator dependent and has limited applicability in obese patients or those with overlying bowel gas. Furthermore, uniform criteria for the diagnosis of RAS have not yet been established. Those commonly used include a peak systolic velocity >200 cm per second in the main renal artery associated with poststenotic turbulence. A side-to-side difference in the resistive index of more than 0.05 is a useful indirect duplex parameter.

Computed Tomographic Angiography

CTA is often used to detect RAS. Isotropic pixels obtained during a single breath-hold provide data of sufficient fidelity to reconstruct three-dimensional (3D) images (Fig. 10.32). Accessory renal arteries are almost always detected with CTA. Renal artery stenoses, in either the main or an accessory renal artery, are also detected with a high degree of accuracy. The sensitivity and specificity of CTA in detecting RAS of 50% or more are approximately 90% and 97%, respectively. When only stenoses of 75% or greater are considered, the sensitivity is even higher. Because many of the false-positive and false-negative results are from accessory arteries, the accuracy of detecting stenoses in the main renal arteries is nearly as good as catheter arteriography.

CT urine attenuation ratios have been used as an adjunct sign in the detection of RAS. The hyperconcentration of excreted contrast material in the ischemic kidney can be seen as an increased density on unenhanced CT images.

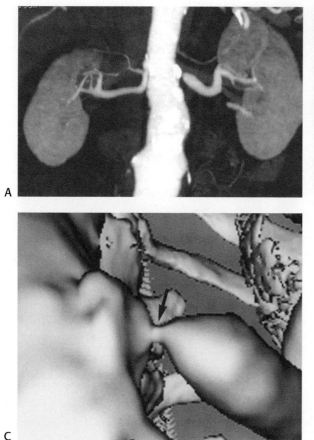

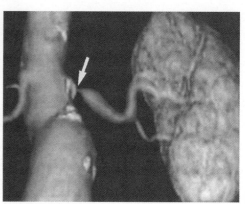

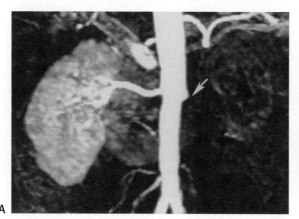

FIGURE 10.32. Renal artery stenosis. **A:** Extensive vascular disease is seen in the abdominal aorta on this CT angiogram, but the origin of the left renal artery is not well visualized. **B:** An oblique view demonstrates a high-grade stenosis of the proximal left renal artery (*arrow*). **C:** The stenosis (*arrow*) is also demonstrated on a shaded surface display image.

Magnetic Resonance Angiography

MRA has been used to detect RAS using a variety of pulse sequences. In addition to being a noninvasive test, ionizing radiation is not involved. However, gadolinium-based contrast media must be avoided in patients with compromised renal function to avoid the development of nephrogenic sclerosing fibrosis.

The results of clinical studies in this rapidly evolving field have been encouraging. When compared with angiography, the sensitivities and specificities of MRA for the detection of RAS are around 95%, similar to CTA.

MRA may be used to detect stenoses involving the proximal portion of the renal artery, the most common site of involve-ment by atherosclerosis. Evaluation of branch or accessory renal arteries is more difficult. It is also not clear how well this technique will detect FMD. The renal parenchyma is seen on both MRA (Fig. 10.33), CTA (Fig. 10.34) and CT (Fig 10.35) images, which help to assess the likelihood of return of function after revascularization.

Radionuclide Renography

Radionuclide renography coupled with the administration of an angiotensin-converting enzyme (ACE) inhibitor, captopril, has been used to screen patients with normal renal function for renovascular

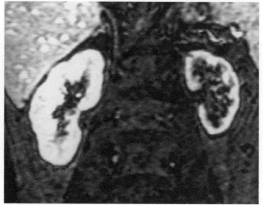

FIGURE 10.33. High-grade renal artery stenosis. **A:** MRA demonstrates complete occlusion of the proximal left renal artery (*arrow*). **B:** A delayed image demonstrates enhancement of an atrophic left kidney from col-lateral vessels.

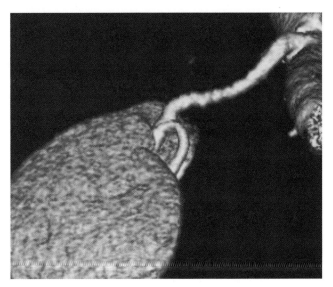

FIGURE 10.34. FMD. The string of beads appearance of FMD is seen on this CTA examination.

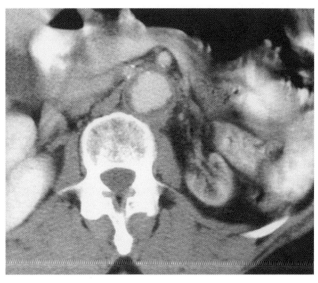

FIGURE 10.35. Atrophic left kidney. Chronic RAS has resulted in a severely atrophic left kidney.

hypertension. However, it has lost popularity because it provides no visualization of the renal arteries and has little predictive value for response to treatment.

Arteriography

Digital subtraction catheter arteriography remains the gold standard for the detection of RAS. The hemodynamic significance may be assessed by the severity of the stenosis and by the presence or absence of collateral vessels. Lesions must occlude at least 50% of the vessel diameter to be considered significant.

However, this measurement is imprecise and does not assess the cross-sectional area or, more importantly, flow. Collateral vessels indicate that the lesion is significant because alternate pathways to provide flow have developed. Epinephrine may further restrict flow to the kidneys and may make these collaterals more apparent (Fig. 10.36).

The most appropriate treatment may often be determined by the nature and location of the stenosis. A focal stenosis of the main renal artery often responds to PTA, whereas a long stenosis, orifice lesion, or bilateral disease does not do as well. In most centers, PTA with or without stenting is the treatment of choice for a RAS.

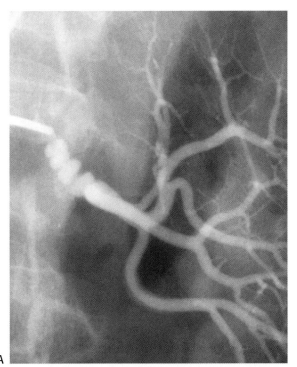

A

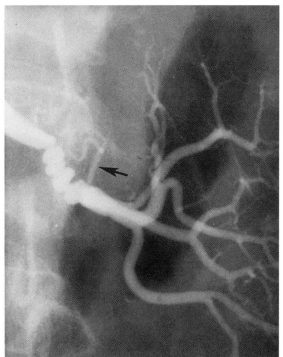

B

FIGURE 10.36. Renal artery stenosis with collateral vessels. **A:** A conventional left renal arteriogram demonstrates FMD. **B:** Repeat arteriogram after the intra-arterial injection of 5 mg of epinephrine shows collateral vessels (*arrow*) not seen on the initial run.

However, surgery may be selected for lesions that will be technically difficult for PTA, or for lesions at the renal orifice, which may be caused by atherosclerosis of the aorta, rather than by the renal arteries.

Renin Measurement

Because renovascular hypertension is renin mediated, peripheral renin levels are elevated more often in patients with renovascular hypertension than in patients with essential hypertension. Selective renal vein sampling measures the renin level secreted by each kidney. Samples from the main renal veins and IVC are usually sufficient. If a renin-producing tumor or branch RAS is suspected, more selective samples may be needed. An ipsilateral/contralateral renal vein renin ratio of 1.5 or greater is generally considered lateralizing and predictive of renovascular hypertension. Such patients are likely to be cured by correction of the RAS. Unfortunately, even captopril-stimulated renal vein renin measurements are not sufficiently sensitive to enable prediction of which patients will respond to revascularization or are not sufficiently specific to exclude patients who do not have renovascular hypertension.

Treatment

PTA has been used to treat RAS in patients with renovascular hypertension since its initial report by Dotter and Judkins in 1964. Advances on that initial technique have resulted in sophisticated balloon catheters and vascular stents that are now in common use (Fig. 10.37). Although these interventions are designed to improve or cure hypertension, they often improve or stabilize renal function.

Among patients with renovascular hypertension due to atherosclerosis, treatment with stent-supported angioplasty results in cure or response in 60% to 80% of patients. Although FMD accounts for <10% of patients with renovascular hypertension, it affects a younger population. The cumulative clinical success of PTA among this population approaches 90%.

RENOVASCULAR HYPERTENSION IN CHILDREN

The incidence of hypertension in children of 1% to 2% is much lower than the incidence in the adult population. The majority of these hypertensive children have a secondary cause.

Acquired renal parenchymal disease is the most common cause of hypertension among children. Other causes include the hemolytic uremic syndrome, renal trauma, nephrotic syndrome, and chronic pyelonephritis. Both acute glomerulonephritis and congenital malformation account for approximately 20% of cases of renal hypertension. In approximately 10%, it is renovascular hypertension. Children with renovascular hypertension tend to be younger and have higher levels of blood pressure than children with essential hypertension. Creatinine and urinalysis are usually normal in both groups.

The most common etiology of renovascular hypertension among children is FMD, which is seen more commonly among boys than among girls. As in adults, the proximal portion of the renal artery is seldom involved, but unlike the adult population, the classic string of beads appearance is seldom seen in children (Fig. 10.38).

RAS due to neurofibromatosis type I is the next most common etiology for renovascular hypertension in children. The proximal renal artery is involved, and an associated hypoplasia of the abdominal aorta may also be involved.

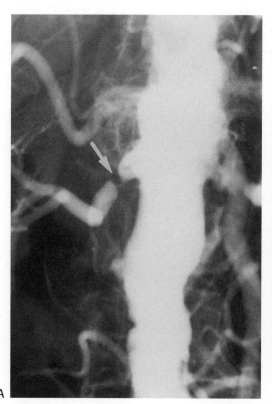
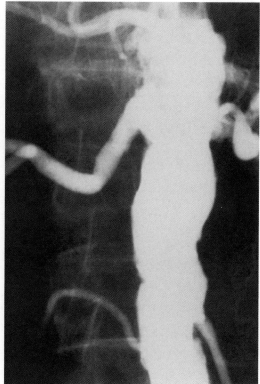

FIGURE 10.37. Transluminal angioplasty. **A:** Preliminary arteriogram demonstrates generalized atherosclerotic changes as well as a tight RAS (*arrow*). **B:** The lumen is widely patent after PTA.

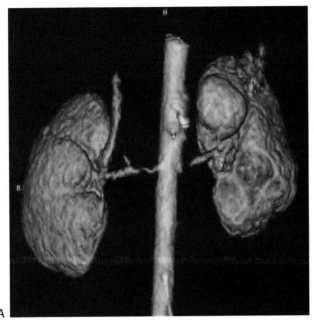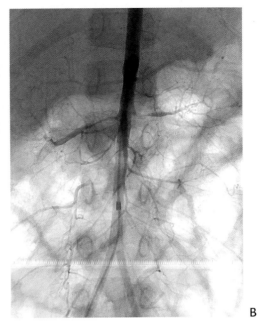

FIGURE 10.38. FMD in a child. **A:** Volume-rendered CT scan demonstrates narrowing of both main renal arteries. **B:** Bilateral RAS is confirmed on catheter angiography.

Vasculitides are a common cause of renovascular hypertension in children. Takayasu disease is often the etiology in patients from India and South Africa. The middle aortic syndrome due to nonspecific aortitis was responsible for 4 of the 30 cases of renovascular hypertension reported by Stanley et al. (1984). An irregular narrowing of the aorta with stenosis of the proximal renal artery is seen in these patients, and bilateral involvement is usual.

In view of the high incidence of a secondary cause of hypertension, children suspected of renovascular hypertension often go directly to intra-arterial digital angiography. Children are increasingly examined with cross-sectional imaging, especially MRA, which provides anatomic information about the kidneys as well as the main renal arteries.

The treatment of RAS causing renovascular hypertension in children has traditionally been surgical; however, PTA has become the treatment of choice in adults and is being used with increasing frequency in children.

The success rate for PTA in children is lower than in adults for two reasons. The smaller size of the vessel and more frequent arterial vasospasm make children more difficult to angiogram and dilate. The most common etiologies of RAS in adults, atherosclerosis and FMD, respond well to PTA, whereas many children have a more fibrotic process that cannot be adequately dilated.

RENAL VEIN THROMBOSIS

Thrombosis of the renal vein is usually caused by an underlying abnormality of hydration, the clotting system, or the kidney itself. Occasionally, extrinsic compression may occlude the IVC or the renal vein and may cause clot formation because of absent or slow flow. Renal or left adrenal tumors may grow along the veins, resulting in tumor thrombus in the renal vein. Renal vein thrombosis is more common on the left side, presumably reflecting the longer left renal vein compared with the right.

The clinical manifestations of renal vein thrombosis depend on the age of the patient, the specific disease process, and the speed with which it occurs. In infants, renal vein thrombosis is often an acute event incited by dehydration because of a volume-depleting

illness such as severe diarrhea. The kidney swells and renal function deteriorates. If the venous occlusion is not relieved, the kidney will infarct and atrophy.

In adults, the most common underlying abnormality is membranous glomerulonephritis. Approximately 50% of patients with membranous glomerulonephritis have renal vein thrombosis. Thrombosis occurs less frequently in lipoid nephrosis, immunoglobulin A (IgA) nephropathy, or minimal change disease. Although patients with renal vein thrombosis often present with the nephrotic syndrome, the protein loss is caused by the underlying renal disease rather than the venous thrombosis. In patients with no renal disease and renal vein thrombosis, little or no proteinuria is seen.

Masses that produce extrinsic compression on the renal vein may also induce renal vein thrombosis. Retroperitoneal fibrosis, a tumor mass, acute pancreatitis, trauma, and retroperitoneal surgery may each incite renal vein thrombosis. Thrombocytosis, elevated clotting factors, or dehydration may also induce renal vein thrombosis. When thrombosis is gradual in onset, symptoms may be mild. If sufficient collateral vessels exist, renal function may be unaffected. If thrombosis occurs more acutely, collateral vessels are less likely to develop and clinical symptoms such as back pain are common. Laboratory abnormalities are nonspecific; the marked proteinuria seen in these patients is caused by the underlying nephrotic syndrome rather than by the renal vein thrombosis. Pulmonary embolism is a common associated problem.

The radiographic findings also depend on the underlying disease process and the extent of collateral venous flow. If collateral veins are unable to drain the kidney adequately, the kidney will be enlarged. A persistent nephrogram is seen on excretory urography, and the collecting system is attenuated. However, because renal function is impaired, retrograde pyelography may be required to exclude obstruction. Sharp calyces, however, are usually seen well enough on an excretory urogram to exclude obstruction.

Ultrasound is often used to exclude ureteral obstruction but also may demonstrate an enlarged, relatively hypoechoic kidney. In some cases, renal vein thrombosis can be imaged. With Doppler ultrasound, an arterial wave form is detected proximal to the venous

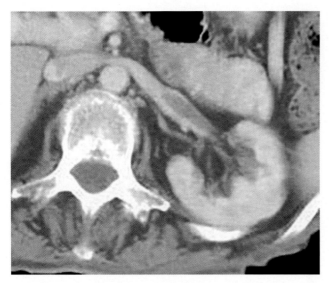

FIGURE 10.39. Renal vein thrombosis. Thrombus is seen in the left renal vein on an enhanced CT scan.

clot. There is a shift in the antegrade systolic frequency and reversal of flow during diastole. These findings, however, are not specific for renal vein thrombosis because they may also be seen with acute tubular necrosis or transplant rejection.

CT is highly sensitive in detecting renal vein thrombosis and may be used to exclude a renal mass such as a carcinoma growing into the renal vein. Renal enlargement with diminished opacification reflecting impaired function is seen. Edema in the renal sinus space and venous collaterals may be identified (Fig. 10.39). Intravenous contrast should opacify the renal veins; absence of enhancement of a kidney that has arterial flow implies venous thrombosis.

Magnetic resonance imaging (MRI) is proving to be even more accurate than CT for vascular imaging, because it does not rely on good cardiac function to propel a bolus of contrast medium to the renal veins. It is often used to detect and delineate venous extension of renal adenocarcinoma but can also be applied to renal vein or caval thrombosis. Rapidly acquired gradient-recalled echo images can be obtained without intravascular contrast media. This is especially valuable in patients with a contraindication to iodinated contrast media (Fig. 10.40).

Anticoagulation is the standard therapy for renal vein thrombosis. This prevents clot propagation, whereas endemic enzyme

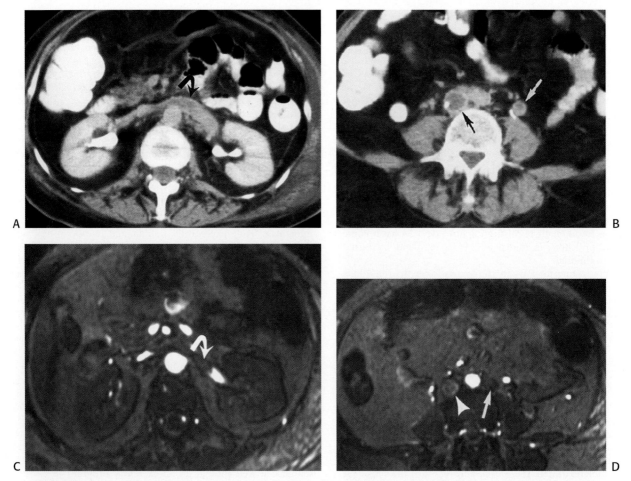

FIGURE 10.40. Renal vein thrombosis. **A:** A CT scan through the level of the left renal vein demonstrates thrombosis (*curved arrow*) by the absence of enhancement. **B:** Below the kidneys, thrombosis of the IVC (*black arrow*) and left gonadal vein (*white arrow*) can be seen. **C:** MRI confirms the renal vein thrombosis by the absence of signal (*curved arrow*). **D:** At a lower level, thrombosis of the IVC (*arrowhead*) and left gonadal vein (*arrow*) are also seen.

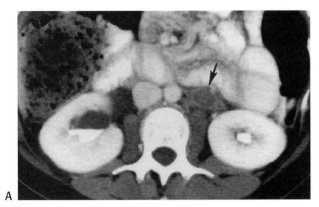 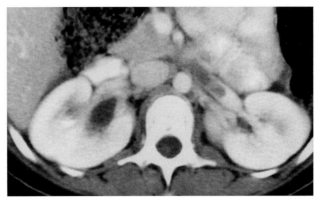

FIGURE 10.41. Ovarian vein thrombosis. **A:** Thrombosis of the left ovarian vein (*arrow*) is demonstrated on this enhanced CT scan. **B:** More cephalad images demonstrate thrombus extension into the left renal vein. Incidentally, note the hydronephrosis of pregnancy involving the right kidney in this recently postpartum female.

systems lyse or recanalize the thrombosed vessel. Pulmonary embolism is a common complication of renal vein thrombosis. Lytic therapy may be used in patients in whom the thrombosis is more acute and in whom the clinical manifestations are more severe.

GONADAL VEIN THROMBOSIS

Thrombosis of the gonadal veins unrelated to tumor thrombus is most commonly seen in women during the postpartum period. Stasis of blood, increased levels of circulating clotting factors, and damage to the vessel wall are contributing factors. Postpartum ovarian vein thrombosis is more common on the right; the left side may be spared by reflux of blood into the gonadal vein. Ovarian vein thrombosis may also be seen as a consequence of gynecologic surgery or pelvic inflammatory disease. Yassa and Ryst (1999) reported finding ovarian vein thrombosis in 40 (80%) of 50 patients who had undergone total abdominal hysterectomy and bilateral

salpingo-oophorectomy with retroperitoneal lymph node dissection. The predilection for involvement of the right side was also present in this group of patients.

Abdominal radiographs and excretory urography are unrevealing, although hydronephrosis of pregnancy may be evident. Gray-scale and Doppler ultrasound may demonstrate an echogenic thrombus in an enlarged ovarian vein. However, much of the ovarian vein may be hidden by overlying bowel gas. MR and CT are the preferred imaging modalities. A low-density thrombus is easily detected on an enhanced abdominal CT examination (Fig. 10.41). Reconstructed images in the coronal or sagittal planes may help demonstrate the thrombus. MRI demonstrates ovarian vein thrombus (Fig. 10.42) as an absence of enhancement after gadolinium administration.

Patients with gonadal vein thrombosis are often treated with antibiotics and anticoagulation, although asymptomatic patients, such as those with prior gynecologic surgery, may not require treatment.

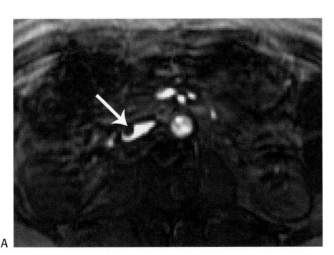 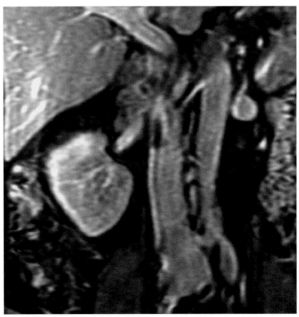

FIGURE 10.42. Gonadal vein thrombosis. **A:** A nubbin of clot (*arrow*) is seen in the IVC at the site of entry of the right gonadal vein. **B:** The vertical orientation of the thrombus is better demonstrated on this coronal image.

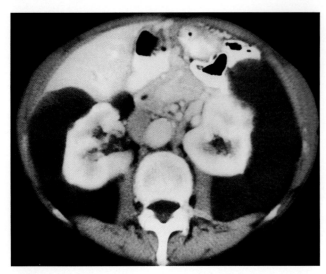

FIGURE 10.43. Lymphangiomatosis. Multiple, bilateral thin-walled cysts are seen in the perinephric space.

RENAL LYMPHANGIOMATOSIS

Renal lymphangiomatosis is a rare disorder in which lymphatic tissue fails to develop a normal communication with the rest of the lymphatic system. Cystic masses develop, usually in the perinephric space immediately adjacent to the kidney, as a result of obstruction of larger lymphatics that drain through the renal pelvis.

Patients may present with a palpable abdominal mass, or perinephric cystic masses may be found incidentally on cross-sectional imaging studies. The condition is usually bilateral and may be hereditary. Pregnancy may exacerbate the condition. Renal function is normal.

Abdominal radiographs and excretory urography will likely appear normal. Multiple cystic masses are seen with sonography. In some cases, debris from previous hemorrhage may be seen. Multiple, thin-walled cystic masses are seen on CT (Fig. 10.43). The density of the cystic masses approximates that of water, unless hemorrhage has occurred, in which case the density is elevated.

Renal lymphangiomatosis must be distinguished from autosomal-dominant polycystic kidney disease (ADPKD). Patients with ADPKD have innumerable parenchymal cysts, whereas the cysts are perinephric in lymphangiomatosis.

Because lymphangiomatosis is benign and most patients are asymptomatic, there is no treatment.

SUGGESTED READINGS

Anatomy

Beckmann CF, Abrams HL. Idiopathic renal vein varices: incidence and significance. *Radiology.* 1982;143:649.

Hohenfellner M, Steinbach F, Schultz-Lampel D, et al. The nutcracker syndrome: new aspects of pathophysiology, diagnosis and treatment. *J Urol.* 1991;146:685.

Lautin EM, Haramati N, Frager D, et al. CT diagnosis of circumcaval ureter. *AJR Am J Roentgenol.* 1988;150:591.

Reed MD, Friedman AC, Nealy P. Anomalies of the left renal vein: analysis of 433 CT scans. *J Comput Assist Tomogr.* 1982;6(6):1124.

Vasculitis

Bateman H, Rehman A, Valeriano-Marcet J. Vasculitis-like Syndromes. *Curr Rheumatol Rep.* 2009;11:422.

Fauci AS, Haynes BF, Katz P, et al. Wegener's granulomatosis: prospective clinical and therapeutic experience with 85 patients for 21 years. *Ann Intern Med.* 1983;98:76.

Greco BA, Cooper LT. Congenital and inflammatory arteritides. In: Lerman LO, Textor SC, eds. *Renal Vascular Disease.* London: Springer-Verlag; 2014.

Halpern M, Citron BP. Necrotizing angiitis associated with drug abuse. *AJR Am J Roentgenol.* 1971;3:663.

Litvak AS, Lucas BA, McRoberts JW. Urologic manifestations of polyarteritis nodosa. *J Urol.* 1976;115:572.

Luqmani RA, Suppiah R, Grayson PC, et al. Nomenclature and classification of vasculitis—update on the ACR/EULAR diagnosis and classification of vasculitis study (DCVAS). *Clin Exp Immunol.* 2011;164(suppl 1):11.

Nosher JL, Chung J, Brevetti LS, et al. Visceral and renal artery aneurysms: a pictorial essay on endovascular therapy. *Radiographics.* 2006;26:1687.

Platt JF, Rubin JM, Ellis JH. Lupus nephritis: predictive value of conventional and Doppler US and comparison with serologic and biopsy parameters. *Radiology.* 1997;203:82.

Weyand CM, Goronzy JJ. Medium- and large-vessel vasculitis. *N Engl J Med.* 2003;349:160.

Radiation Nephritis

Cassady JR. Clinical radiation nephropathy. *Int J Radiat Oncol Biol Phys.* 1995;31:129–1256.

Krochak RJ, Baker DG. Radiation nephritis. *Urology.* 1986;27:389–393.

Renal Embolism and Infarction

Gasparini M, Hofmann R, Stoller M. Renal artery embolism: clinical features and therapeutic options. *J Urol.* 1992;147:567.

Hélénon O, Rody FE, Correas J, et al. Color Doppler US of renovascular disease in native kidneys. *Radiographics.* 1995;15:833–854.

Lessman RK, Johnson SF, Coburn JW. Renal artery embolism—clinical features and long-term follow-up of 17 cases. *Ann Intern Med.* 1978;89(4):477.

Malmed AS, Love L, Jeffrey RB. Medullary CT enhancement in acute renal artery occlusion. *J Comput Assist Tomogr.* 1992;16:107.

Renal Artery Aneurysm

DuBrow RA, Patel SK. Mycotic aneurysm of the renal artery. *Radiology.* 1981;138:577.

Tham G, Ekelund L, Herrlin K, et al. Renal artery aneurysms: natural history and prognosis. *Ann Surg.* 1983;197(3):348.

Arteriovenous Fistula

Crotty KL, Orihuela E, Warren MM. Recent advances in the diagnosis and treatment of renal arteriovenous malformations and fistulas. *J Urol.* 1993;150:1355.

Maruno M, Kiyosue H, Tanoue S, et al. Renal arteriovenous shounts: clinical features, imaging appearance, and transcatheter embolization based on angioarchitecture. *Radiographics.* 2016;36:580–595.

Renal Vein Thrombosis

Gatewood OMB, Fishman EK, Burrow CR, et al. Renal vein thrombosis in patients with nephrotic syndrome: CT diagnosis. *Radiology.* 1986;159:117.

Grant TH, Schoettle BW, Buchsbaum MS. Post partum ovarian vein thrombosis: diagnosis by clot protrusion into the IVC at sonography. *AJR Am J Roentgenol.* 1993;160:551.

Jacoby WT, Cohan RH, Baker ME, et al. Ovarian vein thrombosis in oncology patients: CT detection and clinical significance. *AJR Am J Roentgenol.* 1990;155:291.

Tempany CMC, Morton RA, Marshall FF. MRI of the renal veins: assessment of nonneoplastic venous thrombosis. *J Comput Assist Tomogr.* 1992;16:929.

Yassa N, Ryst E. Ovarian vein thrombosis: a common incidental finding in patients who have undergone total abdominal hysterectomy and bilateral salpingo-oophorectomy with retroperitoneal lymph node dissection. *AJR Am J Roentgenol.* 1999;172:45.

Yun SJ, Lee JM, Narn DH, et al. Discriminating renal nutcracker syndrome from asymptomatic nutcracker phenomenon using multidetector computed tomography. *Abdom Radiol.* 2016;41:1580–1588.

Renal Lymphangiomatosis

Leder RA, Frederick MG, Hall BP, et al. Genitourinary case of the day. *AJR Am J Roentgenol.* 1995;165:197–200.

Meredith WT, Levine E, Ahlstrom NG, et al. Exacerbation of familial renal lymphangiomatosis during pregnancy. *AJR Am J Roentgenol.* 1988;151:965–966.

Renal Parenchymal Hypertension

Amparo EG, Fagan CJ. Page kidney. *J Comput Assist Tomogr.* 1982;6(4):839.

Bonsib SM, Meng RL, Johnson FP Jr. Ask-Upmark kidney with contralateral renal artery fibromuscular dysplasia. *Am J Nephrol.* 1985;5:450.

Dunnick NR, Hartman DS, Ford KK, et al. The radiology of juxtaglomerular tumors. *Radiology.* 1983;147:321.

Haab F, Duclos JM, Guyenne T, et al. Renin secreting tumors: diagnosis, conservative surgical approach and long-term results. *J Urol.* 1995;153:1781–1784.

Sonda LP, Konnak JW, Diokno AC. Clinical aspects of nonvascular renal causes of hypertension. *Urol Radiol.* 1982;3:257.

Renovascular Hypertension

Baumgartner I, Lerman LO. Renovascular hypertension: screening and modern management. *Eur Heart J.* 2011;32:1590–1598.

Boudewijn G, Vasbinder C, Nelemans PJ, et al. Diagnostic tests for renal artery stenosis in patients suspected of having renovascular hypertension. *Ann Intern Med.* 2001;135:404–411.

Boulduc JP, Oliva VL, Therasse E, et al. Diagnosis and treatment of renovascular hypertension: a cost-benefit analysis. *AJR Am J Roentgenol.* 2005;184:931–937.

Lewis VD, Meranze SG, McLean GK, et al. The midaortic syndrome: diagnosis and treatment. *Radiology.* 1988;167:111.

Rountas C, Vlychou M, Vassiou K, et al. Imaging modalities for renal artery stenosis in suspected renovascular hypertension: prospective intraindividual comparison of color Doppler US, CT angiography, CD-enhanced MR angiography, and digital subtraction angiography. *Inf Healthcare.* 2007;29(3):295–302.

Soulez G, Oliva VL, Turpin S, et al. Imaging of renovascular hypertension: respective values of renal scintigraphy, renal Doppler US, and MR angiography. *Radiographics.* 2000;20:1355–1368.

Textor S. Renovascular hypertension in 2007: where are we now? *Curr Cardiol Rep.* 2007;9:453–461.

Tullus K, Roebuck DJ, McLaren CA, et al. Imaging in the evaluation of renovascular disease. *Pediatr Nephrol.* 2010;25:1049–1056.

Radionuclide Renography

Boubaker A, Prior JO, Meuwly JY, et al. Radionuclide investigations of the urinary tract in the era of multimodality imaging. *J Nucl Med.* 2006;47:1819–1836.

Fine EJ, Blaufox D. Renal scintigraphy: an update. *Appl Radiol.* 2001;19–25.

Doppler Ultrasound

Hélénon O, Rody FE, Correas JM, et al. Color Doppler US of renovascular disease in native kidneys. *Radiographics.* 1995;15:833–854.

Kliewer MA, Tupler RH, Carroll BA, et al. Renal artery stenosis: analysis of Doppler waveform parameters and tardus-parvus pattern. *Radiology.* 1993;189:779.

Lee HY, Grant EG. Sonography in renovascular hypertension. *J Ultrasound Med.* 2006;21:431–441.

Computed Tomographic Angiography

Sung CK, Chung JW, Kim SH, et al. Urine attention ratio: a new CT indicator of renal artery stenosis. *AJR Am J Roentgenol.* 2006;187:532–540.

Urban BA, Ratner LE, Fishman EK. Three-dimensional volume-rendered CT angiography of the renal arteries and veins: normal anatomy, variants, and clinical applications. *Radiographics.* 2001;21:373–386.

Magnetic Resonance Angiography

Herborn CU, Watkins DM, Runge VM. Renal arteries: comparison of steady-state free precession MR angiography and contrast-enhanced MR angiography. *Radiology.* 2006;239:263–268.

Morita S, Masukawa A, Suzuki K, et al. Unenhanced MR angiography: techniques and clinical applications in patients with chronic kidney disease *Radiographics.* 2011;31(2):E13–E33.

Schoenberg SO, Rieger JR, Michaely HJ, et al. Functional magnetic resonance imaging in renal artery stenosis. *Abdom Imaging.* 2006;31:200–212.

Willoteaux S, Faivre-Pierret M, Moranne O, et al. Fibromuscular dysplasia of the main renal arteries: comparison of contrast-enhanced MR angiography with digital subtraction angiography. *Radiology.* 2006;241:922–929.

Renin Measurement

Harrington DP, Whelton PK, Mackenzie EJ, et al. Renal venous renin sampling: prospective study of techniques and methods. *Radiology.* 1981;138:571.

Roubidoux MA, Dunnick NR, Klotman PE, et al. Renal vein renins: inability to predict response to revascularization in patients with hypertension. *Radiology.* 1991;178:819.

Renovascular Hypertension in Children

Lacombe M. Surgical treatment of renovascular hypertension in children. *Eur J Vasc Endovasc Surg.* 2011;41:770–777.

Tullus K, Brennan E, Hamilton G, et al. Renovascular hypertension in children. *Lancet.* 2008;371:1453–1463.

Urolithiasis and Nephrocalcinosis

Calcifications can be found in the kidneys and renal collecting systems and ureters for a number of reasons. This includes urolithiasis, nephrocalcinosis, and dystrophic calcification. *Urolithiasis* is defined as stone formation within the renal collecting systems or ureters. Most stones are formed in the pelvocalyceal system and then may be passed distally. Urolithiasis in the kidneys is termed nephrolithiasis. Occasionally, stones may form in a cavity that communicates with the collecting system, such as in a calyceal diverticulum, in the bladder, or in a urethral diverticulum. *Nephrocalcinosis* is defined as calcifications that form in the renal parenchyma, outside of the renal collecting systems. Most patients who develop urolithiasis do not and will not develop nephrocalcinosis; however, many patients who have nephrocalcinosis will also have urolithiasis. *Dystrophic calcification* is calcification of abnormal tissue such as in tumors, cyst walls, inflammatory masses, or vessels. Dystrophic renal calcification should be distinguished from urolithiasis and nephrocalcinosis.

Because calcification is readily detected on abdominal radiography, patients with urolithiasis and nephrocalcinosis may often have abnormalities detected with conventional urography. When supplemented with ultrasonography (US) and computed tomography (CT), even the vast majority of radiolucent stones are easily detected. Because of its ability to detect both urologic and nonurologic causes of abdominal pain, CT has become the primary imaging modality for evaluating patients with suspected acute ureteral obstruction from a ureteral calculus. In this chapter, common causes and the imaging appearances of urolithiasis and nephrocalcinosis will be reviewed.

UROLITHIASIS

Urolithiasis in Adults

Urolithiasis, which refers to the formation of stones in the urinary tract and which includes both stones in the kidneys or nephrolithiasis and stones in the ureters or ureterolithiasis, is a common problem among people who live in temperate climates. In the United States, it is estimated that more than 10% of men and 7% of women will develop a urinary tract stone in their lifetime. The peak age for the onset of renal stone disease is 20 to 30 years, but the tendency for stone formation is often lifelong. The incidence of urolithiasis appears to be increasing for reasons that are not understood. While most patients who develop urolithiasis have isolated episodes, it has been estimated that approximately 10% of affected patients will have another episode within 2 years and nearly 40% within 15 years.

A low urinary output is believed to aid in urinary tract stone formation, yet people from areas with hot climates such as Africa, where dehydration and diminished urinary output may be more common, have a low incidence of stone disease. Perhaps people living in hot climates are genetically less likely to form stones.

In the United States, the Southeastern States often are called the *stone belt* because they have the highest incidence of stone disease. Patients in the Southeastern States are nearly twice as likely to have a history of stone disease compared to patients living elsewhere in the United States. Certain dietary habits are also associated with a higher risk of urolithiasis, including reduced fluid intake; decreased intake of fruits, fiber, and vegetables; and increased consumption of high-fructose foods, sugar-sweetened juice, and animal protein. Interestingly, although most urinary tract stones are composed of calcium oxalate, a diet rich in oxalate has not been strongly correlated with stone formation.

The presence of urolithiasis has also correlated positively with the presence of a number of other diseases. Patients with urinary tract stones are overall more likely to have metabolic syndrome (obesity, diabetes mellitus, and hypertension), coronary artery disease, and chronic kidney disease.

It has also been shown that obese patients who have undergone Roux-en-Y gastric bypass surgery are more than twice as likely to develop urinary tract stones as are similarly obese women who have not undergone this surgery. In contrast, it is not clear that the risk of urolithiasis increases in patients who have had other types of weight reduction surgery, including laparoscopic band insertions or sleeve gastrectomies. This difference is probably because patients who have had Roux-en-Y procedures have a component of fat malabsorption, while patients who have had other types of weight reduction surgery do not. Fat remaining in the gastrointestinal tract lumen (due to malabsorption) precipitates with calcium. There is, therefore, less calcium available to precipitate with oxalic acid. The oxalate, therefore, remains water soluble and is resorbed back into the blood stream in the ileum, possibly increasing the risk of calcium oxalate stone formation.

The most common presenting symptom of urolithiasis is renal colic, which is usually caused by an obstructing ureteral stone. Controversy remains regarding whether calyceal stones cause pain. Most calyceal stones are asymptomatic, but occasionally, their removal is associated with relief of pain.

Renal colic is abrupt in onset, most frequently beginning in the flank and radiating to the groin. Men may complain of testicular pain, whereas women may feel discomfort radiating to the labia majora. Patients with stones in the distal ureter may present with symptoms of bladder irritability. Typically, patients suffering renal colic cannot find a comfortable position in which the pain is relieved.

Hematuria is present in most, but not all, patients with urolithiasis. So, the detection of gross or microscopic hematuria in a patient with flank pain is very suggestive of the diagnosis; however, the absence of hematuria cannot exclude the diagnosis. In one study, up to 33% of patients with documented ureteral stones had five or fewer red cells per high-powered field on microscopic examination, while 11% had no hematuria whatsoever.

Types of Stones
Radiopaque Stones

There are many different types of urinary tract stones. While some stones have pure chemical composition, many stones contain mixed components. Some of the different chemical components of common urinary tract stones are listed in Table 11.1. Analysis of stone composition is very important, as it may help to determine an etiology for the stone formation, the efficacy of treatment, and future management.

Calcium Oxalate and Calcium Phosphate The most common urinary tract stones are calcium oxalate stones, accounting for approximately 70% of all calculi. Calcium phosphate stones are much less frequently encountered, accounting for up to 15% of all urinary tract stones. The most common cause of calcium stones is believed to be hypercalciuria. Ionized calcium is filtered by the glomerulus, but most of this free calcium is reabsorbed by the tubules. However, there is a maximum reabsorption that can occur. Most calcium stone formers have idiopathic hypercalciuria, without hypercalcemia. There are many less common causes of hypercalciuria. An abnormally large amount of calcium may be absorbed from the digestive tract. This occurs in patients with hypervitaminosis D, sarcoidosis, and the milk–alkali syndrome. Too much calcium may also be mobilized from the bony skeleton. This may result from immobilization, extensive bone metastases, or hyperparathyroidism. A partial list of factors producing hypercalciuria is provided in Table 11.2.

It is currently believed that most calcium oxalate stones form as a result of the formation of Randall plaques, which consist of deposits of calcium phosphate (hydroxyapatite) that accumulate in the basement membranes of the Henle loop in the renal

TABLE 11.2
Causes of Hypercalciuria

Increased absorption
Idiopathic hypercalciuria
Hypervitaminosis D
Milk–alkali syndrome
Sarcoidosis
Beryllium poisoning

Increased mobilization from bone
Hyperparathyroidism
Immobilization
Bone metastases
Multiple myeloma
Hyperthyroidism
Cushing syndrome

Decreased tubular reabsorption
RTA
Fanconi syndrome
Wilson disease
Amphotericin B toxicity

papillae, just deep to the urothelium, perhaps as a result of hypercalciuria. Randall plaques eventually break through the urothelium, with subsequent calcium oxalate deposition and renal stone formation. These plaques can be seen during ureteroscopy and can produce increased attenuation of the renal papillae on unenhanced CT. In one study, for example, more than 50% of patients with no history of stone disease whose renal papillae measured >43 HU went on to develop renal stones (usually calcium stones) within 7 years. In comparison, none of the patients whose renal papillae measured <32 HU developed renal stones within this time period.

There are two different types of calcium oxalate stones: the more common calcium oxalate dihydrate (weddellite) and calcium oxalate monohydrate (whewellite). While both types of stones are generally quite radiopaque and easily seen on abdominal radiographs, calcium oxalate monohydrate stones are typically the most radiopaque of the calcium stones. While calcium oxalate dihydrate and calcium phosphate stones are usually easily fragmented by extracorporeal shock wave lithotripsy (ESWL), calcium oxalate monohydrate stones are generally harder to fragment.

TABLE 11.1
Common Chemical Composition of Urinary Tract Stones

Type	Percentage of Stones	Visible on CT	Visible on US	Visible on x-ray
Calcium oxalate and phosphate, mixed	34	++	++	++
Calcium oxalate, pure	33	++	++	++
Calcium oxalate dehydrate				
Calcium oxalate dihydrate				
Calcium phosphate, pure	6	++	++	++
"Triple phosphate" (struvite + apatite)	15	++	++	++
Uric acid	8	++	++	—
Cystine	3	++	++	+
Xanthene	<1	++	++	—
Matrix	<1	—	++	—
Metabolic (including protease inhibitor and triamterene)	<1	—	++	—

There are also two different types of calcium phosphate stones: the more common calcium phosphate (apatite stones) and calcium hydrogen phosphate stones (brushite). Some investigators have speculated calcium phosphate stones may develop via a different mechanism than calcium oxalate stone formation. One study has speculated that these may result from precipitation of plugs of calcium phosphate in dilated ducts of Bellini and in collecting ducts.

Magnesium Ammonium Phosphate Magnesium ammonium phosphate (struvite) stones, which are seen in 5% to 15% of all urinary tract stone patients, form when the urine pH is high, exceeding 7.2. Alkalinized urine is most commonly found in the setting of a urinary tract infection with a urea-splitting, gram-negative enteric organism, such as *Proteus mirabilis*. Thus, struvite calculi are also commonly referred to as *infection stones*. Because women have more urinary tract infections, struvite stones are seen more frequently in women than in men.

Pure struvite stones, which are rare, are radiolucent. Typically, however, struvite is found mixed with calcium phosphate (apatite) to form so-called triple phosphate stones, which are easily seen on plain radiographs. These calcium–magnesium–ammonium phosphate stones are seen in association with infected urine. They account for approximately 70% of staghorn calculi (Fig. 13.6), with the remainder being composed of cystine or uric acid.

Cystine Cystine stones are encountered in approximately 1% of adult and 8% of pediatric urinary tract stone patients. Patients with cystinuria have a defect in renal tubular reabsorption of dibasic amino acids, which includes cystine. The defect is inherited as an autosomal recessive trait and is present in the intestinal mucosa as well as in the renal tubular cells. The only manifestation in most patients is nephrolithiasis. Excess cystine excreted in the urine exceeds its solubility, and as a result, cystine stones are produced. The opacity of cystine stones depends on how much contamination with calcium is present. However, many, even pure cystine stones, are still easily seen on abdominal radiographs.

Radiolucent Stones

Uric Acid Unlike other mammals, humans lack the enzyme uricase, which converts uric acid into allantoin. In the urine, uric acid exists either freely or as the much more soluble salt, sodium urate. Acidic urine contributes to an increased concentration of less soluble free uric acid.

Overall, about 5% to 10% of patients with urinary tract stones develop uric acid stones; however, the reported incidence varies by country. Patients with urate calculi have hyperuricosuria and a low urine pH, but do not necessarily have hyperuricemia. This situation is encountered in patients who take medications to acidify their urine, but it may also be present in patients with chronic diarrhea or after an ileostomy.

Inborn errors of metabolism may result in hyperuricemia and uric acid lithiasis. Patients with gout or Lesch–Nyhan syndrome are prone to form uric acid stones. Similarly, overindulgence in foods high in purine and proteins metabolized to uric acid may lead to hyperuricemia, hyperuricosuria, and uric acid stones. The ingestion of uricosuric drugs such as salicylates and thiazides may increase the urine uric acid concentration sufficiently that uric acid stone formation is promoted.

Xanthine These very rare stones may be seen in patients with hereditary xanthinuria, but may also be present in patients treated with allopurinol, which blocks the conversion of xanthine to uric acid. Xanthine stones are relatively radiolucent because their density is similar to uric acid stones.

Matrix Matrix stones are composed primarily of coagulated mucoids and have very little crystalline component. They are found most commonly in patients with alkaline urine, which occurs more commonly in patients with urease-producing infections such as those caused by *Proteus* species.

Other Protease inhibitors, such as indinavir and atazanavir, are utilized in combination with other drugs to treat patients with human immunodeficiency virus type I (HIV-1) infection. These drugs are partially excreted in the urine, where they have low solubility and are prone to precipitate out as crystals, particularly in urine that is less acidic. Protease inhibitor crystals are flat, rectangular plates that may be found in the urine in a variety of patterns. While they are radiolucent on abdominal radiographs and do not have high attenuation on CT, they have been detected as echogenic foci on ultrasound examinations. Over time, these crystals may calcify and become dense enough to be seen in CT. There are other low-attenuation metabolic stones as well, such as triamterene stones.

Imaging of Urolithiasis

Stones may cause obstruction of an infundibulum or obstruction at any point along the ureter. The most obvious sign of obstruction is delayed opacification of the renal collecting system after contrast material administration. The nephrogram is also delayed, compared with the normal contralateral side, but may show increasing intensity with time (increasingly dense nephrogram). It should be noted, however, that even a large staghorn calculus may not obstruct urine flow. Ureteral calculi tend to lodge at three specific locations in the ureter—(1) the ureteropelvic junction (UPJ), (2) where the ureter crosses the iliac vessels at the pelvic brim, and, most commonly, (3) at the ureterovesical junction. The probability of stone passage is related to the size of the stone as well as its location. Approximately 90% of stones 4 mm or less in diameter pass spontaneously. Stones measuring 5 mm or more in maximal diameter and/or located more proximally in the ureter are much less likely to pass.

On occasion, an obstructed renal collecting system can decompress itself by leakage of urine, typically from one or more calyceal fornices, into the renal sinus. This is known as pyelosinus extravasation and is most commonly associated with acute high-grade obstruction and a sudden abrupt rise in the pressure in the renal collecting system and ureter; however, it can occur with only mild degrees of acute obstruction and, rarely, with chronic obstruction. Pyelosinus extravasation is not unusual in patients with an acute obstruction from ureteral stones and has no associated morbidity if the urine is not infected. From the renal sinus, extravasated urine may track through the renal hilum and surround the renal pelvis and proximal ureter.

Abdominal Radiography

The plain abdominal radiograph is a useful examination in evaluating patients suspected of having urolithiasis. While up to 90% of urinary tract calculi are radiopaque, as many as 50% of urinary tract stones may not be detected on conventional abdominal radiographs, due to overlying bowel gas and stool, as well as overlying bones (ribs, lumbar spine, iliac bones, and sacrum). The lateral tips of the transverse processes can be especially confusing because their cortical margin may mimic a ureteral stone.

Calcium oxalate and phosphate, magnesium ammonium phosphate, and cystine stones are generally well seen on plain abdominal radiographs (Figs. 11.1 and 11.2). Calcium oxalate monohydrate stones are the most radiopaque (Fig. 11.3), while most cystine stones are often only faintly opaque. Uric acid stones are insufficiently radiopaque to be seen on an abdominal radiograph and account for the majority of radiolucent stones. Xanthene, matrix, and metabolic stones are also radiolucent.

Many common calcifications in the abdomen must be distinguished from urinary tract stones. Hepatic or splenic calcifications are seldom a problem because they rarely overlie the kidneys. However, stones in a low-lying gallbladder may overlie the right

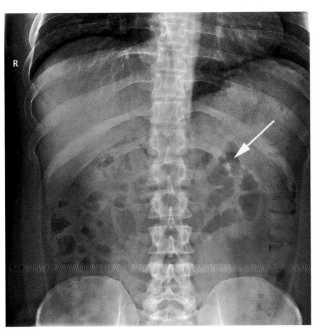

FIGURE 11.1. Calcium oxalate stone. An abdominal radiograph shows a small radiopaque stone in the upper pole of the left kidney (*arrow*).

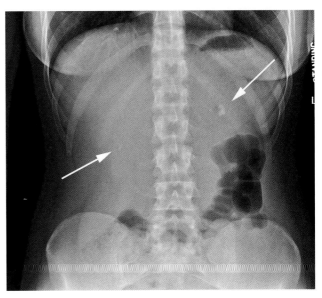

FIGURE 11.3. Calcium oxalate monohydrate stone. An abdominal radiograph shows multiple stones in both kidneys (*arrows*). The stones are very radiopaque, a finding characteristic of calcium oxalate monohydrate stones. On chemical analysis, the stone consisted of 70% calcium oxalate monohydrate and 30% calcium phosphate.

renal collecting system. In most cases, gallstones are larger than kidney stones and have a characteristic rounded or ovoid shape. This allows them to be distinguished from renal calculi. However, renal calculi in an obstructed portion of the collecting system or within a calyceal diverticulum (Fig. 11.4) may mimic gallstones. On an oblique radiograph, gallstones should rotate anteriorly, whereas renal stones remain in a more posterior location.

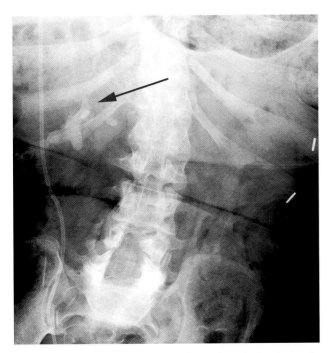

FIGURE 11.2. Magnesium ammonium phosphate stone. An abdominal radiograph in a patient with chronic urinary tract infection shows a large calculus composed of magnesium ammonium phosphate in the lower pole of the right kidney (*arrow*).

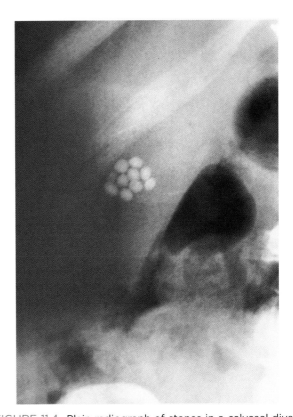

FIGURE 11.4. Plain radiograph of stones in a calyceal diverticulum. A conventional abdominal radiograph shows a cluster of multiple small rounded stones in the right upper quadrant. These were subsequently confirmed to reside within a renal calyceal diverticulum. Most renal stones are ovoid or triangular in shape rather than round. In fact, these calcifications could be confused with gallstones.

Pancreatic calcification is most frequently seen in patients with chronic pancreatitis. These usually affect the entire pancreas and cross from one side of the abdomen to the other. The involvement of the entire gland helps distinguish these calcifications from renal stones. Calcification of the costal cartilage of the lower thoracic ribs and arterial calcifications are usually linear, which helps differentiate them from renal stones. Furthermore, arterial and rib calcifications lie in predictable locations.

The calcifications most often confused with urinary tract calculi are phleboliths and calcified mesenteric lymph nodes. Typically, phleboliths, which are calcifications that form in thrombosed portions of pelvic veins, are rounded, have a central lucency, and are seen in the true pelvis, often caudal to the level of the distal ureter. However, in some instances, central lucency may not be apparent, and these may be impossible to distinguish from ureteral stones without opacification of the ureter. Calcified mesenteric lymph nodes typically have a mottled calcific pattern. Oblique films may show calcified mesenteric lymph nodes to lie anterior to the retroperitoneum.

Excretory Urography

Excretory urography is no longer routinely used in evaluating patients with suspected stone disease; it has been largely supplanted by unenhanced CT as the modality of choice. For this reason, there will be no further discussion of this once frequently performed procedure.

Ultrasound

Urinary tract calculi can be identified on ultrasound as highly echogenic foci, which demonstrate posterior acoustic shadowing (Fig. 11.5). These features, which are observed with both radiopaque and radiolucent stones, can be useful in distinguishing lucent renal stones from other renal collecting system filling defects, such as blood clots or tumors. When the kidney is well seen, renal stones as small as 0.5 mm may be detected. On color Doppler imaging, many stones demonstrate an artifact consisting of rapidly alternating areas of red and blue color (Fig. 11.6). This "twinkling artifact" has been detected immediately deep to any strong rough surface, most commonly calcification. Identification of a "twinkling artifact" has facilitated identification of renal stones; however, it has also been shown that reliance on twinkle artifact alone can be problematic. In fact, isolated twinkle artifact in the kidney has a sensitivity of only

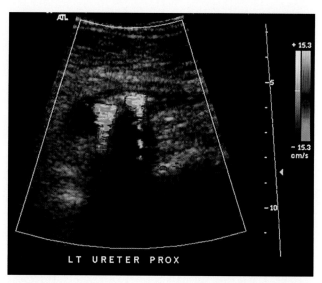

FIGURE 11.6. Ultrasound in a patient with a urinary tract calculus. A longitudinal color Doppler image shows an echogenic focus in the proximal left ureter. Extensive twinkling artifact is identified.

80% in detecting urinary tract stones. In contrast, the specificity of this finding is substantially lower, at only 40%, when thin-section unenhanced CT is used as a gold standard. That is, most isolated twinkle artifact in the kidneys is not produced by renal stones. This sign is, therefore, best utilized in conjunction with other ultrasound findings, including identification of an echogenic focus producing the artifact and posterior shadowing behind the echogenic focus. Requiring combinations of findings to be present before urolithiasis is diagnosed improves specificity, but this occurs at the cost of reduced sensitivity (to only about 30%).

Ultrasound is also helpful in demonstrating obstruction of the collecting system. Although the degree of pelvocaliectasis and ureterectasis from an acute ureteral obstruction due to a stone is often mild, it can still usually be distinguished from the normal collecting system (Fig. 11.7). Furthermore, the dilated ureter can sometimes be followed to the point of obstruction and the stone identified (Fig. 11.8).

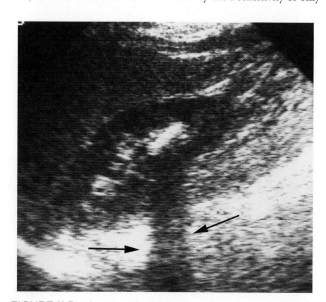

FIGURE 11.5. Ultrasound in a patient with a urinary tract calculus. A longitudinal ultrasound image demonstrates a highly echogenic structure in the lower pole of the right kidney, which demonstrates pronounced posterior acoustic shadowing (*arrows*).

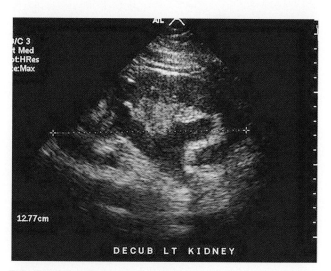

FIGURE 11.7. Ultrasound in a patient with a urinary tract calculus. A longitudinal image through the left kidney shows separation of the normal renal sinus fat due to the presence of a dilated intrarenal collecting system and renal pelvis, as a result of an obstruction.

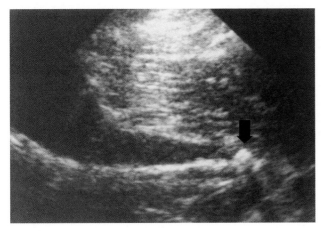

FIGURE 11.8. Ultrasound in a patient with a urinary tract calculus. A longitudinal image reveals pronounced proximal ureterectasis that continues to the site of an echogenic focus in the proximal ureter (*arrow*). Findings are diagnostic of an obstructing ureteral calculus.

Ultrasound has been used to identify obstruction on color Doppler imaging by assessing the bladder for absence of normal intermittent jets of flowing contrast from the obstructed ureter. A ureteral jet consists of color Doppler detected flow of urine from peristalsing nonobstructed ureters into the bladder (Fig. 11.9). This may require interrogation of the ureterovesical junction regions for several minutes, as ureteral peristalsis is intermittent. Both sides should be examined, as asymmetry in flow facilitates identification of an absent or asymmetrically decreased jet, a finding that strongly suggests obstruction.

Computed Tomography

Unenhanced CT for Detection of Urinary Tract Calculi CT is extremely accurate in detecting or excluding urinary tract calculi, as nearly all calculi have high attenuation on CT.

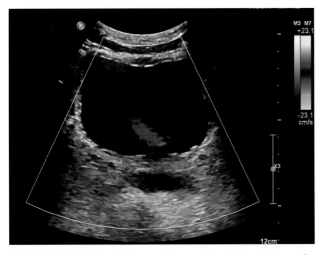

FIGURE 11.9. Ureteral jet on ultrasound. A transverse color Doppler image shows a jet of urine entering the bladder from the left ureter. After several minutes, no jet was identified on the right, a finding consistent with a right ureteral obstruction.

For renal stone CT, images are obtained using 1.25- to 5-mm-thick helical scans from the top of the kidneys to the base of the bladder during suspended respiration. Most stones are detected as high-attenuation foci at both ranges of thickness, although smaller stones can sometimes be missed when only thicker images are obtained (Fig. 11.10). Renal stone CT is typically performed without intravenous contrast material. Oral contrast material is also not needed. The patient is usually placed in the supine position. While some have suggested the examination be performed routinely in the prone position to aid in differentiating stones lodged in the ureterovesical junction from those that have passed into the bladder, such a distinction is usually easily made in supine patients, because most stones located in the region of the ureterovesical junction can be presumed to reside within the distal ureter and not the bladder. Coronal reconstructions are often useful in facilitating accurate long-axis measurements of ureteral stone size (Figs. 11.11 and 11.12). Also, intrarenal calculi are often more easily seen on coronal

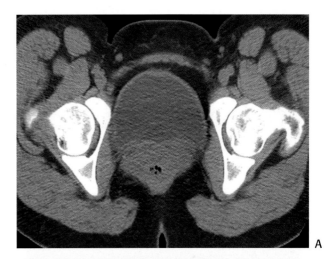

A

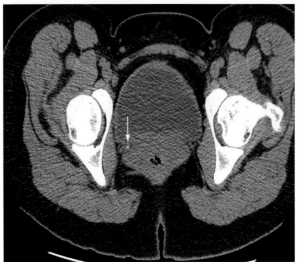

B

FIGURE 11.10. Distal ureteral calculus better seen on thin-section images. **A:** An unenhanced axial CT image obtained using an image collimation of 5 mm fails to demonstrate a tiny calculus at the right ureterovesical junction. **B:** The stone is conspicuous on a 2.5-mm-thick image reconstructed from the same image dataset (*arrow*).

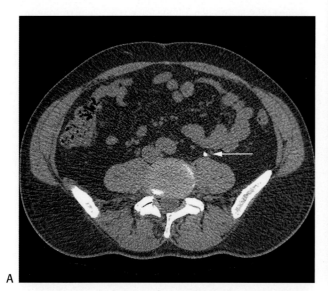

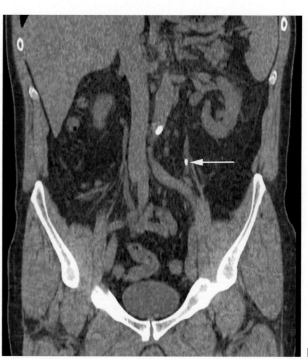

FIGURE 11.11. Value of coronal reformatted images. **A:** An unenhanced axial CT image shows a small stone in the mid left ureter (*arrow*). The stone was measured to be 3 mm in maximal diameter. **B:** A coronally reformatted image shows that the stone's dimension is longest in the *z*-axis. The stone was measured to be 6 mm in maximal diameter on this image (*arrow*). As is the case with many ureteral calculi, this stone's maximal size would have been underestimated had only the axial images been reviewed.

than on axial images. Calcium, struvite, cystine, and even the radiolucent stones, such as uric acid calculi, are seen on CT because the density of all of these stones is far greater than that of urine or soft tissue. Only matrix and metabolic stones (including those that form in patients on protease inhibitors) are not identified on unenhanced CT (Fig. 11.13).

Detection of Urinary Tract Calculi on Contrast-Enhanced CT Although it has been traditionally believed that noncontrast CT is superior to contrast-enhanced CT in detecting urinary tract calculi, few studies have compared the relative sensitivities of these two types of scans. In fact, many stones can be

detected on contrast-enhanced CT obtained prior to contrast material excretion into the renal collecting systems, with the stones most likely to be missed being small (Fig. 11.14). In one study, for example, 95% of all stones measuring at least 3 mm in maximal diameter and 99% of stones measuring at least 4 mm in diameter were detected on contrast-enhanced portal venous, or corticomedullary phase, CT images. In comparison, tiny stones (measuring <3 mm and <2 mm in maximal diameter) were identified only 72% and 61% of the time, respectively. The clinical utility of missing tiny renal stones in many patients is arguable. Even if these should enter and obstruct the ureter at some point, they would be likely to pass spontaneously.

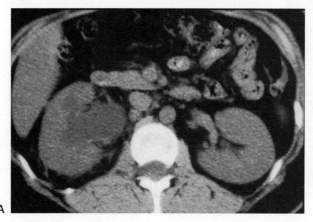

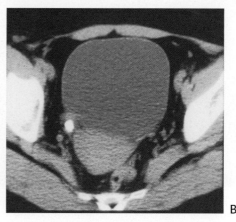

FIGURE 11.12. Value of reformatted images. **A:** An unenhanced axial CT image through the kidneys shows right pelvocaliectasis. **B:** A more caudal image demonstrates a large ureteral stone impacted at the ureterovesical junction.

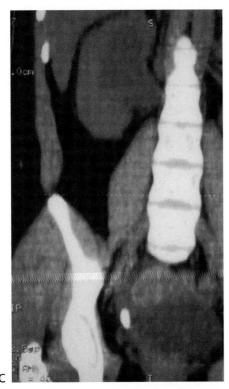

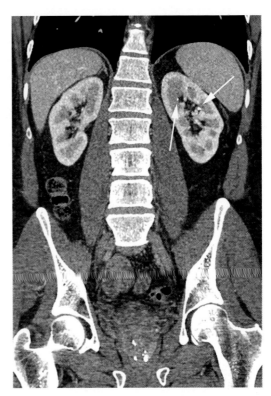

FIGURE 11.12. (continued) Value of reformatted images. **C:** The coronal reformatted image shows the dilated ureter extending to the stone at the ureterovesical junction. The maximal stone diameter can be seen to be longest on this image.

FIGURE 11.14. Nephrolithiasis on portal venous phase contrast-enhanced CT. A single contrast-enhanced coronally reformatted CT image shows two small stones in the midportion to upper pole of the left kidney (*arrows*).

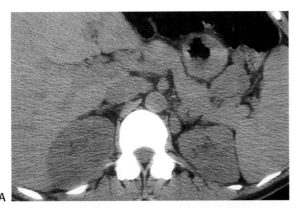

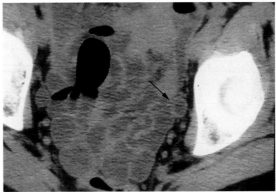

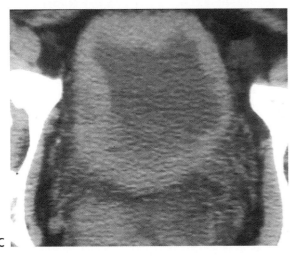

FIGURE 11.13. Indinavir stone on unenhanced CT. An HIV-infected patient developed sudden left flank pain. **A–C:** Images through the entire left renal collecting system show that there is left pelvocaliectasis and ureterectasis (*arrow*) to the level of the ureterovesical junction. No high-attenuation stone is demonstrated.

Analysis of Stone Composition on Unenhanced CT A number of studies have been published attempting to differentiate among the different types of urinary tract calculi using CT attenuation measurements. Most of these have shown that, overall, uric acid stones tend to have much lower attenuation values than the other stones (with uric acid stone attenuation measurements often being between 100 and 500 HU). One investigation found that a combination of stone attenuation and urine pH can be used to identify uric acid stones with a high positive predictive value (provided that the stone is large enough to measure accurately [>4 mm]). A stone of this size measuring <500 HU in a patient with a urine pH of 5.5 or less has a 90% chance of being a uric acid stone. In contrast, most other stones measure considerably higher, with calcium stones having the highest attenuation. Many calcium stones measure more than 800 to 1,000 HU. Magnesium ammonium phosphate and cystine stones tend to have intermediate attenuation values, although there is much overlap. For example, in one review, cystine stones were found to cluster into two groups, with the majority having attenuation values of <550 HU (thereby overlapping with uric acid stones), but a minority having attenuation values of >850 HU (thereby overlapping with calcium stones).

The consensus of opinion is that standard CT stone attenuation measurements are not sufficiently accurate to allow for stone characterization in most patients. This is because many stones are too small to measure reliably, and there is too much overlap in the attenuation measurements for stones of different chemical compositions, including between uric acid and nonuric acid stones. Furthermore, many stones contain mixed components. For example, some stones will contain uric acid and calcium components together. Thus, at the present time, CT is not widely used for attempted distinction among urinary tract calculi.

Analysis of Stone Composition on Dual-Energy CT More recently, investigators have studied the ability of dual-energy CT to characterize the chemical composition of urinary tract calculi. With dual-energy CT, scans are obtained using both low-energy (i.e., 80 kV) and high-energy (i.e., 140 to 150 kV) x-rays. The differences in stone attenuation between the low- and high-energy scans can then be used to provide additional information about stone content. It has been shown that dual-energy CT can be performed in most patients without exposing them to any significant increase in the total radiation dose.

Dual-energy CT has been demonstrated to be much more effective than standard CT in characterizing urinary stones. In some studies, dual-energy CT has allowed for differentiation of uric acid from nonuric acid stones with more than 90% accuracy. With dual-energy CT, specific calcium material density and uric acid material density images can be created. The former depict calcium, but not uric acid stones as having high attenuation, and the latter vice versa (Figs. 11.15 and 11.16).

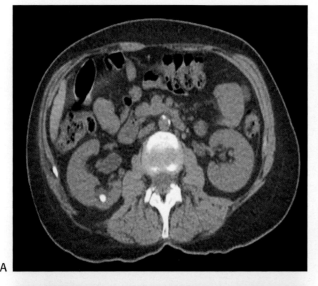

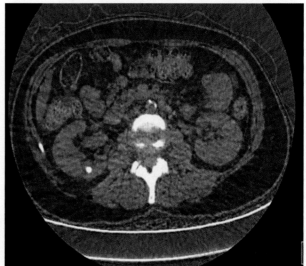

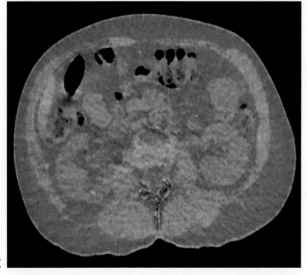

FIGURE 11.15. Dual-energy CT of a predominantly calcium containing stone. (Courtesy of Ravi Kaza, M.D.) **A:** A reconstructed monochromatic unenhanced axial CT image at 75 keV shows a calculus in the right kidney. **B:** A calcium material density image again demonstrates the stone. **C:** The stone is barely visible on the uric acid material density images reconstructed from the same dataset.

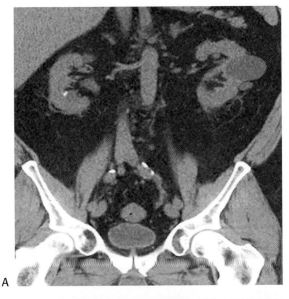

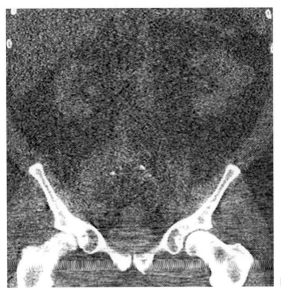

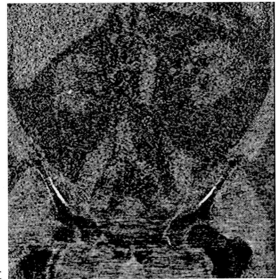

FIGURE 11.16. Dual-energy CT of a uric acid stone. (Courtesy of Ravi Kaza, M.D.) **A:** A reconstructed monochromatic unenhanced axial CT image at 75 keV shows a calculus in the right kidney. **B:** A calcium material density image again does not demonstrate the stone. **C:** This stone is clearly visible on the uric acid material density images reconstructed from the same dataset.

There are some problems with dual-energy CT, however. Differentiation among all of the different types of nonuric acid stones is still not possible, due to measurement overlap and inaccuracy of measurements of small stones (<3 to 5 mm), and many stones containing mixed components may be classified erroneously. Furthermore, some researchers have also observed measurement variability when different dual-energy scanners are used.

Unenhanced CT in Patients with Acute Flank Pain In 1995, Smith et al. compared unenhanced CT with excretory urography in the evaluation of patients with acute flank pain. The authors found that unenhanced helical CT was better than excretory urography in identifying ureteral stones in patients with ureteral colic. Since that time, CT has become the method of choice for evaluation of patients with acute flank pain. Current data suggest that CT has a sensitivity of 97%, a specificity of 96%, a positive predictive value of 96%, a negative predictive value of 97%, and an overall accuracy of 97% in detecting urinary tract stones.

CT diagnosis of a ureteral stone can be made by assessment for both *primary* and *secondary* findings. The primary finding is the detection of a stone within the renal collecting system or ureteral lumen (Fig. 11.17). Although this is seemingly straightforward, distinguishing stones from extraurinary calcifications can at times be difficult, particularly in the pelvis, where phleboliths may be especially problematic. This can be a substantial problem, especially in thin patients with little extraperitoneal fat. As previously mentioned, on plain radiographs, many phleboliths have radiolucent centers, allowing them to be correctly identified. Unfortunately, this finding is much less commonly seen on CT.

Sometimes, the gonadal vein can be confused with the ureter. At the level of the renal hilum, the ureter is located medial to the gonadal vein; as the ureter descends into the pelvis, these two structures cross so that the ureter becomes located lateral to the vein (Fig. 11.18). The gonadal vein also tends to be located somewhat more anteriorly than the ureter. On occasion, a calcified phlebolith can form in the gonadal vein. This can be confused with a midureteral calculus (Fig. 11.19).

Secondary findings indicate the presence of a urinary tract obstruction and are almost always identified in patients with obstructing urinary tract calculi. A variety of secondary findings have been described. These include, most commonly, dilation of

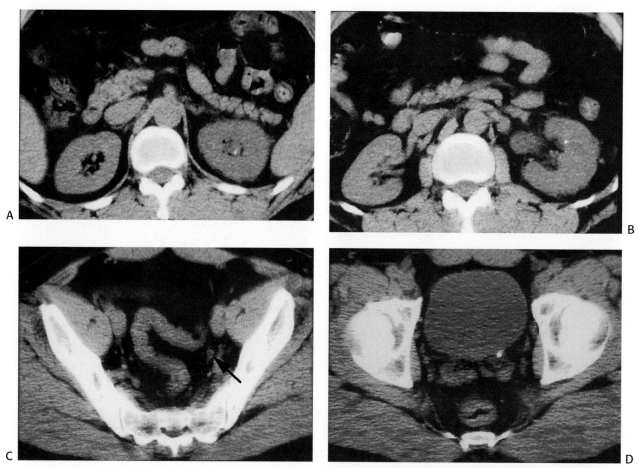

FIGURE 11.17. CT in a patient with acute left flank pain. **A:** An unenhanced axial CT image through the upper pole of the kidney shows left caliectasis with effacement of the pericalyceal fat. A small calyceal calculus is also seen. **B:** An image at the level of the midkidney shows distension of the renal pelvis. An additional calyceal calculus is present. **C:** The dilated left ureter (*arrow*) can be followed into the pelvis. **D:** A stone is seen impacted at the left ureterovesical junction.

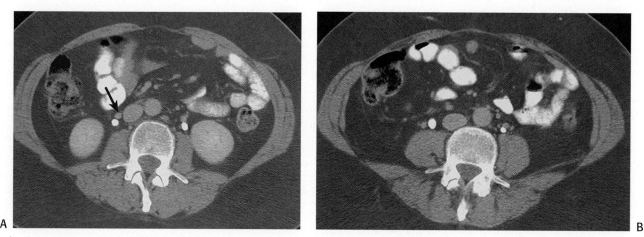

FIGURE 11.18. Relationship of the gonadal vein to the ureter on CT. **A:** An axial excretory phase contrast-enhanced CT image obtained at the level of the lower pole of the kidney shows the gonadal vein (*arrow*) to be medial and anterior to the ureter. **B:** More inferiorly, the vein can be seen lateral to the ureter.

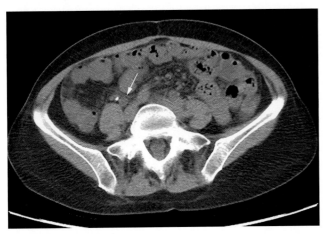

FIGURE 11.19. CT of a calcified gonadal vein phlebolith. An axial unenhanced CT image shows a calcified phlebolith in the right gonadal vein. The ureter (*arrow*) is seen medially.

the collecting system and/or the ureter and perinephric and/or perinephric edema and fluid. Perinephric edema and fluid can produce, mild, moderate, or severe stranding in the perinephric space and renal sinus (Fig. 11.20). Less well-publicized signs include enlargement and slightly diminished attenuation of the obstructed kidney (such that the obstructed renal parenchyma measures approximately 5 HU lower than that of the nonobstructed contralateral kidney).

The earliest sign of acute ureteral obstruction is effacement of the pericalyceal fat as a result of acute obstruction. The ureter will also quickly dilate and be visible to the point of obstruction by careful review of sequential images. Experimental data suggests that ureteral dilation can occur in as quickly as 10 minutes after the onset of acute obstruction. Smith et al. found that ureteral dilation was present in 90% of patients with ureterolithiasis and was absent in a similar percentage of patients without an acute calculus. Ureteral dilation alone should not be relied on as the only evidence of acute obstruction, however, as patients with a recently passed stone, infection, older previous episodes of obstruction, and vesicoureteral

reflux may also have this finding. Smith et al. have shown, however, that a combination of pelvocaliectasis and ureterectasis with perinephric and/or periureteric edema/stranding together has a positive predictive value for ureteral stone disease of about 99%.

Residual perinephric edema and dilation of the collecting system from a recently passed a stone should be suggested when the typical findings of acute obstruction are present on CT, but no stone is identified (Fig. 11.21), especially if these findings are present in a patient's whose flank pain has recently improved or resolved. It must be emphasized, however, that perinephric stranding, too, is not specific for current or recent ureteral obstruction. This finding may also be present in patients with acute pyelonephritis, renal vein thrombosis, renal infarction, and other nonspecific renal conditions (Fig. 11.22). Thus, CT scans in which secondary signs are present, but no definite ureteral stone is identified, must be interpreted with caution, especially in patients presenting with a fever or other evidence of an acute urinary infection.

In the few patients with stones in whom secondary signs are absent, a correct diagnosis of urolithiasis may be much more difficult, when the ureter cannot be followed along the entirety of its course. Imaging characteristics of abdominal and pelvic calcifications that might allow for differentiation of urinary from extraurinary calcifications (primarily distinguishing ureteral stones from phleboliths) are the "rim" and the "comet-tail" signs.

The "rim" sign refers to a thin rim of soft tissue that can be seen around a stone lodged in the ureter, but that is not present around a phlebolith (Fig. 11.23). This can only be used when there is sufficient fat around the circumference of the stone so that it can be seen separately from other surrounding soft tissues. When present, the "rim" sign suggests that a pelvic calcification is overwhelmingly likely to be a ureteral calculus. The rim sign is more likely to be present around smaller stones and absent around larger stones. It is felt to represent the edematous wall of the ureter surrounding a small stone.

The "comet-tail" sign describes a linear or curvilinear soft tissue density that extends from a pelvic calcification. It likely represents the vein in which the calcified phlebolith has formed (Fig. 11.24). When present, the "comet-tail" sign indicates that a pelvic calcification is overwhelmingly likely to be a phlebolith. Care must be taken, however, to distinguish a tortuous ureter containing a stone (pseudo tail) from a vein containing

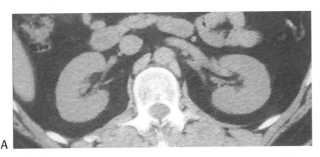

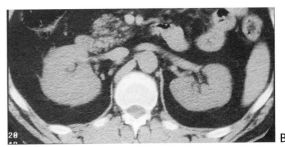

FIGURE 11.20. CT of perinephric stranding. **A:** An unenhanced axial CT image shows normal perinephric fat bilaterally, without any stranding. **B:** An unenhanced axial CT image in another patient shows mild stranding surrounding the right kidney. **C:** An unenhanced axial CT image in a third patient demonstrates more pronounced (moderate to severe) left perinephric stranding.

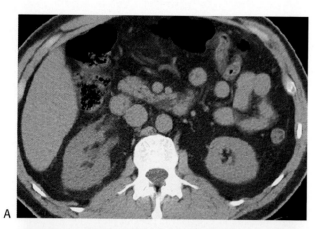

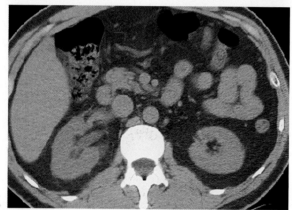

FIGURE 11.21. CT of the kidneys in a patient with a recently passed stone. **A, B:** Two unenhanced axial CT images show mild right perinephric edema in a patient who had recently passed a stone. There were no calcifications noted in the right ureter on the more caudally obtained images.

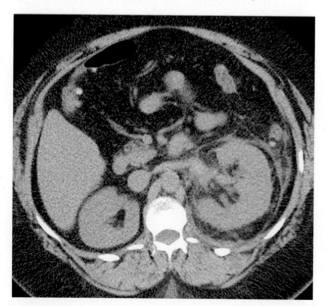

FIGURE 11.22. CT of renal vein thrombosis. An unenhanced axial CT image demonstrates mild dilation of the left renal collecting system and increased perinephric stranding and fluid. These are typical secondary signs of a urinary tract obstruction due to a ureteral calculus. This patient, however, had acute renal vein thrombosis.

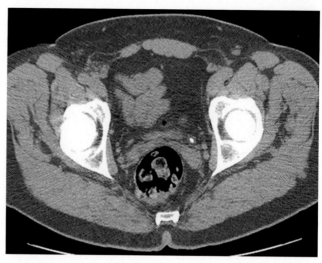

FIGURE 11.23. CT of a "rim" sign. An unenhanced axial CT image shows a circumferential rim of soft tissue attenuation surrounding a stone in the distal left ureter. This finding has been encountered only around calculi (and not phleboliths).

a phlebolith (true tail). Some authors have questioned the utility of the rim and tail signs, as they point out that there is great intraobserver variability in their detection and that they are rarely found in patients who do not have sufficient secondary signs of obstruction, already making it obvious whether or not a calcification is in the ureter.

One important additional benefit of the use of CT for evaluation of patients with suspected urolithiasis is that it may allow for alternate diagnoses, which may be the cause of the patient's symptoms, to be made. Studies have suggested that an alternate diagnosis requiring therapy may be present in 15% to 25% of patients undergoing CT for suspected renal colic. Such conditions include renal cell carcinomas (Fig. 11.25), hemorrhagic renal cysts (Fig. 11.26), renal vein thrombosis (Fig. 11.22), ruptured abdominal aortic aneurysms (Fig. 11.27), enlarged lymph nodes, and gynecologic abnormalities.

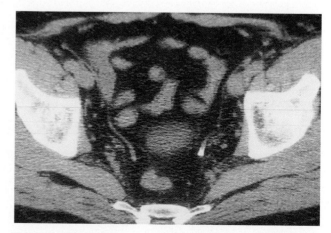

FIGURE 11.24. CT of a "comet-tail" sign. An unenhanced axial CT image shows a linear area of soft tissue attenuation leading up to a calcified phlebolith in the left hemipelvis. This likely represents a portion of the thrombosed vein in which the phlebolith has formed. This finding is believed to be seen only adjacent to phleboliths (and not ureteral stones).

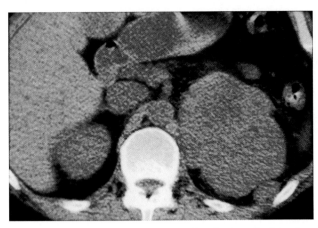

FIGURE 11.25. Alternate diagnosis for flank pain found on noncontrast CT: renal cancer. An unenhanced axial CT image shows a large irregular mass in the upper pole of the left kidney. This was subsequently diagnosed as a renal cancer.

Radiation Exposure from Renal Stone CT Increased use of CT in the past 30 years has led to a dramatic rise in patient radiation exposure. Patients with a history of known or suspected recurrent urinary tract calculi are particularly susceptible to radiation exposure, because multiple renal stone CTs may be requested by emergency department physicians over even short periods of time. Some patients can have dozens of examinations performed within a few years. These patients are felt to be at increased risk of developing a radiation induced cancer. This is especially the case, because many patients with renal stone disease are young and more radiosensitive. They also have longer life expectancies.

Efforts have been made in recent years to reduce the number of ordered CT examinations and the dose of all CT examinations should a CT be requested. One recent study by Smith-Bindman and colleagues has demonstrated that initial triage of patients with suspected urolithiasis to ultrasound reduced patient radiation exposure, with no significant difference in the number of subsequent serious adverse events. Of course, many, but not all, patients assigned to the ultrasound first groups went on to have CT scans anyway.

A number of hardware and software CT dose-saving techniques have been implemented in the past few years. These

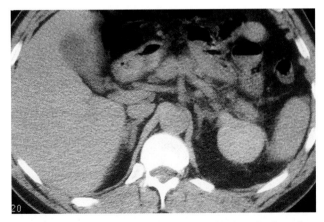

FIGURE 11.26. Alternate diagnosis for flank pain found on noncontrast CT: hemorrhagic cyst. An unenhanced axial CT image shows a high-attenuation mass in the upper pole of the left kidney. A small amount of increased perinephric stranding is noted, likely representing hematoma.

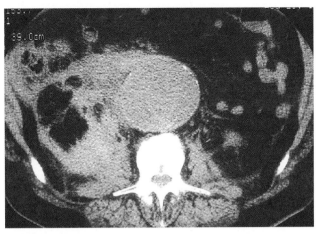

FIGURE 11.27. Alternate diagnosis for flank pain found on noncontrast CT: ruptured abdominal aortic aneurysm. An unenhanced axial CT image shows a large ruptured abdominal aortic aneurysm with extensive adjacent hematoma.

include decreasing the mA exposure for renal stone CT in thin patients (e.g., from 120 to 80 kVp) and the use of automated dose modulation, whereby the scanner automatically reduces the dose when thinner and less dense portions of the body are being scanned. Iterative reconstruction techniques such as ASIR (Adaptive Statistical Iterative Reconstruction) and MBIR (Model-Based Iterative Reconstruction) by General Electric Healthcare (Milwaukee, WI) have also been adopted, which allow for scans to be acquired while exposing patients to substantially lower doses of radiation. Patient radiation exposure can thereby be reduced to <1 mSv, a dose similar to that of an abdominal radiograph. This is particularly feasible with renal stone CT, since the contrast between the high-attenuation stone and adjacent soft tissues is high. Such a distinction between a urinary tract stone and adjacent tissue can usually be made easily, even on noisier low-dose CT images.

Of course, increased image noise is the price that must be paid for substantial dose reduction. Low-dose images (especially those obtained using MBIR) tend to be noisier and less aesthetically pleasing (Fig. 11.28). Additionally, evaluation of structures that are of similar soft tissue attenuation may be more limited. This could lead to a reduced ability to identify other abnormalities that may have produced symptoms mimicking those of urolithiasis.

Magnetic Resonance Imaging

Magnetic resonance imaging is not commonly used for detection of urinary tract calculi; however, on occasion, stones are detected incidentally in patients being imaged for other reasons. Since calcium emits no signal, urinary tract stones appear on MRI as areas of signal void and thus as filling defects (Fig. 11.29).

Treatment of Urinary Tract Calculi

Because approximately 80% of all urinary tract stones pass spontaneously, intervention in patients with urolithiasis is often not needed. In fact, more than 90% of stones <4 mm in diameter and 50% of stones 4 to 7 mm in diameter pass spontaneously. Conversely, stones 8 mm or larger rarely pass through the ureter and into the bladder, and intervention is usually required.

Almost all urinary tract stones in either the native or the reconstructed urinary tract are treated with ESWL or endourologic procedures, regardless of size, location, or hardness. The success of

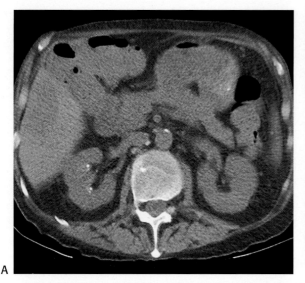 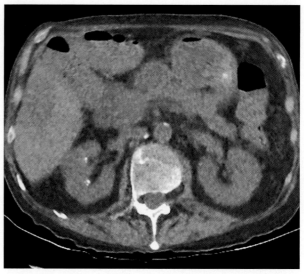

FIGURE 11.28. Radiation dose CT reconstruction techniques. **A:** ASIR unenhanced axial CT image shows several small stones in the right kidney. The estimated absorbed radiation dose to the patient for this study would be 2.4 mSv. **B:** MBIR image at the same level again shows the right renal calculi. The images, which are not as sharply marginated, are not considered to be as aesthetically pleasing. The estimated radiation dose to the patient for this study would be 0.6 mSv.

these techniques is so great that open surgical procedures are now exceedingly unusual.

ESWL, which removes urinary tract calculi by fragmentation and spontaneous passage, has eliminated the need for a percutaneous nephrostomy in most patients and has become the primary treatment for symptomatic nephrolithiasis. Many patients will have residual stone fragments after ESWL, however, with fragments more likely and more numerous in patients with larger initial stone burdens. These fragments often pool in the lower pole collecting systems, due to gravity. In fact, residual stone fragments are seen in nearly 50% of patients treated with ESWL. While stones are easily treated with ESWL, some are more resistant to fragmentation. This includes the very radiopaque calcium oxalate monohydrate stones and those cystine stones that display smooth rather than rough surface contours.

Some patients still require percutaneous treatment to supplement ESWL or to treat complications arising from incomplete stone passage, while others, with large stones, including staghorn calculi may be treated entirely with percutaneous techniques.

Imaging studies have been used to predict the likelihood of stone-free success rates following treatment with ESWL. It has been found that plain radiography can be used to predict the ability of ESWL to fragment urinary tract calculi. For example, urinary tract stones in the renal pelvis that measure <1.5 cm in maximal diameter are less likely to be effectively fragmented when they are more radiopaque than bone, homogeneous, or when they have smooth irregular outlines, with only a 50% to 60% success rate for each of these features, compared with about 90% when these features are not present. Stone attenuation measurements on CT can also be used to predict ESWL fragmentation success, with higher attenuation stones (such as those exceeding 976 HU) being much more resistant to fragmentation. Several other imaging features have also been found useful in

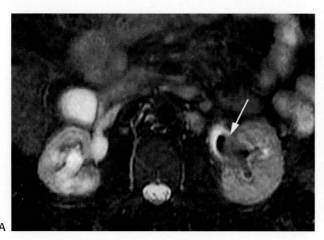 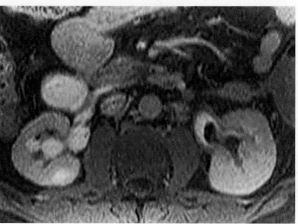

FIGURE 11.29. MRI of nephrolithiasis. **A:** A T2-weighted axial MR image shows a large filling defect in the left renal collecting system (*arrow*), corresponding to a staghorn calculus. **B:** The stone is better visualized on an excretory phase gadolinium-based contrast material-enhanced T1-weighted fat-suppressed axial MR image.

predicting ESWL success rates, with the unsuccessful fragmentation much more likely for larger stones, stones with larger surface areas (which is a similar feature to stone irregularity), and in patients who have large skin to stone distances (due to large patient body habitus).

Attempts have also been made to predict the effectiveness of percutaneous nephrostolithotomy based upon imaging study findings, in achieving a stone- and fragment-free outcome. A number of scoring systems have been suggested, none of which has been universally accepted; however, these have identified a number of factors that predict treatment effectiveness. These include stone location (with upper pole stones being more difficult to remove), stone CT attenuation (with higher attenuation stones again being more difficult to fragment), stone multiplicity (with success less likely when there are more stones), abnormal anatomy (such as with stones in calyceal diverticula), the presence of partial or complete staghorn calculi, longer tract lengths, the presence of obstruction, preexisting spinal disease (spina bifida or spinal injury), and a history of prior surgery. One system even incorporates the volume of cases being handled at the center where nephrostolithotomy is to be performed as a predictor.

Imaging studies, particularly CT, are utilized to assess patients for complications after stone removal. One such complication is collecting system obstruction by stone fragments in the ureter. These fragments are more likely to be problematic when moderate- or large-sized stones have been treated. They can accumulate on top of one another in the distal ureter, a condition known as *steinstrasse* (street of stones), with resulting obstruction (Fig. 11.30). Urologic intervention may be needed in patients who develop a steinstrasse that is prolonged. Other complications seen after ESWL include

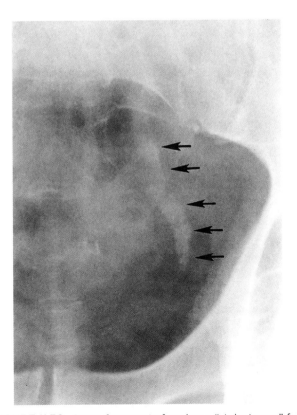

FIGURE 11.30. Stone fragments forming a "steinstrasse" following extracorporeal shock wave lithotripsy. After ESWL, a row of multiple stone fragments (steinstrasse) are seen in the distal ureter (*arrows*).

subcapsular and perinephric hematomas and, less commonly, adjacent organ injuries (to the liver, spleen, or pancreas, with the latter resulting in pancreatitis). Additional complications may result from percutaneous stone removal, including persistent renal collecting system injury, bowel perforation, pneumothorax, and pleural effusion.

Urolithiasis in Pregnant Women

Urolithiasis is a common nonobstetric cause of abdominal pain in pregnant patients. It is usually encountered in the second and third trimesters of pregnancy. Interestingly, in comparison to other adult patients, most pregnant women develop calcium phosphate rather than calcium oxalate stones. Diagnosis of urolithiasis in pregnant women is more difficult than in the general population due primarily to concerns about exposing the fetus to ionizing radiation. Additionally, the anatomy in the lower abdomen and pelvis is distorted by the presence of an enlarged uterus and the fetus, making evaluation more difficult.

Imaging evaluation of pregnant women with suspected urinary tract stones should begin with US. Stones can be seen directly in the kidneys and distal ureters near the ureterovesical junctions; however, much of the ureter cannot be visualized. All patients can be assessed for the signs of acute urinary tract obstruction, including pelvocaliectasis, asymmetrically increased resistive indices (with a resistive index on the symptomatic side of >0.70 highly predictive of obstruction), and absence of a ureteral jet on the suspected side of obstruction on color Doppler imaging (which should be evaluated by viewing this region for at least 5 minutes). Unfortunately, most pregnant patients develop "physiologic" dilation of their intrarenal collecting systems and ureters, most commonly on the right. This dilation is probably caused by a combination of fetal compression and hormonal changes. In patients with acute flank pain, it can be difficult to distinguish between renal colic and physiologic dilation with ultrasound, unless an obstructing stone is demonstrated directly. Some investigators have advocated performance of heavily T2-weighted unenhanced MRI as a second-line study. Gadolinium-based contrast material should be avoided, however, if possible, since there are theoretical risks of its administration to the fetus. Low-dose noncontrast CT could also be obtained for further assessment, after obtaining consent from the patient and the referring service.

Urolithiasis in Children

Although urinary tract stones are rarely seen in children, the incidence is increasing, particularly in adolescents. As with adults, most urinary tract stones in children are composed of calcium oxalate; however, calcium phosphate stones are more common. In developing countries, bladder calculi are common in children. They are most often uric acid stones and are unrelated to obstruction or infection. In industrialized countries, pediatric urinary tract calculi are found much more frequently in the upper urinary tract, as in adults.

The male preponderance of stones seen in adults does not occur in children; boys and girls are equally likely to be affected. Hematuria is the most common presenting symptom, and rather than the severe pain of ureteral colic seen in adults, children often complain of more diffuse abdominal pain. The vast majority of pediatric patients have an underlying predisposing factor. Thus, children with urolithiasis must be carefully evaluated for metabolic, anatomic, or infectious causes. Another major etiology of childhood stones is immobilization, such as may occur after a bone fracture or other illness. Urolithiasis is rare in very young children, but has been reported in premature infants who have received furosemide.

STONES IN CALYCEAL DIVERTICULA AND MILK OF CALCIUM STONES

Calyceal diverticula are congenital urothelial-lined cystic structures which communicate with the renal collecting systems usually via a neck. Diverticular necks are variable, and while they can be large, most are narrow and short or narrow and long. Occasionally, the neck may become occluded.

Calyceal diverticula do not secrete urine; however, they often opacify on excretory phase imaging, due to reflux of excreted contrast from the renal collecting system into the diverticulum. Two types of calyceal diverticula have been described: the more common small polar type (type I) and the less common and larger centrally located type (type II). Calyceal diverticula are often asymptomatic; however, complications may occur. Stones may form within them, sometimes resulting in symptoms of pain and/or hematuria.

Stones within calyceal diverticula can often be seen on conventional radiography or ultrasound, as well as on CT (Figs. 11.4 and 11.31). The calyceal diverticula themselves can be detected on all cross-sectional imaging studies; however, communication with the renal collecting systems can only be confirmed if excretory phase images are obtained, in which case they will opacify (Fig. 11.31). On ultrasound, unenhanced CT or MRI, or early enhanced CT or MRI, they can be confused with renal cortical or parapelvic cysts.

On occasion, milk of calcium, which is a viscous suspension of calcium salts in fluid, may form in calyceal diverticula. Identification of milk of calcium in a cystic renal mass is not absolutely diagnostic of a calyceal diverticulum, however, as it can also sometimes be found in renal cysts and in obstructed and dilated intrarenal collecting systems. Milk of calcium can contain various combinations of calcium oxalate, calcium phosphate, and/or calcium carbonate.

On plain radiography, milk of calcium often appears as a hazy radiopacity overlying the kidney. On ultrasound, the stone material is often echogenic, while on CT, the milk of calcium can be seen as a dependent layer of high-attenuation material within the dependent aspect of a diverticulum or other cavity in which it has formed. This results in a fluid–fluid level with nondependently located water attenuation material (Fig. 11.32). Patients with milk of calcium stones are sometimes, but not always, symptomatic, as they may develop pain and/or hematuria. Milk of calcium may also become infected. Persistent symptoms indicate the need for treatment.

When treatment of stones or milk of calcium in calyceal diverticula is necessary, percutaneous techniques must be performed When stones are present, fragmentation with ESWL does not ensure stone passage, due to the inability of fragments to pass easily through the neck, at least when the necks are thin or occluded. When milk of calcium is present, ESWL is not necessary, since no actual focal stones are present to begin with. Percutaneous nephrostolithotomy or laparoscopic removal is performed, usually preceded by dilation of the neck, to facilitate subsequent drainage of the stone material or milk of calcium into the renal collecting system.

NEPHROCALCINOSIS

Nephrocalcinosis refers to calcification within the renal parenchyma and outside of the renal collecting systems. Calcifications form in the kidneys when the solubility product of calcium and phosphate or oxalate in the extracellular fluid is exceeded. There are a number of causes of nephrocalcinosis. It is not surprising that many of these are the result of abnormally high levels of serum or excreted calcium. Certain diseases have a predilection to produce calcifications in specific anatomic areas of the kidneys (Table 13.1). Thus, metastatic nephrocalcinosis may be further

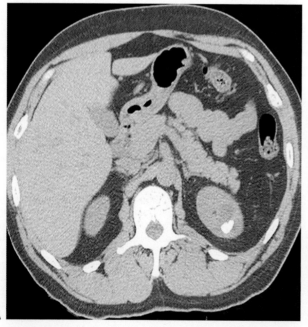
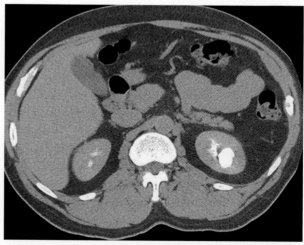

FIGURE 11.31. CT of a stone in a calyceal diverticulum. **A:** An unenhanced axial CT image shows a large calcification in the upper pole of the left kidney. A small water attenuation mass is noted anterior to the calcification. It is not certain whether or not the calcification is within or adjacent to the mass. **B:** An excretory phase contrast-enhanced axial CT image obtained several minutes later shows that excreted contrast material has accumulated within the mass and also surrounds the stone, allowing for a diagnoses of a stone in a calyceal diverticulum to be made.

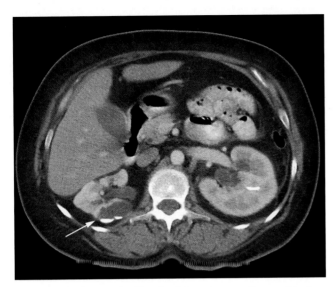

FIGURE 11.32. CT of milk of calcium in a cystic renal lesion. A corticomedullary phase axial CT image demonstrates calcification layering dependently in a low-attenuation left renal lesion (*arrow*). The calcification has a horizontal anterior margin, as it forms a fluid–fluid level with more anteriorly located simple fluid.

subdivided into two types according to the predominant location: the more common medullary nephrocalcinosis and cortical nephrocalcinosis.

Medullary Nephrocalcinosis

Causes

Most calcification in the renal parenchyma occurs in the renal medulla and, hence, is termed medullary nephrocalcinosis. Medullary nephrocalcinosis is usually bilateral. The most common exception is medullary sponge kidney, which may be unilateral or segmental.

The most common etiologies to produce medullary nephrocalcinosis are hyperparathyroidism, distal (type I) renal tubular acidosis (RTA), and renal tubular ectasia; however, recent research has indicated that nephrocalcinosis may also occur in other patients without any systemic disease. Medullary nephrocalcinosis is also a known neonatal complication of premature delivery, with a correlation between its prevalence and gestational age at delivery. Other less common causes include milk–alkali syndrome, sarcoidosis, vitamin D intoxication, other hypercalcemic states, hypophosphatasia, William syndrome, Bartter syndrome, primary hyperaldosteronism, and as a complication of administration of a variety of nephrotoxic drugs such as furosemide and amphotericin B. A brief discussion of each of the most common causes of medullary nephrocalcinosis is provided in the paragraphs that follow.

Idiopathic Medullary Nephrocalcinosis (in the Absence of Systemic Disease)

Radiologists have difficulty distinguishing between nephrolithiasis and medullary nephrocalcinosis on imaging studies. Recent studies have demonstrated that many patients who have undergone stone fragmentation and extraction procedures and who are believed to have residual fragments in their renal collecting system, as a result of imaging studies, do not have any stones present in their collecting systems when subsequent endourologic procedures are performed. In fact, many remaining calcifications actually represent medullary nephrocalcinosis. Thus, a substantial number

of patients with nephrolithiasis without systemic disease actually have medullary nephrocalcinosis or a combination of nephrolithiasis and nephrocalcinosis. This is particularly true in patients who form calcium phosphate stones. In one study, by Bhojani and colleagues, for example, 10 (71%) of 14 patients with hydroxyapatite kidney stones and 11 (58%) of 19 patients with brushite stones were also found to have nephrocalcinosis. In comparison, only 6 (18%) of 34 patients with calcium oxalate stones had nephrocalcinosis. This observation is not surprising, as many stones begin as plugs and/or plaques in the renal pyramids, with the mechanism of stone precipitation likely being different for calcium phosphate and calcium oxalate stone formers. It is now believed by some that nephrolithiasis and nephrocalcinosis represent a spectrum of disease.

Hyperparathyroidism

While primary hyperparathyroidism may be caused by a parathyroid adenoma, carcinoma, or hyperplasia of the chief cells of the parathyroid gland, it is most commonly due to a single adenoma. Typically, serum calcium levels are high and serum phosphate levels are low, a finding which helps distinguish primary from the secondary hyperparathyroidism seen in patients with chronic kidney disease (in which serum phosphate levels are also elevated).

Renal Tubular Acidosis

Patients with RTA have a defect in the tubules that prevents the kidney from producing acidic urine. The risk of stone formation and nephrocalcinosis is increased in these patients, as calcium salts are less soluble in alkaline urine than in acid urine. Primary RTA is caused by an inherited enzymatic defect. The manifestations of primary RTA, which include urolithiasis, osteomalacia, and hypokalemia, can be treated with alkalinizing salts. Secondary RTA occurs as a result of a diminished ability of the distal tubule to excrete hydrogen ions. Disease processes that cause secondary RTA by impairing hydrogen ion excretion by the distal tubule include Fanconi syndrome, Wilson disease, and amphotericin B toxicity.

RTA is divided into proximal and distal forms. The proximal variety (type II) of RTA does not produce nephrocalcinosis and does not have radiographic manifestations. In the distal form (type I), the distal renal tubule can no longer secrete hydrogen ions. This defect results in bicarbonate loss, reduced acid excretion, secondary aldosteronism, and hypokalemia. Nephrocalcinosis occurs in approximately 75% of these patients and commonly appears as dense clusters of calcifications in the medullary pyramids.

Medullary Sponge Kidney

Renal tubular ectasia is believed to represent a congenital abnormality that causes cystic dilation of the renal collecting tubules. This dilation can result in urinary stasis with a subsequent tendency to develop medullary nephrocalcinosis and nephrolithiasis. Many reserve the term medullary sponge kidney for those patients in whom both renal tubular ectasia and medullary nephrocalcinosis develop together. The calcifications found in medullary sponge kidney can be composed of either calcium oxalate or calcium phosphate. They are usually small and asymptomatic, but they may cause colic if they migrate into the collecting system, enlarge, and begin to pass down the ureter.

Milk–Alkali Syndrome

Nephrocalcinosis may occur in patients who consume large quantities of antacids and milk. This has been termed the *milk–alkali syndrome*. As previously mentioned, alkaline urine facilitates precipitation of calcifications in the renal parenchyma (as well as of urinary tract stones).

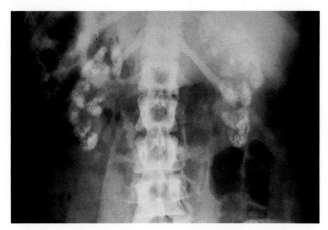

FIGURE 11.33. Plain radiograph of medullary nephrocalcinosis. An abdominal radiograph demonstrates extensive bilateral renal medullary calcification in this patient with hyperparathyroidism.

Imaging of Medullary Nephrocalcinosis

Medullary nephrocalcinosis is often easily identified on plain radiography as it results in the formation of multiple renal medullary calcifications (Fig. 11.33). Unlike extensive nephrolithiasis, the calcifications in nephrocalcinosis do not conform to the shapes of the renal calyces and infundibula as they get larger. Nonetheless, differentiation between nephrolithiasis and nephrocalcinosis can be difficult, particularly since many patients have both. In fact, endourology may be required to determine whether a renal calcification is in the collecting system or parenchyma in some instances. As previously discussed, many calcifications presumed to be parenchymal on imaging studies have subsequently been confirmed to be within the renal collecting systems during endourology (and vice versa). Nephrocalcinosis can also be identified on ultrasound, with highly echogenic foci detected in the renal pyramids, beyond which acoustic shadowing may or may not be detected, depending on the size of the calcifications (Fig. 11.34). CT also clearly shows the high-attenuation calcifications in the medulla (Fig. 11.35).

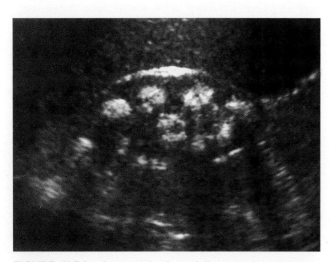

FIGURE 11.34. Ultrasound of medullary nephrocalcinosis. A longitudinal ultrasound image in a patient with medullary nephrocalcinosis shows highly echogenic material in the renal pyramids, much of which demonstrates posterior acoustic shadowing.

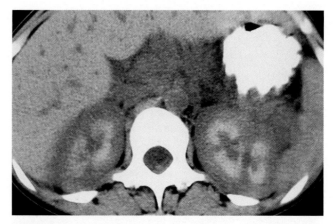

FIGURE 11.35. CT of medullary nephrocalcinosis. An unenhanced axial CT image shows subtle bilateral renal medullary high-attenuation material (calcification) in this patient with medullary nephrocalcinosis.

CT and MR urography can be used to identify renal tubular ectasia/medullary sponge kidney as a specific cause of medullary nephrocalcinosis, because these modalities can depict the dilated renal collecting tubules in the renal papilla after contrast material administration, which produce a brushlike appearance in the renal pyramids (Fig. 11.36). Additionally, the systemic diseases that cause nephrocalcinosis usually result in the development of diffuse bilateral disease, while renal tubular ectasia, which consists of an anatomic rather than a metabolic defect, can be bilateral, unilateral, or even segmental. Unilateral or segmental nephrocalcinosis should, therefore, suggest the diagnosis of medullary sponge kidney, as should a linear configuration of medullary calcifications, resulting from their location within the thin dilated collecting tubules.

Cortical Nephrocalcinosis

Cortical nephrocalcinosis refers to renal parenchymal calcification that is located along the periphery of the kidneys. The medullary pyramids are spared in most patients with cortical nephrocalcinosis.

Causes

The most common entities to produce cortical nephrocalcinosis are oxalosis, acute cortical necrosis, and chronic glomerulonephritis. Another cause of cortical nephrocalcinosis is transplant rejection. Also, infection with *Pneumocystis carinii*, *Mycobacterium avium-intracellulare* (MAI), and cytomegalovirus can result in multiple stippled calcifications in the renal cortex in HIV-infected patients.

Oxalosis

Increased excretion of oxalic acid may be due to an inborn error of metabolism (primary) or may be secondary to other disorders. Hyperoxaluria may cause nephrocalcinosis and may also result in calcium oxalate stone formation. The term *oxalosis* is used to indicate precipitation of oxalate crystals in extrarenal tissues such as the kidneys, myocardium, lung, spleen, or arterial walls. Calcium oxalate crystals may precipitate in the renal tubules, which become obstructed and lead to tubular necrosis and atrophy. The crystals may stimulate an immune response in the kidney, causing an interstitial nephritis. This then results in progressive renal parenchymal atrophy and renal failure.

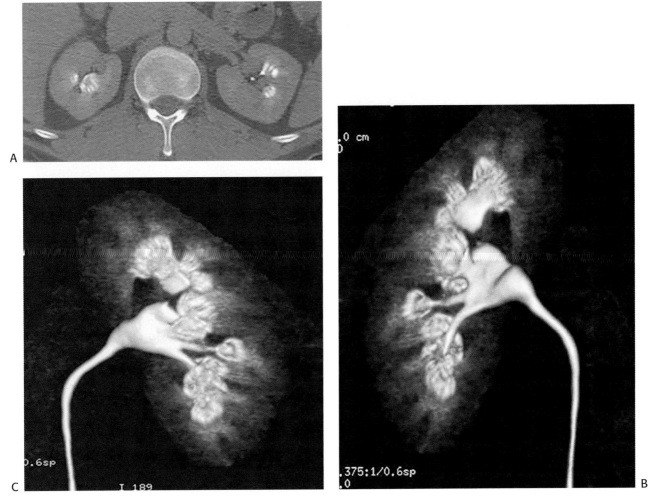

FIGURE 11.36. CT of medullary sponge kidney. **A:** An unenhanced axial CT image demonstrates linear calcifications in multiple renal pyramids. The calcifications have a linear configuration, consistent with their being located in dilated collecting tubules. **B, C:** Coronal reformatted volume-rendered excretory phase contrast-enhanced images of both kidneys show that all of the renal pyramids have a brushlike appearance, consistent with diffuse bilateral renal tubular ectasia.

Primary oxaluria is a rare autosomal recessively inherited inborn error of metabolism. There is no gender predilection. There are now three identified biochemical forms (caused by three different enzymatic defects, all of which lead to overproduction of oxalate). The most common defect is low or absent activity of liver peroxisomal alanine: glyoxylate aminotransferase, which accounts for nearly 80% of cases. Other mutations produce abnormalities of other enzymes, including glyoxylate/reductase/hydroxypyruvate reductase or 4-hydroy2-oxaglogluterate aldolase. All of these mutations also lead to excess oxalate in the urine. The urine then becomes supersaturated with calcium and oxalate, with these ions precipitating into crystals within renal tubular cells including in proximal nephrons and the collecting tubules.

Patients with primary oxalosis present with renal stones early in life, with a median age of presentation and of diagnosis being approximately 5 and 10 years, respectively. Patients can present with nephrolithiasis and/or nephrocalcinosis, with the latter being characteristically of the cortical type, in which dense calcification of the entire kidney develops. In one recent series, about 60% of patients with primary oxalosis had nephrolithiasis, 34% nephrocalcinosis, and 24% of patients both nephrolithiasis and nephrocalcinosis.

Oxalosis patients with nephrocalcinosis appear to be at a much higher risk for developing end-stage kidney disease than are patients who only develop nephrolithiasis.

The most common cause of secondary oxalosis is small bowel disease, such as after small bowel resections, and patients with celiac disease or Crohn disease. All of these patients have increased absorption of oxalate by the colon because of increased solubility of oxalate. Other causes of secondary hyperoxaluria include pyridoxine deficiency, methoxyflurane anesthesia, or increased consumption of leafy green vegetables high in oxalic acid.

Acute Cortical Necrosis

Acute cortical necrosis most commonly develops as a result of a severe vascular insult. It has been seen in severely ill hypotensive patients. One typical, classically described clinical situation that occurs during pregnancy is placental abruption with hemorrhage. Acute cortical necrosis may also be caused by ingestion of toxins such as ethylene glycol (antifreeze). The acute insult results in necrotic renal cortical tissue, which then becomes fibrotic (Fig. 11.37). Over the long term, calcifications occur in the renal cortex.

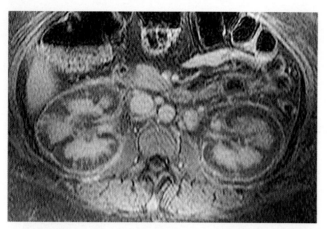

FIGURE 11.37. MRI of acute cortical necrosis. A T1-weighted fat-suppressed contrast-enhanced axial MR image in a patient who has been severely ill demonstrates nearly uniform absent perfusion of a rim of tissue along the periphery of both kidneys.

Chronic Glomerulonephritis

Patients with chronic glomerulonephritis can develop cortical nephrocalcinosis. One syndrome, which is known to be associated with chronic glomerulonephritis, is Alport syndrome. Alport syndrome is characterized by glomerulonephritis and interstitial fibrosis and is frequently also associated with nerve deafness and, in a minority of patients, cataracts. It is inherited as an autosomal dominant trait with variable penetrance. The disease is transmitted to both sons and daughters, but it is incompletely expressed in women. Hematuria in patients with Alport syndrome often begins in childhood. Mild proteinuria may also be present. Progression to renal failure is slow, with death often encountered by the third to fifth decade.

Imaging

The imaging appearance of cortical nephrocalcinosis is quite different from that of medullary nephrocalcinosis or nephrolithiasis. The calcifications in cortical nephrocalcinosis outline the entire renal contour. These calcifications throughout the renal cortex can often be seen on plain radiography or CT (Figs. 11.38 and 11.39).

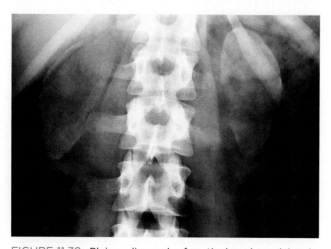

FIGURE 11.38. Plain radiograph of cortical nephrocalcinosis. An abdominal radiograph shows small kidneys with dense bilateral cortical calcification.

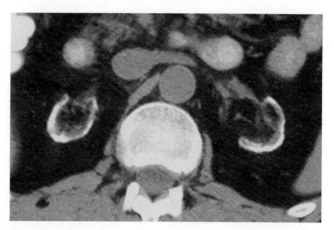

FIGURE 11.39. CT of cortical nephrocalcinosis. An unenhanced axial CT image of a patient with Alport syndrome shows dense bilateral cortical calcification in small kidneys, findings characteristic of cortical nephrocalcinosis resulting from chronic glomerulonephritis.

They are either identified as distinct structures or they can be small and diffuse, producing an appearance that mimics that of a persistent nephrogram (following contrast media administration). On ultrasound, the cortex is typically echogenic, but there is usually no posterior acoustic shadowing (which may be due to the frequently small size of the calcifications).

Nephrocalcinosis in Children

Because urinary calcium excretion varies directly with urinary sodium excretion, furosemide, which increases sodium excretion, also results in hypercalciuria. This is especially marked in preterm babies, because the increase in volume of amniotic fluid during the last trimester of pregnancy results from an increased excretion of sodium and water by the fetal kidney. Thus, premature babies have a higher urinary calcium level at birth and are more prone to nephrocalcinosis than are full-term children. This nephrocalcinosis is typically medullary, resulting in echogenic renal pyramids. Another cause of this finding in children is treatment with vitamin D for hypophosphatemic rickets or hypophosphatemic bone disease. Pyramidal hyperechogenicity in a pattern mimicking nephrocalcinosis can also occur in some children with autosomal recessive polycystic kidney disease.

SUGGESTED READINGS

Urolithiasis

Blake SP, McNicholas MM, Raptopoulous V. Nonopaque crystal deposition causing ureteric obstruction in patients with HIV undergoing indinavir therapy. *AJR Am J Roentgenol.* 1998;171:717–720.

Bove P, Kaplan D, Dalrymple N, et al. Reexamining the value of hematuria testing in patients with acute flank pain. *J Urol.* 1999;162:685–687.

Ciudin A, Luque MP, Salvador R, et al. The evolution of CT diagnosed papillae tip microcalcifications: can we predict the development of stones. *J Endourol.* 2014;28:1016–1021.

Daudon M, Bazin D, Letavernier E. Randall's plaque as the origin of calcium oxalate kidney stones. *Urolithiasis.* 2015;43:S5–S11.

Gleeson MJ, Griffith DP. Struvite calculi. *Br J Urol.* 1993;71:503–511.

Kim SH, Lee SE, Park IA. CT and US features of renal matrix stones with calcified center. *J Comput Assist Tomogr.* 1996;20:404–406.

McLeod RS, Churchill DN. Urolithiasis complicating inflammatory bowel disease. *J Urol.* 1992;148:974–978.

Moore CL, Daniels B, Singh D, et al. Ureteral stones: implementation of a reduced-dose CT protocol in patients in the emergency department with moderate to high likelihood of calculi on the basis of STONE score. *Radiology.* 2016;280(3):743–751.

Schwartz BF, Schenkman N, Armenakas NA, et al. Imaging characteristics of indinavir calculi. *J Urol.* 1999;161:1085.

Shoag J, Tasian GE, Goldfarb DS, et al. The new epidemiology of nephrolithiasis. *Adv Chronic Kidney Dis.* 2015;22:273–278.

Wang LC, Osterberg EC, David SG, et al. Recurrent nephrolithiasis associated with atazanavir use. *BMJ.* 2014; doi:10.1136/bcr-2013-201565.

Ultrasound Evaluation of Stone Disease

Burge HJ, Middleton WD, McClennan BE, et al. Ureteral jets in healthy subjects and in patients with unilateral ureteral calculi: comparison with color Doppler US. *Radiology.* 1991;180:437–442.

Kamaya A, Tuthill T, Rubin JM. Twinkling artifact on color Doppler sonography: dependence on machine parameters and underlying cause. *AJR Am J Roentgenol.* 2003;180:215–222.

Laing FC, Benson CB, DiSalvo DN, et al. Distal ureteral calculi: detection with vaginal US. *Radiology.* 1994;192:545–548.

Masch WR, Cohan RH, Ellis JH, et al. Clinical effectiveness of prospectively reported sonographic twinkling artifact for the diagnosis of renal calculus in patients without known urolithiasis. *AJR Am J Roentgenol.* 2016;206:326–331.

Unenhanced CT for Detection of Urinary Tract Calculi

Ciaschini MW, Remer EM, Baker ME, et al. Urinary calculi: radiation dose reduction of 50% and 75% at CT—effect on sensitivity. *Radiology.* 2009;251(1):105–111.

Deshmukh S, Kambadakone A, Sahani DV, et al. Hounsfield density of renal papillae in stone formers: analysis based pm stone composition. *J Urol.* 2015;193:1560–1563.

Dym RJ, Duncan DR, Spektor M, et al. Renal stones on portal venous phase contrast-enhanced CT: does intravenous contrast interfere with detection. *Abdom Imaging.* 2014;39:525–532.

Grosjean R, Daudon M, Chammas MF, et al. Pitfalls in urinary stone identification using CT attenuation values: are we getting the same information on different scanner models? *Eur J Radiol.* 2013;83:1201–1206.

Metser U, Ghai S, Ong YY, et al. Assessment of urinary tract calculi with 64 MDCT: the axial versus coronal plane. *AJR Am J Roentgenol.* 2009;192(6):1509–1513.

Patel SR, Wagner LE, Lubner MG, et al. Radiopacity and Hounsfield attenuation of cystine urolithiasis: case series and review of the literature. *J Endourol.* 2014;28:472–475.

Rucker CM, Menias CO, Bhalla S. Mimic of renal colic: alternative diagnoses at unenhanced helical CT. *Radiographics.* 2004;24:S11–S33.

Spettel S, Shah P, Sekhar K, et al. Using Hounsfield unit measurement and urine parameters to predict uric acid stones. *Urology.* 2013;82:22–26.

Williams JC Jr, Lingerman JE, Coe FL, et al. Micro-CT imaging of Randall's plaques. *Urolithiasis.* 2015;43:S13–S17.

Unenhanced CT in Patients with Acute Flank Pain

Abramson S, Walders N, Applegate KE, et al. Impact on the emergency department of unenhanced CT on diagnostic confidence and therapeutic efficacy in patients with suspected renal colic. A prospective study. *AJR Am J Roentgenol.* 2000;175:1689–1695.

Al-Nakshabandi NA. The soft tissue rim sign. *Radiology.* 2003;229:239–240.

Ather MH, Faizullah K, Achakzai I, et al. Alternate and incidental diagnoses on noncontrast-enhanced spiral computed tomography for acute flank pain. *Urol J.* 2009;6(1):14–18.

Boridy IC, Nikolaidis P, Kawashima A, et al. Ureterolithiasis: value of the tail sign in differentiating phleboliths from ureteral calculi at nonenhanced helical CT. *Radiology.* 1999;211:619–621.

Goldman SM, Faintuch S, Ajzen SA, et al. Diagnostic value of attenuation measurements of the kidney on unenhanced helical CT of obstructive ureterolithiasis. *AJR Am J Roentgenol.* 2004;182:1251–1254.

Guest AR, Cohan RH, Korobkin M, et al. Assessment of the clinical utility of the rim and comet-tail signs in differentiating ureteral stones from phleboliths. *AJR Am J Roentgenol.* 2001;177:1285–1291.

Heneghan JP, Dalrymple NC, Verga M, et al. Soft tissue "rim" sign in the diagnosis of ureteral calculi with use of unenhanced helical CT. *Radiology.* 1997;202:709–711.

Hoppe H, Studer R, Kessler TM, et al. Alternate or additional findings to stone disease on unenhanced computed tomography for acute flank pain can impact management. *J Urol.* 2006;175:1725–1730.

Kawashima A, Sandler CM, Boridy IC, et al. Unenhanced helical CT of ureterolithiasis: value of the tissue rim sign. *AJR Am J Roentgenol.* 1997;168:997–1000.

Levine J, Neitlich J, Smith RC. The value of prone scanning to distinguish ureterovesical junction stones from ureteral stones that have passed into the bladder: leave no stone unturned. *AJR Am J Roentgenol.* 1999;172:977.

Smith RC, Verga M, Dalrymple N, et al. Acute ureteral obstruction: value of secondary signs on helical unenhanced CT. *AJR Am J Roentgenol.* 1996;167:1109–1113.

Smith RC, Verga M, McCarthy S, et al. Diagnosis of acute flank pain: value of unenhanced helical CT. *AJR Am J Roentgenol.* 1996;166:97–101.

Dual Energy CT

Ascenti G, Siragusa C, Racchiusa S, et al. Stone targeted dual energy CT: a new diagnostic approach to urinary calculus. *AJR Am J Roentgenol.* 2010;195(4):953–958.

Bonatti M, Lombardo F, Zamboni G, et al. Renal stones composition in vivo determination: comparison between 100/Sn140 kV dual-energy CT and 120 kV single-energy CT. *Urolithiasis.* 2017;45(3):255–261. doi:10.1007/s00240-016-0905-6.

Hidas G, Eliahou R, Duvdevani M, et al. Determination of renal stone composition with dual-energy CT: in vivo analysis and comparison with X-ray diffraction. *Radiology.* 2010;257(2):394–401.

Kaza RK, Platt JF. Renal applications of dual-energy CT. *Abdom Radiol.* 2016;41:1122–1132.

Kaza RK, Platt JF, Cohan RH, et al. Dual-energy CT with single- and dual-source scanners: current applications in evaluating the genitourinary tract. *Radiographics.* 2012;32:353–369.

Motley GK, Dalrymple N, Keesling C, et al. Hounsfield unit density in the determination of urinary stone composition. *Urology.* 2001;58:170–173.

Radiation Exposure from Renal Stone CT

Andrabi Y, Piankh O, Agrawal M, et al. Radiation dose considerations in kidney stone examinations: integration of iterative reconstruction algorithms with routine clinical practice. *AJR Am J Roentgenol.* 2015;204:1055–1063.

Chen TT, Wang C, Ferrandino MN, et al. Radiation exposure during the evaluation and management of nephrolithiasis. *J Urol.* 2015;194:878–885.

Jepperson MA, Cernigliaro JG, Ibrahim EH, et al. In vivo comparison of radiation exposure of dual-energy CT versus low-dose CT versus standard CT for imaging urinary calculi. *J Endourol.* 2015;29:141–146.

Jin DH, Lamberton GR, Broome DR, et al. Effect of reduced radiation CT protocols on the detection of renal calculi. *Radiology.* 2010;255(1):100–107.

Katz DS, Venkataramanan N, Napel S, et al. Can low dose unenhanced multidetector CT be used for routine evaluation of suspected renal colic? *AJR Am J Roentgenol.* 2003;180:313–315.

Liu W, Esler SJ, Kenny BJ, et al. Low dose nonenhanced helical CT of renal colic: assessment of ureteric stone detection and measurement of effective dose equivalent. *Radiology.* 2000;215:51–54.

Smith-Bindman R, Aubin C, Bailitz J, et al. Ultrasonography versus computed tomography for suspected nephrolithiasis. *N Eng J Med.* 2014;371:1100–1110.

Tack D, Sourtzis S, Delpierre I, et al. Low dose unenhanced multidetector CT of patients with suspected renal colic. *AJR Am J Roentgenol.* 2003;180:302–311.

Treatment of Urolithiasis

Celik S, Bozkurt O, Kaya FG, et al. Evaluation of computed tomography findings for success prediction after extracorporeal shock wave lithotripsy for urinary tract stone disease. *Int Urol Nephrol.* 2015;47:69–73.

Eisner BH, McQuaid JW, Hyams E, et al. Nephrolithiasis: what surgeons need to know. *AJR Am J Roentgenol.* 2011;196:1274–1278.

Hussein A, Anwar A, Abol-Nasr M, et al. The role of plain radiography in predicting renal stone fragmentation by shockwave lithotripsy in the era of noncontrast multidetector computed tomography. *J Endourol.* 2014;28:850–853.

Lee HY, Yang YH, Lee YL, et al. Noncontrast computed tomography factors that predict the renal stone outcome after shock wave lithotripsy. *Clin Imaging.* 2015;39:845–850.

Marinkovic SP, Marinkovic CM, Xie D. Spleen injury following left extracorporeal shockwave lithotripsy (ESWL). *BMC Urol.* 2015;15:(4):1–3.

Motamedinia P, Okhunov A, Okeke Z, et al. Contemporary assessment of renal stone complexity using cross-sectional imaging. *Curr Urol Rep.* 2015;16(4):18. doi: 10.1007/s11934-015-0494-x.

Tarplin S, Ganesan V, Monga M. Stone formation and management after bariatric surgery. *Nat Rev Urol.* 2015;12:263–270.

Stones in Calyceal Diverticula and Milk of Calcium Stones

El-Shazly M. Milk of calcium stones: radiological signs and management outcome. *Urolithiasis.* 2015;43:221–225.

Hewitt MJ, Older RA. Calyceal calculi simulating gallstones. *AJR Am J Roentgenol.* 1980;134:507–509.

Matlaga BR, Kim SC, Watkins SL, et al. Pre-percutaneous nephrolithotomy opacification for caliceal diverticular calculi. *J Endourol.* 2006;20:175–178.

Sejiny M, Al-Qahtani S, Elhaous A, et al. Efficacy of flexible ureterorenoscopy with holmium laser in the management of stone-bearing caliceal diverticula. *J Endourol.* 2010;24:961–967.

Urolithiasis in Pregnancy

Masselli G, Weston M, Spencer J. The role of imaging in the diagnosis and management of renal stone disease in pregnancy. *Clin Radiol.* 2015;70:1462–1471.

Urolithiasis in Children

Nimkin K, Lebowitz RL, Share JC, et al. Urolithiasis in a children's hospital: 1985–1990. *Urol Radiol.* 1992;14:139–143.

Nephrocalcinosis

Bhojuani N, Paonessa JE, Hameed TA, et al. Nephrocalcinosis in calcium stone formers who do not have systemic disease. *J Urol.* 2015;194:1308–1312.

Boyce AM, Shawker TH, Hill SC, et al. Ultrasound is superior to computed tomography for assessment of medullary nephrocalcinosis in hypoparathyroidism. *J Clin Endocrinol Metab.* 2013;98:989–994.

Hsi RS, Stoller ML. A spectrum: nephrocalcinosis-nephrolithiasis. *J Urol.* 2015;194:1188–1189.

Katz ME, Karlowicz MG, Adelman RD, et al. Nephrocalcinosis in very low birth weight neonates: sonographic patterns, histologic characteristics, and clinical risk factors. *J Ultrasound Med.* 1994;13:77.

Koraishy FM, Ngo TTT, Israel GM, et al. CT urography for the diagnosis of medullary sponge kidney. *Am J Nephrol.* 2014;39:165–170.

Miller NL, Humphreys MR, Coe FL, et al. Nephrocalcinosis: redefined in the era of endourology. *Urol Res.* 2010;38:421–427.

Schell-Feith EA, Kist-van Holthe JE, van der Heijden AJ. Nephrocalcinosis in preterm neonates. *Pediatr Nephrol.* 2010;25:221–230.

Tang X, Bergstralh EJ, Mehta RA, et al. Nephrocalcinosis is a risk factor for kidney failure in primary hyperoxaluria. *Kidney Int.* 2015;87:623–631.

Pelvicalyceal System and Ureter

PHYSIOLOGY

The intrarenal collecting system and ureter serve as conduits for transport of urine from the kidney to the bladder. The ureter transports urine from the renal pelvis to the bladder through a series of peristaltic contraction waves. The frequency of these waves is proportional to the rate of urine output from the kidney and is probably mediated by the degree of distention of the renal pelvis. In the normal ureter, each wave completely coapts the inner surfaces of the wall, so that the bolus of urine inferior to it is propelled ahead of the contraction wave.

The timing of the contraction waves in one ureter is independent of the other, and the ureter is usually empty between boluses; during CT urography, therefore, it is normal to see long segments of ureter completely lacking opacified urine. A bolus of urine expelled into the bladder creates a jet effect since the ureteral lumen at the ureterovesical junction (UVJ) is less distensible than the rest of the ureter and acts as a nozzle; these jets may be seen by Doppler ultrasound, CT (if the ureteral urine is opacified), and MRI. As the rate of urine formation increases, there is an increase in both the frequency and the volume of each peristaltic contraction. During maximal diuresis, the ureter may fill with urine so quickly that individual contraction waves do not form and the ureter fills with urine from the pelvis to the bladder as a continuous column.

With normal rates of urine flow, the renal pelvic pressure stays low and coaptation of the ureteral walls prevents urine from flowing retrograde back into the renal pelvis. The UVJ acts as a one-way valve and keeps urine from flowing from the bladder into the ureter, even when the ureteral musculature is relaxed. The ability of ureteral peristalsis and a competent ureterovesical valve to keep pressure in the renal pelvis low is crucial: elevated renal pelvic pressure reduces renal medullary blood flow, which normally takes place through the relatively low-pressure vasa recta, and thus compromises renal function.

PAPILLARY NECROSIS

Papillary necrosis is a clinical pathologic entity found in association with several diseases that affect the kidney. Each disease is thought to be associated with renal medullary ischemia, which causes necrosis and sloughing of papillary tissue. This sloughing results in characteristic radiologic findings.

Papillary necrosis varies greatly in severity and rate of progression. It may be part of a condition that produces severe acute renal abnormalities with massive sloughing of most papillary tissue accompanied by hematuria and colic or may follow an indolent course, with only minimal radiographic abnormalities and no clinical symptoms. The possible etiologies of papillary necrosis may be recalled using the mnemonic nonsteroidal anti-inflammatory drug (NSAID): NSAIDs, sickle cell hemoglobinopathies, analgesic abuse, infection (such as tuberculosis and pyelonephritis), and diabetes mellitus. The most common etiologies are analgesic use, diabetes mellitus, and sickle cell anemia.

Analgesic Nephropathy

Analgesic nephropathy was first described in 1953 in Sweden, where several patients with interstitial nephritis were found to have consumed large amounts of analgesics, which usually consisted of combinations of aspirin and phenacetin. Although over-the-counter combinations of aspirin and phenacetin have been removed from the market, they have been replaced by combinations of aspirin and acetaminophen. Both in combination and alone, these drugs may, in large doses, also produce renal disease. Similar analgesic nephropathy is caused by NSAIDs. Patients with renal disease resulting from analgesic abuse also have an increased incidence of transitional cell carcinoma (TCC), especially of the upper tracts.

Sickle Cell Disease

Sickle cell disease is the result of the homozygous hemoglobin S gene, which is present in approximately 10% of African Americans and in approximately 30% of black Africans. The abnormal hemoglobin results in the classic sickle cell shape of erythrocytes; these cells are less malleable than normal and tend to occlude capillaries, producing regions of ischemia and infarction in the renal medullae and papillae. Up to 50% of patients with sickle cell disease develop renal papillary necrosis. Papillary necrosis may also occur in patients with sickle cell trait.

Infection

The association of pyelonephritis and papillary necrosis sometimes is confusing. In some cases, the main factor may be a comorbidity such as diabetes. However, when the kidneys are infected by tuberculosis, the bacilli initially lodge in the cortex and move down the nephrons to the medulla, where they cause focal caseating granulomata, which then slough portions of tissue and produce papillary necrosis.

Diabetes Mellitus

This disease produces various renal abnormalities. Ischemia caused by small-vessel disease can cause papillary necrosis, but the abnormalities are not limited to this region. Diabetic nephrosclerosis affects the entire kidney and ultimately may lead to severe renal failure.

Radiology

The plain film is commonly normal; rarely, a sloughed but retained papilla may develop a ring of calcification on its surface and become visible. If the whole papilla is necrotic, the calcifications may be 5 to 6 mm in diameter.

The classic radiologic features of renal papillary necrosis are best shown by pyelography and CTU. There are several patterns of calyceal changes. Small collections of contrast medium may be seen in the papillary region (Figs. 12.1 and 12.2) and may be round, elongated, or irregular in shape. They may extend from the calyceal fornices or directly into the tip of the papillae (Fig. 12.3). Central erosion of the papilla is known as the medullary type of papillary necrosis. Alternatively, the entire papilla may become necrotic and slough; this is known as the papillary type of papillary necrosis. If the sloughed tissue has disappeared from the calyx and has been passed down the ureter, the calyx may be blunted with no remnant of the papilla at all. Alternatively, the entire papilla or large pieces of it may be retained

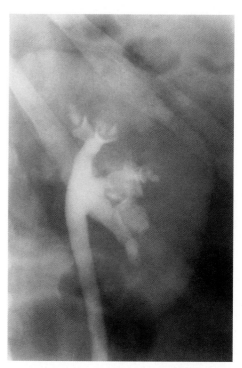

FIGURE 12.1. Papillary necrosis. Collections of contrast medium of varying sizes are present in the papillary regions adjacent to normal calyces.

and may form circular or irregular filling defects (Fig. 12.4); these defects may be calcified on their peripheries (Fig. 12.5).

MEDULLARY SPONGE KIDNEY (BENIGN TUBULAR ECTASIA)

Medullary sponge kidney (MSK) is a condition characterized by dilatation of the renal collecting ducts (of Bellini) in the papillae. When the dilatation is mild, it may produce parallel streaks of contrast in the papillae. This finding is called benign tubular ectasia and can involve only one, a few, or all of the calyces. In more severe cases, small globular regions of dilated tubules may appear, which, in turn, may contain small stones. This is termed *MSK* and is one cause of medullary nephrocalcinosis (Fig. 12.6).

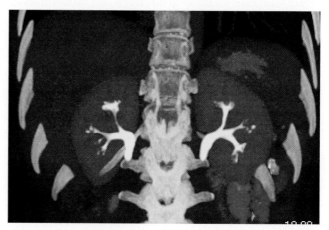

FIGURE 12.2. Papillary necrosis. CT urogram shows small rounded and linear collections of contrast adjacent to the calyces bilaterally.

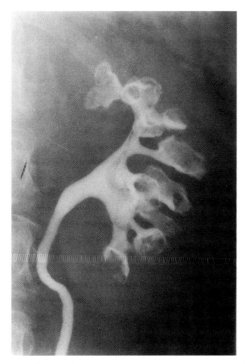

FIGURE 12.3. Papillary necrosis. Retrograde pyelogram shows rounded filling defects in many calyces representing sloughed, but retained, papillae.

Patients with benign tubular ectasia are asymptomatic. Patients with MSK may have microhematuria, and on occasion, stones may erode into the collecting system and produce episodes of renal colic.

CALYCEAL DIVERTICULUM

A calyceal diverticulum is a urothelium-lined cavity connected to the intrarenal collecting system by a narrow neck. It can arise from any part of the collecting system from the renal pelvis to a calyx

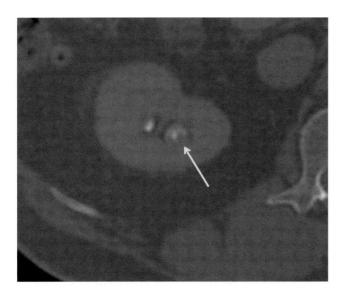

FIGURE 12.4. Papillary necrosis. The contrast-filled papillary tip (*arrow*) is seen on this axial CT image.

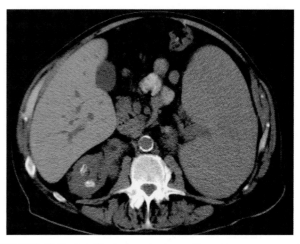

FIGURE 12.5. Calcified sloughed papillae. Noncontrast CT shows ringlike calcifications in the right kidney in this patient with lymphoma (note mass around right renal pelvis and splenomegaly).

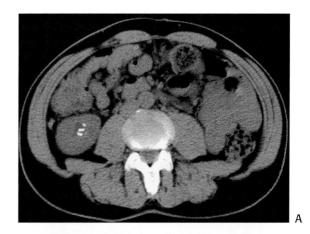

A

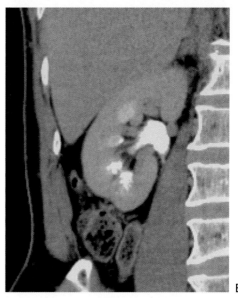

B

FIGURE 12.6. Medullary sponge kidney. **A:** Noncontrast CT shows elongated medullary stones in the right lower kidney (no stones were seen elsewhere). **B:** CT urogram shows coarse striations around right lower pole calyces.

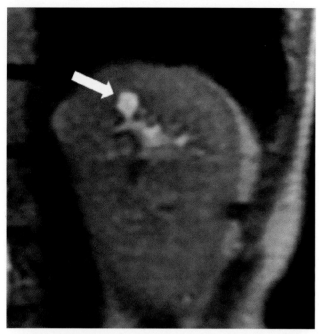

FIGURE 12.7. Calyceal diverticulum. T2-weighted MRI reveals the diverticulum as a spherical outpouching (*arrow*) arising from an upper pole calyx.

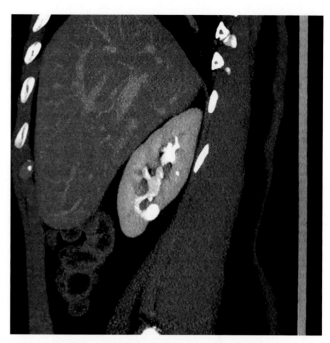

FIGURE 12.9. Calyceal diverticulum; sagittal reconstruction from CT urogram. The contrast-filled structure appears in the posterior portion of the lower pole.

but is most commonly seen extending from the fornix of a calyx (Fig. 12.7). These lesions can range in size from a few millimeters to several centimeters in diameter. They may contain calcified stones, most frequently appearing as a cluster of small stones (Fig. 12.8). Calyceal diverticula, with or without stones, are usually asymptomatic but may cause microhematuria. The stones that form

within them may rarely pass and cause ureteral colic but are usually confined to the diverticulum by the narrow neck.

On imaging studies, a calyceal diverticulum classically appears as a spherical collection of contrast medium adjacent to a papilla but outside the area where calyces typically lie. A cluster of small stones outside the normal topography of the calyces is usually an indicator of a calyceal diverticulum (Fig. 12.8). If the diverticulum is large and arises from the pelvis, it is more likely to cause infundibular or calyceal compression and displacement. The fluid-filled cavity comprising a calyceal diverticulum, together with any stones it contains, may be seen on CT or ultrasound. The diverticulum will typically opacify after the collecting system due to retrograde filling (Figs. 12.9 and 12.10).

RENAL SINUS

Renal Sinus Fat

Fat is normally found in the renal sinus in varying amounts surrounding the pelvicalyceal and vascular structures. This fat is sparse in infancy and childhood, but with advancing age, it increases in volume and becomes detectable. In anatomically normal patients, this change probably reflects the loss of renal parenchymal volume that occurs with age. In patients who are obese, who have excess truncal fat from exogenous steroids or Cushing syndrome, or whose renal parenchymal volume has been reduced by disease, the amount of sinus fat may be considerable and is known as sinus lipomatosis. The extreme of this condition is termed *replacement fibrolipomatosis* and usually accompanies severe loss of renal parenchyma. In these entities, the infundibula may look very attenuated, or thinned, or even slightly bowed, but infundibular obstruction is not a feature of this condition.

As with fat elsewhere, renal sinus fat is echogenic, resulting in the central echo complex in normal kidneys. Enlargement of the central renal echo complex is seen in sinus lipomatosis or replacement fibrolipomatosis, and the parenchyma may be thinned. CT directly reveals the sinus fat (Fig. 12.11), which is usually of the same density as other retroperitoneal fat.

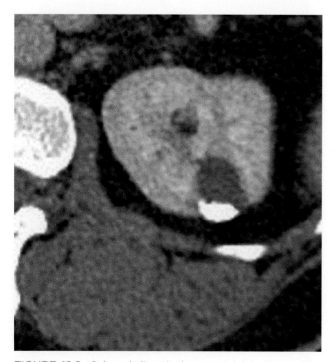

FIGURE 12.8. Calyceal diverticulum containing stones. The diverticulum is not opacified; a layer of small stones is seen in its dependent portion.

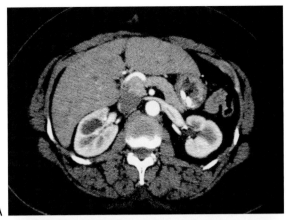

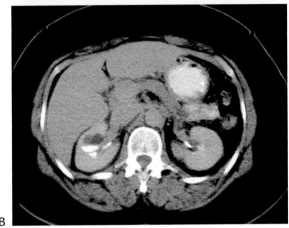

FIGURE 12.10. Large calyceal diverticulum. **A:** Early contrast CT shows large, rounded low-attenuation area in the anterior aspect of the right kidney. **B:** Delayed CT shows contrast-urine level as the diverticulum begins to fill with contrast.

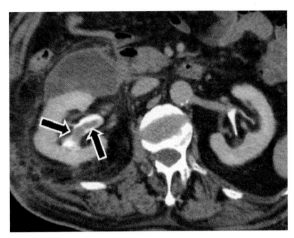

FIGURE 12.12. Clot in collection system, appearing as filling defect (arrows) surrounded by contrast.

Renal Sinus Hemorrhage

Hemorrhage into the renal sinus or collecting system may occur in various clinical circumstances including benign or malignant renal tumors, arteritis, aneurysms, arteriovenous malformations, trauma, coagulation disorders, or other bleeding diatheses. In the central portion of the kidney, bleeding may occur into the renal sinus or the wall or lumen of the collecting system.

The radiologic appearance depends on the compartment into which bleeding has occurred. Blood clots are always accompanied by gross hematuria; they may pass into the ureter and produce acute obstruction. Because the kidney produces urokinase, blood clots often dissolve, although they may reform if bleeding persists. On ultrasound examinations, blood clots have moderate echogenicity, less than that of renal sinus fat. They do not produce the acoustic shadowing seen with stones. CT demonstrates blood clot as an opacity slightly denser than adjacent soft tissues or as a filling defect in an opacified lumen (Figs. 12.12 and 12.13). They can be clearly distinguished from stones, because

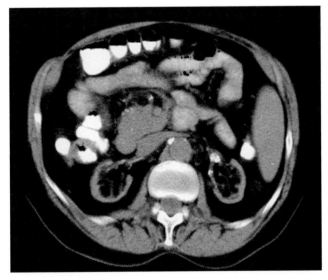

FIGURE 12.11. Replacement fibrolipomatosis. End-stage kidneys with fibrofatty tissue filling the renal sinuses, which are enlarged due to renal parenchymal atrophy.

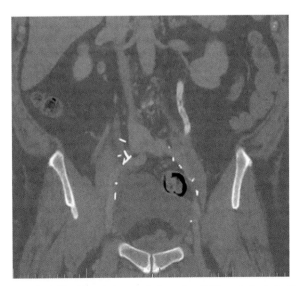

FIGURE 12.13. Blood clots in left ureter. Filling defects in the ureter are due to blood clots.

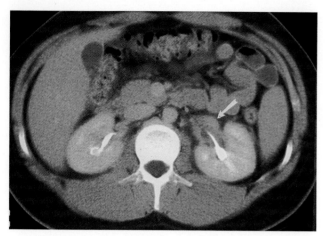

FIGURE 12.14. Suburothelial hemorrhage. CT in this patient with hemophilia shows high-density blood conforming to the shape of the renal pelvis and narrowing its lumen.

even uric acid stones, which are not seen on plain films, have attenuations of 300 to 500 Hounsfield units and are clearly seen on CT. Hemorrhage into the wall of the intrarenal collecting system and/or ureter, first described by Antopol and Goldman in 1948, is seen most frequently in patients with a bleeding disorder or those receiving anticoagulant medication. CT reveals a high-attenuation thickening of the renal pelvic or ureteral wall (Fig. 12.14).

VASCULAR IMPRESSIONS/CROSSINGS

The renal artery and its major branches are in close association with the collecting system and can cause bandlike impressions on the infundibula and renal pelvis; veins are more compressible and less likely to deform adjacent structures. Vessel abnormalities protruding into the renal sinus, such as aneurysms (Fig. 12.15) and arteriovenous malformations, may also indent the collecting system. Tortuosity or aneurysms of the iliac vessels or aorta may deflect the ureters. Occasionally, patients with severe renal artery stenosis may form collaterals that produce vascular notching on the ureter; retroperitoneal branches from the aorta supply the ureteral artery, which enlarges and becomes tortuous before supplying flow that enters the renal artery distal to the stenosis. Venous collaterals associated with inferior vena cava or renal vein obstruction may also produce an irregular notching of the ureter. At several well-defined points between the calyces and the bladder, vessels crossing the collecting system may actually result in obstruction to the normal flow of urine; these are discussed in the following paragraphs.

Fraley Syndrome

Nonobstructive bandlike indentations of the infundibula or renal pelvis are the typical findings when a renal vessel lies immediately adjacent to the collecting system. This most frequently involves the upper pole infundibulum or anterior surface of the renal pelvis. On rare occasions, the upper pole infundibulum may be scissored between two vessels resulting in hydrocalyx and pain. Alternatively, the pressure from a single crossing vessel can also result in the finding of an isolated hydrocalyx (Fig. 12.16). Either is known as Fraley syndrome.

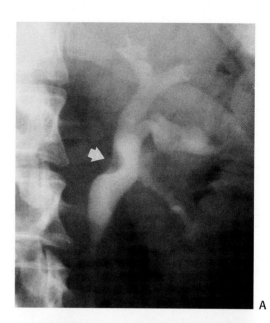

A

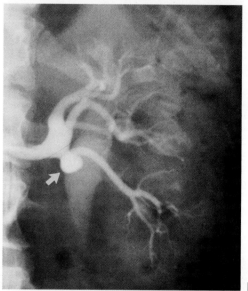

B

FIGURE 12.15. **A:** Renal artery aneurysm. Urography shows a renal pelvic defect (*arrow*). **B:** Selective renal arteriography shows a renal artery aneurysm (*arrow*) in the exact position of the renal pelvic defect.

Crossing Vessels in Ureteropelvic Junction Obstruction

Ureteropelvic junction (UPJ) obstruction is typically caused by a deficiency or derangement of the smooth muscle at the UPJ, preventing transmission of a normal peristaltic wave. However, a crossing vessel, almost always the renal artery or a major branch, may cause extrinsic compression and varying degrees of obstruction of the UPJ. These vessels may exacerbate an intrinsic obstruction and can complicate endoscopic treatment of the UPJ obstruction by excessive bleeding or reduced treatment success rates. It is therefore necessary that accurate preoperative imaging be performed to allow for appropriate treatment planning, since a crossing vessel is an indication for open or laparoscopic

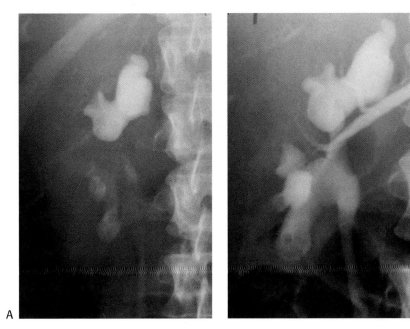

A

B

FIGURE 12.16. Renal artery partially obstructing upper pole infundibulum. **A:** Urography reveals dilated upper pole calyces. **B:** Renal arteriography shows a branch of the renal artery compressing upper pole infundibulum.

repair for many surgeons. During pyeloureterography, a vascular impression may be seen at the UPJ in these patients (Fig. 12.17). CT angiography can usually identify the presence of a crossing vessel.

Retrocaval (Circumcaval) Ureter

The origin of this anomaly is discussed in Chapter 1. Cross-sectional imaging, especially CT (Fig. 12.18) or MR, is useful to delineate the retrocaval course of the ureter.

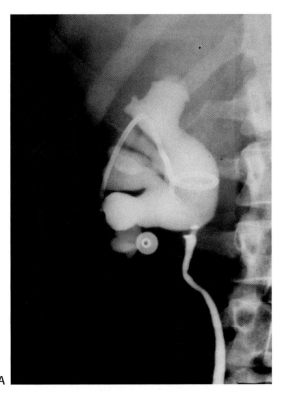

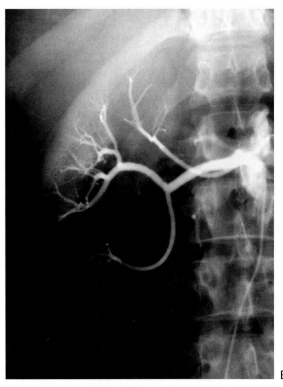

A

B

FIGURE 12.17. Hydronephrosis secondary to crossing vessel at UPJ. **A:** Retrograde ureteropyelogram shows an extrinsic impression on the UPJ and an associated hydronephrosis. A percutaneous nephrostomy tube is in place. **B:** Selective right renal arteriogram shows a branch of the renal artery curving around the renal pelvis and crossing the UPJ.

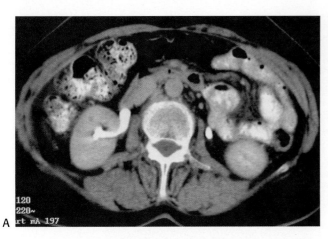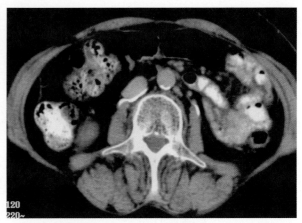

FIGURE 12.18. Retrocaval ureter. **A:** Contrast CT shows mildly dilated right renal pelvis. **B:** Right ureter can be seen crossing behind IVC.

Ovarian Vein Syndrome

The right ovarian vein crosses the ureter at approximately the level of L3. It seldom causes a distinct vascular impression, but cases of mild ureteral dilation and hydronephrosis proximal to the level where the ovarian vein is presumed to cross the ureter have been reported, sometimes in association with pyelonephritis. These been attributed to thrombosis of the vein. The syndrome typically occurs in young women who have had one or more pregnancies and is known as the ovarian vein syndrome (Fig. 12.19).

BENIGN COLLECTING SYSTEM AND URETERAL MASSES

Papillomas

Papillomas are benign tumors of the transitional epithelium that may appear in the collecting system, ureter, or bladder; they are rare in the upper tract. Some pathologists do not make a clear distinction between papillomas and low-grade TCCs. Papillomas appear as polypoid filling defects which may have recognizable stalks. Inverted papillomas are extremely unusual lesions that have a central core composed of transitional epithelium rather than of connective tissue and are covered with the normal layer of transitional cell epithelium. They are small and intrinsically benign, but a few

patients have been described in whom urothelial malignancy has been found near the inverted papilloma or elsewhere in the urinary tract.

Connective Tissue Tumors

Connective tissue tumors of the collecting system are rare; both malignant and benign tumors originating from muscular, vascular, fibrous, and neural tissues have been described. They present as masses arising from the calyceal, renal pelvic, or ureteral walls. As a group, their surfaces may be less irregular than those of epithelial malignancies, but their specific diagnoses cannot be established radiologically.

Fibroepithelial Polyps

The *fibroepithelial polyp* is the most common, albeit infrequently encountered, benign tumor of the collecting system and ureter. The lesion consists of a core of fibrous and vascular tissue covered with normal transitional epithelium. It is usually solitary, but multiple lesions have been reported. These polyps may bleed slightly or cause obstruction and flank pain. They are not premalignant.

Imaging may reveal the lesion to be mobile, owing to its long stalk. The polyps vary in size from a few millimeters to many

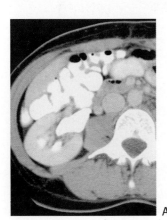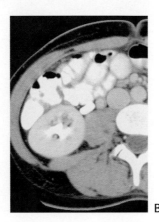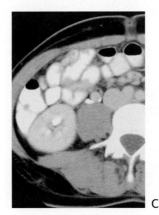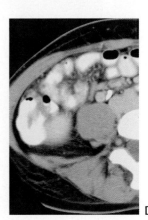

FIGURE 12.19. Ovarian vein syndrome in a multiparous woman with recurrent right-sided pyelonephritis. **A:** Contrast CT shows mild right hydronephrosis. **B:** The right ureter is dilated and adjacent to the prominent right ovarian vein. **C:** The ureter crosses behind the ovarian vein. **D:** The ureter lies medial to the ovarian vein.

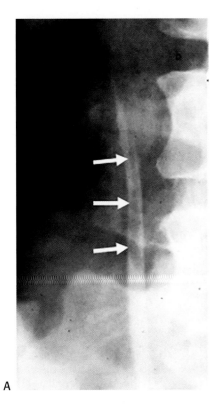
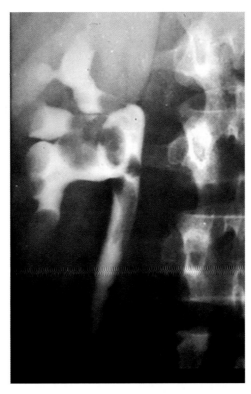

A   B

FIGURE 12.20. Fibroepithelial polyp: two cases. **A:** The polyp is a long thin structure (*arrows*) in the lumen of the ureter. **B:** The polyp has multiple blunt projections, which form filling defects in the renal pelvis and proximal ureter.

centimeters in length. Most fibroepithelial polyps have a smooth cylindrical appearance (Fig. 12.20A), but multitentacled or frond-like appearances (Fig. 12.20B) have been reported. Unlike primary malignant tumors, these polyps are most commonly found in the proximal one-third of the ureter and typically occur in children and young adults. They should be distinguished from vermiform (wormlike) clots in the ureteral lumen.

MALIGNANT TUMORS

Primary Urothelial Tumors

Urothelial tumors of the bladder are much more common than are tumors of the upper urinary tract. Of primary renal malignancies, only about 7% develop in the collecting system, and tumors of the ureter are three to four times less common than those occurring in the renal pelvis. Most urothelial malignancies are TCCs; squamous cell carcinomas are unusual, and adenocarcinomas are rarer still. The histologic types are not distinguishable radiologically. TCCs have a tendency to be multiple, so that both synchronous (Figs. 12.21 and 12.22) and metachronous lesions may be seen; having had a prior upper tract TCC is a strong risk factor for developing another one. For this reason, complete nephroureterectomy, including resection of a generous cuff of bladder around the ipsilateral ureteral orifice is the standard therapy for upper tract lesions that are resectable at the time of diagnosis. Other predisposing factors that place patients at risk for developing TCC include analgesic abuse, exposure to aniline dyes or petroleum derivatives, administration of cyclophosphamide, and a long history of heavy smoking. Long-standing upper tract stone disease may be a risk factor for squamous cell carcinoma; whether leukoplakia or upper urinary tract cholesteatomas increase the risk is debatable.

Any upper urinary tract tumor may present with gross or microscopic hematuria. The patients may have pain, especially if

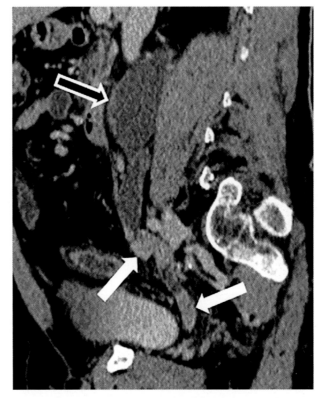

FIGURE 12.21. Synchronous ureteral tumors. Sagittal reconstruction of CT reveals two soft tissue ureteral masses (*solid arrows*) producing obstructive ureteral dilatation (*bordered arrow*).

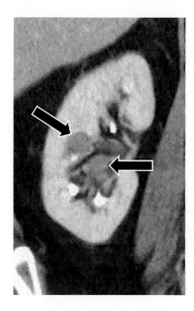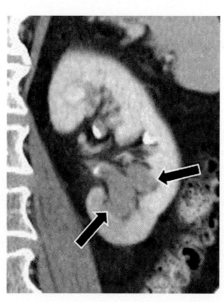

FIGURE 12.22. Bilateral synchronous collecting system urothelial tumors. The lesions appear as poorly-enhancing soft tissue masses (*arrows*) within expanded calyces.

the tumors have caused hydronephrosis, and voided urine may contain exfoliated malignant cells that are detectable on cytologic examination.

Small carcinomas of the collecting system may be detected by CT (Fig. 12.23), MRI (Fig. 12.24), or pyelography (Fig. 12.25). Tumors may appear as intraluminal filling defects, which may be polypoid or flat; their surface is usually fronded or irregular (Fig. 12.26); occasionally, calcification may occur and is usually found on the surface of the tumor. A tumor growing within the ureteral lumen may stretch the surrounding ureteral wall, unlike other intraluminal pathology. If the ureter distal to such a tumor is opacified with contrast during retrograde ureterography, the focally dilated ureter and the inferior convex margin of the tumor may produce a characteristic luminal shape called a goblet or champagne-glass sign (Fig. 12.27).

The most common conditions to cause a filling defect in the lumen of an opacified upper urinary tract are tumor, blood clot,

and stone. The differential diagnostic possibilities also include rarer conditions, such as a sloughed papilla, fungus ball, and even invasion of the collecting system by a renal parenchymal tumor. The diagnosis of blood clot is supported by a CT density consistent with clot or by a subsequent examination which shows the filling defect has lysed and disappeared; conversely, a blood clot can be virtually excluded if there is no gross hematuria. On CT, stones—even uric acid stones—are much denser than any other natural intraluminal object. Sloughed intact papillae are rare; sometimes they may look like polypoid tumors and are usually associated with blunted

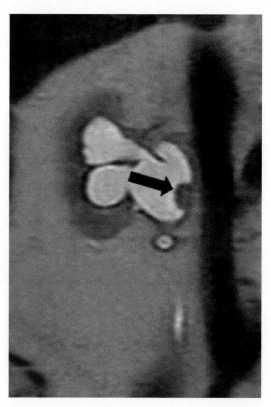

FIGURE 12.23. Small renal pelvic transitional cell tumor (*arrow*) is shown at the medial aspect of the renal pelvis by CTU.

FIGURE 12.24. T2-weighted MRI reveals small mass (*arrow*) protruding into dilated renal pelvic lumen.

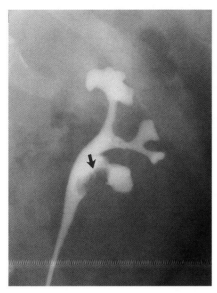

FIGURE 12.25. TCC of the renal pelvis. Retrograde pyelography reveals a solitary renal pelvic filling defect (*arrow*).

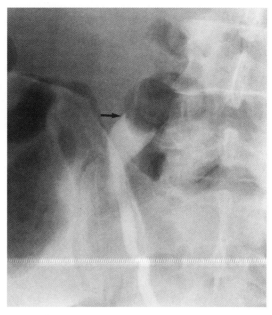

FIGURE 12.27. Retrograde ureteropyelogram shows a filling defect in the ureter representing the tumor (*arrow*). A classic goblet sign is demonstrated.

calyces at the sites from which the papillae detached. Fungus balls (mycetomas) are also rare; they are usually accompanied by signs of fungal pyelonephritis and may be diagnosed by finding hyphae in the urine. Ultrasound is not sufficiently sensitive for small tumors to have a place in tumor detection but may be useful in differentiating stones from other intraluminal structures. Larger tumors may be visible as hypoechoic structures (Fig. 12.28) and even may be specifically differentiated from other lesions by demonstrating Doppler flow.

Small TCCs may have growth patterns in addition to forming polypoid intraluminal structures. Like carcinomas in other tubular structures, they may infiltrate the wall of the collecting system or

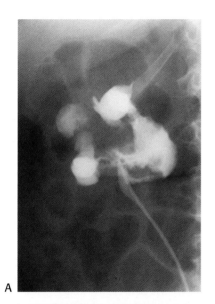

A

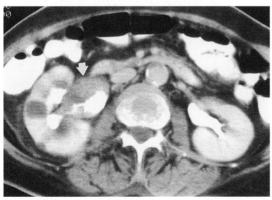

B

FIGURE 12.26. Transitional cell carcinoma. **A:** Retrograde pyelography demonstrates a large, irregular filling defect in the renal pelvis. **B:** The soft tissue mass (*arrow*) is shown on this enhanced CT examination.

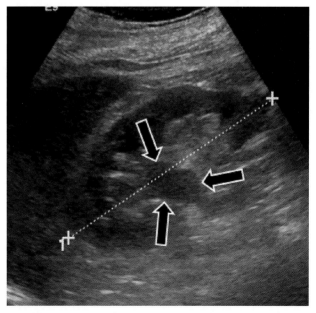

FIGURE 12.28. Transitional cell carcinoma. Ultrasound examination showing hypoechoic discrete mass (*arrows*) in the renal sinus.

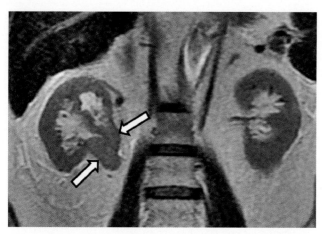

FIGURE 12.29. Renal pelvic urothelial tumor. MRI reveals thickening of the walls of the right renal pelvis.

ureter and appear on images as local regions of mural thickening (Fig. 12.29). As they continue to enlarge, they often cause obstruction. A variety of appearances may be encountered: the tumor itself may be visible on CT or MRI; the tumor may be outlined by contrast in a pyeloureterography phase (Fig. 12.30) and may be detected by focal enhancement if early postcontrast views are obtained. There may be evidence of obstruction of an infundibulum renal pelvis or ureter, with varying severity of hydronephrosis demonstrable by ultrasound, CT, MRI, and retrograde pyeloureterography (Figs. 12.21 and 12.31).

This wall thickening and obstruction present another differential diagnostic problem. Focal mural thickening may be produced by local intramural hemorrhage; this can be identified by gross hematuria, increased density on noncontrast CT and spontaneous resolution. Endometriosis occasionally occurs within the wall of the

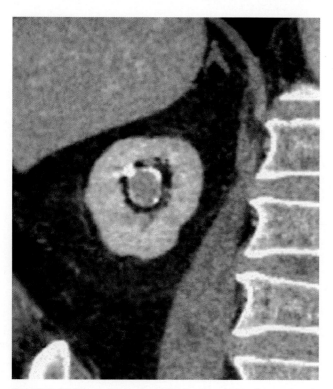

FIGURE 12.30. Low-stage TCC. In this CTU, the tumor is clearly seen outlined by contrast.

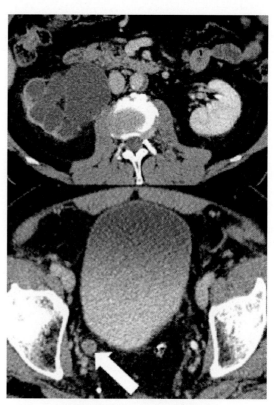

FIGURE 12.31. Right distal ureteral TCC (*arrow*) obstructing ureter and producing hydronephrosis.

distal ureter, though the more common form of ureteral involvement is a periureteral mass. Patients with this condition usually have more widespread pelvic disease and characteristic symptoms. Leukoplakia (see section Inflammatory Conditions) and cholesteatoma may be impossible to distinguish from neoplasm on morphologic or clinical grounds but are rare.

Intramural tumors, with or without circumferential infiltration, may obstruct and appear as strictures. Like esophageal and colon tumors, these lesions often have abrupt shelflike edges (Fig. 12.32) and may produce an apple-core appearance. Often the mass of the tumor permits distinction from benign strictures, but sometimes the appearance overlaps that of benign disease. Tuberculosis often produces local strictures but is usually accompanied by calcification and renal parenchymal destruction, which indicates the real etiology. Retroperitoneal fibrosis may infiltrate the wall of any part of the upper urinary tract, but the characteristic appearance of the associated retroperitoneal mass usually leads to the correct diagnosis.

Finally, urothelial tumors in the kidney may grow to a degree at which they appear as large central renal sinus masses (Fig. 12.33). These can be detected by any tomographic imaging technique. Ultrasound reveals them to be hypoechoic masses with Doppler flow. CT and MRI demonstrate them as soft tissue masses, which enhance slightly with contrast. The pyelographic phase of CT urography may demonstrate a severely distorted collecting system or, if there has been obstruction by the mass, no opacification of the collecting system at all and reduced enhancement of the surrounding renal parenchyma.

Urothelial tumors frequently metastasize initially to local lymph nodes. Size is an important criterion in determining whether a node contains a metastasis; no specific diameter permits simultaneously high sensitivity and specificity, but a short-axis diameter of 5 mm. is a commonly used threshold. Diffusion-weighted MR imaging is useful; restricted diffusion is a relatively reliable indicator of a metastasis in a borderline-sized node.

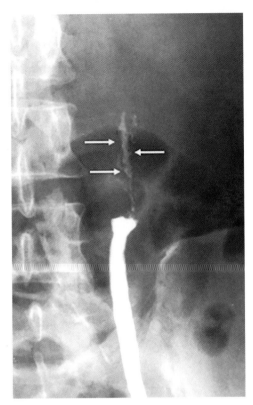

FIGURE 12.32. Circumferential ureteral TCC. Retrograde ureterogram reveals shelflike edge of narrowed segment; the narrow portion (*arrows*) has an irregular margin reflecting the inner surface of the encircling tumor.

Usually, renal cell carcinomas and renal urothelial tumors can be distinguished without difficulty, but when a mass involves both the parenchyma and structures in the renal sinus, differential diagnosis may be harder. A mass whose center is in or near the renal sinus, or which primarily occupies the collecting system lumen,

is likely to be urothelial (Fig. 12.33). A mass that is centered more peripherally, even if part of it grows into the collecting system, is likely to be renal cell. If the collecting system is distorted by a central renal mass but remains patent and smooth-walled, the mass is probably renal cell. Finally, urothelial carcinomas usually enhance only faintly; floridly enhancing masses are almost always renal cell.

CTU is highly sensitive and specific in detecting upper tract urothelial cancer. It usually demonstrates the mass in the renal pelvis or the ureter and also depicts any associated hydronephrosis. The mass is usually of soft tissue density and may enhance slightly with intravenous contrast administration. Large tumors in the renal pelvis may contain low-density necrotic regions that do not enhance.

MR urography can demonstrate upper tract urothelial tumors in much the same way as CTU, using both strongly T2-weighted techniques and urine enhancement with gadolinium, but is technically suboptimal more often: motion artifact interferes more frequently than it does with CT, and the intensity of gadolinium-enhanced urine within the collecting system is more difficult to manage.

Staging

In most cases, CT or MRI of the abdomen and pelvis suffice for initial staging; chest CT may be indicated if there are localizing symptoms or if there is advanced subdiaphragmatic disease.

Upper tract urothelial cancers are staged by a system similar to those used for staging epithelial cancers in muscular tubes elsewhere. Ta and Tis are limited to the urothelium; T1 connotes invasion of the lamina propria, T2 is invasion into the muscularis, T3 connotes invasion completely through the muscularis into the intrarenal or periureteral fat, and T4 indicates invasion of adjacent organs (for the ureter) and invasion completely through the kidney into the perinephric fat. Ta, Tis, T1, and T2 are difficult to distinguish since the muscular wall is thin and incomplete invasion through it is almost impossible to demonstrate with current technology (Figs. 12.23, 12.24, and 12.30). Stage T3 can be identified in cases in which the wall underlying the tumor cannot be seen at all and when the advancing edge of the tumor can be seen to be inseparable from peripelvic (Fig. 12.33) or periureteral fat. In stage 4 disease, the tumor invades through the kidney into perirenal fat (Fig. 12.34) or from the ureter into adjacent organs. In N0 disease,

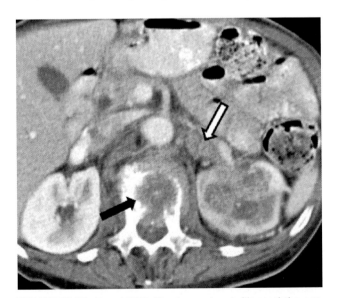

FIGURE 12.33. Renal TCC. The tumor has infiltrated the center of the left kidney (and hence is stage T3) and expanded to invade a large part of the organ. It has metastasized to a local node (*bordered arrow*) and a vertebral body (*black arrow*).

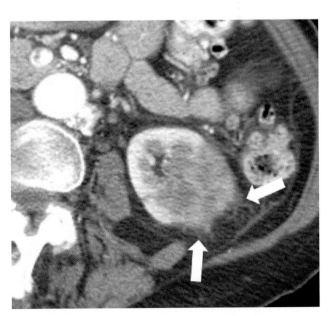

FIGURE 12.34. Renal TCC. The tumor has invaded completely through the renal cortex into perirenal fat (*arrows*) and is thus stage T4.

there is no nodal involvement; N1 tumors demonstrate a single abnormal node smaller than 2 cm in diameter, N2 tumors have several enlarged nodes but none larger than 5 cm, and N3 is identified when there is a nodal mass larger than 5 cm. M0 disease has no metastases; any metastasis is stage M1 disease.

Follow-up for urothelial tumors should be frequent and may include any modality that allows a detailed look at the lining of the remaining urinary tract, such as CT urography or retrograde ureteropyelography. Following nephroureterectomy, CT or MRI is useful for evaluating the renal bed for recurrences. Second primary urothelial tumors often occur in the bladder; although imaging is often capable of detecting these recurrences, small flat lesions are hard to identify, so that serial cystoscopy is routinely performed along with upper tract imaging.

Secondary Urothelial Tumors

Extrinsic neoplasms involving the ureter are much more common than primary ureteral neoplasms, because the latter are relatively uncommon and because the ureter is near many structures that frequently harbor malignancies. In many cases, obstruction of the ureter results from direct extension of the neoplasm from primary sites such as the cervix, prostate, and bladder. Ureteral obstruction may also occur because of adjacent retroperitoneal lymph node enlargement due to lymphoma or metastases from other primary tumors.

The ureter may also be indirectly obstructed from malignant disease because some tumors, such as breast cancer, invoke an intense periureteral desmoplastic reaction. In such cases, imaging studies may demonstrate extrinsic compression of the ureter by a soft tissue mass (Fig. 12.35); this is known as *malignant retroperitoneal fibrosis*. This may be difficult to diagnose by needle biopsy since there are relatively few malignant cells scattered throughout the

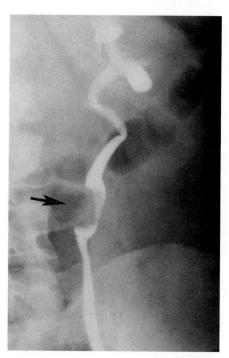

FIGURE 12.36. Malignant melanoma metastatic to the left ureter (*arrow*).

fibrotic obstructing plaque. Much less commonly, hematogenous metastases to the ureter may present as solitary filling defects simulating primary ureteral tumors (Fig. 12.36); melanoma; carcinomas of the kidney, breast, lung, and prostate; and multiple myeloma may be responsible.

Patients who experience ureteral obstruction after radiation therapy should not be assumed to have a benign radiation-induced stricture. The ureter is relatively resistant to radiation, so that postradiation ureteral obstruction often means that the tumor had involved the ureteral wall before therapy or has recurred.

VESICOURETERAL REFLUX

Primary vesicoureteral reflux is caused by an abnormality limited to the UVJ (Fig. 12.37) and is congenital and familial. It is more commonly unilateral than bilateral. Although the prevalence of this condition is not known, it is found in as many as one-half of infants and children with urinary tract infections.

Reflux may also be secondary, that is, associated with a disease that alters the anatomy of the UVJ. A bladder diverticulum immediately adjacent to the UVJ may facilitate reflux. Male infants with posterior urethral valves have a high incidence of reflux. Bladder inflammatory processes, such as tuberculosis or schistosomiasis, may produce reflux and neurogenic bladders may be associated with reflux as well. Ureteral duplication anomalies, imperforate anus, and other congenital urinary tract abnormalities are frequently accompanied by reflux. When a renal transplant is accompanied by a transplanted ureter, reflux often occurs. If the kidney that supplies a ureter becomes anuric or is resected, the nonfunctional ureter may demonstrate reflux.

Secondary changes in the urinary tract may be produced by the reflux. If the reflux is intermittent and mild, no changes may occur, but with more severe reflux, anatomic, physiologic, and pathologic changes may appear. The bladder may be affected by high-volume reflux. During voiding, the detrusor contraction expels most of the urine into the refluxing ureter rather than through the urethra. This ureteral urine refills the bladder immediately after voiding, so that

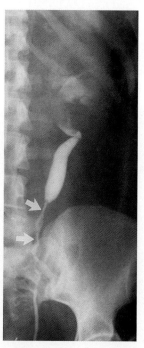

FIGURE 12.35. Metastatic retroperitoneal carcinoma involving the left ureter. The midureter is irregularly encased and narrowed (*arrows*); the proximal ureter is dilated. Insufficient contrast agent has been injected in this retrograde study to completely opacify the intrarenal collecting system. (From Amis ES Jr, Newhouse JH. *Essentials of Uroradiology*. Boston, MA: Little, Brown & Co.; 1991:282, with permission.)

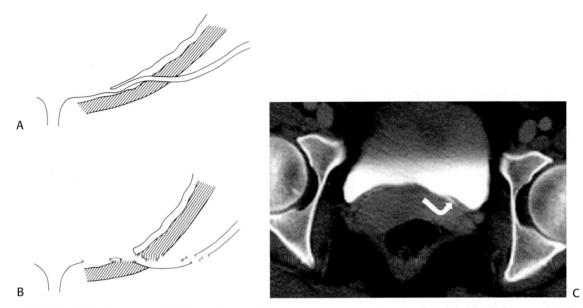

FIGURE 12.37. Diagram of UVJ. **A:** Normal—the ureter traverses the muscle wall (*shaded*) at an angle and courses submucosally before emerging at the orifice. This anatomy produces a competent valve. **B:** Refluxing—there is no submucosal ureteral course; vesicoureteral reflux occurs. (From Amis ES Jr, Newhouse JH. *Essentials of Uroradiology*. Boston, MA: Little, Brown & Co.; 1991:246, with permission.) **C:** Normal left ureterovesical junction. In this CT urogram, the *arrow* shows the lumen of the submucosal portion of the left ureter, corresponding to **(A)**.

the additional urine produced before the next voiding distends the bladder to an abnormal degree.

The ureter itself may become abnormal. During voiding, a large-volume retrograde bolus travels up the ureteral lumen, stretching the ureter, which becomes dilated and tortuous. The muscular wall thins, peristalsis becomes less effective, and the ureter may become chronically distended. Hydronephrosis of any degree may appear. Children with severe bilateral ureteral caliectasis and a bladder distended by the mechanism described above have a condition known as the megaureter–megacystis syndrome. It has been ascribed to bladder outlet obstruction and may be associated with posterior urethral valves, but severe vesicoureteral reflux may produce the syndrome without any obstruction.

A correlation exists between vesicoureteral reflux and urinary tract infection. In patients with bacilluria, the concentration of bacteria within the urine reflects a balance between the reproduction rate of the organisms and the rate at which they are washed out during voiding. If the ureters and bladder are normal, they are nearly empty at the end of micturition so that sterile urine subsequently produced (assuming the kidneys are not infected) dilutes the small amount of remaining urine quickly and reduces the concentration of bacteria. This process becomes ineffective if a large volume of urine persists in the ureters and bladder after voiding. Also, in some patients, especially very young patients with high-pressure reflux, bacterial cystitis or pyelitis may become pyelonephritis if infected urine is forced retrograde into renal tubules by reflux. For these reasons, urinary tract infections in young children often prompt investigation for vesicoureteral reflux.

Vesicoureteral reflux may be asymptomatic and resolve spontaneously during childhood without changes to the upper urinary tracts; alternatively, it may persist and cause permanent damage to the kidneys. Low grades of reflux often produce no pyelocalyceal changes at all. However, at the instant in which reflux occurs, there may be varying degrees of pyelocalyceal distention, the morphology of which may be indistinguishable from obstructive hydronephrosis. Depending on the duration and severity of the reflux, the distention may or may not persist between episodes of reflux or after the reflux has resolved.

Persistent and severe reflux may cause focal renal parenchymal scarring. This may be unilateral or bilateral and may involve a very small portion of a kidney or nearly the entire organ. The scarring has a predilection to appear in the poles, especially the upper poles, and is felt to be related to the occurrence of intrarenal reflux of urine into the collecting tubules (Fig. 12.38). When severe, it may produce chronic renal failure of any degree, as may the hydronephrosis that often accompanies severe reflux.

Because the scarring involves focal thinning of the renal parenchyma that extends from the renal capsule to the level of the papilla, inward retraction of the renal margin and outward expansion of the calyx appear. The normal concave surface of the papilla becomes flattened or even convex. Focal calyceal blunting, usually referred to as *calyceal clubbing*, with adjacent parenchymal thinning resulting

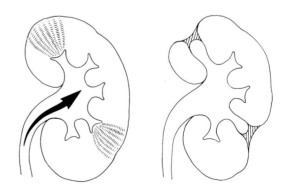

FIGURE 12.38. Intrarenal reflux. Diagram showing pattern of intrarenal reflux followed by scar formation, with focal parenchymal thinning and focal calyceal blunting. (From Amis ES Jr, Newhouse JH. *Essentials of Uroradiology*. Boston, MA: Little, Brown & Co.; 1991:252, with permission.)

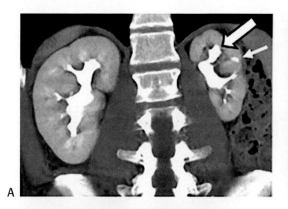
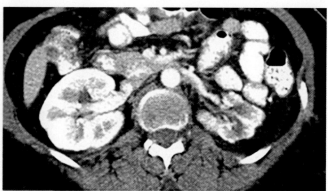
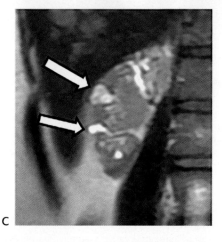

FIGURE 12.39. Three cases of reflux nephropathy. **A:** CT urogram shows blunted upper pole calyx (*large arrow*); an adjacent calyx is associated with cortical thinning (*small arrow*). **B:** Scarring from reflux. CT shows overall shrinking and focal atrophy of the left kidney. **C:** T2-weighted MRI reveals blunted calyces in several sites (*arrows*); the associated parenchyma is so thin that only the renal capsule separates the calyces from the perinephric fat.

from reflux is a relatively specific set of imaging findings associated with reflux and is called chronic atrophic pyelonephritis or reflux nephropathy (Fig. 12.39). When the entire kidney is involved, the renal contour may be grossly irregular due to the multiplicity of scars, or the kidney may actually be small and relatively smooth due to the diffuseness of the scarring. Focal scarring, with findings similar to that of reflux nephropathy, can be produced by a stone impacted in an infundibulum, resulting in an isolated hydrocalyx and atrophy of the adjacent parenchyma. If reflux is severe, parenchymal thinning may be accompanied by hydronephrosis (Fig. 12.40).

Screening for Vesicoureteral Reflux

The most common reason for seeking reflux in a pediatric patient is urinary infection. Which modality to use, and in which circumstances, continues to be a complicated issue. Benefits must be evaluated in terms of utility of acquired information in guiding management; the risks include radiation exposure and the discomfort of urethral catheterization. Treatment is, of course, tailored for each patient; short courses of antibiotics are used for acute infections, lengthy periods of antibiotic prophylaxis are sometimes indicated to suppress infection and possibly to ameliorate progressive scarring, and transurethral or open reflux-correcting surgery may be chosen to reduce the chances of subsequent infection and to reduce progressive scarring and hydronephrosis. Debate continues regarding the utility of long-term antibiotics and the indications for surgery. Most authorities agree that even a single urinary infection should prompt screening in very young infants and in young boys, in whom posterior urethral valves are sufficiently frequent and dangerous that voiding cystourethrography should not be postponed. In young girls older than 2 years, urinary infections are so frequent that there is some difference of opinion regarding whether all patients should be screened. Some

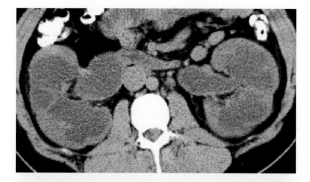
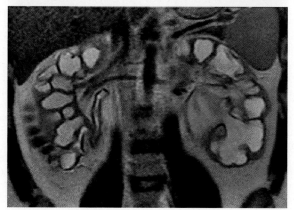

FIGURE 12.40. Severe reflux nephropathy. There is widespread parenchymal thinning with hydronephrosis demonstrated by CT **(top)** and T2-weighted MRI **(bottom)**.

authorities believe that the first infection should prompt a search for reflux, whereas others think that only a series of infections indicate workup. Screening young adult women with urinary infection reveals reflux in only a small number.

Reflux is demonstrated by either radiographic or radionuclide cystourethrography. Radionuclide cystourethrography has the highest sensitivity for reflux and lowest radiation dose but fails to reveal intrinsic urethral or bladder wall abnormalities. Urethral abnormalities are rare in girls, so radionuclide cystography is a good choice. In boys, who might have posterior urethral valves, radiographic cystourethrography is necessary. Whichever method is used, several points are worth emphasizing. First, a voiding study is necessary; cystography alone is not sufficient to exclude reflux. The patient should be awake in order to void as normally as possible. A small urethral catheter will permit the patient to void around the catheter, so that the bladder can be filled and voiding can be observed more than once if necessary. For radiographic cystourethrography, fluoroscopy is needed, as transient reflux, functional details of micturition, and urethral abnormalities are easily missed without fluoroscopic control.

Whatever the examination type, vesicoureteral reflux is diagnosed by observing contrast medium or isotope in the ureter and/ or collecting system after it has been instilled into the bladder. A patient may demonstrate low-pressure reflux (reflux that occurs during the early stage of bladder filling) or high-pressure reflux (reflux that occurs during voiding). The international classification (Fig. 12.41) of vesicoureteral reflux was developed to quantify the degree of reflux (Table 12.1).

Radionuclide cystography demonstrates reflux as streaks of activity extending from the bladder into the ureters and collecting systems. The international classification of reflux is not commonly applied to radionuclide studies, but the amount of activity that appears in the upper urinary tracts can be quantified and can produce a measurement useful in serial follow-up examinations.

Another approach, sometimes termed the "top-down" workup, involves imaging the kidneys first, on the assumption that if they are normal, reflux severe enough to need surgical intervention is unlikely. Investigating the kidneys by excretory urography has been almost completely abandoned, and CT urography is rarely recommended, probably because of its relatively high radiation dose. DMSA renal scintigraphy has a comparatively low radiation dose and is sometimes used as the first imaging test; hydronephrosis and severe scarring are reliably demonstrated but minor scarring

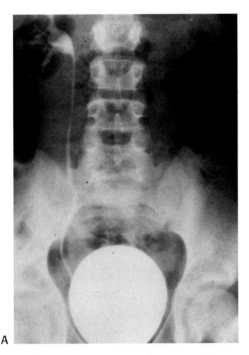

A

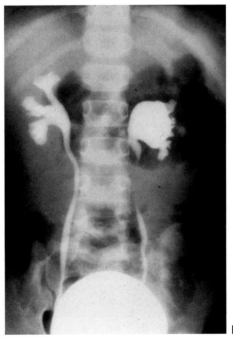

B

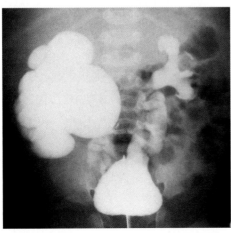

C

FIGURE 12.41. Various grades of reflux. **A:** Grade II vesicoureteral reflux. In this cystogram, contrast flowed from the bladder into the entire ureter collecting system but has not caused dilation. (Courtesy of Robert Cleveland, MD.) **B:** Grade III vesicoureteral reflux (bilateral). Cystography reveals bilateral opacification of the ureters and collecting systems with mild pyelocaliectasis. (Courtesy of Robert Cleveland, MD.) **C:** Grade V vesicoureteral reflux on the right; grade III to IV on left. Cystography demonstrates reflux and severe upper tract dilation, especially on the right. (From Amis ES Jr, Newhouse JH. *Essentials of Uroradiology.* Boston, MA: Little, Brown & Co.; 1991:251–252, with permission.)

TABLE **12.1**	
International Classification of Vesicoureteral Reflux	
Grade	Extent
I	Reflux only into ureter
II	Reflux into collecting system, without dilation
III	Reflux into collecting system, with mild dilation
IV	Reflux into collecting system, with moderate dilation
V	Reflux into collecting system, with severe dilation

may be missed. Renal ultrasound is freely used because of its lack of ionizing radiation, low cost, and patient comfort, but it, like scintigraphy, may miss small scars. If either test reveals renal anatomic abnormalities that might have been produced by reflux, voiding cystourethrography may then be employed.

"One-stop shopping" evaluation could be achieved by imaging techniques, which can evaluate renal anatomy and the bladder and ureters together. Ultrasound, using microbubble contrast agents instilled via a urethral catheter, and MRI have both been tried, but the absence of approved ultrasound contrast agent in the United States has hindered development of sonography for this task, and MR urography, although promising, is still being investigated.

URETERAL OBSTRUCTION

Acute Obstruction

Pathophysiology

Acute obstruction of the ureter leads almost immediately to an increase in urine pressure proximal to the obstruction. A transient increase in renal blood flow may occur but is quickly followed by reductions in renal blood flow, glomerular filtration, and renal concentrating ability.

High-grade acute obstruction may sufficiently increase calyceal pressure to rupture a calyceal fornix, with escape of urine into the renal sinus. This urine may dissect through the sinus, escape through the renal hilus, and diffuse along periureteral and other planes in the retroperitoneum, from which it is usually absorbed into capillaries or lymphatics and returned to the circulation. In most cases, the resorption is complete, but in rare instances the urine may form a discrete collection, become encapsulated, and persist as a urinoma. Rarely, usually in very young children, the urine may flow into the peritoneal cavity and form urinary ascites.

Peristalsis of the collecting system and ureter is diminished proximal to the site of acute obstruction. Distention of these structures is limited in acute obstruction, even when severe. Only long-standing elevation of intraluminal pressure leads to marked dilation of the ureter and collecting system.

If acute obstruction is relieved within a few days, the anatomy and physiology usually return to normal. The ureter and collecting system reverse their distention and reacquire a normal peristaltic pattern. There is little or no persistent renal anatomic abnormality, and blood flow and urine formation return to normal. The precise length of time that the kidney can tolerate acute obstruction without permanent loss of function is not known. In patients suffering iatrogenic ureteral injury, however, return of at least some renal function has been described with periods of obstruction ranging from weeks to months. Acute severe or complete ureteral

obstruction may, if not relieved, lead to a small poorly functioning kidney with little or no hydronephrosis.

The most common cause of acute ureteral obstruction is a calculus that becomes lodged in the ureter. Calculi can obstruct the ureter at any point; larger stones tend to lodge in the upper ureter and small ones at the UVJ, which is the narrowest part of the collecting system. UVJ stones may produce focal edema of the intramural ureter, which presents as a round filling defect in the bladder and is sometimes called a *pseudoureterocele*. When an obstructing stone is passed, the clinical and imaging signs of obstruction frequently resolve immediately, although in some cases, the UVJ edema may prolong the obstruction.

Blood clots that form in the kidney may cause acute ureteral obstruction similar to that produced by calculi. The findings are identical to those produced by nonopaque calculi. Sloughed papillae and fungus balls may rarely cause acute ureteral obstruction.

Imaging of Acute Obstruction

Retrograde Studies

Retrograde ureteropyelography may be helpful in diagnosing completely obstructing lesions of the ureter. When the obstructing ureteral lesion permits contrast medium to flow superiorly past it, the collecting system and ureter proximal to the obstructing lesion may be seen to be slightly dilated. Various types of backflow may be seen during retrograde pyelography due to transient elevation of pressure within the collecting system caused by vigorous injection of contrast medium. Each has a typical radiographic appearance. Filling of the collecting ducts (pyelotubular backflow) is seen as streaks of contrast extending from the calyces into the parenchyma of the kidney (Fig. 12.42) while in pyelosinus backflow, the collecting system *leak* or rupture typically occurs at the fornix of one or more calyces, and contrast tracks through the renal sinus around the collecting system and can extend through the renal

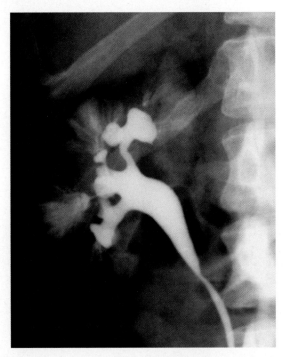

FIGURE 12.42. Pyelotubular backflow. Retrograde pyelogram shows streaks of contrast extending from all but the lower pole calyces. The mild distention of the collecting system attests to the exuberant pressure exerted during the contrast injection.

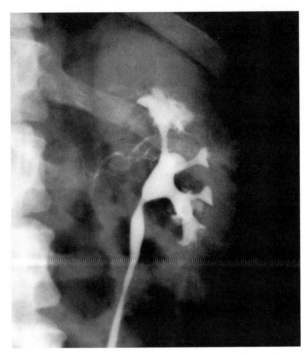

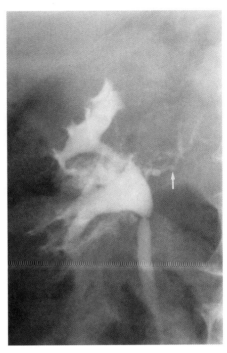

FIGURE 12.43. Pyelosinus backflow. Retrograde pyelogram demonstrates an irregular collection of contrast in the region of the upper pole calyx, indicating rupture of the calyceal fornix and extravasation of contrast into the renal sinus. Also seen is pyelolymphatic backflow.

FIGURE 12.45. Pyelolymphatic backflow. Retrograde pyelogram demonstrating filling of lymphatic channels (*arrow*). Pyelosinus backflow is also seen.

hilum and surround the proximal ureter and lower pole of the kidney (Fig. 12.43). Contrast medium may also be seen in the veins (pyelovenous backflow; Fig. 12.44) or lymphatics (pyelolymphatic backflow; Fig. 12.45). Great caution is urged in performing retro-

grade studies when infection is present, as the increased pressure exerted on the infected urine proximal to an obstruction during an injection can force it into the systemic circulation via pyelovenous backflow, resulting in a generalized septicemia.

Computed Tomography

Unenhanced CT performed during acute obstruction often shows a slightly enlarged kidney whose parenchyma is slightly less dense (Fig. 12.46) than that of the normal kidney. The perinephric fat adjacent to the kidney may reveal edema and jagged interstitial lines, or "stranding" (Fig. 12.47), and there may be a thin layer of perinephric fluid representing extravasated urine; these abnormalities may extend along the renal pelvis and proximal ureter. There is usually mild ureteral and pyelocalyceal dilation. In unusual cases in which a large amount of escaped urine forms a urinoma, CT may reveal a fluid collection (Fig. 12.48) near the kidney. If contrast is

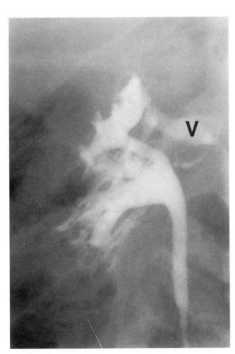

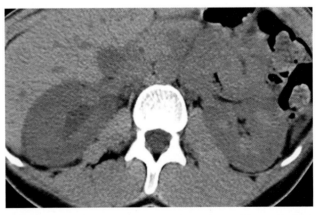

FIGURE 12.44. Pyelovenous backflow. Contrast medium is seen in the renal vein (*V*) as well as the lymphatics and renal sinus during this retrograde pyelogram.

FIGURE 12.46. Noncontrast CT of a patient with acute right distal ureteral obstruction. The right renal parenchyma is more lucent than the normal left side.

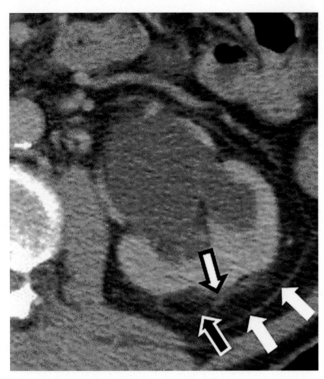

FIGURE 12.47. Ureteral obstruction. There is slight thickening of the posterior pararenal fascia (*white arrows*) and there is a small amount of pericapsular fluid and edema ("stranding") (*bordered arrows*).

used, the parenchymal opacification of the obstructed side occurs more slowly than normal (Fig. 12.49). Delayed images may reveal intense parenchymal opacification, the "obstructive nephrogram" (Fig. 12.50). Opacified urine flows into the collecting system more slowly than on the normal side; delayed views may show this urine to have leaked into the perinephric or periureteral fat (Fig. 12.51).

Radionuclide Studies

The mechanism of excretion of diethylenetriaminepentaacetic acid (DTPA) is identical to that of urographic contrast agents, so that renal

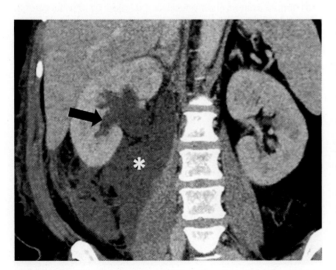

FIGURE 12.48. Acute right distal ureteral obstruction. There is moderate dilatation of the intrarenal collecting system (*arrow*) with a large urinoma (*asterisk*).

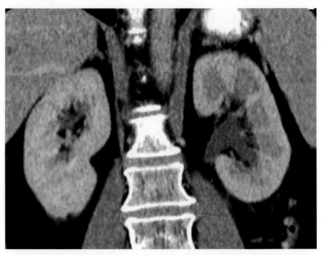

FIGURE 12.49. Contrast-enhanced CT; left ureteral obstruction. The left intrarenal collecting system is slightly dilated; the left nephrogram is delayed in evolution: it is still in the corticomedullary phase with unenhanced medullary pyramids, whereas the normal right side demonstrates nephrographic opacification to have included the medullary regions.

scintigraphy reveals abnormalities that reflect those seen on CT. The activity in the renal parenchyma increases more slowly in an acutely obstructed kidney than in a normal one and maintains its peak intensity longer. The peak intensity may or may not be greater than the peak of the normal side. The isotope appears in the collecting system more slowly than on the normal side, the peak calyceal activity is protracted, and its greatest intensity is variable. The advancing margin of isotope moves slowly along the ureter to the point of obstruction and displays a protracted washout. If forniceal rupture has occurred, the isotope may be seen in the perinephric space.

Ultrasonography

The demonstration of calyceal dilation by ultrasound remains the most useful screening test for acute ureteral obstruction in

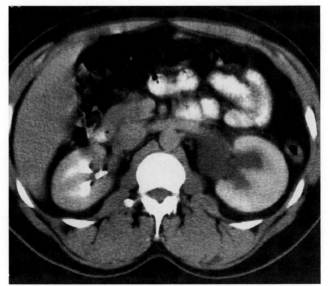

FIGURE 12.50. Obstructive nephrogram. CT showing an obstructive nephrogram on the left with nonopacified urine filling the calyces and renal pelvis.

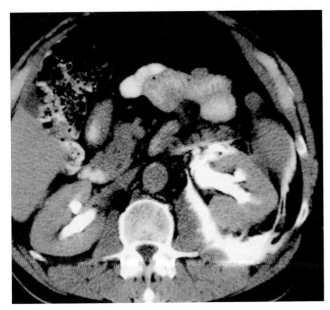

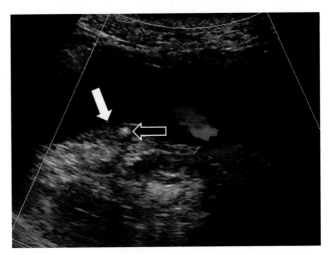

FIGURE 12.53. Color Doppler ultrasound of the bladder in a patient with an obstructing right UPJ stone. The small stone (*bordered arrow*) is seen within a mound of edema (*white arrow*), which often forms around stones impacted at this site. A ureteral jet is displayed as red on the nonobstructed side; there was no jet from the obstructed ureter.

FIGURE 12.51. Pyelosinus extravasation. Delayed contrast CT shows extravasated contrast around the left renal pelvis and in the medial and posterior perirenal space. The patient had bilateral ureteral obstruction secondary to bladder outlet obstruction by an enlarged prostate.

patients whose clinical picture suggests it. An echo-free area in the renal sinus (*splitting* of the central echo complex) corresponding to a mildly dilated renal pelvis may be observed (Fig. 12.52). With more significant hydronephrosis, coronal views will show the dilated infundibula and calyces as well. Although ultrasound is generally accurate in excluding hydronephrosis, it may produce both false-positive and false-negative results. The ranges of volumes of normal and acutely obstructed pyelocalyceal systems significantly overlap. False-negative results may occur when a small, acutely obstructed collecting system has not sufficiently dilated to be recognized as abnormal or when pyelocalyceal decompression occurs because of forniceal rupture. Other fluid-filled structures may mimic dilated collecting systems, including renal hilar vessels (which may be identified by demonstrating flow using color Doppler), renal sinus cysts (which may be suspected from the inability to demonstrate dilated infundibula connecting with a dilated pelvis), and a normal collecting system that has become

slightly distended because of an extremely full bladder (reexamination after voiding will show resolution of such distention). Dilation caused by obstruction usually involves the entire ureter proximal to the obstruction. The most proximal ureter may be seen while the kidney is examined, but the middle portion of the ureter is often obscured by overlying bowel. Color Doppler ultrasound may demonstrate a jet of urine expelled into the bladder by a peristaltic wave (*ureteral jet*). Although such jets may be seen in cases of proximal partial ureteral obstruction, when prolonged observation fails to demonstrate any jet, the ipsilateral kidney is assumed to be anuric due to high-grade or complete ureteral obstruction (Fig. 12.53). However, a jet may be seen in cases of partial proximal ureteral obstruction and may be absent in a dilated aperistaltic ureter without obstruction.

Pulsed Doppler ultrasound of intrarenal arteries may demonstrate abnormalities of arterial flow of kidneys affected by acute ureteral obstruction. In many acutely obstructed kidneys, diastolic flow velocity undergoes a relatively greater decrease than does systolic flow, with a consequent increase in the resistive index. Measurement of resistive indices alone cannot be used to diagnose obstruction; a chronically obstructed kidney may not have an elevated resistive index, and kidneys with various intrinsic parenchymal or small-vessel diseases may have elevated resistive indices without obstruction. However, when resistive index measurements are combined with other ultrasound findings and when symmetry is analyzed, the measurement is of considerable aid in distinguishing obstructed from nonobstructed kidneys.

Magnetic Resonance Imaging

The renal enlargement that accompanies acute ureteral obstruction can obviously be seen in MR examinations, and T2-weighted images elegantly reveal the perirenal edema and fluid (Fig. 12.54) that usually accompany it. Pyeloureteral distention may be visualized and, because the pharmacokinetics of the gadolinium compounds most frequently used for abdominal imaging are the same as those of iodinated contrast media, acute obstruction is manifested by delayed parenchymal enhancement and slow enhancement of urine in the upper tracts. It is less sensitive than CT in detecting small stones but may serve as a diagnostic technique when CT is contraindicated and ultrasound is inconclusive.

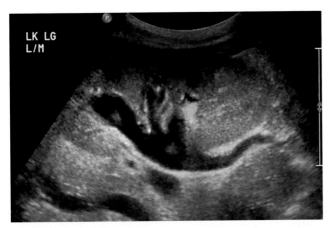

LK LG
L/M

FIGURE 12.52. Hydronephrosis. Longitudinal renal ultrasound shows a dilated collecting system.

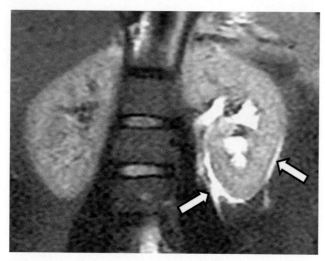

FIGURE 12.54. Acute left ureteral obstruction; T2-weighted MRI. Leaked urine has formed a thin layer (*arrows*) adjacent to the renal capsule.

Chronic Obstruction

Long-standing, complete ureteral obstruction progressively reduces renal blood flow and glomerular filtration. As obstruction continues, there is a progressive atrophy of the renal parenchyma as a result of increased calyceal—and presumably interstitial—pressure. If the obstruction is of sudden onset, complete and unrelieved, the kidney does not become hydronephrotic but atrophies (Fig. 12.55). Persistent, incomplete obstruction causes changes that are quantitatively and qualitatively different. Some tubular atrophy appears, but glomeruli usually remain. Concentrating capacity is diminished,

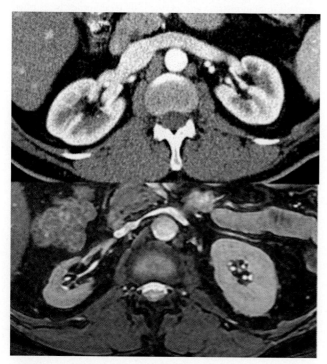

FIGURE 12.55. Postobstructive atrophy. **Top:** CT reveals normal kidneys. **Bottom:** T2-weighted MRI reveals atrophy of the right kidney; there had been inadvertent ligation of the right ureter, which was subsequently diagnosed and repaired.

and urine flow tends to decrease. Initial loss of renal tissue is more severe in the medulla, so that even though the parenchyma thins, the outer dimensions of the kidney may not diminish and may even increase. The greatest degree of cortical thinning and renal expansion takes place with moderately severe obstruction that has been present since birth.

There are multiple causes of chronic ureteral obstruction. In general, the dilation increases both with the duration of obstruction and as a direct function of the intraluminal pressure. The most severe dilation, therefore, does not happen with very mild obstruction or with complete obstruction (after which urine formation tends to cease) but at an intermediate state in which the degree of obstruction increases intraluminal pressure but does not cause immediate severe oliguria.

If a lesion causing chronic obstruction resolves, the dilation tends to decrease. Parenchymal atrophy recovers little, if at all, but the collecting system and ureter may diminish in diameter. They do not, however, return to normal if significant stretching of their walls has occurred.

Urinary obstruction at the level of the bladder outlet may cause abnormalities of the kidneys, collecting systems, and ureters similar to those produced by chronic partial ureteral obstruction. This process occurs when bladder pressure increases above the level at which ureteral peristalsis can completely expel each bolus into the bladder lumen; ureteral pressure begins to increase and the ureteral, pyelocalyceal, and renal changes, described previously, begin to appear. Hydronephrosis is usually bilaterally symmetrical when it is caused by bladder outlet obstruction.

Imaging of Chronic Obstruction

Radiography

If chronic obstruction has produced severe hydronephrosis, the kidney may be visible as a soft tissue mass in the renal fossa. Radiography may reveal any opaque stones that might be responsible for the obstruction.

Retrograde Pyelography

Retrograde pyelography demonstrates the morphology of the dilated collecting system and ureter. As with acute obstruction, increased volume of these structures, along with oliguria, may produce delayed washout of the contrast medium introduced by retrograde injection.

Computed Tomography

CT reflects the anatomic findings described above. The overall renal dimensions may be abnormal; varying degrees of renal parenchymal thinning and calyceal and renal pelvic dilation may be seen (Fig. 12.56). The dense obstructive nephrogram seen with acute ureteral occlusion is not demonstrated with chronic obstruction; instead, the parenchyma poorly opacifies on the nephrographic phase and the calyces fill abnormally slowly with opacified urine. The collecting system may be shown to opacify first in the dependent portion of the collecting system (Fig. 12.57), because contrast medium is heavier than urine and there is no active peristaltic mixing. If the collecting system is not opacified, cysts in the renal sinus may look like dilated calyces and pelvis and mimic hydronephrosis (Fig. 12.58) (the same pitfall occurs with ultrasound).

Ultrasonography

Sonography is highly reliable in the detection of chronic ureteral obstruction by demonstrating pyelocaliectasis; sensitivities ranging from 93% to 100% have been reported. Pyelocaliectasis appears as echo-free regions conforming to the anatomy of the collecting system in the central echo complex of the kidney (Fig. 12.59), and, as with acute obstruction, ureteral dilation may also be shown.

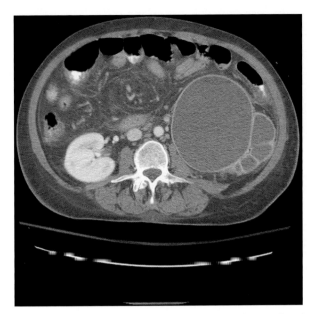

FIGURE 12.56. Severe obstructive atrophy. The pyelocalyceal system of the left kidney is grossly hydronephrotic, and the renal parenchyma has been markedly thinned.

Abnormal resistive indices may be seen but are less reliable in chronic than acute obstruction because chronically obstructed kidneys may lack the elevated intracalyceal pressure associated with abnormal Doppler measurements. False-positive ultrasound findings may occur; the collecting system may appear dilated in patients who are not obstructed but who have extrarenal pelves, vesicoureteral reflux, or persistent changes due to obstruction that has been relieved.

Radionuclide Studies

As in cases of acute obstruction, radionuclide examinations in chronic obstruction display findings similar to those seen on urography or CT as long as a compound is used that is excreted by the kidney in the same way as contrast medium. The uptake of activity in the renal parenchyma may be slowed; its peak may be delayed when compared with that of the normal kidney, but the intensity of isotope in the parenchyma never exceeds that seen on the normal

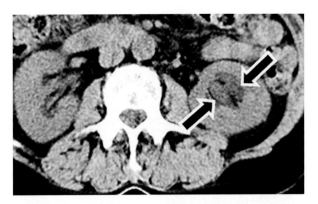

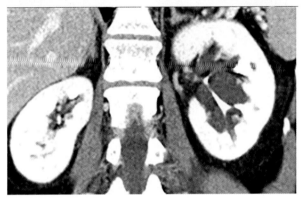

FIGURE 12.58. Pseudohydronephrosis. In noncontrast CT image **(top)**, fluid-filled structures within the renal sinus (*arrows*) mimic dilated calyces. In the pyelogram phase, they are seen to be cysts that compress the infundibula.

side. Activity appears within the collecting system more slowly than normal, by nature of the increased collecting-system volume; however, the total amount of activity seen within it may, at its peak, be considerably greater than that ever seen on the normal side. Washout from the collecting system is prolonged and progression of the leading edge of isotope down the ureter may be slow.

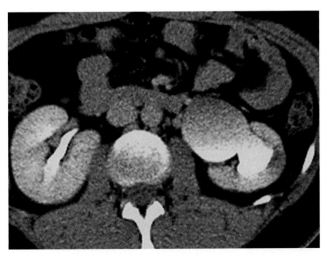

FIGURE 12.57. CT urogram in a patient with unilateral pyelectasis. Contrast first layers in the dependent portion of the left renal pelvis.

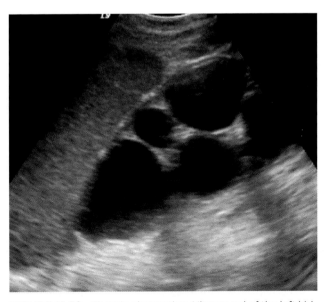

FIGURE 12.59. Chronic obstruction. Ultrasound of the left kidney reveals markedly dilated calyces and parenchymal atrophy.

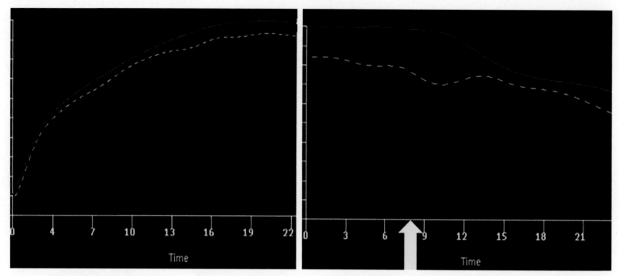

FIGURE 12.60. Renogram in a patient with bilateral obstruction. **Left:** The activity of each kidney (*red* and *green lines*) rises slowly and reaches a peak at about 20 minutes. **Right:** Lasix was administered at the time indicated by the *yellow arrow*; activity decreases very slowly bilaterally.

Although in many patients with upper tract dilation it is easy to determine whether the abnormalities are associated with ongoing obstruction, some cases with varying degrees of pyelocaliectasis or ureterectasis may not be accompanied by a partially obstructing lesion. These patients may have previously experienced ureteral obstruction that has subsequently been relieved but the dilation has not completely resolved. Alternatively, patients may have upper tract dilation caused by vesicoureteral reflux that has resolved or been repaired or may even have innate ureteral abnormalities such as the prune belly syndrome. In these patients, diagnosis or exclusion of concomitant obstructing lesions is important. If the ureters are obstructed, the offending lesion may need surgical correction to prevent deterioration of renal function. If the ureters are not obstructed, unnecessary surgery can be avoided. In these cases, a diuretic renogram may be used to distinguish obstructed from nonobstructed systems.

To perform the diuretic renogram, a diuretic is administered (usually furosemide, 1 mg/kg, maximum 20 mg intravenously) either at the beginning of the study or when a large amount of isotope has accumulated within the affected collecting system. If the isotope in the collecting system remains at a high level or even increases in amount (Fig. 12.60), ureteral obstruction is presumed to be present. If the isotope washes out very rapidly after the diuretic is administered, the system is not obstructed (Fig. 12.61). The distinction is not always easy; multiple methods of interpretation have been proposed, including analysis of time to peak activity and fraction of peak activity remaining at the end of the study and analysis of the washout curve, including shape, slope and time to half maximum activity, effect of bladder distention, and patient position.

Nuclear medicine studies are also useful in conditions in which a severely hydronephrotic kidney may be considered for resection versus having its obstructing lesion repaired. CT and ultrasound may contribute to this decision as well; each of these studies is able to provide an estimate of the volume of remaining parenchyma and provide at least a semiquantitative estimate of the maximum amount of function an affected kidney might have.

Magnetic Resonance Imaging

Chronically obstructed kidneys may be demonstrated by MRI. Static images—that is, strongly T2-weighted images with fat saturation resembling those obtained for MRCPs—display the dilated upper

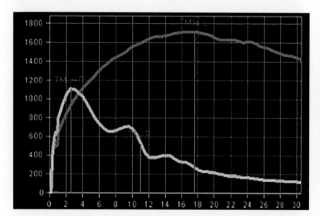
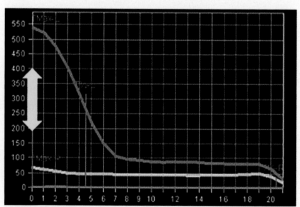

FIGURE 12.61. Nonobstructive pyelocaliectasis. **Left:** Renogram reveals slow rise, delayed and elevated peak, and slow washout in the abnormal kidney; the other kidney's time–activity curve is normal. **Right:** Lasix was administered at the time indicated by the *yellow arrow*; the abnormal kidney activity diminishes rapidly with a normal half-time, a pattern consistent with absence of obstruction.

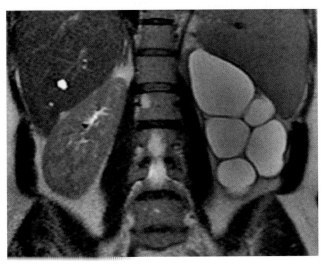

FIGURE 12.62. UPJ obstruction on MRI. T2-weighted axial image shows high-signal dilated left collecting system.

tract very well (Fig. 12.62). Excretory MR urography has advantages and limitations similar to those of CT urography: although the enhancement patterns of the kidney and collecting system offer valuable information regarding function, oliguric or anuric kidneys may fail to produce enhancement of urine down to the obstructing point.

URETERAL DILATION

Ureteral Spindle

Normal peristalsis produces changes in ureteral diameter; a bolus of urine in a noncontracted portion of ureter may expand the ureteral lumen up to a diameter of 8 mm. In some patients, a segment of the middle one-third of the ureter superior to the crossing iliac vessels may be slightly dilated; this appearance is called the *ureteral spindle*.

Primary Megaureter

Dilated ureters are almost always caused by obstruction or reflux, but there are unusual conditions in which dilatation occurs without either; primary megaureter (sometimes referred to by the phrase ureteral achalasia) is such an abnormality. The most distal part of the ureter, a segment typically about 2 cm. long, is not dilated. Proximal to this, the ureter is dilated to varying degrees (Fig. 12.63). Dilation of the ureter occurs proximal to this segment more severely in the distal than proximal part of the ureter. The dilated portion may be short or extend almost to the UPJ and tapers in diameter as it is closer to the kidney; rarely, the dilation may extend to involve the calyces (Fig. 12.64). Primary megaureter may be seen in either children or adults. It is commonly asymptomatic, more usually unilateral than bilateral, and not progressive.

Ureteral dilatation without obstruction may also be seen in certain congenital abnormalities, such as the Eagle–Barrett (prune-belly) syndrome (Fig. 12.65), or in circumstances with chronically high urine flow, such as occurs in patients with untreated diabetes insipidus.

URETERAL COURSE

The normal ureter begins at its junction with the renal pelvis, leaves the kidney through the hilus, and descends to the pelvis within the perirenal space. The proximal ureter often lies lateral to the psoas muscle and begins lateral to the gonadal vessels; as it descends,

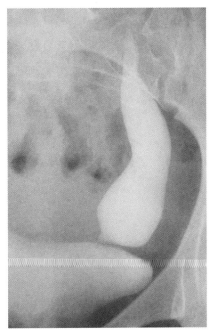

FIGURE 12.63. Primary megaureter. Dilation of the distal left ureter is seen on this excretory urogram.

it courses first posterior and then medial to these vessels (this relationship is useful to remember when it is necessary to trace a normal unopacified ureter from the kidney to the pelvis). It then descends anterior and then medial to the psoas. It emerges from Gerota fascia at approximately the L4 to L5 level, where it crosses anterior to the common iliac artery. Within the true pelvis, the ureter takes a gentle posterolateral course approximately to the level of the iliac spine and then runs anteromedially to enter the bladder.

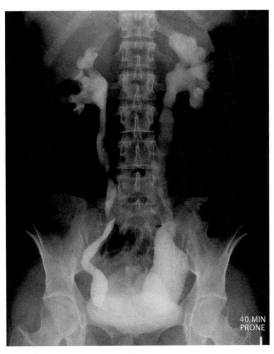

FIGURE 12.64. Primary megaureter. This excretory urogram shows grade II megaureter on the right and grade III megaureter on the left.

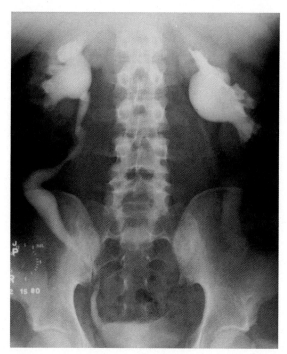

FIGURE 12.65. Prune-belly syndrome. Excretory urography reveals tortuous dilated ureters.

Any adjacent mass or fluid collection may displace the ureter in almost any direction. There are a few reliable directions of displacement, however: midretroperitoneal lymphadenopathy usually pushes the ureter laterally, pelvic lymphadenopathy usually pushes it medially, and a bladder diverticulum may insinuate itself lateral to the pelvic ureter and displace it medially (Fig. 12.66).

Herniation of the ureter is rare but can cause significant deviation of one or both ureters from their normal course. Ureteral

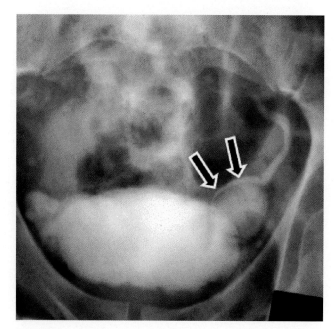

FIGURE 12.66. The distal ureter (arrows) courses along the surface of a bladder diverticulum and is displaced superiorly and medially.

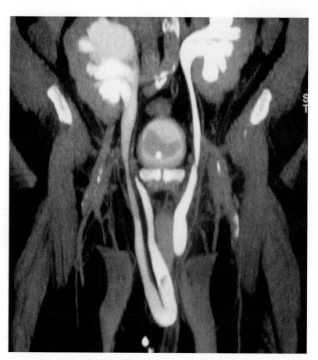

FIGURE 12.67. Bilateral inguinal herniation of the ureters. The kidneys have become ptotic due to traction on the ureters. (From Akpinar E, Turkbey B, Ozcan O, et al. Bilateral scrotal extraperitoneal herniation of ureters. Computed tomography urographic findings and review of the literature. J Comput Assist Tomogr. 2005;29:790–792, with permission.)

herniations usually can be recognized on CT or urography. The ureter accompanies hernias into the groin or scrotum only rarely and, of these cases, only a few are obstructed (Fig. 12.67).

INFLAMMATORY CONDITIONS

Leukoplakia (Squamous Metaplasia)

Squamous metaplasia is a rare inflammatory condition, usually associated with chronic infection and/or stone disease, which may occur in the collecting system, ureter, or bladder. When found in the ureter, it usually involves the proximal third and is almost always associated with involvement of the renal pelvis. The term leukoplakia refers to a white patch seen on the surface of an area of squamous metaplasia; when the keratinized epithelium forms a soft tissue mass, the condition is referred to as a cholesteatoma. Although there is an association between squamous metaplasia and squamous cell carcinoma in the bladder, whether there is such an association in the upper urinary tract is not clear. Imaging typically reveals the lesion as a flat mass or region of thickening of the renal pelvic or ureteral wall; the thickening may give a corduroy appearance.

Malacoplakia

Malacoplakia is an uncommon inflammatory condition of the urinary tract that is usually associated with chronic urinary tract infection, often Escherichia coli. It is not a premalignant condition and is more common among immunocompromised patients. The lesions consist of smooth yellow or brown subepithelial plaques composed of inflammatory cells (histiocytes) that contain basophilic staining inclusions known as Michaelis–Gutmann bodies. The bladder is the most common site of urinary tract involvement, followed

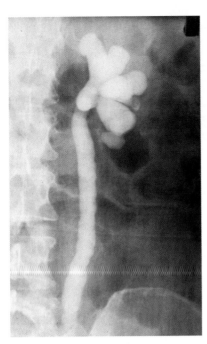

FIGURE 12.68. Ureteral malacoplakia. A retrograde pyelogram reveals a slightly dilated ureter with scalloped margins throughout its length. (Courtesy of Richard C. Pfister, MD.; From Amis ES Jr, Newhouse JH. *Essentials of Uroradiology*. Boston, MA: Little, Brown & Co.; 1991:275, with permission.)

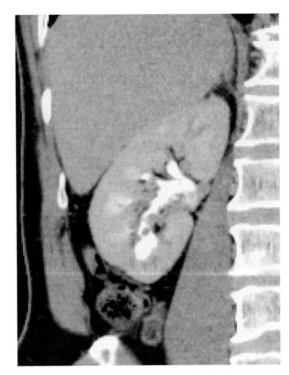

FIGURE 12.69. Pyelitis cystica. Coronal CT shows multiple, discrete, rounded lesions arising from the inferior wall of the renal pelvis. Collection of contrast in the lower pole is focal MSK.

in frequency by the ureter, the renal pelvis, and the urethra. On imaging, the lesions are demonstrated as a series of flat filling defects that characteristically involve the distal ureter but may involve long segments of any part of the ureter (Fig. 12.68). Ureteral obstruction may or may not be present. The lesions are usually multiple and may coalesce, producing a cobblestone appearance.

Pyelitis and Ureteritis Cystica

This condition consists of multiple, small, subepithelial fluid-filled cysts in the wall of the renal pelvis and/or ureter. Pyelitis and ureteritis cystica are usually asymptomatic but may be accompanied by hematuria and symptoms of urinary tract infection. They do not cause obstruction and are not premalignant. They may be unilateral or bilateral and appear slightly more frequently in women. Although these conditions have been reported in all age groups, they are usually found in patients between 50 and 60 years of age.

The typical radiographic appearance is that of multiple, small (2- to 3-mm) radiolucent filling defects in the renal pelvis (Fig. 12.69) or ureter. In the ureter, they have a slight predilection for the proximal third and cause scalloping or even a ragged appearance of the ureteral margins when seen in profile during urography (Fig. 12.70) or retrograde pyelography. The differential diagnosis includes hemorrhage into the ureteral wall (which usually produces filling defects that are not perfectly hemispheric and that resolve quickly), papillary neoplasms (which are rarely as numerous as the cysts of ureteritis cystica), and prolonged ureteral stenting (which may cause protrusion of the urothelium into the side holes of the stent and produce circular filling defects when the stent is removed). However, the radiographic appearance of ureteritis cystica is usually sufficiently characteristic to allow a confident diagnosis. The conditions may regress or disappear with treatment of the underlying inflammatory condition but may also persist after successful treatment.

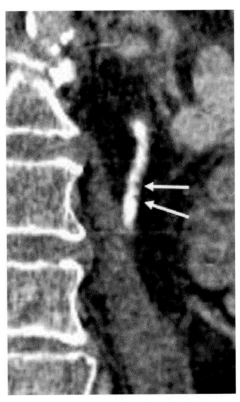

FIGURE 12.70. CTU of ureteritis cystica. The lesions (*arrows*) are small hemispherical filling defects that protrude into the ureteral lumen.

Ureteral Diverticulosis

Ureteral diverticulosis (or pseudodiverticulosis) consists of one or more small (4-mm or less) outpouchings of the ureter. The lesions are hyperplastic buds of ureteral epithelium that project from the ureteral lumen into, but not entirely through, the muscular layers of the ureteral wall.

Ureteral pseudodiverticulosis may be associated with hematuria and urinary tract infection; it has also been found to coexist with a wide range of urinary tract conditions, including calculi, benign prostatic hypertrophy, and TCC.

Ureterography reveals small outpouchings of the ureteral lumen (Fig. 12.71); the ureter may be otherwise normal, or there may be mild narrowing at the site of the diverticula. The condition does not cause ureteral obstruction.

The association of ureteral pseudodiverticulosis and malignancy, usually TCC, warrants careful evaluation of these patients. Urothelial malignancy has been reported as occurring in 46% of patients with ureteral pseudodiverticula. The most common site of malignancy was the bladder. In some patients, the malignant tumors developed several years after demonstration of ureteral diverticulosis.

Schistosomiasis

Schistosomiasis of the urinary tract most commonly involves the bladder but can involve the ureter. The responsible fluke, *Schistosoma haematobium*, is endemic in areas where the specific type of snail necessary for asexual reproduction of the organism is present. Endemic regions include parts of the Middle East, India, Puerto Rico, and a number of African countries, especially Egypt, Nigeria, South Africa, Tanzania, and Zimbabwe. (The life cycle of the fluke is described in Chapter 13.)

The condition usually affects patients younger than 30 years of age and is more common in males than females. Symptoms of ureteral involvement may be absent or limited to flank pain. Ureteral

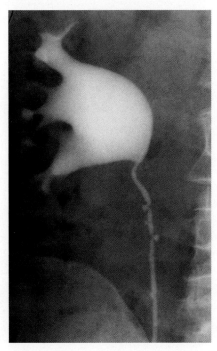

FIGURE 12.71. Ureteral pseudodiverticulosis. The small diverticula are well demonstrated; notice the minimal ureteral narrowing at the site of the larger diverticula.

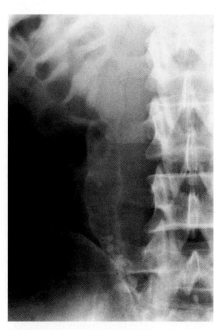

FIGURE 12.72. A diffusely calcified right ureter is seen in this patient with urinary schistosomiasis.

disease is almost always bilateral but is usually asymmetric. The disorder most commonly involves the distal ureters. This infestation results in varying degrees of ureteral stenosis, thickening, wall calcification, and dilation. The ureter may also be obstructed by schistosomal involvement of the bladder wall adjacent to the distal ureter.

Radiologic findings of urinary bilharziasis are characteristic. Calcification, most commonly involving the pelvic portions of the ureters, is present in 75% of the cases. Calcification is usually linear (Fig. 12.72) or *tram-track*, but it may also be patchy, curvilinear, or diffuse. There are varying degrees of dilation and stenosis. In early stages of the disease, only mild distention of the distal ureters may be seen, but in more advanced cases, a beaded appearance of the ureters secondary to multiple strictures may appear; this is similar to the abnormalities found in tuberculous ureteritis. Although the ureters are dilated, they are not tortuous; they tend to be straightened, especially in the midportions. Involvement of the UVJ commonly leads to vesicoureteral reflux. Solitary or multiple ureteral filling defects (bilharzial polyps) tend to appear in the early inflammatory stages of the disease rather than in the later calcified stages. Although *Bilharzia* of the bladder predisposes to bladder carcinoma, this complication is very rare in the ureter.

Tuberculosis

Urinary tract infection with *Mycobacterium tuberculosis* is a result of hematogenous dissemination of the organisms to the kidney from other sites, usually the lungs. Although both kidneys are thought to receive the organisms, the disease usually progresses in only one. Renal tuberculosis seeds the intrarenal collecting system and then descends through the ureters to the lower urogenital system. Hematuria, sometimes gross, may be the first sign, but symptoms of lower urinary tract disease (frequency, dysuria, suprapubic pain) may also herald urinary tract involvement.

Radiographically demonstrable collecting system and ureteral abnormalities are found in approximately half of patients with renal tuberculosis. The findings may be demonstrated on CT if renal function is sufficient; otherwise, retrograde or antegrade pyelography may be necessary.

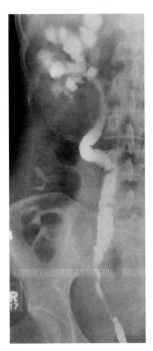

FIGURE 12.73. Ureteral tuberculosis. Retrograde ureteropy-elogram shows multiple strictures, as well as the characteris-tic calyceal changes.

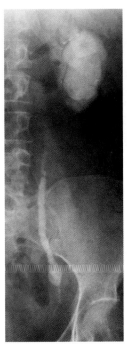

FIGURE 12.74. Urinary tract tuberculosis. A plain abdominal radiograph reveals putty-like calcification in the kidney and ureter.

The typical lesions of tuberculosis are collecting system and ureteral strictures, often occurring at multiple levels (Fig. 12.73), and usually are unilateral. The epithelial lining of the calyces, infundibula, pelvis, and ureter may become inflamed and ulcerated from tuberculous infection. After this phase resolves, reactive fibrosis may cause strictures at any level and produce obstruction. Fibrosis in and around the superior part of the renal pelvis may result in narrowing of the pelvis. Fibrosis of an infundibulum can result in a hydrocalyx. Fibrosis at the UPJ may result in caseous pyonephrosis, which may calcify and produce the classic appearance of tubercu-lous autonephrectomy.

In the ureter, multiple strictures may produce alternating seg-ments of dilation and narrowing; the resulting beaded appearance is characteristic of ureteral tuberculosis. The ureter is shortened and straightened owing to periureteral fibrosis (*pipestem* ureter). Calcification of the ureters is considerably less common in tubercu-lous ureteritis than in bilharzial ureteritis and also is less common than calcification in the kidneys; when present, it may be linear or may appear as a faint, putty-like calcification of inspissated material that fills the ureteral lumen (Fig. 12.74).

Tuberculosis should be the primary diagnosis when strictures are seen at multiple levels throughout the intrarenal collecting sys-tem and ureter.

MISCELLANEOUS CONDITIONS

Amyloidosis

Amyloidosis is a disorder characterized by infiltration of the affected organ by various insoluble proteins or protein–polysac-charide complexes. The disease is usually systemic and may accom-pany another systemic disorder, such as multiple myeloma. Ureteral amyloidosis is extremely rare. The radiographic features are non-specific; a localized ureteral stricture (Fig. 12.75), often in the dis-tal ureter and often indistinguishable from neoplasm, is the usual finding.

Endometriosis

Endometriosis is a condition of women of childbearing age in which endometrial tissue develops outside the endometrial cav-ity of the uterus. Ectopic endometrium undergoes the same cyclic changes as orthotopic tissue, and the periodic necrosis and hemorrhage that occur produce hemorrhagic cystic lesions or masses. The ectopic endometrial tissue may represent embryonic rests or an acquired condition in which retrograde menstruation

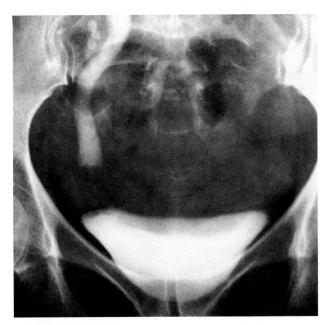

FIGURE 12.75. Amyloidosis of the ureter. (Courtesy of John Hodson, MD.)

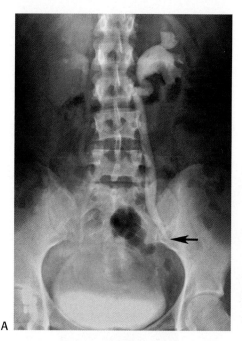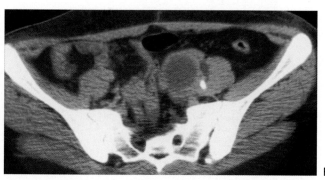

FIGURE 12.76. Endometriosis. **A:** Upright radiograph from an excretory urogram shows extrinsic compression of the left ureter at the pelvic brim (*arrow*). **B:** CT scan through the pelvis shows the ureter to be encased by a multilocular cystic mass proven to be an endometrioma.

through the fallopian tubes deposits endometrial tissues on the peritoneal surfaces. The lesions most commonly occur within the myometrium; on the surface of the uterus, ovaries, or fallopian tubes; and on the peritoneal surfaces of other pelvic organs and the pelvic side walls; they may also involve the bladder or ureters. Although the active disease and associated symptoms usually resolve with menopause, the lesions may persist in postmenopausal women.

Two forms of ureteral endometriosis have been described—intrinsic and extrinsic—both involving the distal ureter. Extrinsic involvement is more common than intrinsic disease. Extrinsic disease compresses the ureter or involves the ureteral adventitia, whereas with the intrinsic form, there is direct invasion of the ureter by endometrial tissue that may lie within the lamina propria or muscular layers of the ureter. Ureteral involvement may result in obstruction due to narrowing of the pelvic ureter and, occasionally, intraureteral masses. Patients most commonly present with infertility and severe pelvic pain with menstruation.

In only a small minority of patients is the urinary tract affected by endometriomas; the bladder is more frequently involved than the ureter. Ureteral involvement generally occurs in cases with widespread pelvic disease, although cases involving just the ureter have been reported. When the ureter is involved, flank pain and hematuria (which may or may not be cyclic) are clues to the disease. The endometriomas may be difficult to visualize by noninvasive techniques if they are small; when they are larger, they display the characteristics of hemorrhagic cystic lesions or soft tissue masses, whether they are imaged by ultrasound, CT, or MR (Fig. 12.76). Retrograde ureterography usually reveals a short or medium-length ureteral stricture in the distal segment; the involved segment is usually within a few centimeters of the inferior aspect of the sacroiliac joint. The stricture is usually smooth but abruptly tapered, and there may be sharp medial angulation of the ureter in the region of the narrowed segment. The ureter distal to the site of involvement is normal.

Inflammatory Bowel Disease

Genitourinary complications may occur in up to 25% of patients with inflammatory bowel disease. Urolithiasis is a common complication; obstruction due to direct ureteral involvement with inflammatory bowel processes is the second most frequent complication. In most patients, urinary tract involvement appears after the gastrointestinal disease has been present for years.

Ureteral involvement by Crohn disease usually occurs distally on the right. The process may involve the ureter by direct extension of bowel inflammation to the pericolic or retroperitoneal regions, or by fistulae that extend from an involved bowel segment to the retroperitoneum, with periureteral inflammation that may or may not involve a flank abscess. Rarely, the left ureter may be involved in patients with granulomatous colitis or with Crohn disease that involves the jejunum.

On imaging, the involved ureter usually displays a sharply tapered smooth area of narrowing over several centimeters, which may cause varying degrees of obstruction (Fig. 12.77). A soft tissue inflammatory mass can usually be demonstrated by CT or MRI, which may simultaneously display the narrowing and wall thickening of the terminal ileum characteristic of Crohn disease. When ureteral narrowing and obstruction have been caused by an acute exacerbation of inflammatory bowel disease, the obstruction usually diminishes with resolution of active bowel inflammation or surgical bypass of the abnormal segment. When the process has become chronic, however, dense periureteral fibrosis requiring ureterolysis may be present.

A small fraction of patients with diverticulitis have involvement of the ureter, usually on the left. As in patients with Crohn disease, a focus of inflammation or frank abscess appears adjacent to the involved bowel and includes the ureter; the ureter itself may be displaced, compressed, or surrounded by the mass, and the specific diagnosis depends on the clinical or imaging diagnosis of diverticulitis.

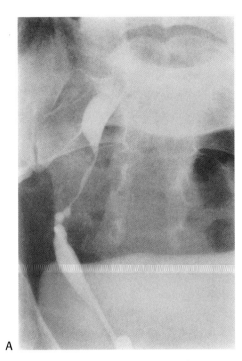 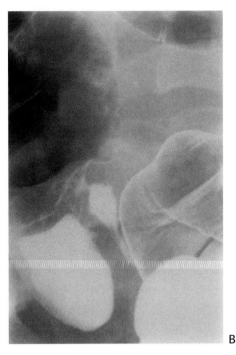

FIGURE 12.77. Crohn disease. **A:** Retrograde ureteropyelogram shows a long ureteral stricture involving the right ureter at the level of the pelvic brim. **B:** Barium enema shows characteristic changes of Crohn disease involving the terminal ileum.

Rarely, appendicitis and periappendiceal abscesses may involve and narrow the ureter. The appearance of the ureter on urography often does not offer a specific diagnosis of appendicitis, but if the clinical and imaging studies provide other indications of appendiceal inflammation or abscess formation, the diagnosis becomes apparent.

Pelvic Inflammatory Disease

Pelvic inflammatory disease and tuboovarian abscesses may produce extrinsic ureteral obstruction by surrounding the ureter with inflammation or by producing an abscess that compresses the ureter. This complication is more likely to occur in cases of chronic or recurrent pelvic inflammation than in the acute stages of the disease. The obstruction usually occurs at the pelvic brim, and its radiologic appearance is similar to that produced by inflammatory bowel disease. In some cases, the ureteral obstruction resolves after conservative therapy, but when scarring and fibrosis are present, ureterolysis may be necessary.

Retroperitoneal Fibrosis

Retroperitoneal fibrosis is a disease in which a mass of fibrous tissue develops in the retroperitoneum. It most frequently appears between the kidneys and the pelvic brim and, by involving the ureters, becomes a disease primarily of urologic importance (see Chapter 4).

Ureteral Dilation in Pregnancy

The physiologic dilation of the upper urinary tract that occurs during the third trimester of pregnancy extends from the kidney to the site at which the ureters are compressed between the enlarged uterus and the iliac arteries. The proximal two-thirds of the ureters are dilated with more pronounced changes seen on the

right (Fig. 12.78). The distal ureters are normal in caliber. Slight differences in the angles at which the arteries and ureters cross may be responsible for the asymmetric degrees of dilation between the right and the left ureter. The changes usually resolve after delivery but may persist to a varying degree.

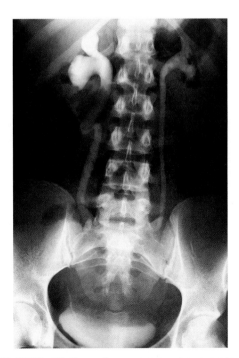

FIGURE 12.78. Dilation of pregnancy. An excretory urogram shows bilateral ureterectasis, worse on the right, in this recently pregnant patient. The soft tissue mass in the pelvis is the still enlarged uterus.

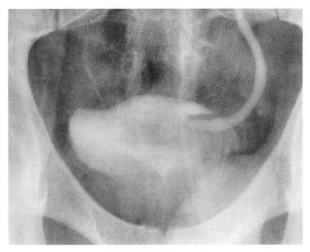

FIGURE 12.79. Pseudoureterocele. A dilated left ureter with a *halo sign* surrounding the ureteral orifice is seen in this patient with a calculus impacted at the ureterovesical junction.

Pseudoureterocele

The edema associated with impaction of a ureteral calculus at the UVJ or recent passage of a ureteral calculus may produce a filling defect in the bladder that mimics a ureterocele when the bladder urine is opacified (Fig. 12.79). Such patients should be evaluated carefully to exclude the possibility of a TCC that has arisen at the UVJ, partially obstructing the ureter and causing distal dilation and protrusion into the bladder lumen.

Procidentia

Procidentia of the uterus is an uncommon cause of bilateral ureteral obstruction; in severe cases, it has led to hydronephrosis and progressive renal failure. The patients are usually elderly females with severe uterine prolapse. The ureters descend through the pelvic floor (Fig. 12.80) and may or may not be accompanied by

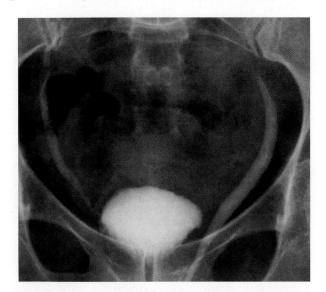

FIGURE 12.80. Prolapsed bladder and distal ureter. This urogram reveals the nonprolapsed portion of the bladder; the prolapsed portion was not included on the film. The left ureter descends through the pelvic floor toward the prolapsed segment of the bladder.

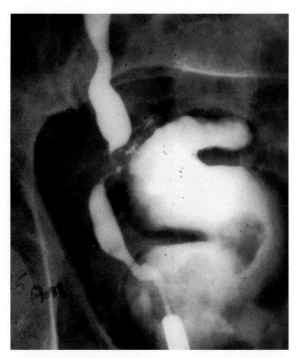

FIGURE 12.81. Ureterocolic fistula. Retrograde ureterogram shows fistula to sigmoid colon secondary to diverticulitis.

imaging signs of associated bladder prolapse. The mechanism of ureteral obstruction is poorly understood; ureteral kinking, obstruction produced by the uterine artery, pressure from the levator ani muscles, and mechanical deformity of the UVJs have all been proposed.

Ureteral Fistulae

Ureteral fistulae may develop as a result of penetrating trauma or as a complication of surgery involving or adjacent to the urinary tract (Fig. 12.81). They may also develop as a result of adjacent malignant or inflammatory disease. Most ureteral fistulae present with associated urinary tract infection or with clinical evidence of urine flow through the fistula. Rarely, fistulae between the ureter and a blood vessel may result in massive gross hematuria.

The diagnosis of a ureteral fistula is usually established by ureterography. Direct antegrade or retrograde injection of contrast medium into the ureter is more likely to demonstrate the fistula than CT because of the higher contrast concentration and greater intraureteral pressures that can be achieved (Fig. 12.81). Rarely, contrast studies of the gastrointestinal tract in patients with ureteroenteric fistulae may demonstrate the communication with the ureter. CT urography may demonstrate the primary lesion and movement of contrast medium through the fistula to or from the ureteral lumen.

SUGGESTED READINGS

General

Potenta SE, D'Agostino R, Sternberg KM, et al. CT urography for evaluation of the ureter. *Radiographics.* 2015;35(3):709–726.

Papillary and Collecting System Abnormalities

Ginalski JM, Portmann L, Jeager P. Does medullary sponge kidney cause nephrolithiasis? *AJR Am J Roentgenol.* 1990;155(2):299.

Gong MB, Davidson AJ. Development and progression of renal papillary necrosis in SA hemoglobinopathy. *Urol Radiol.* 1980;2:55.

Jung DC, Kim SH, Jung SI, et al. Renal papillary necrosis: review and comparison of findings at multi-detector row CT and intravenous urography. *Radiographics.* 2006;26:1827–1836.

Koraishy FM, Ngo TT, Israel GM, et al. CT urography for the diagnosis of medullary sponge kidney. *Am J Nephrol.* 2014;39(2):165–170.

Lang EK, Macchia RJ, Thomas R, et al. Detection of medullary and papillary necrosis at an early stage by multiphasic helical computerized tomography. *J Urol.* 2003;170:94.

Lin C-C, Shih B-F, Shih S-L, et al. Potential role of Tc-99m DTPA diuretic renal scan in the diagnosis of calyceal diverticulum in children. *Medicine.* 2015;94(24):e985.

Lin N, Xie L, Zhang P, et al. Computed tomography urography for diagnosis of calyceal diverticulum complicated by urolithiasis: the accuracy and the effect of abdominal compression and prolongation of acquisition delay. *Urology.* 2013;82(4):786–790.

Oza KN, Rezvan M, Moser R. Subepithelial hematoma of the renal pelvis (Antopol-Goldman lesion). *J Urol.* 1996;155:1032.

Zawada ET, Sica DA. Differential diagnosis of medullary sponge kidney. *South Med J.* 1984;77:686.

Renal Sinus

Fishman MC, Pollack HM, Arger PH, et al. Radiographic manifestations of spontaneous renal sinus hemorrhage. *AJR Am J Roentgenol.* 1984;142:1161–1164.

Gayer G, Zissin R. The renal sinus—transitional cell carcinoma and its mimickers on computed tomography. *Semin Ultrasound CT MR.* 2014;35(3):308–319.

Hammond NA, Lostumbo A, Adam SZ, et al. Imaging of adrenal and renal hemorrhage. *Abdom Imaging.* 2015;40(7):2747–2760.

Rha SE, Byun JY, Jung SE, et al. The renal sinus: pathologic spectrum and multimodality imaging approach. *Radiographics.* 2004;24:S117.

Subramanyam BR, Bosniak MA, Horii SC, et al. Replacement lipomatosis of the kidney: diagnosis by computed tomography and sonography. *Radiology.* 1983;148:791.

Vascular Impressions/Crossings

Fraley EE. Vascular obstruction of superior infundibulum causing nephralgia. *N Engl J Med.* 1966;275:1403.

Herkanwal SK, Platt JF, Cohan RH, et al. Helical computed tomography for identification of crossing vessels in ureteropelvic junction obstruction—comparison with operative findings. *Urology.* 2003;62:35.

Lawler LP, Jarret TW, Corl FM, et al. Adult ureteropelvic junction obstruction: insights with three-dimensional multi-detector row CT. *Radiographics.* 2005;25:121.

Parikh DR, Hammer MR, Kraft KH, et al. Pediatric ureteropelvic junction obstruction: can magnetic resonance urography identify crossing vessels? *Pediatr Radiol.* 2015;45(12):1788–1795.

Pienkny AJ, Herts B, Streem SB. Contemporary diagnosis of retrocaval ureter. *J Endourol.* 1999;13:721.

Quillin SP, Brink JA, Heiken JP, et al. Helical (spiral) CT angiography for identification of crossing vessels at the ureteropelvic junction. *AJR Am J Roentgenol.* 1996;166:1125.

Ritter L, Gotz G, Sorge I, et al. Significance of MR angiography in the diagnosis of aberrant renal arteries as the cause of ureteropelvic junction obstruction in children. *RoFo: Fortschritte auf dem Gebiete der Rontgenstrahlen und der Nuklearmidizin.* 2015;187(1):42–48.

Tumors of the Collecting Systems and Ureters

Caoili EM, Cohan RH, Inampudi P, et al. MDCT urography of upper tract urothelial neoplasms. *AJR Am J Roentgenol.* 2005;184:1873.

Dillman JR, Caoili EM, Cohan RH, et al. Detection of upper tract urothelial neoplasms: sensitivity of axial, coronal reformatted, and curved-planar reformatted image-types utilizing 16-row multi-detector CT urography. *Abdom Imaging.* 2008;33:707–716.

Honda Y, Goto K, Sentani K, et al. T categorization of urothelial carcinomas of the ureter with CT: preliminary study of new diagnostic criteria proposed for differentiating T2 or lower from T3 or higher. *AJR Am J Roentgenol.* 2015;204(4):792–797.

Hughes FA, Davis CS. Multiple benign ureteral fibrous polyps. *Radiology.* 1976;126(4):723.

Kirkali Z, Tuzel E. Transitional cell carcinoma of the ureter and renal pelvis. *Crit Rev Oncol Hematol.* 2003;47:155.

Leder RA, Dunnick NR. Transitional cell carcinoma of the kidney and ureter. *AJR Am J Roentgenol.* 1990;155:713.

Oldbring J, Glifberg I, Mikulowski P, et al. Carcinoma of the renal pelvis and ureter following bladder carcinoma: frequency of risk factors and clinicopathologic findings. *J Urol.* 1989;141:1311.

Takeuchi M, Konrad AJ, Kawashima A, et al. CT urography for diagnosis of upper urinary tract urothelial carcinoma: are both nephrographic and excretory phases necessary? *AJR Am J Roentgenol.* 2015;205(3):w320–w327.

Urban BA, Buckley J, Soyer P, et al. CT appearance of transitional cell carcinoma of the renal pelvis: part 1. Early-stage disease. *AJR Am J Roentgenol.* 1997;169:157.

Urban BA, Buckley J, Soyer P, et al. CT appearance of transitional cell carcinoma of the renal pelvis: part 2. Advanced-stage disease. *AJR Am J Roentgenol.* 1997;169:163.

Vikram R, Sandler CM, Ng CS. Imaging and staging of transitional cell carcinoma: part 2, upper urinary tract. *AJR Am J Roentgenol.* 2009;192(6):1488–1493.

Wang J, Wang H, Tang G, et al. Transitional cell carcinoma of upper urinary tract vs. benign lesions: distinctive MSCT features. *Abdom Imaging.* 2009;34:94–106.

Williams TR, Wagner BJ, Corse WR, et al. Fibroepithelial polyps of the urinary tract. *Abdom Imaging.* 2002;27:217.

Winalski CS, Lipman JC, Tumeh SS. Ureteral neoplasms. *Radiographics.* 1990;10:271–283.

Wong-You-Cheong JJ, Wagner BJ, Davis CJ Jr. Transitional cell carcinoma of the urinary tract: radiologic-pathologic correlation. *Radiographics.* 1998;18(1):123–142.

Xu AD, Ng CS, Kamat A, et al. Significance of upper urinary tract urothelial thickening and filling defect seen on MDCT urography in patients with a history of urothelial neoplasms. *AJR Am J Roentgenol.* 2010;195(4):959–965.

Yousem DM, Gatewood OM, Goldman SM, et al. Synchronous and metachronous transitional cell carcinoma of the urinary tract: prevalence, incidence and radiographic detection. *Radiology.* 1988;167:613.

Vesicoureteral Reflux

Darge K, Riedmiller H. Current status of vesicoureteral reflux diagnosis. *World J Urol.* 2004;22:88.

Newhouse JH, Amis ES Jr. The relationship between renal scarring and stone disease. *AJR Am J Roentgenol.* 1988;151:1153.

Riccabona M. Imaging in childhood urinary tract infection. *Radiol Med.* 2016;121(5):391–401.

Shaikh N, Spingarn RB, Hum SW. Dimercaptosuccinic acid scan or ultrasound in screening for vesicoureteral reflux among children with urinary tract infections. *Cochrane Database Syst Rev.* 2013;(7):CD010657

Strife JL, Bisset GS III, Kirks DR, et al. Nuclear cystography and renal sonography: findings in girls with urinary tract infection. *AJR Am J Roentgenol.* 1989;153:115.

Ureteral Obstruction and Dilatation

Berrocal T, Lopez-Pereira P, Arjonilla A, et al. Anomalies of the distal ureter, bladder, and urethra in children: embryologic, radiologic, and pathologic features. *Radiographics.* 2002;22:1139.

Grattan-Smith JD, Jones RA. MR urography: Technique and results for the evaluation of urinary obstruction in the pediatric population. *Magn Reson Imaging Clin N Am.* 2008;16(4):643–660.

Hamilton S, Fitzpatrick JM. Primary non-obstructive megaureter in adults. *Clin Radiol.* 1987;38:181.

Kamholtz RG, Cronan JJ, Dorfman GS. Obstruction and the minimally dilated renal collecting system: US evaluation. *Radiology.* 1989;170:51.

King LR. Megalouretere: definition, diagnosis and management. *J Urol.* 1980;123:222.

Platt JF, Rubin JM, Ellis JH. Acute renal obstruction: evaluation of intrarenal duplex Doppler and conventional ultrasound. *Radiology.* 1993;186:685.

Riccabona M. Obstructive diseases of the urinary tract in children: lessons from the last 15 years. *Pediatr Radiol.* 2010;40(6):947–955.

Sudah M, Vanninen RL, Partanen K, et al. Patients with acute flank pain: comparison of MR urography with unenhanced helical CT. *Radiology.* 2002;223(1):98–105.

Zhang S, Shang Q, Ji C, et al. Improved split renal function after percutaneous nephrostomy in young adults with severe hydronephrosis due to ureteropelvic junction obstruction. *J Urol.* 2015;193(1):191–195.

Ureteral Course

Apkinar E, Turkbey B, Ozcan O, et al. Bilateral scrotal extraperitoneal herniation of ureters. Computed tomography urographic findings and review of the literature. *J Comput Assist Tomogr.* 2005;29:790.

Bree RL, Green B, Keiller DL, et al. Medial deviations of the ureters secondary to psoas muscle hypertrophy. *Radiology.* 1976;118:691.

Cunat JS, Goldman SM. Extrinsic displacement of the ureter. *Semin Roentgenol.* 1986;21(3):188.

Pollack HM, Popky GL, Blumberg ML. Hernias of the ureter: an anatomic-roentgenographic study. *Radiology.* 1975;117:275.

Collecting System/Ureter Infections/Inflammation

Becker JA. Renal tuberculosis. *Urol Radiol.* 1988;10:25.

Goldman SM, Fishman EK, Hartman DS, et al. Computed tomography of renal tuberculosis and its pathological correlates. *J Comput Assist Tomogr.* 1985;9:77.

Jorulf H, Lindstedt E. Urogenital schistosomiasis: CT evaluation. *Radiology.* 1985;157:745.

Premkumar A, Lattimer J, Newhouse JH. CT and sonography of advanced urinary tract tuberculosis. *AJR Am J Roentgenol.* 1987;148:65.

Shebel HM, Elsayes KM, Abou El Atta HM, et al. Genitourinary schistosomiasis: life cycle and radiologic-pathologic findings. *Radiographics.* 2012;32(4):1031–1046.

Wasserman NF. Inflammatory disease of the ureter. *Radiol Clin North Am.* 1996;34(6):1131–1156.

Young SW, Khalid KH, Farid Z, et al. Urinary tract lesions of Schistosoma haematobium. *Radiology.* 1974;111:81.

Miscellaneous Collecting System and Ureteral Conditions

Balleyguier C, Roupret M, Nguyen T, et al. Ureteral endometriosis: the role of magnetic resonance imaging. *J Am Assoc Gynecol Laparosc.* 2004;11:530.

Banner MP. Genitourinary complications of inflammatory bowel disease. *Radiol Clin North Am.* 1987;25(1):199.

Benson RC Jr, Swanson SK, Farrow GM. Relationship of leukoplakia to urothelial malignancy. *J Urol.* 1984;131:507.

Comiter CV. Endometriosis of the urinary tract. *Urol Clin North Am.* 2002;29:625.

Cozar Olmo JM, Carcamo P, Gaston de Iriarte E, et al. Genitourinary malakoplakia. *Br J Urol.* 1993;72(1):6–12.

Hertle L, Androulakakis R. Keratinizing desquamative squamous metaplasia of the upper urinary tract: leukoplakia-cholesteatoma. *J Urol.* 1982;127:631.

Iosca S, Lumia D, Bracchi E, et al. Multislice computed tomography with colon water distention (MSCT-c) in the study of intestinal and ureteral endometriosis. *Clin Imaging.* 2013;37(6):1061–1068.

Kottra JJ, Dunnick NR. Retroperitoneal fibrosis. *Radiol Clin North Am.* 1996;34(6):1259–1275.

Menendez B, Sala X, Alvarez-Vigande R, et al. Cystic pyeloureteritis: review of 34 cases. Radiology aspects and differential diagnosis. *Urology.* 1997;50(1):31–37.

Silver TM, Vinson RK. Ureteroceles vs pseudoureteroceles in adults *Radiology.* 1977;122:81.

Sillou S, Poiree S, Millischer AE, et al. Urinary endometriosis: MR imaging appearance with surgical and histological correlations. *Diagn Interv Imaging.* 2015;96(4):373–381.

Wasserman NF. Pseudodiverticulosis: unusual appearance for metastases to the ureter. *Abdom Imaging.* 1994;19(4):376.

Wasserman NF, Zhang G, Posalaky IP, et al. Ureteral pseudodiverticula: frequent association with uroepithelial malignancy. *AJR Am J Roentgenol.* 1991;157:69.

Willis JS, Pollack HM, Curtis JA. Cholesteatoma of the upper urinary tract. *AJR Am J Roentgenol.* 1981;136:941.

Yohannes P. Ureteral endometriosis. *J Urol.* 2003;170:20.

The Urinary Bladder

THE NORMAL BLADDER

The normal urinary bladder serves as a reservoir for urine. It consists of a muscular sac, lined by mucosa (which includes urothelial cells), submucosa/lamina propria, a muscular layer (the muscularis propria, which is made up of superficial and deep muscles), and a serosal/adventitial layer. The bladder is bordered by the extraperitoneal spaces along its anterior and lateral aspects and by the peritoneal space at the dome.

The muscle in the bladder wall, the detrusor muscle, consists of numerous interlacing smooth muscle bundles forming a complex meshwork of muscle. The anatomic arrangement is such that when the detrusor contracts, the bladder reduces size equally in all dimensions, resulting in efficient emptying. The muscle fibers of the detrusor continue through the bladder neck and surround the proximal urethra, forming the internal sphincter. The detrusor muscle and the internal sphincter are smooth muscles, but unlike other types of smooth muscle, they are under voluntary control. The external urethral sphincter, composed of striated muscle, surrounds the urethra where it passes through the urogenital diaphragm. This sphincter is composed of both slow- and fast-twitch muscle fibers. The slow-twitch fibers allow a more sustained contraction than normal striated muscle. The external sphincter is able to close the urethra acutely and can serve as a passive continence mechanism for prolonged periods. Because the internal and external sphincters have different nerve supplies, their continence functions are independent of each other. However, the primary continence mechanism in both men and women is the smooth muscle internal sphincter at the bladder neck.

During filling, the normal bladder may hold up to 1,000 mL of urine at a relatively low pressure, in part because of its intrinsic properties but also because the normal individual retains voluntary control of the bladder at the level of the cerebral cortex. During normal bladder filling, there is an unconscious inhibition of the micturition reflex in the cerebral cortex. In other words, healthy individuals do not have to consciously think about their bladder to keep it from emptying. However, as the bladder distends toward capacity, the cerebral cortex becomes aware of the need to void, and micturition can be consciously activated.

Coordinated voiding occurs in a well-defined order: relaxation of the external urethral sphincter, detrusor contraction, and, finally, funneling (opening) of the internal sphincter. At the completion of voiding, the external sphincter is voluntarily contracted, resulting in reflex inhibition of detrusor contraction. The internal sphincter then milks any urine remaining in the proximal urethra back into the bladder. Figure 13.1 diagrams the neuroanatomical pathways governing voiding.

BENIGN BLADDER CONDITIONS

Filling Defects

Filling defects in the bladder must be differentiated from contour defects. A filling defect is an area of incomplete opacification on cystography or excretory phase CT or MRI and denotes something lying free within the bladder lumen. Contour defects are mural or mucosal lesions that alter the contour of the contrast-filled bladder; examples include urothelial tumors, metaplastic and inflammatory masses, and wall thickening from any cause. The most common filling defects in the bladder are stones and blood clots.

Bladder Calculi

Most urinary tract stones form in the kidneys. They may migrate down the ureter into the bladder and are quickly passed via the urethra. Calculi remain in the bladder only when there is some degree of outlet obstruction or when they form on a foreign body within the bladder. Bladder outlet obstruction is the most common cause of bladder stones, and 70% of adults with bladder stones have a component of bladder outlet obstruction. For this reason, bladder stones are much more common in men, due

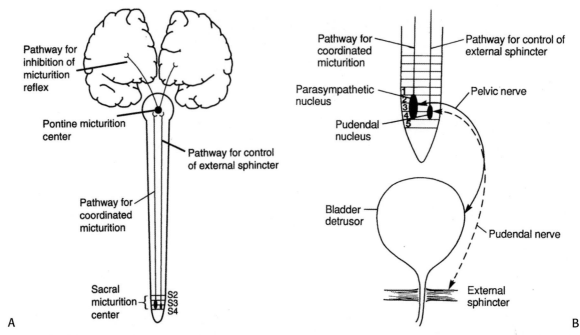

A

B

FIGURE 13.1. Neuroanatomy of voiding. **A:** Upper tract neuroanatomy. Centers in the cortex inhibit micturition and also provide conscious control of the external sphincter. The pontine micturition center integrates these central control functions. Pathways for control of the bladder and external sphincter travel through the spinal cord from the pontine micturition center to the sacral micturition center. **B:** Lower tract neuroanatomy. A pelvic nerve connects the parasympathetic nucleus in the sacral micturition center to the bladder detrusor. The pudendal nerve connects the pudendal nucleus in the sacral micturition center to the external sphincter. (From Amis ES Jr, Blaivas JG. Neurogenic bladder simplified. *Radiol Clin North Am.* 1991;29:571, with permission.)

to the high incidence of benign prostatic hyperplasia. Additional causes of bladder outlet obstruction include neurogenic bladders and urethral strictures. Most bladder stones due to obstruction are comprised of calcium oxalate, calcium phosphate, or a mixture of both.

Rarely, there are other causes of bladder stones, which include infections with urea-splitting organisms (magnesium ammonium phosphate or triple phosphate stones), cystinuria (cystine stones), and hyperuricosuria (uric acid stones). In some cases, there may be more than one cause, such as bladder infection associated with outlet obstruction or obstruction with the need for catheterization. Intermittent clean catheterization may introduce pubic hairs into the bladder that can also act as nidi for calcareous deposits resulting in stone formation. Even more unusual causes of bladder calculi are sutures in the bladder wall, which can act as a foreign body on which stones may form, and foreign bodies (usually self-introduced into the urethra), which may also form a nidus for stone formation.

Many bladder stones are asymptomatic and are discovered incidentally. Symptomatic patients present with bladder pain, which may be a dull ache suprapubically. Referred pain to the penis, buttock, perineum, or scrotum may also occur. Microscopic hematuria in bladder stone disease may result from chronic irritation of the bladder mucosa. Gross hematuria is rare. Bladder stones are more common in men than in women, which is likely in part due to the high frequency of benign prostatic hyperplasia.

Bladder stones may be visualized directly with plain radiography, ultrasound, and CT and indirectly, as areas of signal void, with MRI. Bladder stones vary from very dense to radiolucent on plain films and vary in size from a few millimeters in diameter to large stones that fill the entire bladder. Calcified stones over a few millimeters in diameter are usually apparent on plain

radiographs. However, they may be obscured by overlying fecal material or they may overlie the sacrum and coccyx, where they may be difficult to identify.

Bladder calculi may assume various configurations, as seen on conventional radiographs and other imaging studies. A laminated appearance is not unusual in bladder stones. These can grow to quite large sizes and can be single or multiple. On conventional radiography, stones with multiple spicules are termed "jackstones" (Fig. 13.2), and those with a bumpy margin are known as "mulberry

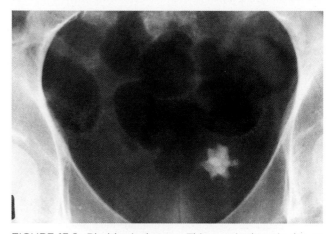

FIGURE 13.2. Bladder jackstone. This terminology is due to the multiple spiculations. (From Amis ES Jr, Newhouse JH. *Essentials of Uroradiology.* Boston, MA: Little, Brown and Company; 1991:226, with permission.)

stones" (Fig. 13.3). Stones associated with bladder outlet obstruction may be numerous, and they are usually small and round. Multiple stones may have a faceted configuration (Fig. 13.4).

Pure uric acid stones are radiolucent on plain film studies and are not seen. Bladder calculi composed of struvite or cystine may be only faintly radiopaque.

Ultrasound demonstrates bladder stones as echogenic foci with acoustic shadowing (Figs. 13.5 and 13.6). Radiolucent or poorly calcified stones on radiography are well seen on ultrasound and are not significantly different in appearance from well-calcified stones. The mobility of a shadow-producing lesion within the bladder distinguishes a stone from a calcified bladder tumor.

CT shows essentially all bladder calculi, whatever their composition, as highly attenuating (Fig. 13.7). Tumors with calcification are easily distinguished from stones. On MRI, bladder stones typically demonstrate signal void (due to calcification) on all sequences.

Small bladder stones seen at cystoscopy can be easily grasped by forceps and removed through the cystoscope. Larger stones

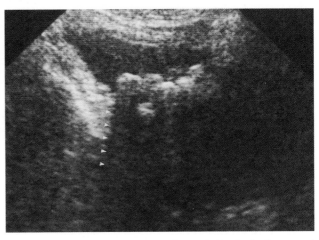

FIGURE 13.5. Bladder stones. Transabdominal ultrasound in a patient shows multiple bladder stones seen as bright echoes with acoustic shadowing (*arrowheads*).

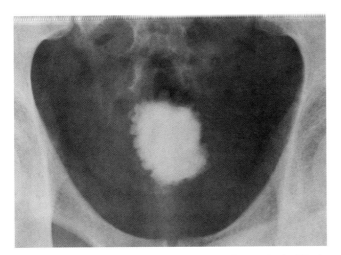

FIGURE 13.3. Mulberry bladder stone. (From Amis ES Jr, Newhouse JH. *Essentials of Uroradiology*. Boston, MA: Little, Brown and Company; 1991:226, with permission.)

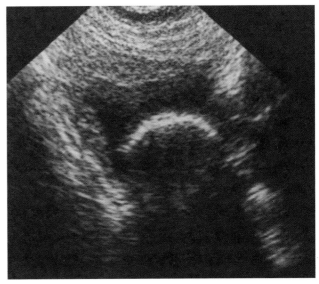

FIGURE 13.6. Bladder stone. A single large bladder stone is present producing acoustic shadowing.

must be crushed or must be disintegrated into small fragments using lithotripsy. Fragments are washed out through the urethra by continuous irrigation throughout the procedure. Very large stones are usually removed surgically. Pure uric acid stones too large for simple cystoscopic removal may be dissolved by systemic urinary alkalinization.

Blood Clots

Blood clots in the bladder may have a vermiform or wormlike appearance, particularly if bleeding has occurred in the upper urinary tract and a clot has formed in the ureter. Blood clots will not be detected on conventional radiography but will appear as filling defects during conventional cystography. Ultrasound shows that the blood clot is quite echogenic, a bladder tumor, which often has an echogenicity similar to the bladder wall. CT may help to distinguish a blood clot from a tumor or stone by demonstrating the typical high, but not extremely high, attenuation of blood on unenhanced images (60 to 80 Hounsfield units [HU]) (Fig. 13.8).

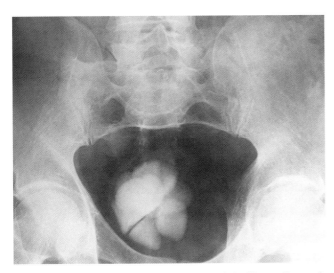

FIGURE 13.4. Faceted bladder stones. Plain film radiograph of the pelvis shows multiple multifaceted stones lying to the right of midline. (From McCallum RW, Colapinto V. *Urological Radiology of the Adult Male Lower Urinary Tract*. Springfield, IL: Charles C. Thomas; 1976:264–265, with permission.)

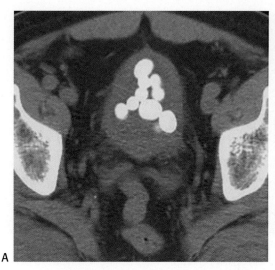
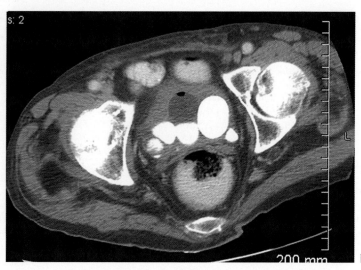

FIGURE 13.7. Bladder stones. **A:** Unenhanced axial CT image demonstrates multiple small rounded stones in this patient with bladder outlet obstruction from an enlarged prostate. **B:** Multiple large calculi, some of which appear faceted, are identified on this contrast-enhanced axial CT image in another patient. The balloon of an indwelling Foley catheter can be identified anterior to one of the stones.

On MRI, blood clot may have a variety of appearances, due to its age; however, unlike other bladder-filling defects, it can have suggestive high T1 and low T2 signal. Blood clot does not demonstrate increased attenuation or signal intensity on contrast-enhanced CT or MR images, unless there is active bleeding. On occasion, a clot may be so large as to essentially fill the bladder (Fig. 13.9).

Foreign Bodies

Foreign bodies within the bladder are most commonly inserted by the patient. Among other items, pens, pencils, matches, wire, tubing, and string can be seen within the bladder lumen (Fig. 13.10). Foreign bodies may also be iatrogenic (e.g., broken or shorn catheter fragments) or may result from penetrating trauma (e.g., bullets). A rare complication of bladder catheterization is the introduction of pubic hairs into the bladder, which may become encrusted with calcium.

Edema

Mucosal edema may develop around a ureteral orifice, most often caused by a stone impacted at the ureterovesical junction, but it may also be seen in patients who have recently passed a ureteral stone. Focal mucosal edema in the bladder itself may result from bladder irritation by extravesical conditions such as acute appendicitis, Crohn disease, or sigmoid diverticulitis. Another cause of focal bladder wall edema is an indwelling catheter, whose tip may irritate the bladder wall, most commonly near the dome. In some instances, generalized bullous edema of the bladder wall may accompany acute cystitis.

Cystography in patients with focal bladder wall edema shows the irregularity of the bladder wall and, often, a contour defect. Ultrasound or CT can show an extravesical cause for localized bladder edema, such as an appendiceal or peridiverticular abscess or other bowel abnormality. If no localized extravesical mass is seen, focal thickening can also indicate a bladder tumor. Fortunately,

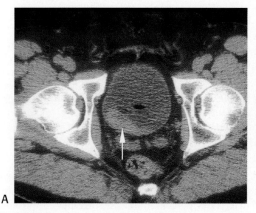
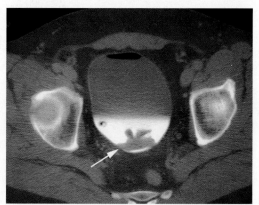

FIGURE 13.8. Blood clot. **A:** Unenhanced axial CT image demonstrates a soft tissue attenuation structure in the posterior aspect of the bladder (*arrow*), subsequently confirmed to represent a blood clot at cystoscopy. **B:** Contrast-enhanced axial CT image obtained during the excretory phase shows a blood clot to have an irregular vermiform appearance (*arrow*). There was no evidence of enhancement, confirming the likelihood that this filling defect represents a blood clot and not a tumor.

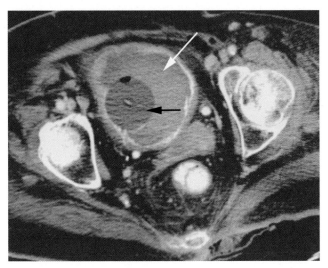

FIGURE 13.9. Blood clot. Contrast enhanced axial CT image shows a thin rim of contrast in the bladder surrounding a high-attenuation clot filling the entire bladder (*white arrow*). The bladder also contains a Foley catheter balloon (*black arrow*). The patient was bleeding from a renal cell carcinoma.

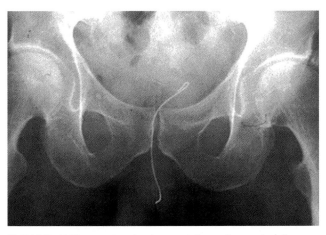

FIGURE 13.10. Foreign body. A plain radiography demonstrates a thin tubular metallic structure extending from the urethra to the bladder. This was a pipe cleaner inserted by the patient in an attempt to self-treat voiding difficulty.

many bladder neoplasms have been shown on CT and MRI to enhance to a greater extent on portal venous/corticomedullary phase images than an edematous bladder wall.

Infectious Conditions

Virtually all severe acute infections of the bladder can result in diffuse bullous edema of the urothelium, leading to a nodular irregular contour of the bladder on imaging studies. In many instances, this acute pattern will resolve with treatment in a matter of days and the bladder will return to its normal smooth appearance. However, severe acute infections can progress to a chronic phase, in which the bladder capacity is significantly reduced by fibrosis and contraction of the bladder wall. Changes of chronic cystitis from many of the inflammatory (irritative) bladder processes are all similar. It is usually not possible to distinguish among the different etiologies based upon the imaging appearance of a chronically inflamed and fibrotic bladder. Specific types of cystitis are discussed in the paragraphs that follow.

Acute Bacterial Cystitis

Several factors contribute to a natural resistance of the bladder to infection. These include an intrinsic resistance of the bladder mucosa, washing of organisms out of the bladder by normal voiding, trapping of organisms entering the bladder through the urethra by mucous secretions from the periurethral glands, and a bactericidal effect of prostatic secretions. Bladder infection seldom develops unless there is interference with one or more of these factors. For example, infection is more common when the bladder mucosa has been damaged by trauma, stone, or tumor; when outlet obstruction prevents bacteria from being completely washed out; and when bladder catheterization or instrumentation introduces infection by bypassing the protective mechanisms of the urethra and prostate.

Acute cystitis is diagnosed when more than 100,000 bacteria are present in 1 mL of urine. Most bacteria causing cystitis enter the bladder through the urethra. *Escherichia coli* is the most commonly encountered offending organism, but other common agents are often encountered, including species of *Staphylococcus, Streptococcus, Proteus, Pseudomonas, Aerobacter,* and *Candida*. In contrast to the other bacterial infections, tuberculosis typically infects the bladder by descending down the ureter from a granulomatous focus that develops in one or both kidneys (as a result of hematogenous seeding from the lungs).

Acute cystitis usually responds well to antibiotic therapy and in uncomplicated cases does not progress to chronic disease. Although cystitis may recur two or three times a year in sexually active women, more frequent recurrence of acute cystitis and cases that are resistant to antibiotic therapy suggest that there are other underlying risk factors, including urinary stone disease, bladder diverticula, colovesical fistulae, or perivesical infection/abscess. In such cases, imaging of the entire urinary tract and cystoscopic evaluation of the bladder are indicated to assess affected patients for any of these or other predisposing abnormalities.

Cystitis due to tuberculosis is an interstitial process initially associated with mucosal edema and later progressing to bladder wall thickening and fibrotic contraction, with reduced bladder capacity and a predisposition to vesicoureteral reflux. Rarely, there can be associated calcification of the bladder wall.

Emphysematous Cystitis

Emphysematous cystitis is a rare condition nearly always found in diabetic or immunocompromised patients. This infectious cystitis is most often due to *E. coli*. The gas is produced as a result of glucose fermentation with subsequent production of carbon dioxide and hydrogen. The gas initially is formed in the bladder wall and subsequently transgresses the mucosa into the lumen of the bladder. Emphysematous cystitis is associated with the same type of irritative symptoms as is any other acute bladder infection. While gas within the bladder wall and lumen together is nearly always the result of emphysematous cystitis, gas within the bladder lumen, but not in the bladder wall, is almost always the result of catheterization or instrumentation (during which air is introduced into the bladder) or fistula to the colon, small bowel, or vagina.

In patients with emphysematous cystitis, the plain film typically shows gas within the bladder and irregular streaky radiolucencies within the bladder wall (Fig. 13.11). Air within the bladder lumen should not be mistaken for rectal air. Air within the bladder conforms to the bladder shape, that is, ovoid with the long-axis horizontal (like an egg on its side) and in central position low in the pelvis (Fig. 13.12). Gas within the rectum has a vertical orientation, and the rectal folds often may be recognized. A lateral radiograph often distinguishes the anterior position of the bladder from the posterior location of the rectum. CT clearly shows the mural and, if present, the luminal locations of the gas (Fig. 13.13).

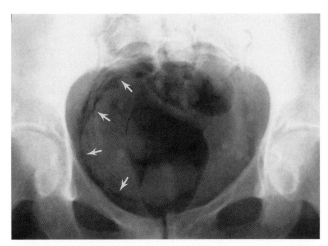

FIGURE 13.11. Emphysematous cystitis. Linear collections of gas within the bladder wall (*arrows*) indicate infection in this patient with diabetes mellitus.

Emphysematous cystitis responds rapidly to appropriate antibiotic therapy and control of underlying diseases such as diabetes. If untreated, however, the disease can be fatal. It does not progress to a chronic condition.

Alkaline Encrustation Cystitis

Alkaline encrustation cystitis is a rare chronic inflammatory bladder condition. It often occurs in association with bladder infection, including *Corynebacterium*. It is also frequently encountered in chronically ill and immunocompromised patients, often developing after instrumentation. Urea-splitting bacteria in these patients may cause a virulent cystitis, resulting in areas of necrosis and sloughing of the mucosa and a severe inflammatory reaction in the muscularis propria and adventitia. An alkaline urine is produced by the release of ammonia from urea, which then leads to calcium salt deposition in necrotic areas of the mucosa. As a result, calcification can develop

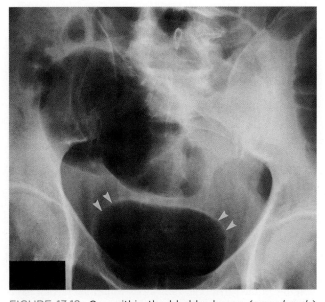

FIGURE 13.12. Gas within the bladder lumen (*arrowheads*) resulting from colovesical fistula. (Modified from McCallum RW, Colapinto V. *Urological Radiology of the Adult Male Lower Urinary Tract.* Springfield, IL: Charles C. Thomas; 1976:302, with permission.)

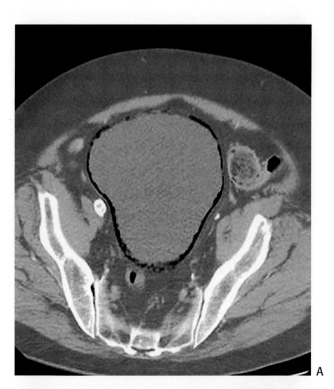

A

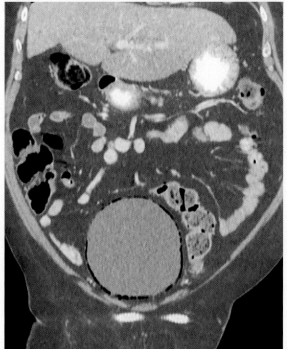

B

FIGURE 13.13. Emphysematous cystitis. Axial **(A)** and coronal contrast-enhanced **(B)** CT images of a patient with emphysematous cystitis show a characteristic thin rim of gas in the bladder wall. There is no air within the bladder lumen.

in the bladder wall (Fig. 13.14). Treatment usually consists of appropriate antibiotics and cystoscopic removal of the encrustations.

Schistosomiasis

Schistosomiasis (Bilharzia) is one of the most common parasitic infections in the world but is especially prevalent in the Nile

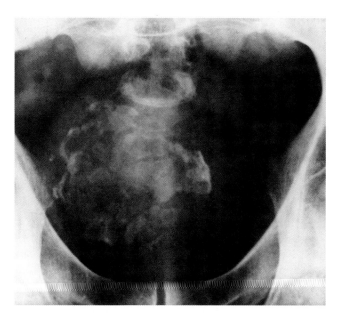

FIGURE 13.14. Alkaline encrustation cystitis. Plain radiograph of the pelvis in a patient with alkaline encrustation cystitis reveals irregular sheetlike calcification in the region of the bladder.

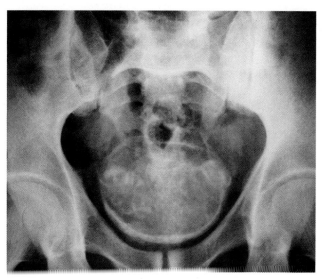

FIGURE 13.15. Schistosomiasis. Dense calcification is seen within the bladder wall. Seminal vesicle calcification can also be seen through the bladder (Courtesy of S. Sejeni, M.D.).

Valley. Only *Schistosoma haematobium* affects the urinary tract. The definitive host is a human, and the intermediate host is a freshwater snail. Because the disease typically involves the intestines and bladder, eggs escape the human host in the feces and urine. These eggs, when deposited in freshwater, hatch into miracidia, which infest snails, develop, and emerge as cercariae. These cercariae infect humans directly through the skin, when humans enter infested waters. After the skin is penetrated, the cercariae enter peripheral capillaries, drain to the lung, squeeze through the alveolar capillaries, and enter the systemic circulation. The cercariae that survive enter the mesenteric arteries and subsequently pass through the portal venous system. They develop into adolescent flukes in the portal system and then migrate against the flow in the portal system using two suckers, which they alternately attach to the wall of a vein. They eventually reach the smallest venules in the wall of the bladder, probably through the hemorrhoidal plexus. From there, millions of eggs enter the urine or are trapped in the bladder walls where they die, producing a severe granulomatous reaction. The granulomas calcify, causing linear streaks of calcium in the bladder wall. Large conglomerations of eggs in the bladder wall produce masses known as bilharzioma, which may also eventually calcify.

The clinical presentation of patients with schistosomiasis haematobium infection is typically hematuria. In initial stages, the bladder mucosa is edematous and hemorrhagic. Later, the bladder becomes fibrotic often with a reduced volume and calcified wall. Cystoscopic examination of patients with schistosomiasis is mandatory to exclude squamous cell carcinoma of the bladder, which has a markedly increased incidence. Biopsy may be necessary to distinguish bilharzioma from carcinoma, although carcinoma usually presents as a later complication. Schistosomiasis rarely affects the kidneys or renal collecting systems and ureters, except by obstruction due to bladder disease or involvement of the distal ureter. In contrast to tuberculosis, if schistosomiasis does involve the upper tracts, such involvement is the result of retrograde spread of infection from the bladder.

As the disease progresses, plain film radiography may show dense calcification of the bladder wall or bladder stones (Fig. 13.15).

Calcification of the distal ureter may also be seen but is rarely present without bladder involvement. A bladder tumor should be suspected when follow-up studies show absence of wall calcification in areas that were previously calcified (Fig. 13.16). Although there are other causes of bladder calcification, including tuberculosis, radiation cystitis, alkaline-encrusted cystitis, and, rarely, bladder cancer, none is as common or as dramatic as schistosomiasis. Additionally, patients with schistosomiasis may develop wall calcifications in normal-sized bladders or contracted bladders. In contrast, patients with other types of cystitis nearly always develop calcifications in their bladder only after it has become contracted and fibrotic, thus appearing small in capacity. In patients with schistosomiasis, the

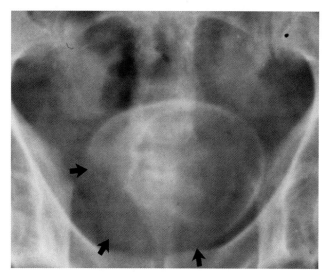

FIGURE 13.16. Schistosomiasis with squamous cell carcinoma. Plain film radiograph of the pelvis reveals a faintly calcified wall in a patient with schistosomiasis. Note that the right inferolateral wall of the bladder is not calcified (*arrows*). This loss of calcification in a previously calcified bladder indicates the development of a tumor in this region.

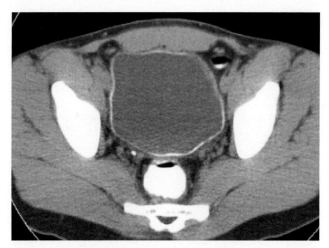

FIGURE 13.17. Schistosomiasis. Unenhanced axial CT image shows a thin rim of calcification in an otherwise normal-appearing bladder wall. Note that, in comparison to patients with other types of cystitis who develop bladder wall calcification, the bladder capacity appears normal in this patient.

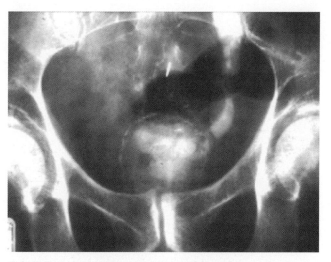

FIGURE 13.18. Radiation cystitis. Cystogram in a patient who had previously received external beam radiation for treatment of prostate cancer. The bladder capacity is decreased, and there is calcification in the bladder wall. Reflux is also noted into a dilated left ureter.

ureterovesical junction may be partially obstructed by the changes in the bladder wall, resulting in ureteral dilation. Schistosomiasis may also affect the prostate and urethra. The disease may also result in urethral fistula formation, producing a pattern similar to that seen with advanced tuberculosis. Fistulae may drain into the perineum, scrotum, suprapubic skin, or buttocks.

CT is more sensitive than plain radiographs in visualizing faint calcifications in the walls of the ureters and bladder in patients with suspected schistosomiasis (Fig. 13.17).

Candidiasis

Candidiasis of the bladder is most typically seen in poorly controlled diabetic patients. It also causes fermentation of sugars in the urine, forming gas in the bladder lumen. It may present with the development of fungus ball in the bladder lumen. These fungus balls may be single or multiple and are seen as laminated, gas-containing filling defects within the bladder.

Inflammatory Noninfectious Conditions

Radiation Cystitis

Usually seen after external beam irradiation doses of 30 Gray (3,000 rads) or more, the acute form of radiation cystitis is associated with edema and hemorrhage. This acute phase is usually self-limiting and resolves completely. However, it may progress to mucosal ulceration, fibrosis, and a small capacity bladder. Rarely, calcification of the bladder wall may occur. Hemorrhage in the acute phase may be severe, and angiographic embolization may be necessary to control bleeding. Cystography and CT show contour irregularity of the bladder wall due to edema that is indistinguishable from other causes of bladder mucosal edema. Over time, a fibrotic reaction may occur, resulting in chronic bladder wall thickening, reduced bladder capacity, and the appearance of calcification, findings which are easily seen on CT and/or MRI (Fig. 13.18). Fortunately, severe acute or chronic cystitis as a complication of radiation therapy is uncommon.

Hemorrhagic Cystitis

Many patients treated with the alkylating chemotherapeutic and immunosuppressive agents such as cyclophosphamide and

ifosfamide have developed an acute hemorrhagic cystitis after treatment. The inflammatory change in the bladder is caused by exposure of the bladder mucosa to the metabolic end products of these agents (including acrolein), resulting in marked bladder edema with hemorrhage. Massive bleeding has sometimes occurred and has required aggressive measures for control, including angiographic embolization or cystectomy.

The acute form of hemorrhagic cystitis, usually after high-dose intravenous injections of cyclophosphamide and ifosfamide, has tended to resolve with symptomatic therapy with no adverse sequelae; however, a chronic form sometimes may occur after many months of oral cyclophosphamide therapy, progressing to a thick-walled contracted bladder, which is easily detected on cross-sectional imaging studies (Fig. 13.19). Bladder wall calcification is a rare, occasionally encountered, finding in these patients (Fig. 13.20). There is also an increased incidence of bladder carcinoma in patients being treated with cyclophosphamide (Fig. 13.21) or ifosfamide.

In recent years, chemoprotective agents have been utilized in patients treated with alkylating chemotherapeutic agents, with one of these, mesna, having been observed to reduce the incidence of hematuria by binding to and inactivating acrolein (via sulfhydryl groups in the mesna molecule). Administration of mesna may also result in a decrease in the likelihood of subsequent development of bladder cancer, although data here are limited.

Interstitial Cystitis

Interstitial cystitis is seen almost exclusively in women, usually after menopause. A cluster of cystoscopic findings is required for diagnosis. This includes hemorrhagic bladder mucosa and characteristic, but not commonly found, ulcerations near the bladder dome that crack and bleed with bladder distention (Hunner ulcers). Infiltration of the bladder wall with chronic inflammatory cells results in fibrosis and a very small capacity bladder, often with a capacity of no more than 30 to 50 mL (Fig. 13.22). Now, interstitial cystitis is often grouped together with a number of other abnormalities that can result in bladder pain (bladder pain syndromes), some of which are present in the absence of inflammation. In comparison to interstitial cystitis, many of

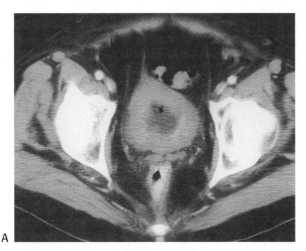

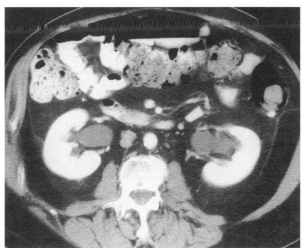

FIGURE 13.19. Hemorrhagic cystitis. **A:** Marked thickening of the bladder wall is demonstrated on this contrast-enhanced axial pelvic CT image. **B:** The markedly thickened bladder wall has caused bilateral ureteral obstruction, which has produced bilateral pelvocaliectasis, as seen on a more cephalad axial CT image.

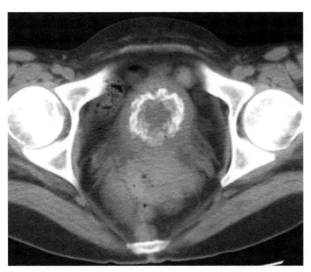

FIGURE 13.20. Hemorrhagic cystitis. Unenhanced axial CT image demonstrates a markedly thick-walled and contracted bladder, with dense calcification along the entire inner wall.

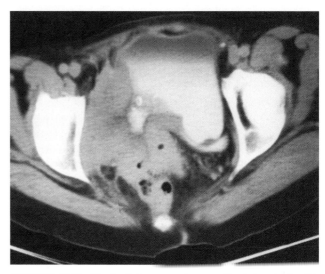

FIGURE 13.21. Urothelial cancer in a patient treated with cyclophosphamide. Contrast-enhanced axial CT image demonstrates a large right-sided urothelial cancer extending through the bladder wall to the right pelvic sidewall.

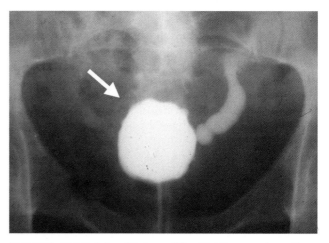

FIGURE 13.22. Interstitial cystitis. Voiding cystourethrogram shows small capacity bladder with bilateral reflux and thickened wall (*arrow*). The patient could not tolerate further bladder distention.

these other bladder pain syndromes are more commonly seen in younger patients.

Patients with interstitial cystitis and bladder pain syndromes present with severe pelvic pain, which often, but not always, worsens as the bladder fills, resulting in the need for frequent bladder emptying. There is no known etiology, although some affected patients may have other diagnoses, including fibromyalgia, chronic fatigue syndrome, and anxiety or depression. These conditions may all be extremely debilitating because of the small bladder capacity and the pain associated with overfilling. Treatment of interstitial cystitis usually consists of ablation or corticosteroid injection of any Hunner ulcerations, with a high success rate. Treatment of other bladder pain syndromes can be more problematic. In the past, bladder augmentation has been used to treat some patients who develop small capacity bladders.

Cystitis Cystica

Cystitis cystica is a benign condition, most commonly found in women with recurrent or chronic cystitis secondary to *E. coli* infection. Cystic lesions 1 to 2 cm in diameter tend to occur in the bladder base and on the trigone. These lesions result from degeneration of subepithelial clusters of transitional cells known as von Brunn nests. Radiographically, the bladder base shows multiple small or large rounded contour defects (Fig. 13.23), a finding suggestive of, but not specific for, cystitis cystica.

Cystitis Glandularis

Cystitis glandularis occurs with further metaplasia of the von Brunn nests into glandular structures resembling intestinal epithelium. It is seen with chronic or recurrent infections. An association with pelvic lipomatosis has also been suggested. These lesions are considered premalignant or, at the least, associated with malignancy, as patients with cystitis glandularis may develop bladder adenocarcinomas. On cystoscopy, there are typically one or more irregular mucosal lesions grossly resembling bladder cancer. Radiographically, these lesions cannot be clearly differentiated from cancer (Fig. 13.24) and often require biopsy to establish the diagnosis. On occasion, areas of cystitis glandularis can be suggested on imaging studies when cystic areas are noted within a bladder mass.

Eosinophilic Cystitis

Eosinophilic cystitis occurs in patients with severe allergic conditions and is more common in women. Eosinophilic infiltration of the bladder mucosa and submucosa results in edema, hemorrhage, and ulceration. Imaging of the bladder shows mucosal irregularity associated with focal or diffuse wall thickening. The appearance can occasionally mimic that of urothelial cancer. The condition usually responds well to steroids (Fig. 13.25).

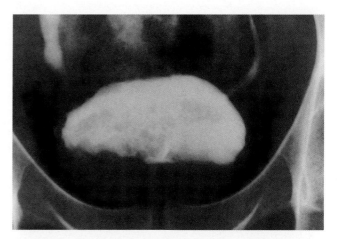

FIGURE 13.24. Cystitis glandularis. Anteroposterior radiograph of the pelvis obtained during an excretory urogram shows irregular, frondlike defects within and along the inferior aspect of the bladder. Biopsy would be required to differentiate this metaplastic process from urothelial carcinoma.

Malacoplakia

Malacoplakia of the bladder is of unknown etiology but is associated with conditions such as pulmonary tuberculosis, chronic osteomyelitis, and long-standing malignant disease elsewhere in the body. The bladder mucosa is involved with multiple, yellow-gray plaques that tend to occur in the bladder base. The histology of these plaques shows histiocytes, lymphocytes, and plasma cells. Michaelis–Gutmann bodies in the biopsy specimen are diagnostic and are thought to result from phagocytized bacteria. Radiographically, rounded contour defects, predominantly in the region of the bladder trigone, may be difficult to differentiate from cystitis, especially cystitis cystica or cystitis glandularis. Occasionally, this benign process may resemble a tumor. Biopsy is required for diagnosis.

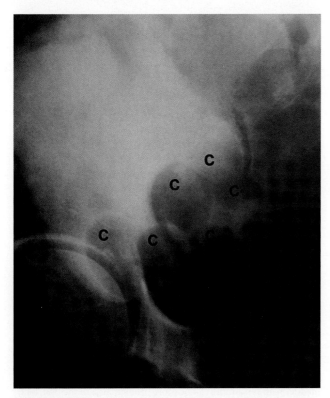

FIGURE 13.23. Cystitis cystica. Oblique radiograph of the pelvis obtained during an excretory urogram shows multiple large smooth rounded contour defects in the bladder base (C) representing cysts. The appearance would be identical on cystography.

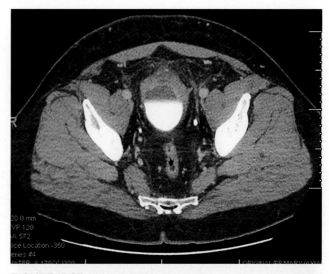

FIGURE 13.25. Eosinophilic cystitis. Contrast-enhanced axial CT image through the pelvis demonstrates lobulated thickening along the anterior aspect of the bladder. The appearance is concerning for urothelial neoplasm; however, biopsy revealed eosinophilic cystitis. The thickening resolved completely within 3 months of corticosteroid treatment.

Uncommon Inflammatory Noninfectious Conditions

Nephrogenic Adenoma

Nephrogenic adenoma is a very rare proliferative response of the bladder epithelium to chronic infection or irritation. It is more commonly encountered in men. The name derives from the histologic appearance of the lesions, which have characteristics similar to those of the proximal tubules of the nephron. This lesion is more common in the bladder than in other locations in the urinary tract. The lesions range from mucosal irregularities to large malignant-appearing masses arising from the bladder wall (Figs. 13.26 and 13.27). No specific imaging findings allow for differentiation of nephrogenic adenoma from bladder cancer. Distinction from cancer may also be difficult at cystoscopy, and biopsy is necessary to establish the diagnosis. Although this condition is not considered premalignant, it can involve the bladder extensively and is difficult to eradicate.

Endometriosis

Although uncommon, the bladder is the most frequent site in the urinary tract to be involved with endometriosis. Endometrial tissue may infiltrate through the bladder muscle and produce mural masses projecting into the bladder lumen. This condition results in cyclic hematuria that is more prominent at menstruation. Ultrasound, CT, and MRI may be helpful in showing a mural mass protruding into the bladder, typically near the dome (blue dome cyst), as a direct extension of an extrauterine endometrial mass (Fig. 13.28).

Amyloidosis

Amyloidosis of the bladder is extremely rare. It may be primary or secondary and may be associated with amyloidosis elsewhere. Affected patients present with hematuria and urinary frequency. Cystoscopy shows irregular infiltrating lesions in the mucosa and submucosa that bleed readily. Biopsy is necessary for diagnosis. Ultrasound, CT, and MRI may show multiple contour defects projecting into the bladder from the bladder wall. The bladder base is often spared. Rarely, bladder wall calcification develops within the submucosal infiltrations. The appearance is nonspecific and cannot be distinguished from that of other mucosal bladder lesions.

Perivesical Infectious and Noninfectious Inflammatory Lesions

Inflammatory lesions in the pelvis can produce reactive thickening of the adjacent bladder wall as well as mucosal irregularities. Focal mucosal changes in the bladder wall may at times be so severe as to

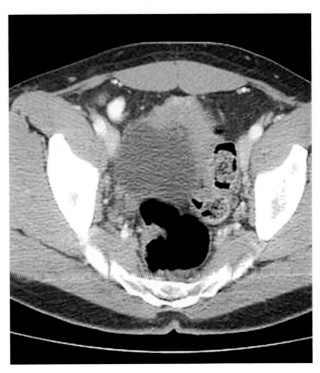

FIGURE 13.27. Nephrogenic adenoma. Contrast-enhanced axial CT image through the pelvis demonstrates asymmetrically increased lobular wall thickening along the left anterior aspect of the bladder. A diagnosis of nephrogenic adenoma was confirmed during cystoscopic biopsy.

mimic tumors. Conversely, urothelial tumors can occasionally be mistaken for secondary bladder inflammation produced by adjacent inflammatory conditions, since locally advanced (stage T4) bladder cancers can extend directly through the bladder wall to involve adjacent organs. Fortunately, in many cases, the patient's clinical presentation will suggest the correct diagnosis. Typical conditions that can involve the bladder include appendiceal (Fig. 13.29), diverticular, and tuboovarian abscesses.

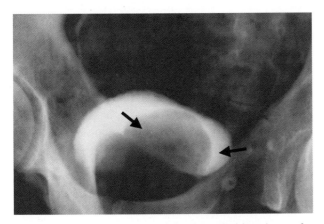

FIGURE 13.26. Nephrogenic adenoma. Bladder phase of an excretory urogram shows a polypoid mass (*arrows*) atop the enlarged prostate. Biopsy showed a nephrogenic adenoma. Note the similarity to a polypoid transitional cell carcinoma.

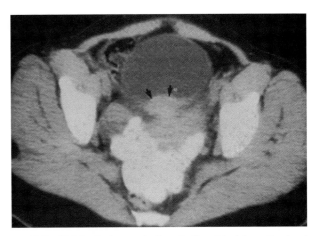

FIGURE 13.28. Endometriosis of the bladder. Contrast-enhanced axial CT image through the pelvis shows a soft tissue mass involving the bladder wall (*arrows*) and extending directly from an irregular pelvic mass. This proved to be endometriosis. (From Amis ES Jr, Newhouse JH. *Essentials of Uroradiology.* Boston, MA: Little, Brown and Company; 1991:297, with permission.)

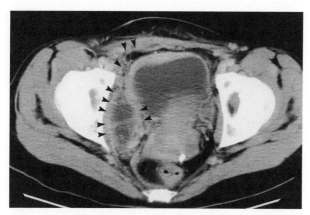

FIGURE 13.29. Perivesical abscess. Contrast-enhanced axial CT image of the pelvis shows an extensive thick-walled peri-appendiceal abscess on the right (*arrowheads*). Note that there is marked adjacent reactive bladder wall thickening, which could be mistaken for a bladder neoplasm.

Bladder Diverticula

Bladder diverticula are most commonly acquired, developing as a result of functional or mechanical bladder outlet obstruction. Functional bladder outlet obstruction is usually seen in patients with neurogenic bladders. Neurogenic dysfunction of the bladder often results in the formation of multiple diverticula in children and adults. Mechanical obstructions are most commonly due to prostatic enlargement. Bladder diverticula due to mechanical outlet obstruction are rare in children but may be seen in boys with posterior urethral valves. Often, acquired bladder diverticula are multiple, usually arising from the lateral walls and rarely arising near the bladder dome. Obstructive diverticula are acquired and are pseudodiverticula, as they do not contain the normal muscular layer of the bladder wall.

Rarely, some patients can have a congenital deficiency in bladder musculature adjacent to the ureterovesical junction, leading to diverticulum formation (Fig. 13.30). Congenital diverticula are true diverticula, containing all layers of the bladder wall. These are referred to as Hutch diverticula. Hutch diverticula are commonly associated with ipsilateral vesicoureteral reflux.

Bladder diverticula have either wide or narrow necks. A wide-necked diverticulum empties readily, but a narrow-necked diverticulum empties slowly and is more likely to have residual urine after voiding. A large bladder diverticulum may displace the bladder to the opposite side of the pelvis and may be larger than the bladder. In most such cases, the bladder can be identified on cross-sectional imaging studies by its thickened wall, whereas the diverticulum has a smooth thin wall (due to the lack of muscular layer).

There are a variety of complications of bladder diverticula. Urinary stasis tends to occur in diverticula, which may increase the risk of urinary tract infection. Stones may develop within diverticula as a result of stasis, as well. There may also be a higher incidence of tumor in comparison to the normal bladder lumen, due to prolonged exposure of the urothelium to carcinogens in urine. It has been estimated that diverticular tumors account for about 1% to 1.5% of all bladder tumors.

Tumors in acquired bladder diverticula are more problematic than tumors in the normal bladder or true diverticula. This is because there is a higher risk of perforation when transurethral resection is performed, due to the lack of a muscular layer. Staging of these tumors is also different, since there is no such thing as a stage T2 tumor (in the absence of muscularis propria). As a result of the thin wall of a false bladder diverticulum, tumors here spread outside the bladder more rapidly than do those in the bladder lumen.

Cross-sectional studies are often easily able to image bladder diverticula and their complications. Ultrasound is very

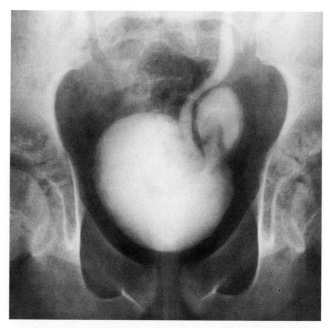

FIGURE 13.30. Hutch diverticulum. A cystogram demonstrates a large left-sided bladder diverticulum, located near the left ureterovesical junction. There is reflux into the left ureter.

effective. Echo-free outpouchings from the bladder are readily seen (Fig. 13.31), and filling defects within a diverticulum such as stones or tumors can also be visualized. Tumors within a diverticulum present as soft tissue masses in the diverticulum or only as thickening of the diverticulum wall, whereas stones often produce shadowing. Tumors may on occasion obstruct the mouth of the diverticulum or can completely fill the diverticulum (Fig. 13.32).

CT is an excellent method of assessing bladder diverticula. Diverticula will opacify on delayed contrast-enhanced images, provided that the neck of the diverticulum is not obstructed (Fig. 13.33).

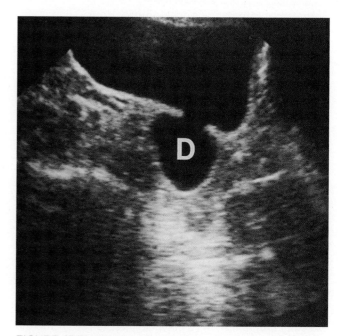

FIGURE 13.31. Bladder diverticulum. Transabdominal ultrasound shows a urine-filled bladder with a urine-filled, wide-necked diverticulum (*D*).

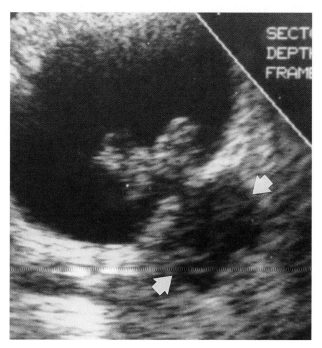

FIGURE 13.32. Bladder diverticulum containing a urothe-lial neoplasm. Transabdominal ultrasound shows a papil-lary urothelial neoplasm projecting into the bladder lumen. Echogenic tissue (representing infiltrative tumor) can also be seen almost completely filling an adjacent posteriorly located bladder diverticulum (arrows).

Stones are easily seen on unenhanced CT images as high-attenuation filling defects, whereas a tumor presents as a soft tissue mass aris-ing from the diverticulum wall. Again, tumors may appear as focal masses protruding into the lumen of the diverticulum (Fig. 13.34) or as infiltrative masses thickening the wall or the neck of the diverticu-lum (Fig. 13.35) (and sometimes obstructing the neck). MRI is also useful in evaluating tumors arising in bladder diverticula (Fig. 13.36).

Bladder Herniation

Patients with herniation of the bladder into or through the inguinal canal present with swelling in the groin or scrotum that increases as

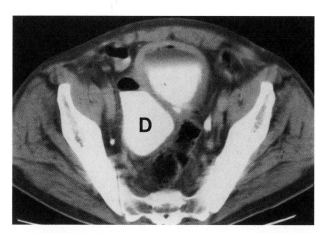

FIGURE 13.33. Bladder diverticulum. Contrast-enhanced axial CT image shows a large bladder diverticulum (D) in the right hemipelvis. Air within the diverticulum and bladder is due to recent instrumentation.

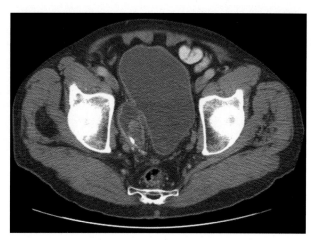

FIGURE 13.34. Urothelial neoplasm in bladder diverticulum. A small soft tissue mass is seen in the middle of a large diver-ticulum along the right posterolateral aspect of the bladder. An area of high attenuation located more posteriorly repre-sents calcification within the tumor.

the urinary bladder fills and subsides as the patient voids. Bladder herniation most commonly is paraperitoneal in location, with the bladder remaining extraperitoneal and medial to a true inguinal her-nia sac. Herniation of the bladder also can be within a true hernia sac or can occur totally extraperitoneally with the peritoneum remaining in the abdomen. The bladder also may herniate through the femoral canal into the thigh or through various incisional hernias.

Bladder herniation can occur in varying degrees and can usu-ally be easily seen when the bladder is filled with contrast medium during cystography (Fig. 13.37) although an upright film is occasionally necessary to make the diagnosis. Bladder herniation

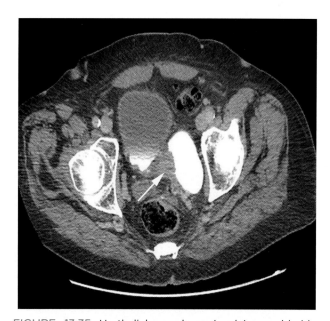

FIGURE 13.35. Urothelial neoplasm involving a bladder diverticulum. An excretory phase contrast-enhanced axial CT image demonstrates a large, lobulated, soft tissue mass located between the posterolateral aspect of the bladder and the medial aspect of an adjacent diverticulum (arrow). Despite the large size of the mass, the neck of the diver-ticulum is not obstructed, since the diverticulum is opacified with excreted contrast material.

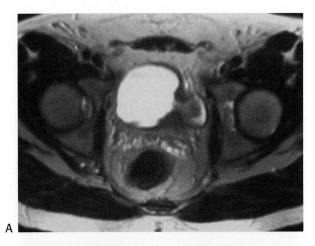

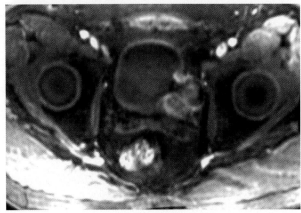

FIGURE 13.36. Urothelial neoplasm in a bladder diverticulum. **(A)** T2-weighted and **(B)** fat-suppressed T1-weighted gadolinium-enhanced axial MR images demonstrate a small diverticulum extending laterally from the left side of the bladder. A soft tissue mass is identified within the diverticulum. The mass can be seen to enhance on the enhanced MR image.

may occasionally be seen as an incidental finding on CT and is usually easy to detect when the bladder lumen contains contrast material (Fig. 13.38). However, in some cases, this condition may be quite subtle (Fig. 13.39).

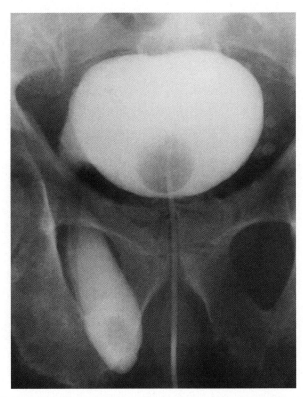

FIGURE 13.37. Bladder herniation. Cystogram shows part of the bladder to have herniated into the right inguinal canal and into the scrotum.

Cystocele and Stress Incontinence

A cystocele is defined as prolapse of the bladder into the anterior portion of the vagina and is seen radiographically as descent of the bladder below the symphysis pubis. A cystocele results from laxity of the pelvic floor muscles and is usually only one component of pelvic floor dysfunction, which may include a cystocele, vaginal vault prolapse, rectocele, enterocele, sigmoidocele, or rectoanal intussusception. Conditions that predispose to pelvic floor dysfunction include multiparity, obesity, prior pelvic surgery, excessive straining, connective tissue disorders, neuropathy, and advancing age. MRI is useful for evaluating the pelvic floor without the need for bladder or rectal opacification.

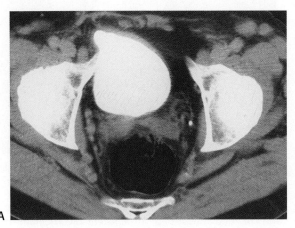

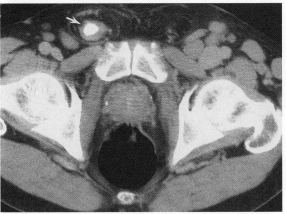

FIGURE 13.38. Bladder herniation. **A, B:** The right anterior aspect of an opacified bladder can be seen to herniate into the right inguinal canal (*arrow*) on this contrast-enhanced axial CT image. This herniation was detected as an incidental finding.

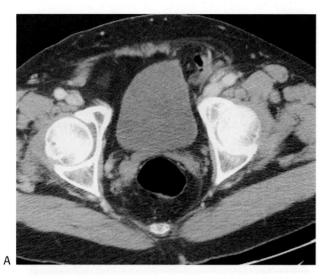

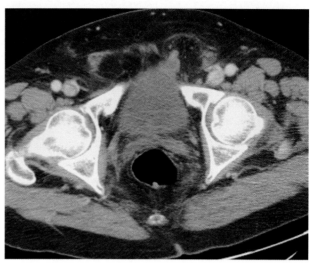

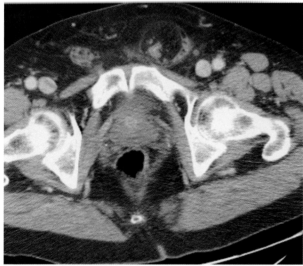

FIGURE 13.39. Subtle bladder herniation. **A:** The left antero-lateral bladder wall points toward the left inguinal canal on this corticomedullary-phase contrast-enhanced axial CT image. Note that the bladder lumen is not yet opacified with excreted contrast material. **B:** The tip of the bladder can be seen entering the inguinal hernia on an image obtained slightly more caudally. **C:** The soft tissue in the hernia on this even more caudal image is the tip of the bladder.

Bladder Fistulae

Enterovesical and Colovesical Fistulae

Patients may develop fistulae between the bladder and bowel as a result of inflammatory, traumatic, or neoplastic processes. Inflammatory etiologies include infection (including due to tuberculosis and schistosomiasis), inflammatory bowel disease, diverticulitis, appendicitis, pelvic inflammatory disease, and previous radiation therapy. Traumatic etiologies include injuries at surgery and penetrating trauma. Occasionally, bladder and bowel malignancies can spread locally into adjacent organs and produce fistulae.

When small bowel is involved, the term enterovesical fistula is preferred. Such fistulae are usually caused by Crohn disease. When the colon is involved, the term colovesical fistula is preferred. The rectosigmoid colon is the most frequently involved segment of large bowel. The most common cause of colovesical fistulae in the United States is diverticulitis. Colon cancer is the second most common cause.

Patients with fistulae from the bladder to the bowel may present with fecaluria, pneumaturia, and/or persistent urinary tract infection. On imaging studies, identification of gas in the bladder lumen is often seen when a fistula to adjacent bowel is present. However, in most instances, detected gas in the bladder lumen on cross-sectional imaging studies has been introduced into the bladder lumen as a result of recent (within 24 hours) instrumentation

(catheterization or cystoscopy). Occasionally, patients with acute cystitis due to *E. coli* may also have air in their bladder lumen in the absence of a fistula. Gas in the bladder wall is found only in emphysematous cystitis.

Cystography demonstrates the actual fistula between bladder and bowel in no more than about 50% of cases. Bowel contrast studies are positive in even fewer cases. However, when the fistulous tract is widely patent, imaging of a contrast-filled bladder or bowel often demonstrates the communication. Cystoscopy may show the actual fistula in some instances; however, in other instances the diagnosis may be difficult. The most typical cystoscopic finding is an isolated area of inflammation of the bladder wall.

CT is the most sensitive imaging study for detection of a bladder fistula, with the most commonly encountered finding being the presence of a small amount of air in the bladder lumen. This diagnosis should be considered in any patients who have intraluminal air and no history of recent instrumentation (Fig. 13.40). Patients may also exhibit focal bladder wall thickening, associated with focal thickening of a loop of small or large bowel adjacent to the bladder (Figs. 13.41 and 13.42). The actual fistula is not identified in many cases. As with cystography and barium enema, CT shows flow of contrast medium through the fistula in no more than 50% of cases. The etiology of the fistula can usually be inferred from the patient's history, other symptoms, and a knowledge of any preexisting medical conditions.

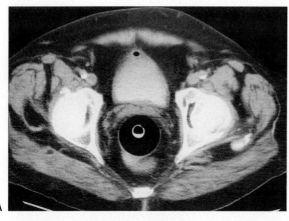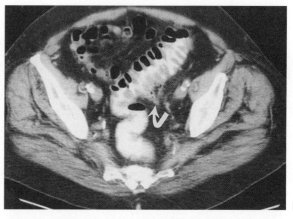

FIGURE 13.40. Colovesical fistula secondary to diverticulitis. **A:** A contrast-enhanced axial CT image through the pelvis shows a small collection of air within the bladder. The patient had no recent instrumentation. **B:** A more cephalad axial CT image shows an area of inflammation extending posteriorly from the sigmoid colon and containing a small amount of oral contrast material (*arrow*). These changes are due to diverticulitis.

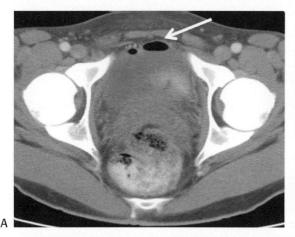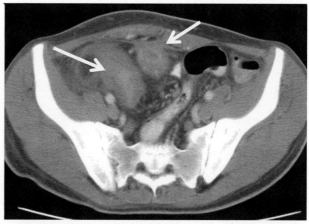

FIGURE 13.41. Enterovesical fistula secondary to Crohn disease. **A:** A contrast-enhanced axial CT image through the pelvis demonstrates a collection of gas within the anterior aspect of the bladder (*arrow*). **B:** A more cephalad scan reveals pronounced thickening of several loops of small bowel in the right lower quadrant (*arrows*).

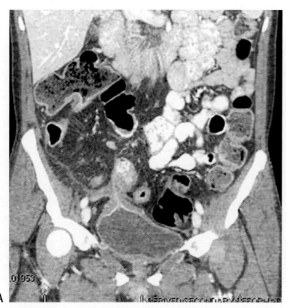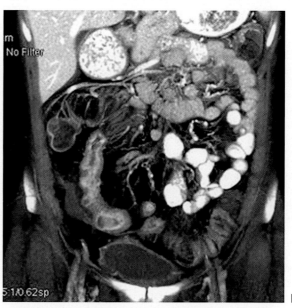

FIGURE 13.42. Enterovesical fistula secondary to Crohn disease. **A:** A contrast-enhanced coronally reformatted image from a CT enterography study shows cephalad tenting of the bladder wall on the right side, with the bladder abutting a loop of thickened small bowel. A punctate collection of gas was noted in the bladder lumen on an adjacent image. **B:** A more anterior image demonstrates a long segment of diseased distal ileum. There is characteristic mural hyperenhancement, indicating the presence of active inflammatory bowel disease.

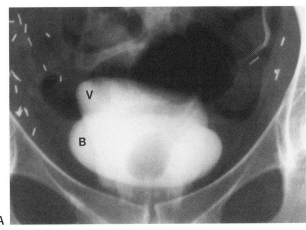

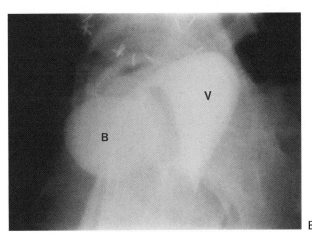

FIGURE 13.43. Vesicovaginal fistula. **A:** Anteroposterior view from a cystogram demonstrates opacification of both the ovoid-shaped bladder (*B*) and the rhomboid-shaped vagina (*V*). **B:** The lateral view demonstrates the fistulous tract between the bladder (*B*) and the vagina (*V*).

Vesicovaginal Fistulae

Vesicovaginal fistulae result in painless constant dribbling of urine from the vagina. They are a known complication in patients undergoing hysterectomy or other pelvic surgery, especially when preoperative radiation was used. Seventy-five percent of cases occur after hysterectomy for a benign condition, with the remainder found after hysterectomy for pelvic malignancy. Vesicovaginal fistulae, because of their typically large size, are usually relatively easy to demonstrate on imaging studies. To visualize the contrast-filled vagina during cystography, oblique, lateral (Fig. 13.43), or postvoiding films may be necessary. Vesicovaginal fistulae may also be detected with CT and MRI (Fig. 13.44).

Bladder Deviations

Various conditions in the pelvis extrinsic to the bladder can focally or circumferentially compress the bladder or deviate the bladder to one side. The etiology of these impressions is not readily identified on fluoroscopic studies (cystography) but is usually readily identified on cross-sectional imaging studies, particularly CT (Fig. 13.45). Common abnormalities that may indent the bladder include enlarged pelvic lymph nodes, tumors arising from the colon, reproductive

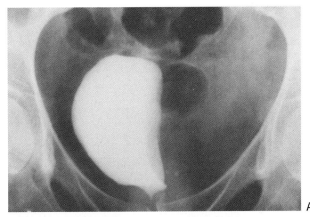

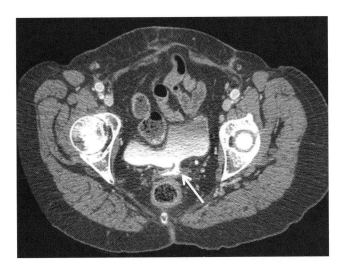

FIGURE 13.44. Vesicovaginal fistula. A contrast-enhanced axial CT image, obtained as part of a CT urogram, demonstrates excreted contrast material in the posterior aspect of the bladder. A linear collection of contrast material continues posterior to the bladder to opacify the vagina, confirming the presence of a fistula (*arrow*).

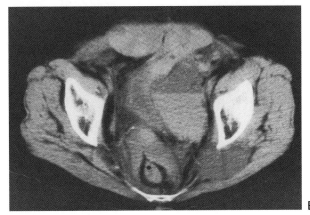

FIGURE 13.45. Pelvic hematoma. **A:** A plain radiograph of the pelvis obtained during cystography shows a large left pelvic mass compressing bladder and displacing it toward the right. **B:** An unenhanced axial CT image demonstrates a large hematoma in the left hemipelvis. There is a fluid–fluid level within the hematoma, due to layering of blood products. The patient had recently undergone surgery for urinary stress incontinence.

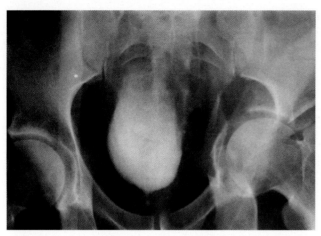

FIGURE 13.46. "Teardrop"/"pear-shaped" bladder due to pelvic hematoma. Bilateral pelvic hematomas from pelvic fractures compress the bladder and create a teardrop configuration of the bladder on this anteroposterior image obtained during a cystogram.

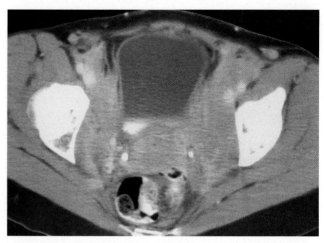

FIGURE 13.47. "Pear-shaped" bladder due to lymphoma. Contrast-enhanced axial CT image shows bilateral external iliac lymph node enlargement compressing the bladder in a patient with lymphoma.

organs, or mesenchymal tissues, presacral teratomas, iliac artery aneurysms, bladder diverticula, hematomas, and abscesses.

An anterior meningomyelocele behind the bladder can deviate the bladder anteriorly. These masses are usually accompanied by pathognomonic changes in the sacrum, including a well-corticated concavity on one side of the sacrum and deviation of the sacrum to the contralateral side (scimitar sacrum). Other cystic lesions that can indent the bladder from behind include seminal vesicle and müllerian duct cysts.

Circumferential compression of the bladder results in a configuration commonly known as a "teardrop" or "pear-shaped" bladder. The etiology of such compression is usually easily determined on cross-sectional imaging studies. Processes that can surround the bladder and alter its contour include the normal variant of a narrow pelvis with prominent iliopsoas muscles, pelvic hematoma (usually seen in the setting of recent surgery or trauma [Fig. 13.46] but also

occasionally encountered in patients with coagulation disorders or who are being anticoagulated), bilateral pelvic lymph node enlargement (often seen in patients with bulky lymph nodes due to lymphoma) (Fig. 13.47), less commonly dilated external iliac arteries or veins, and pelvic sidewall fluid collections (such as lymphoceles following pelvic lymph node dissection).

Another condition resulting in bladder compression is pelvic lipomatosis. This results from a proliferation of mature, unencapsulated fat within the pelvis. No etiology for this condition has been identified. Radiographically, plain films may show a lucency in the pelvis corresponding to the increased fat. The distal ureters are medially deviated, and the midureters may be laterally displaced due to the elevation of the lower urinary tract. Additionally, the ureters may be obstructed in severe cases. On barium enema, the rectosigmoid colon is straightened and narrowed. The excess pelvic fat responsible for compressing the colon and bladder can be easily confirmed with CT or MRI (Fig. 13.48).

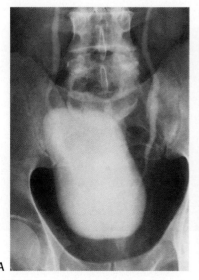
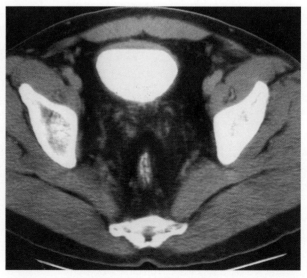

A   B

FIGURE 13.48. "Pear-shaped" bladder due to pelvic lipomatosis. A: An excretory urogram demonstrates the bladder to be vertically oriented and the bladder base is elevated. B: A contrast-enhanced CT image demonstrates excess pelvic fat and absence of soft tissue masses to explain the bladder deformity, findings diagnostic of pelvic lipomatosis.

BLADDER NEOPLASMS

Primary Malignant Neoplasms

Primary neoplasms of the bladder may develop in the muscle wall or urothelium, with tumors of the urothelium comprising approximately 95% of bladder malignancies. Of these urothelial cancers, 90% to 95% contain at least some transitional cell components, while 4% to 8% are entirely composed of squamous cells, and 1% to 2% of only adenomatous cells.

Urothelial Neoplasms Containing Transitional Cell Components

Epidemiology of Bladder Cancer

Bladder cancer is the second most common urinary tract cancer in the United States, following only prostate cancer in frequency. Bladder cancer is much more common in men than women; however, women with bladder cancer tend to present with more advanced disease than men. There is a well-known association of transitional cell containing urothelial carcinomas with chemical carcinogens, including aromatic amines, nitrosamines, and aldehydes, such as acrolein, compounds that are in common use in the textile, rubber, dye, and chemical industries. The latent period between occupational exposure and the development of clinical cancer varies from 15 to 40 years. Other causes of urothelial cancer include smoking, which is felt to be responsible for up to 50% of all bladder cancers, and treatment with cyclophosphamide, a chemotherapeutic agent that results in the excretion of acrolein in the urine. The large proportion of bladder tumors found in cigarette smokers is probably because aromatic amines, nitrosamines, and acrolein are present in cigarette smoke.

Histology of Bladder Cancer

Although it was previously believed that most bladder cancers were composed entirely of transitional cells, it is now known that many of these "transitional cell" neoplasms contain areas with other histologies, including clear cell, glandular, lymphoepithelial, micropapillary, plasmacytoid, sarcomatoid, and squamous cells. Owing to this complicating feature, many pathologists now prefer to refer to these urothelial malignancies as urothelial cancers rather than transitional cell cancers. Some urothelial cancers also contain neuroendocrine or small cell components. In these cases, the tumors are often treated primarily based upon the small cell rather than the transitional cell features (see separate section on neuroendocrine tumors of the bladder).

Presentation and Spread of Bladder Cancer

Patients with transitional cell containing urothelial cancers usually present with hematuria, although irritative symptoms from a secondary infection may be an isolated initial complaint. When the tumor has obstructed one or both ureteral orifices, patients may develop aching loin pain; however, the upper urinary tract obstruction is usually clinically silent because of its slow and insidious onset. It should be noted that many patients with hematuria do not have bladder cancer. In one recent study by Bretlau and colleagues, bladder cancers were ultimately detected in 17% of 395 patients with gross (visible) hematuria and in only 4% of 376 patients with microscopic (nonvisible) hematuria.

Urothelial cancers can occur anywhere in the urinary tract where urothelium is present, but they are most commonly found in the bladder because of its proportionately large surface area (compared with that of the renal collecting systems and ureters) and the fact that the bladder acts as a reservoir for urine. Therefore, any carcinogens in the urine are in contact with bladder urothelium longer than they are with other parts of the urinary tract.

Urothelial cancer spreads by invading the bladder wall, first involving the mucosa, then the muscular layer (muscularis propria), and then completely through the bladder wall into the perivesical tissue. Direct extension into adjacent organs, including the prostatic

urethra, seminal vesicles, and vagina, can occur. Spread of tumor may then occur into pelvic lymph nodes. Hematogenous spread can also occur, most frequently to the liver and lungs. Bone metastases, which may be lytic or sclerotic, are found in a small percentage of cases.

Staging and Grading of Bladder Cancer

Bladder cancer is staged using the tumor, nodes, metastases (TNM) staging classifications (Fig. 13.49). The staging system used for urothelial bladder carcinoma reflects the importance of determining the presence and depth of bladder wall penetration. Approximately 70% of all newly diagnosed urothelial bladder cancer is superficial, 20% to 25% is muscle invasive, and the remaining 5% has metastasized locally, regionally, or distantly.

Detailed evaluation of the upper tracts is essential in patients with bladder cancer in order to exclude multicentric urothelial lesions in the collecting system and ureters. Synchronous or metachronous lesions of the upper urinary tract can be detected in 2% to 7% of patients with bladder cancer. Conversely, approximately 20% of patients with urothelial cancer of the upper urinary tract have a history of bladder tumor.

Cellular grading of bladder cancer is a histologic assessment of the degree of cellular atypia, which predicts tumor aggressiveness. Bladder cancers are usually categorized as belonging to one of two grades: (1) low-grade or well-differentiated tumors or (2) high-grade or poorly differentiated tumors. Grading of bladder carcinoma correlates with staging: High-grade lesions are much more likely to invade into muscle than low-grade lesions.

Both staging and grading are considered in the management of bladder carcinoma. Low-grade and low-stage (Ta, Tis, and T1) bladder cancers are usually managed by local resection. Stage T2 cancers generally require cystectomy. Carcinoma in situ (stage Tis) cancers are more commonly of higher grade than are Ta tumors and are more likely to progress to become invasive.

While cystoscopy remains the gold standard for evaluating the bladder of patients with hematuria, a number of imaging modalities are also used in patients with known or suspected bladder cancer.

Imaging: Abdominal Radiography, Cystography, and Ultrasonography of Bladder Cancer

Plain abdominal radiographs are seldom helpful in imaging bladder cancers. The plain film is usually normal. Stippled or floccular dystrophic calcifications are seen on plain films in bladder cancers

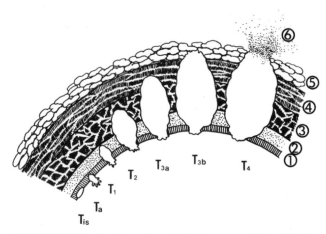

FIGURE 13.49. Staging of urothelial cancer of the bladder using the TNM system. Layers of the bladder wall are as follows: (1) mucosa, (2) submucosa, (3) superficial muscle, (4) deep muscle, (5) perivesical fat, and (6) denoting adjacent organs or distant metastases. (Adapted from Amis ES Jr, Newhouse JH. *Essentials of Uroradiology*. Boston, MA: Little, Brown and Company; 1991:300.)

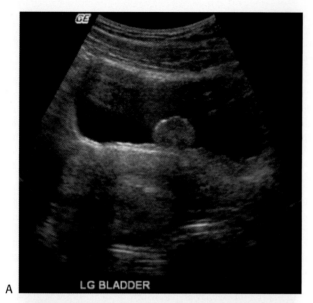

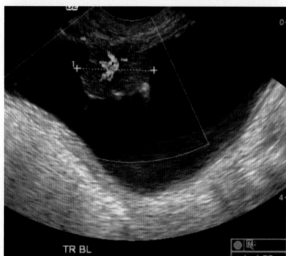

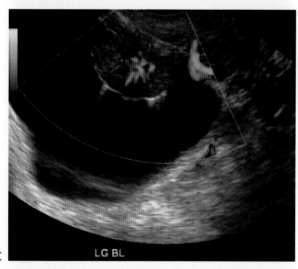

FIGURE 13.50. Urothelial cancer. **A:** A longitudinal image through the bladder demonstrates a small mass protruding into the bladder lumen. **B:** Color Doppler sagittal and **(C)** power Doppler longitudinal images through the lesion demonstrate increased vascularity.

in <1% of cases. Furthermore, such tumor calcification, when present, is much better appreciated on CT. Cystography is insensitive in detecting bladder cancers. When the bladder is filled, its wall is usually well visualized with suprapubic ultrasound. In this setting, an exophytic urothelial bladder cancer may be seen as a soft tissue mass projecting into the lumen from the bladder wall. Bladder cancers may also demonstrate increased vascularity on color Doppler or power Doppler images (Fig. 13.50). Ultrasound has shown little value in the staging of bladder cancer.

Computed Tomography of Bladder Cancer

CT and CT urography have shown excellent sensitivity in detecting bladder cancers. While it was previously thought that CT urographic images obtained during the excretory phase were most sensitive in detecting urothelial neoplasms, recent studies have demonstrated that earlier enhanced images (especially those obtained during the corticomedullary or portal venous phase, beginning at about 60 seconds after the initiation of a contrast injection) may be more sensitive. This is because, on early enhanced images, most urothelial tumors demonstrate brisk enhancement when compared to normal urothelium (Fig. 13.51). On CT, bladder cancers most commonly appear as areas of asymmetric hyperenhancing bladder wall

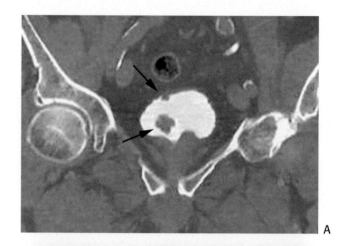

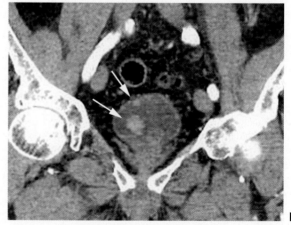

FIGURE 13.51. Two enhancing bladder cancers. **A:** An excretory phase contrast-enhanced coronal reformatted CT image shows two bladder masses, a smaller lesion projecting into the lumen from the superior wall and a larger polypoid lesion located more caudally (*arrows*). **B:** Both masses enhance on the earlier enhanced portal venous–phase images (*arrows*). The degree of enhancement is greater than that of the normal bladder wall.

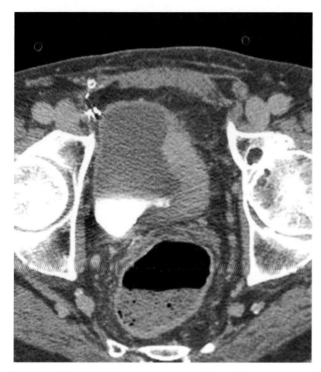

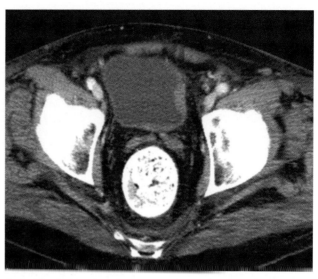

FIGURE 13.53. Bladder cancer presenting with mild asymmetric wall thickening. Portal venous–phase contrast-enhanced axial CT image demonstrates an area of mild wall thickening along the left lateral aspect of the bladder, subsequently confirmed to represent a bladder cancer.

FIGURE 13.52. Bladder cancer presenting with pronounced asymmetric wall thickening. Excretory phase contrast-enhanced axial image from a CT urogram shows a large area of asymmetric wall thickening along the left lateral aspect of the bladder.

thickening. This thickening can be quite pronounced, with masslike areas projecting into the bladder lumen (Fig. 13.52) or it can be mild (Fig. 13.53). Some bladder cancers can be detected on CT when they are quite small. The smaller detected bladder malignancies tend to

be of the papillary type, appearing as tiny filling defects projecting into the bladder lumen (Fig. 13.54). Sometimes, the abnormally increased enhancement of bladder cancers permits their identification on early enhanced images, even when the tumors cannot be seen on the delayed enhanced images (Fig. 13.55). Only rarely does bladder cancer produce diffuse bladder wall thickening (Fig. 13.56), a finding much more suggestive of inflammation/cystitis, neurogenic bladders, or bladder outlet obstruction. On CT urography, the bladder cancers most likely to escape detection are those that are small and flat (carcinoma in situ) and those located at the bladder

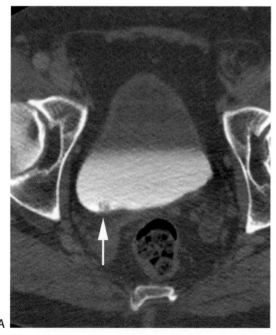

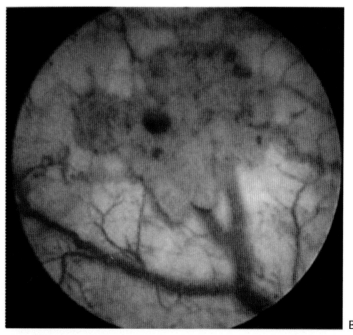

FIGURE 13.54. Bladder cancer presenting as a tiny papillary projection/filling defect. **A:** Excretory phase contrast-enhanced axial image from a CT urogram demonstrates a small irregular mass projecting into the bladder lumen from the right posterior wall (*arrow*). **B:** This was confirmed to represent a papillary cancer at cystoscopy.

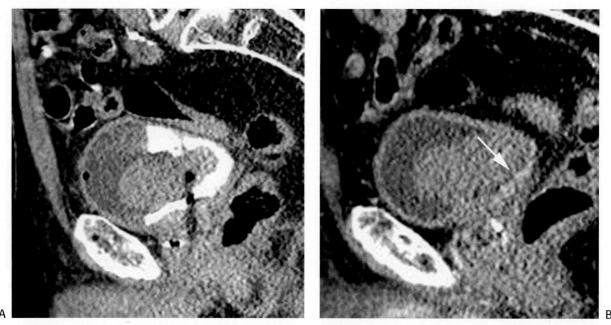

A   B

FIGURE 13.55. Flat bladder cancer with abnormal bladder wall enhancement. **A:** Excretory phase contrast-enhanced sagittal reformatted image demonstrates only a small amount of excreted contrast material in the bladder lumen. Most of the bladder lumen contains blood clot. The urothelial neoplasm cannot be detected. **B:** Corticomedullary phase contrast-enhanced sagittal reformatted image obtained 10 minutes earlier reveals a flat tumor along the posterior wall of the bladder, which is detectable only by its asymmetrically increased enhancement (*arrow*).

base, where volume averaging from adjacent structures, such as the prostate gland, can prevent their recognition.

CT can also be used to assist in the staging of bladder cancer; however, its utility for doing so is limited in the absence of grossly obvious tumor extension. CT cannot determine whether the muscularis propria has been invaded (a feature that distinguishes

stage T1 from T2 tumors). Also, perivesical spread of tumor (stage T3 disease) is difficult to detect unless it is gross. Obstruction of the ureteral orifice can occasionally be identified, however, and suggests that the tumors may have invaded the muscle around the involved ureteral orifice (Fig. 13.57). This is a poor prognostic sign.

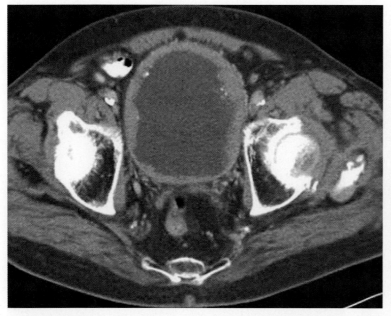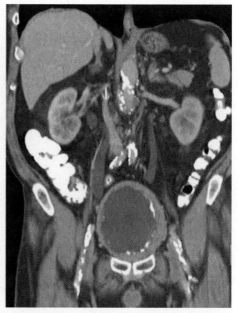

FIGURE 13.56. Bladder cancer producing circumferential wall thickening. Corticomedullary phase contrast-enhanced axial and coronal reformatted CT image demonstrates diffuse lobulated circumferential wall thickening of the bladder, corresponding to a large infiltrative bladder malignancy. Calcifications, which can be seen in some bladder cancers, are noted along the bladder wall surface.

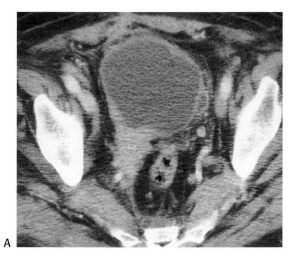

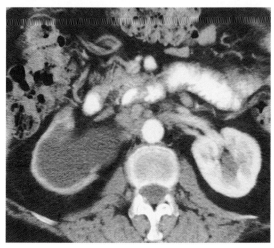

FIGURE 13.57. Bladder cancer obstructing the right ureteral orifice. **A:** A corticomedullary phase contrast-enhanced axial CT image shows a tumor in the right posterolateral aspect of the bladder, involving the right ureterovesical junction. **B:** An axial image obtained at the level of the kidneys demonstrates marked right pelvocaliectasis as a result of the distal ureteral obstruction.

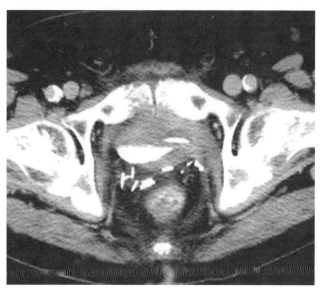

FIGURE 13.59. Urothelial cancer spread to pelvic sidewall. Excretory phase axial CT image through the bladder base shows increased soft tissue along the left bladder wall, representing a bladder cancer. Fat planes between the tumor and the left pelvic sidewall are obliterated indicating gross invasion by tumor. This was locally advanced (stage T4) disease at surgery.

Increased stranding in the perivesical space can be due to either infiltrative tumor or edema (Fig. 13.58). CT can detect pelvic sidewall invasion (stage T4 disease), however, when the fat between the bladder and the pelvic sidewall is obliterated (Fig. 13.59). This is a feature that makes the bladder cancer unresectable. Unfortunately, in some cases, such invasion can be subtle and easily missed (Fig. 13.60).

In recent studies, it has been found that local CT staging of bladder cancer is correct about half the time. Tumors are understaged or overstaged approximately one-quarter of the time.

As previously mentioned, it should be remembered that tumors in bladder diverticula are locally staged differently than those in the bladder itself. Since most bladder diverticula are pseudodiverticula and do not contain a muscular layer, a stage T2 tumor cannot occur in an acquired/pseudodiverticulum.

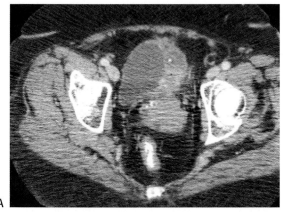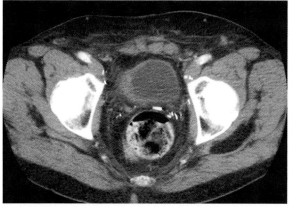

FIGURE 13.58. CT for staging of bladder cancer. Corticomedullary phase contrast-enhanced axial CT images in two different patients. **A:** In the first patient, a large mass is noted along the left lateral bladder wall. There is increased perivesical stranding adjacent to the tumor. At surgery, the stranding was confirmed to represent perivesical tumor (stage T3b disease). **B:** In the second patient, a mass is noted along the right lateral bladder wall. There is increased perivesical stranding adjacent to the tumor, which is quite similar to that noted in the first patient. At surgery, this was confirmed to represent only T2b cancer, with the perivesical stranding due to edema. These two cases show the difficulty that CT may have in local staging of bladder cancer.

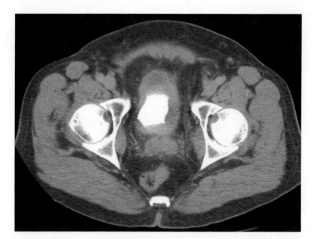

FIGURE 13.60. Urothelial cancer spread to pelvic sidewall. Excretory phase axial CT urographic image shows a large bladder cancer as marked thickening of the bladder wall on the left and posteriorly. There is increased stranding in the left perivesical space; however, much of the perivesical fat is preserved. The tumor was found to be fixed to the left pelvic sidewall (stage T4) at surgery. This case illustrates that CT is effective only in locally staging bladder cancers when obvious tumor spread is detected.

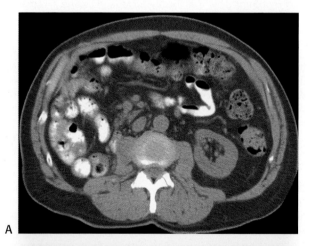

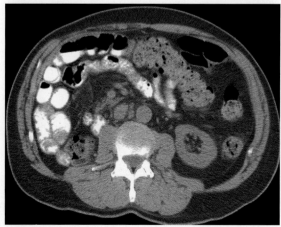

FIGURE 13.61. Lymph node metastases from bladder cancer. **A:** Initial unenhanced axial CT image shows two normal-sized aortocaval lymph nodes in this patient with bladder cancer, who has already had a right nephrectomy for an upper tract lesion. **B:** Two months later, these lymph nodes have enlarged considerably, although they are still normal in size.

CT of the abdomen can be used to assess patients for para-aortic lymph node enlargement and for other sites of regional and distant tumor spread. Bladder cancer usually spreads first to pelvic lymph nodes and then to para-aortic retroperitoneal lymph nodes. When involved lymph nodes are enlarged, CT detection is possible; however, normal-sized lymph nodes may also contain tumor. Thus, as is the case with local staging, lymph node assessment by CT is somewhat limited (Fig. 13.61). Nonetheless, CT has been used to determine the extent of lymph node dissection to be performed at surgery. It has been found that patients with low CT T-stage disease (of T2a or less) are very unlikely at surgery to have positive lymph nodes above the level of the common iliac artery bifurcation. Other sites of metastatic disease can also be detected with CT, including metastases in the liver, lungs, and bones (where either lytic or sclerotic lesions may be produced).

Locally aggressive and metastatic spread of bladder cancer is more commonly seen in patients who have urothelial cancers with atypical histologic features or divergent histologies (with other elements in addition to transitional cells or unusual growth patterns being present). In particular, omental and peritoneal spread of tumor is much more common in these mixed-cell–type subgroups (Fig. 13.62).

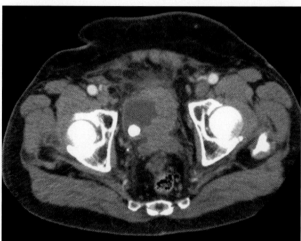

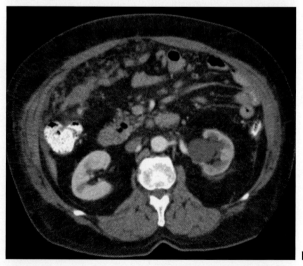

FIGURE 13.62. Urothelial cancer with atypical histologic features. **A:** Corticomedullary phase contrast-enhanced axial CT image demonstrates a large mass along the left lateral aspect of the bladder. Extensive anterior perivesical stranding extends to the anterior abdominal wall. **B:** On a more cephalad image obtained during the same scan, multiple omental nodules are noted. The urothelial cancer had a 40% nested growth pattern.

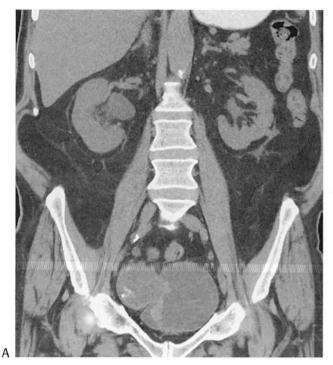
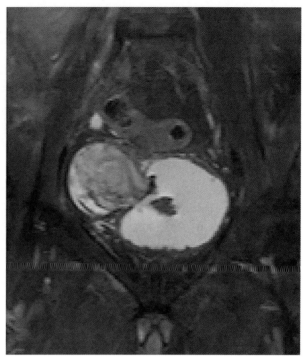

A   B

FIGURE 13.63. Urothelial cancer in a bladder diverticulum. **A:** A noncontrast coronal reformatted CT image shows a large right bladder diverticulum with areas of high attenuation within it (calcification on tumor surface) and in the bladder lumen near the orifice of the diverticulum (clot). **B:** A coronal T2-weighted MRI of bladder clearly shows the large, medium signal intensity mass within the diverticulum extending through the orifice of the diverticulum, as well as lower signal intensity blood clot in the bladder lumen.

Urothelial cancer can be found growing within a bladder diverticulum and even filling its lumen. These tumors can obstruct the orifice of the diverticulum or grow through it into the bladder lumen. Any mural abnormality in a diverticulum during CT scanning should prompt further evaluation for tumor (Fig. 13.63).

Magnetic Resonance Imaging of Bladder Cancer

MRI is able to detect bladder cancer with high sensitivity. Bladder cancers may produce focal asymmetric areas of bladder wall thickening (Fig. 13.64), masslike areas projecting into the lumen (Fig. 13.65), or areas of abnormal hyperenhancement with gadolinium-based contrast material (Fig. 13.66). Recently, a few studies have demonstrated that many bladder cancers can be easily distinguished from normal urothelium on diffusion-weighted MR images, as water molecules in these neoplasms have more restricted diffusion than do water molecules in normal urothelium.

MRI may be able to distinguish high-grade from low-grade bladder tumors, particularly when diffusion-weighted MRI images are obtained. Most high-grade tumors have larger diameters and lower apparent diffusion coefficients than do low-grade tumors. Newer studies have also attempted to assess the ability of other MRI metrics in determining bladder cancer aggressiveness, including changes in region of interest measurement distributions as determined by computer analysis (particularly of skew and kurtosis). To date, there are some promising results, but more work is needed.

The accuracy of MRI for staging of bladder cancer has been assessed in many preliminary studies and has been found to be superior to that of CT. Specifically, MRI has been found to be more accurate than CT in distinguishing bladder cancer, which can be treated topically (stage T1 or less) from that, which requires surgery (stage T2 or more). This is because, unlike CT, MRI is better able

to determine the depth of bladder wall invasion. With superficial noninvasive tumors (stage T1 or less), there is usually preservation of the low signal intensity stripe surrounding the bladder lumen on T2-weighted images, with this stripe including the muscular layer (muscularis propria) of the bladder wall.

The absence of this low-intensity stripe strongly suggests invasion of the bladder wall, including the muscularis propria,

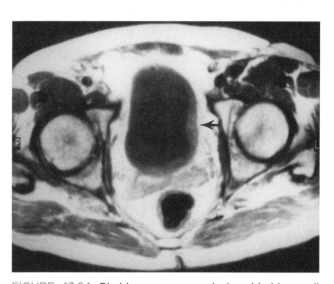

FIGURE 13.64. Bladder cancer producing bladder wall thickening. A T1-weighted axial MRI image shows a left-sided bladder wall mass (*arrow*) extending to the posterior bladder wall.

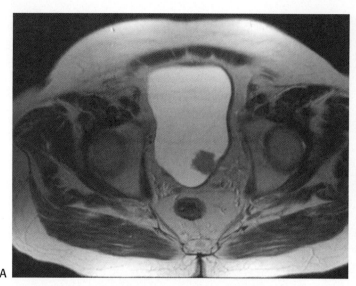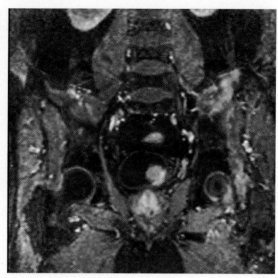

A   B

FIGURE 13.65. Bladder cancer as a papillary mass. **A:** A small papillary neoplasm is easily detected as a filling defect on a T2-weighted unenhanced axial MRI image. **B:** The neoplasm demonstrates brisk enhancement on a subsequent gadolinium-based contrast material–enhanced T1-weighted fat-saturation coronal image.

indicating that at least stage T2 disease is present (Fig. 13.67). Other MRI sequences that have shown promise determining the presence or depth of muscle invasion are diffusion-weighted imaging (where depth of the high signal intensity of the abnormal tumor can be assessed in relation to the lower signal intensity of the bladder wall) and gadolinium-based contrast material–enhanced imaging (where the tumor is readily identified due to its increased enhancement). It is likely that a combination of all of these MR techniques together

FIGURE 13.66. Bladder cancer detectable by its increased enhancement. A flat urothelial cancer could be detected at the left bladder base only on this gadolinium-based contrast material-enhanced T1-weighted fat-saturated coronal MR image, due to its asymmetrically increased enhancement. The cancer is producing minimal, if any, bladder wall thickening.

(now termed multiparametric MRI) is most accurate, with accuracies exceeding 90% in some series.

Preliminary studies have demonstrated that it might be possible to utilize CT or to predict the likelihood of response or the degree of response of bladder cancer and its metastases to subsequent radiation or chemotherapy (based upon initial evaluation of tumor vascularity and diffusion characteristics).

As is the case with CT, MRI can also clearly depict tumors arising within bladder diverticula. Since most bladder diverticula do not have muscularis propria, tumors in bladder diverticula would progress from T1 directly to T3 disease (Fig. 13.63). There is no local stage T2 cancer in most bladder diverticula. As is the case with CT, MRI cannot detect microscopic perivesical spread of tumor.

Positron Emission Tomography of Bladder Cancer

18 fluorodeoxyglucose (FDG)–positron emission tomography (PET) is not used widely for imaging of patients with suspected or known bladder cancer. This is because this radioisotope is excreted normally in the urine and accumulates in the renal collecting systems and bladder. As a result, normal increased bladder activity can obscure detection of bladder cancers, most of which are FDG-avid (Fig. 13.68). In response, many imagers choose to dilute the urine by administering a diuretic at the time of image acquisition.

FDG-PET has been utilized successfully in some patients to detect metastatic disease. Identification of individual lymph node metastases with FDG-PET is superior to CT but is still poor, with high false-negative rates. In contrast, when FDG-avid abnormalities are present, they are very likely to represent tumor. The positive predictive value of FDG-PET is high, at 90% or more.

A number of recent studies have evaluated the utility of newer radiotracers that are not excreted into the urinary tract in patients with bladder cancer. These agents would be preferred over FDG because they would not accumulate in the urine and interfere with image interpretation. Results with C-11 choline or C-11 methionine for PET/CT have been promising but are still preliminary. It remains to be seen whether PET with these or other new radiotracers will have a beneficial effect upon patient survival.

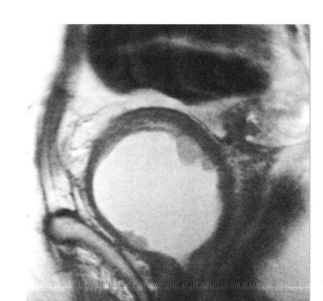
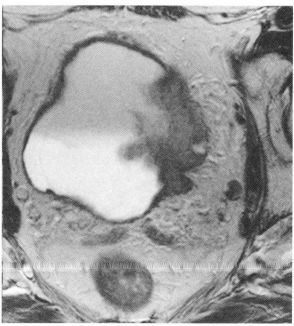

A   B

FIGURE 13.67. Bladder cancer invading the muscularis propria. **A:** A T2-weighted image of the bladder shows multifocal urothelial cancer. There is no disruption of the low-signal intensity stripe, indicating that the bladder wall is intact. **B:** A T2-weighted image of a bladder in another patient showing a large sessile and polypoid urothelial neoplasm. There is disruption of the low signal intensity muscular stripe, indicating that this tumor is muscle invasive. (Cases courtesy of Dr. Jelle Barentsz.)

Treatment of Primary Bladder Cancers

Bladder cancer treatment depends upon the stage and grade of the bladder tumor at the time of detection. Bladder cancers that do not invade the muscle (superficial tumors) may be treated with transurethral resection followed by intravesical instillation of bacillus Calmette–Guerin (BCG) or another topical agent (mitomycin). Many initially superficial bladder tumors recur after treatment, with some of these recurrences being understaged when they are detected. Specifically, bladder wall invasion can be missed in recurrent bladder cancer after topical treatment. Stage T1 tumors and carcinoma in situ (flat tumors) and patients with high-grade

tumors are more likely to develop invasive recurrences, with about half of these having progressed when detected.

Patients with muscle invasive (stage T2) tumors are treated with cystectomy and lymph node dissection (radical cystectomy). Some type of urinary diversion is necessary, an ileal loop with urine drainage to the skin, a continent diversion, or an orthotopic neobladder (see section on Urinary Diversions). Bladder-sparing surgery is performed in some centers but is not widely accepted. Since only about 50% of bladder cancer patients survive 5 years after cystectomy, many patients now receive neoadjuvant chemotherapy prior to surgery, in an attempt to eliminate micrometastatic disease that cannot be detected on imaging studies.

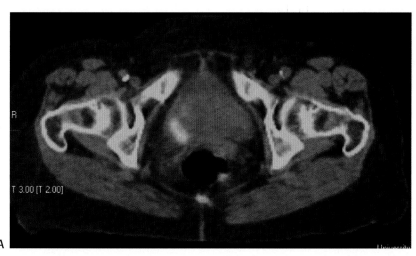
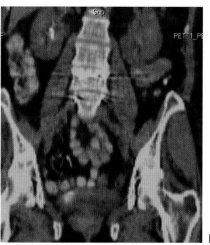

A   B

FIGURE 13.68. Bladder cancer. Axial **(A)** and coronal **(B)** CT/FDG-PET fusion images demonstrate increased FDG uptake in a right-sided bladder cancer. The tumor can be detected even though there is radiotracer in the excreted urine in the bladder lumen.

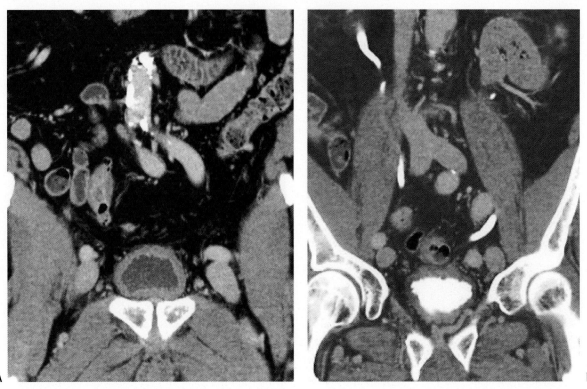

FIGURE 13.69. Bladder wall thickening after treatment of bladder cancer with transurethral resection and BCG. Corticomedullary phase **(A)** and excretory phase **(B)** contrast-enhanced coronal reformatted images from a CT urogram show diffuse circumferential bladder wall thickening due to inflammation. It is difficult to detect recurrent tumors in the setting of such extensive bladder wall thickening. No tumor was found at cystoscopy.

Bladder cancer patients who present with regionally invasive or metastatic disease are treated with chemotherapy. This can be done as neoadjuvant therapy (in patients with T3 disease) or in lieu of surgery (in patients with lymph node involvement or distant metastatic disease). The two first-line chemotherapy regimens that have been shown to prolong survival are MVAC (methotrexate, vinblastine, Adriamycin, and cisplatin) and gemcitabine with cisplatin.

Patients with bladder cancer must be followed for life, since they are at increased risk for developing other urothelial neoplasms and can also develop metastatic disease from their primary cancer. In general, recurrent disease appears in the pelvis in up to 15% of bladder cancer patients within 2 years of cystectomy. Distant metastatic disease, if it will develop after cystectomy, is usually encountered within 2 years, as well with the most commonly affected sites being the lungs, liver, and bones. Treatment of metastatic disease is with chemotherapy.

Imaging After Treatment of Bladder Cancers

CT is often utilized in following bladder cancer patients after topical treatment (transurethral resection and/or bladder instillation of BCG or mitomycin) or after radical cystectomy. Since identification of residual or recurrent bladder tumors can be difficult at cystoscopy in patients treated with transurethral resection and local therapy (due to the development of inflammatory and fibrotic changes in the bladder mucosa), it is not surprising that CT also has difficulty distinguishing benign from malignant changes (Fig. 13.69). It has recently been suggested that corticomedullary phase contrast-enhanced CT may distinguish tumor from inflammation or fibrosis better than excretory phase imaging because tumor tends to enhance to a greater extent than does fibrosis soon after contrast material administration.

As with CT, MRI distinction between inflammation/fibrosis and recurrent tumor in patients who have received topical treatment for noninvasive bladder tumors may be difficult. Both inflammation/fibrosis and recurrent tumor may produce asymmetric areas of bladder wall thickening and abnormal enhancement (Fig. 13.70); however, residual or recurrent tumor tends more often to demonstrate greater restricted diffusion and a greater degree and rate of contrast

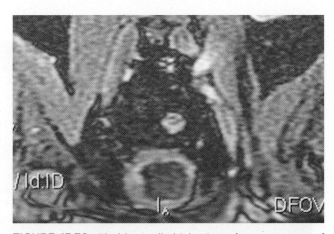

FIGURE 13.70. Bladder wall thickening after treatment of bladder cancer with transurethral resection and BCG. A gadolinium-enhanced T1-weighted, fat-saturated coronal image in a patient who had received topical therapy for bladder cancer shows irregular circumferential bladder wall thickening, with areas of increased enhancement most pronounced at the dome. No tumor was found at cystoscopy.

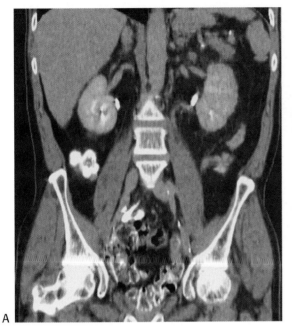 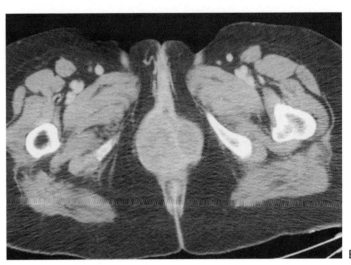

A   B

FIGURE 13.71. Recurrent bladder cancer after cystectomy. **A:** A contrast-enhanced coronal reformatted CT image in a female patient shows the sigmoid colon in the bladder fossa in this patient who has had a cystectomy. **B:** An axial image obtained below the level of the pubic symphysis shows a soft tissue mass in the region of the vulva, which proved to be recurrent tumor.

enhancement than does inflammation or fibrosis. Multifocal abnormalities and masses demonstrating a papillary or frondlike appearance are also more likely to be tumors. Most recurrences that are missed during MRI are low-grade and noninvasive tumors.

Approximately one-third of recurrences following radical cystectomy are at or near the cystectomy site, and two-thirds are in pelvic lymph nodes. CT in such patients not only should include the upper abdomen to evaluate the liver for metastases but also should extend to the deep perineum because this is a common area for recurrence (Fig. 13.71).

Follow-up CT or MR urography is often performed to assess patients who have been treated for bladder cancer for upper tract urothelial cancers, as the incidence of such cancers is increased 2% to 7% in bladder cancer patients. In a recent study, by Sternberg and colleagues, 5.5% of patients with noninvasive bladder cancers developed upper tract cancers within 6 years.

Other Malignant Bladder Neoplasms

Neuroendocrine Carcinomas, Small Cell Cancers, and Paragangliomas

Neuroendocrine tumors include small cell and large cell tumors, carcinoid tumors, and paragangliomas. Although some neuroendocrine tumors may also contain transitional cells, all of these tumors are generally classified within the neuroendocrine group, as the neuroendocrine components have a profound effect on behavior, prognosis, and recommended treatment. In general, small or large cell bladder cancers tend to present as large masses. Extravesical extension and metastatic disease is often detected on imaging studies. Thus, when large aggressive-appearing bladder masses are identified on CT or MRI, the differential diagnosis should include a bladder cancer with atypical histology, including a neuroendocrine tumor.

Paragangliomas are rare neuroendocrine tumors that may arise from chromaffin cells of the sympathetic plexus in or near the bladder wall. Most are found near the trigone. A slight female predilection is reported. While most bladder wall

paragangliomas are benign, up to 30% to 40% have been found to be malignant.

Many patients with bladder paragangliomas are hypertensive. Affected patients may also have characteristic attacks of palpitations, sweating, headache, and blurred vision on micturition. The diagnosis should be suspected by this classic history and can be confirmed by measuring serum catecholamine levels.

Bladder wall paragangliomas produce intramural soft tissue masses on ultrasound, CT, or MRI. Imaging distinction from more common urothelial cancers of bladder is often impossible (Figs. 13.72

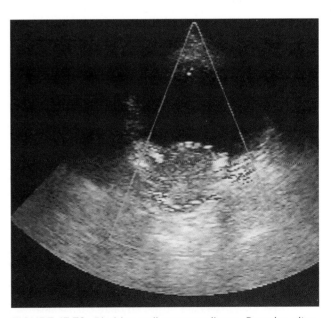

FIGURE 13.72. Bladder wall paraganglioma. Doppler ultrasound shows a vascular mass at the bladder trigone.

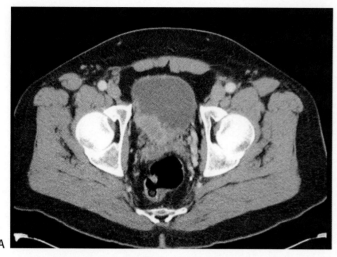
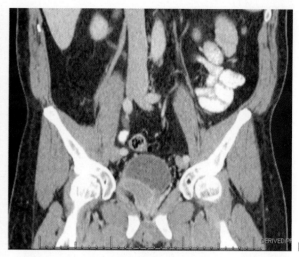

FIGURE 13.73. Bladder wall paraganglioma. Contrast-enhanced axial **(A)** and coronal **(B)** CT images demonstrate an irregular ovoid soft tissue mass along the right posterior aspect of the bladder. This was confirmed to represent a bladder wall paraganglioma. Urothelial cancer could have the same appearance.

and 13.73). However, when small, these masses are often homogeneous and demonstrate brisk enhancement after contrast material administration. Some paragangliomas have a very high signal intensity on T2-weighted MR images. Larger tumors are more likely to be heterogeneous. Calcification may be present. Benign and malignant paragangliomas cannot be distinguished from one another based upon mass imaging characteristics, although the presence of adjacent organ invasion or regional or distant metastatic disease should suggest malignancy (Fig. 13.74).

Pure Squamous Cell Carcinomas

The term squamous cell carcinoma is now reserved for patients who have bladder cancers composed entirely of squamous cells, a histology encountered in about 6% to 8% of patients with bladder cancer. Most patients with pure squamous cell carcinomas have

a history of chronic or recurrent bladder infections, bladder calculi, or both. The incidence of squamous cell tumors is higher in bladder diverticula than in the bladder lumen, probably because stasis and infection are more common in diverticula. Patients with schistosomiasis are also at increased risk for squamous cell tumors.

Squamous cell carcinomas are multifocal in 25% of patients and tend to be poorly differentiated and invasive. The 5-year survival rate for these patients is a dismal 10%. Radiographically, squamous cell carcinoma cannot be differentiated from other bulky urothelial tumors (Fig. 13.75). Due to their propensity to develop in areas of chronic infection and stasis, squamous cell carcinoma should be considered in patients who are predisposed to these conditions and who develop large bladder masses (Figs. 13.76 and 13.77).

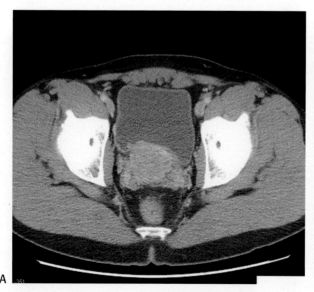
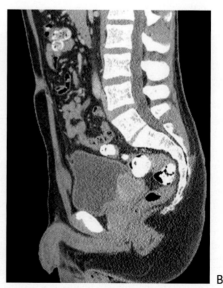

FIGURE 13.74. Bladder wall paraganglioma. Contrast-enhanced axial **(A)** and sagittal **(B)** CT images through the pelvis show a large lobulated mass along the posterior aspect of the bladder. The mass can be seen extending posteriorly into the seminal vesicles. This was found to be a locally invasive malignant paraganglioma.

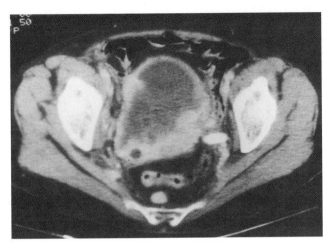

FIGURE 13.75. Bladder squamous cell carcinoma. A contrast-enhanced axial CT image shows irregular thickening of the left posterolateral bladder wall. There is a second focus of tumor on the right, anteriorly. The diffuse nature of the tumor suggests an atypical histology.

Pure Adenocarcinomas

The term adenocarcinoma is now reserved for bladder cancers that are composed exclusively of adenomatous cells. Although pure bladder adenocarcinoma can be an isolated finding, this tumor is typically associated with metaplastic change in patients with bladder exstrophy (Fig. 13.78). It is also seen in patients with cystitis glandularis and in urachal remnants.

Urachal Carcinomas

The urachus is a musculofibrous band 5 to 6 cm long extending from the umbilicus to the anterosuperior surface of the bladder (Fig. 13.79). It lies in the extraperitoneal space of Retzius, between the transversalis fascia anteriorly and the peritoneum posteriorly, and represents a vestigial remnant of the obliterated umbilical arteries and the allantois. It retains a minute lumen lined by transitional epithelium in 70% of adults.

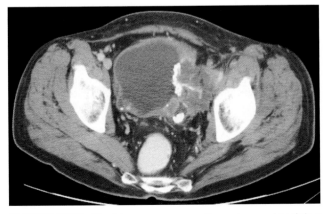

FIGURE 13.76. Bladder squamous cell carcinoma involving a bladder diverticulum. A contrast-enhanced axial CT image shows a tumor arising in a diverticulum from the left lateral wall of the bladder. There are stones in the most dependent portion of the diverticulum, and calcification is present on the tumor surface, where it protrudes into the bladder lumen.

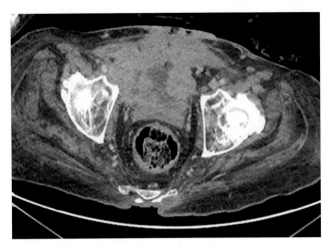

FIGURE 13.77. Bladder squamous cell carcinoma in a patient with a neurogenic bladder. A contrast-enhanced axial CT image in a paraplegic patient with a long-standing history of urinary tract infections demonstrates a large multilobulated mass along the anterior and lateral aspects of the bladder, which extends directly into the anterior abdominal wall. This was an aggressive and extensively invasive squamous cell carcinoma.

The transitional epithelium lining the urachus may undergo metaplasia to glandular epithelium that can produce mucin. Consequently, malignant change can occur in urachal epithelium, with mucin-producing adenocarcinomas most commonly developing (approximately 70%), followed by non–mucin-producing adenocarcinomas (15%), transitional cell carcinomas, squamous cell carcinomas, or sarcomas. Squamous cell carcinomas are also occasionally associated with urachal cysts and calculi in urachal diverticula. About 70% of urachal sarcomas occur in patients younger than 20 years. Urachal carcinomas may occur at any age, but most develop in patients between 40 and 70 years of age. Sixty-five percent of urachal carcinomas occur in male patients, with 90% being juxtavesical rather than being located elsewhere along the course of the urachus.

Patients with urachal carcinoma usually present with hematuria. Mucus is found in the urine in 25% of patients and is strongly suggestive of the diagnosis. Abdominal pain, a lower abdominal palpable mass, and dysuria are also presenting symptoms. An umbilical discharge is rare. Urachal carcinoma may invade the bladder. It is visible cystoscopically in the bladder dome in the large majority of cases.

Imaging can often suggest the diagnosis of urachal cancers. Calcification is common but may be difficult to detect on plain abdominal radiographs. The calcification may be stippled, granular, or curvilinear. Ultrasound may show a complex cystic and solid mass at the dome of the bladder in the midline. CT and MRI are most likely to assist in making a definite preoperative diagnosis, by demonstrating the extravesical location and extent of the tumor. Calcification, which has been reported in 70% of patients, is easily seen on CT. Demonstration of a midline mass immediately cephalad to the anterior aspect of the bladder is highly suggestive of urachal carcinoma (Fig. 13.80). The mass may invade the bladder or extend anterosuperiorly to the umbilicus or both.

The prognosis of patients with urachal carcinoma is poor, with a 5-year survival rate of <15%. The poor prognosis is due to the late

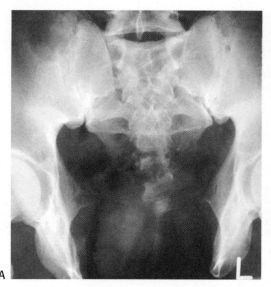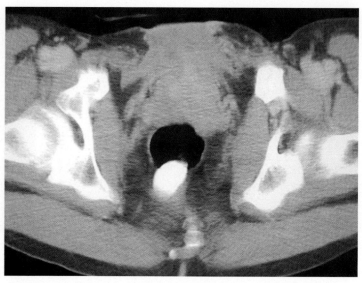

A B

FIGURE 13.78. Adenocarcinoma in a patient with bladder exstrophy. **A:** An anteroposterior abdominal film demonstrates pronounced diastasis of the symphysis pubis. **B:** A contrast-enhanced axial CT image shows extensive soft tissue in the bladder fossa, which extends to the anterior abdominal wall. This tissue corresponds to a large adenocarcinoma.

presentation of symptoms, early local infiltration/invasion, and the early development of lung and bone metastases.

Malignant Mesenchymal Tumors of Bladder Muscle

Malignant mesenchymal tumors of the bladder wall are rare, with the most common being rhabdomyosarcomas and

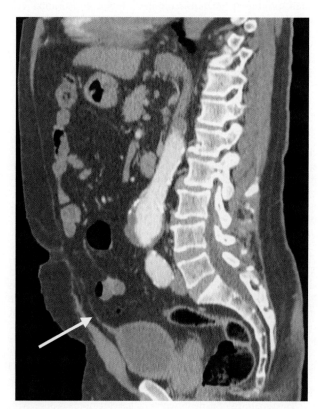

FIGURE 13.79. Urachal remnant. Contrast-enhanced sagittal CT image shows a fibrous cord extending from anterior bladder dome toward the umbilicus (*arrow*).

leiomyosarcomas. Rhabdomyosarcomas have a biphasic age distribution. The embryonal variant of rhabdomyosarcoma occurs during the first few years of life and is quite similar to the rhabdomyosarcoma that arises from the prostate in boys and from the vagina in girls. In fact, it is often very difficult to detect the organ of origin for a rhabdomyosarcoma. The tumors frequently have a lobulated appearance resembling a cluster of grapes, resulting in the term "sarcoma botryoides." Patients with these highly malignant tumors have poor survival rates, even after radical extirpative surgery. Rhabdomyosarcomas and leiomyosarcomas are both seen in older adult patients and tend to be quite large at presentation.

On imaging studies, mesenchymal malignancies of the bladder are usually large, irregular, ulcerating bladder wall masses, unlike the smooth masses that typify benign mesenchymal lesions. They are often heterogeneous, containing areas of low attenuation, corresponding to regions of necrosis. These tumors may grow so large that they almost completely fill the bladder. In most cases, imaging differentiation from other aggressive bladder malignancies is not possible (Fig. 13.81), although a botryoid (cluster of grapes) appearance of a bladder tumor is suggestive of rhabdomyosarcoma. In some cases, extension through the bladder wall into adjacent pelvic organs may even make it difficult, if not impossible, to determine the organ of origin (Fig. 13.82). Biopsy is needed to establish the diagnosis.

Primary lymphoma involving the bladder is rare. When arising in the bladder, lymphoma can appear as a mural-based mass, often in the region of the bladder base, or as lobulated bladder wall thickening (Fig. 13.83). Bladder lymphoma cannot be distinguished from other metaplastic or malignant lesions of the bladder on imaging studies or by gross inspection.

Some aggressive bladder tumors exhibit both sarcomatous and carcinomatous elements and are termed *carcinosarcomas*.

Secondary Bladder Malignancies

Metastases to the bladder constitute only approximately 1% of all malignant bladder lesions. The bladder is involved in only 3% to 4% of patients with terminal carcinomatosis. It is most common for the bladder to be secondarily involved by tumor by direct extension from adjacent pelvic organs, such as prostate,

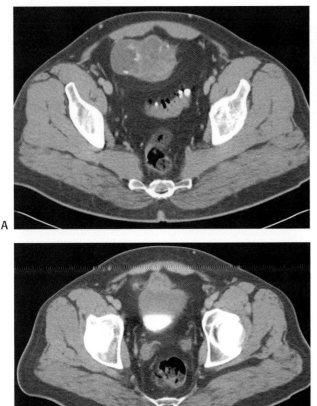

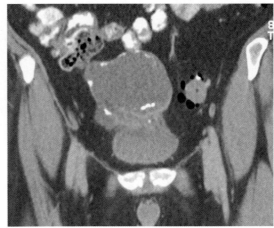

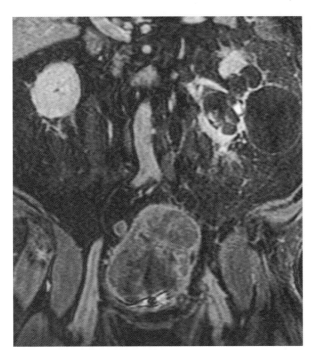

FIGURE 13.80. Urachal cancer. Contrast-enhanced axial **(A, B)** and coronal reformatted **(C)** CT images in a patient with urachal carcinoma demonstrate a complex cystic mass at the anterior aspect of the dome of the bladder. The mass contains areas of fluid and soft tissue attenuation and characteristic foci of calcification.

sigmoid, and cervical cancers. Less frequently, hematogenous seeding of the bladder may occur. The most common secondary tumor to affect the bladder in this fashion is melanoma; however, hematogenous metastases from other malignancies can also be encountered, including from carcinomas of the stomach, colon, pancreas, ovary, breast, kidney, and lung. The bladder can also be secondarily involved in patients with lymphoma. On imaging studies, metastases to the bladder are seen as one or more mural masses projecting into the bladder lumen.

FIGURE 13.81. Bladder leiomyosarcoma. Gadolinium-enhanced T1-weighted, fat saturation, coronal MR image shows a large heterogeneous mass completely replacing the bladder, including the bladder lumen, in this elderly patient. This mass cannot be distinguished from other large aggressive bladder neoplasms.

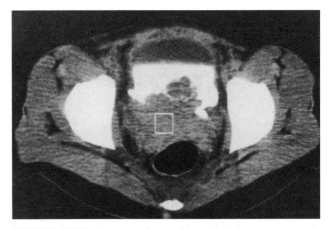

FIGURE 13.82. Sarcoma botryoides (rhabdomyosarcoma). A contrast-enhanced axial CT image shows a large nodular mass in the bladder lumen that also involves the prostate. This was found to arise from the prostate rather than the bladder.

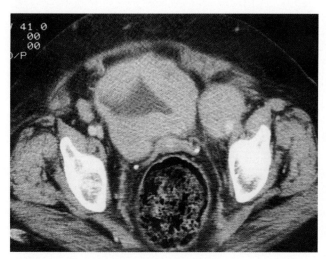

FIGURE 13.83. Lymphoma. A contrast-enhanced axial CT image demonstrates multiple lobulated soft tissue masses in the bladder wall and an enlarged left external iliac lymph node.

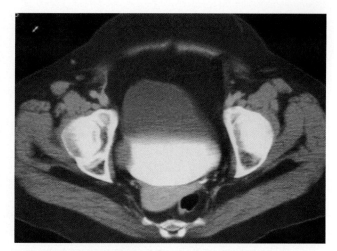

FIGURE 13.84. Bladder leiomyoma. A contrast-enhanced axial CT image through the pelvis demonstrates a small well-defined, smoothly marginated homogeneous mass along the right lateral aspect of the bladder. The mass protrudes slightly into the bladder lumen, although it is also partially exophytic. While the smooth margins of the mass raise the possibility of a bladder leiomyoma, the CT appearance is not diagnostic.

Benign Tumors

Benign bladder tumors are rare, accounting for approximately 1% of bladder neoplasms. The definitive diagnosis is made by biopsy, usually obtained during cystoscopy, and not by radiology, although, on occasion, the correct diagnosis can be suggested on imaging studies. Most benign bladder tumors are mesenchymal in origin and include leiomyomas, neurofibromas, hemangiomas, and pheochromocytomas.

Leiomyomas

Leiomyoma of the bladder is the most common benign bladder tumor. It is usually found in women from 30 to 50 years of age. This lesion usually arises at the trigone but may be found on the lateral or posterior walls. The dome and anterior bladder wall are infrequent sites of involvement. More than 60% of these tumors project intravesically, 30% project extravesically, and the remainder have both intra- and extravesical components. Patients with intravesical leiomyomas commonly present with hematuria and irritative symptoms. Extravesical leiomyomas are usually asymptomatic until they reach a large size, in which case patients will present with a palpable mass.

On imaging studies, an intravesical leiomyoma may be seen as a well-defined mural mass protruding into the bladder lumen. On ultrasound and CT, these lesions appear as soft tissue masses. The smooth nature of the mass can sometimes suggest the correct diagnosis (Fig. 13.84). On MRI, leiomyomas often have low signal intensity on T2-weighted images. They tend to enhance markedly after contrast material administration.

It should be emphasized that whenever a bladder mass is detected on an imaging study, further evaluation with cystoscopy is required. This is because benign lesions cannot be distinguished unequivocally from malignancies in most instances. Owing to the mesenchymal nature of leiomyomas, cystoscopic evaluation will reveal intact urothelium overlying these tumors. Often, there is no urothelial involvement. If there is a large extravesical component, the bladder may be compressed or displaced by the large extrinsic mass. In these cases, it may be difficult to discern that it originates in the bladder wall.

Inverted Papilloma

Inverted papillomas of the bladder are rare urothelial neoplasms comprised of benign urothelial cells. They occur much more commonly in men than women and are usually located in the bladder neck or at the trigone. On imaging studies, these tumors cannot be distinguished from urothelial cancers; however, they usually appear as small polypoid lesions that have a smooth, rather than an irregular papillary, surface. They are most commonly connected to the bladder wall by a stalk.

Fat in the Bladder Wall or Lumen

Rarely, focal fatty masses can be detected in the bladder wall. These are benign lipomas, which are seldom of clinical significance. They have a diagnostic appearance on CT and MRI, due to the presence of macroscopic fat. On CT, they are homogeneous fatty masses, which measure less than −10 HU. On MRI, the masses demonstrate high signal intensity on T1- and T2-weighted images and signal loss on fat-suppressed sequences.

On very rare occasions, a layer of fat can be seen more uniformly within a portion or the entire bladder wall. This finding has little clinical significance and is considered by some to be a normal finding (Fig. 13.85). This should be distinguished from a horizontal linear fat–fluid level within the bladder lumen, a finding which indicates the presence of chyluria (Fig. 13.86). Chyluria, which occurs as a result of an abnormal communication between lymphatics and the urinary tract, is occasionally seen in patients who have had thermal ablations of renal masses or following partial nephrectomy.

URINARY DIVERSIONS

There are several methods for diverting urine from the kidneys above the level of a defunctionalized or surgically absent bladder (Fig. 13.87).

Temporary Diversions

A simple diversion is the end-cutaneous ureterostomy, in which the ureter is transected and the ends brought to the skin. This procedure is rarely used, primarily because ureters that are not

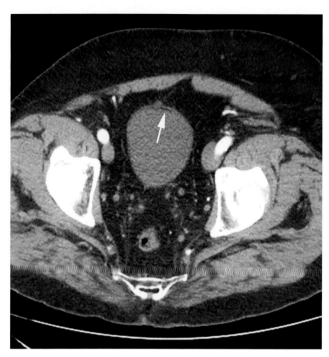

FIGURE 13.85. Benign fat in the bladder wall. An unen-hanced axial CT image demonstrates a thin linear area of fat attenuation within the anterior wall of the bladder (*arrow*). This benign fat, which is of no clinical significance, can be distinguished from chyluria because the interface between the fat and adjacent structures is not a straight horizontal line.

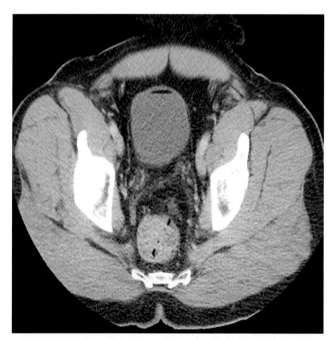

FIGURE 13.86. Chyluria. A contrast-enhanced axial CT image shows a fat–fluid level in the anterior aspect of the bladder lumen. This represents chyluria. The patient had pre-viously had a partial nephrectomy.

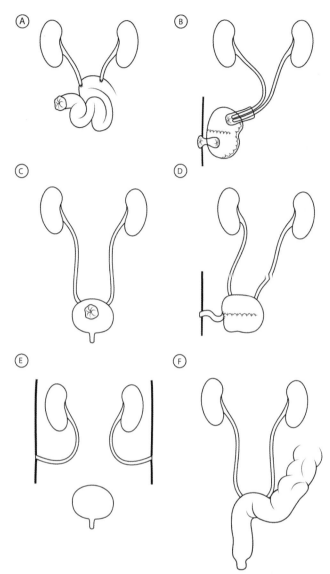

FIGURE 13.87. Types of urinary diversion. **A:** Ileal loop uri-nary diversion (where both ureters are anastomosed to a loop of isolated ileum, which then exits the anterior abdom-inal at an ostomy site). This is a permanent diversion that has been popular since 1950, now most commonly utilized in patients who cannot undergo the more complex urinary diversion procedures. **B:** Continent urinary diversion to ante-rior abdominal wall. The ureters are anastomosed to a tubu-larized loop of small bowel (Kock pouch) or small bowel and colon (Indiana pouch), which is then anastomosed to the anterior abdominal wall via a continent catheteriz-able stoma. **C:** Vesicostomy. An opening is created directly between the bladder and the lower abdominal wall in the midline. **D:** Mitrofanoff technique. The bladder may be aug-mented with a segment of small bowel. The appendix is used as a conduit between the anterior aspect of the augmented bladder and the anterior abdominal wall. **E:** End-cutaneous ureterostomies. These are uncommonly used as they are difficult to keep open unless the ureters are grossly dilated. **F:** Ureterosigmoidostomy. This type of diversion is only rarely performed because of the increased incidence of bowel tumors. (Taken in part from Amis ES Jr, Pfister RC, Hendren WH. Radiology of urinary undiversion. *Urol Radiol.* 1981;3:161, with permission.)

significantly dilated tend to stenose at their anastomoses with the skin. A variation is the loop-cutaneous ureterostomy in which the exteriorized ureter drains into a collecting device. Another relatively simple way of diverting urine is a vesicostomy, in which an opening is created between the anterior aspect of the bladder and the skin. These methods are temporizing measures for patients whose bladder function is suboptimal but can be expected to improve.

Permanent Diversions

Ileal Conduits

A permanent form of supravesical urinary diversion, the ileal conduit, involves isolating an approximately 15 cm length of terminal ileum. The mesentery of this bowel loop is left intact to ensure its viability. The proximal end is closed and the ureters are anastomosed end to side to the loop. The distal open end of the loop is tunneled through the abdominal wall, usually in the right lower quadrant, and a nippled ostomy is formed, over which a collecting device (ostomy bag) can be placed. The ileal conduit is not a reservoir system and drains continuously into the collecting device, which must be worn at all times. Ileal conduits are typically studied by loopography or with CT urography (Fig. 13.88). Because an ileal conduit is a freely refluxing system, it is common to see mild dilatation develop in the upper tracts. Additionally, mucus refluxing into the upper tracts can create multiple filling defects.

If there is no reflux into one or both upper tracts when the loop is filled in a retrograde fashion, there may be a stricture at the ureteroileal anastomosis, which may necessitate an antegrade study such as CT urography or antegrade pyelography to confirm its presence and determine the extent of any obstruction (Fig. 13.89). Such stricturing is usually due to postsurgical

fibrosis, but recurrent tumor can also occur here. Another complication of ileal conduits is fibrosis of the loop with significant narrowing of the ileal lumen.

Continent Diversions

Continent urinary diversions have gained wide acceptance as alternatives to the ileal conduit. There are two types of continent urinary diversions, classified on the basis of the continence mechanism used. Some patients, whose bladders have been removed, are suitable candidates for orthotopic pouches as a direct bladder replacement. These pouches or neobladders are anastomosed to the remaining urethra in men, and the external sphincter becomes the continence mechanism. For those patients in whom direct bladder replacement with a neobladder is inappropriate, a continent pouch, generally known as a cutaneous pouch, can be situated higher in the abdomen and a continent abdominal wall stoma can be created. Both orthotopic and cutaneous pouches are constructed from various bowel segments.

Orthotopic Pouches

Orthotopic bladder replacement is typically used in men who have had a radical cystoprostatectomy for invasive bladder cancer. In such patients, the external sphincter is intact and in many instances is adequate to provide satisfactory urinary continence. This procedure is not used as frequently in women because cystourethrectomy is the desired procedure for invasive bladder cancer.

Procedures for orthotopic bladder replacement continue to evolve. A widely accepted approach is that described by Studer and colleagues. First, a segment of distal ileum is detubularized and reconfigured to form a large reservoir. Detubularization results in interruption of normal bowel continuity, thus preventing organized

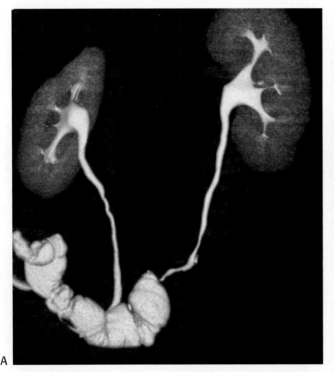
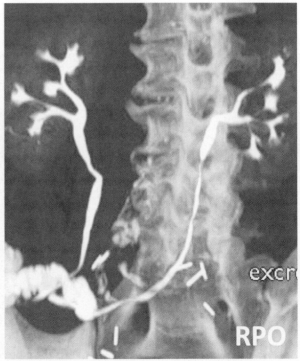

A   B

FIGURE 13.88. Ileal conduits. **A:** Volume-rendered images of an excretory phase coronal image obtained during a CT urogram shows nondilated upper tracts. The ureters are well visualized to the level of the ureteroileal anastomoses and the ileal loop is well opacified. **B:** A three-dimensional reconstructed image from a CT urogram in another patient was obtained in a right posterior oblique orientation. Since the course of the left ureter is elongated, the left ureter and its ileal anastomosis are usually better seen in this projection.

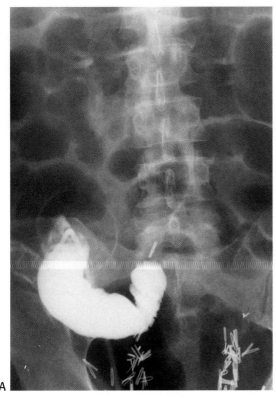 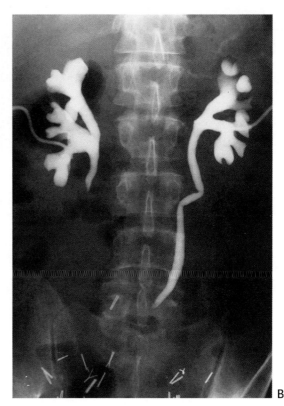

A   B

FIGURE 13.89. Ureteral obstruction after ileal conduit diversion. **A:** The absence of reflux on a loopogram suggests ureteral obstruction. **B:** Bilateral antegrade pyelograms after percutaneous nephrostomy procedures confirm bilateral ureteral obstruction.

contractions that cause intermittent high pressures and which can compromise continence or result in reflux. The detubularized ileal reservoir is then anastomosed distally to the patient's urethra and proximally to an additional isolated single loop (or two loops) of tubular ileum, which is referred to as the afferent limb or "chimney." The ureters are then anastomosed to the afferent limb (with both ureters entering a single limb or one ureter entering one of two limbs) in an end-to-side fashion (Figs. 13.90 to 13.92). Voiding may then be performed by exerting manual pressure in the suprapubic region combined with straining to increase intra-abdominal pressure. In some cases, however, intermittent self-catheterization via the urethra is necessary for emptying. Orthotopic bladders or "neobladders" are quite popular, as they do not require the use of an ostomy bag or catheterization through a stoma on the anterior abdominal wall.

Cutaneous Pouches

Cutaneous pouches are constructed from ileum alone or a combination of terminal ileum and ascending colon. For cutaneous pouches to function properly, they must be of high capacity and must also have low internal pressure. Low pressure in these reservoirs is obtained by detubularizing the bowel segment used. Detubularization is especially important in large bowel reservoirs, which are capable of developing very high pressures. The upper urinary tracts are protected from the effects of reflux or obstruction in these patients by special techniques developed for implanting the ureters into the pouch.

The Kock pouch (Fig. 13.87B) is constructed entirely from a long segment of terminal ileum. Both ends of this isolated ileal segment are intussuscepted. The ureters are attached to the proximal segment, with the intussusception acting as an antirefluxing mechanism. The intussuscepted distal segment acts as a continent

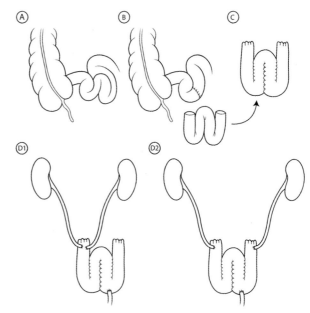

FIGURE 13.90. Creation of an orthotopic neobladder. **A:** A loop of distal ileum is identified. **B:** The loop is removed and isolated and the remaining intact ileum is reanastomosed. **C:** A portion of the isolated loop of ileum is then detubularized and reconstructed to create a larger urinary reservoir. Either one **(D1)** or two **(D2)** remaining portions of ileum that retain their tubular configuration are then used as afferent limbs or "chimneys," with the distal ureters anastomosed to these components.

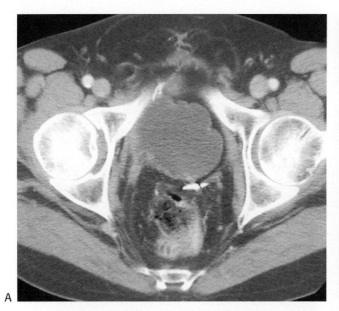
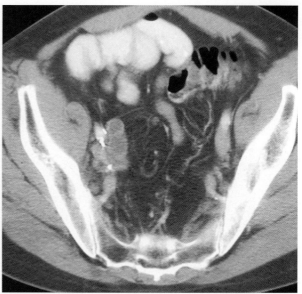

A

B

FIGURE 13.91. Orthotopic ileal neobladder. **A:** Contrast-enhanced axial CT image through the inferior aspect of the pelvis demonstrates the detubularized reservoir in the bladder fossa. **B:** A more cephalad axial image shows the afferent limb of tubularized ileum in the right hemipelvis. This is a normal appearance. The afferent limb should not be mistaken for a necrotic lymph node or abnormal fluid collection.

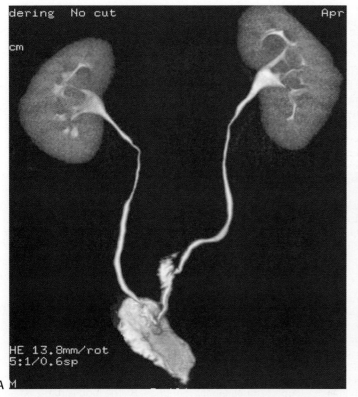
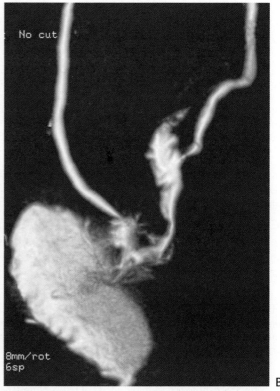

A

B

FIGURE 13.92. Orthotopic ileal bladder. **A, B:** Two volume-rendered coronal plane three-dimensional reconstructed images were obtained in this patient who has had a CT urogram following radical cystectomy with creation of an orthotopic ileal neobladder. The ureters can be seen to anastomose to the tubular afferent limb of ileum (chimney). The afferent limb then connects to the detubularized reservoir.

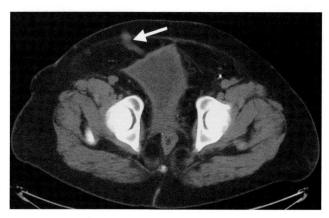

FIGURE 13.93. Cutaneous pouch with a Mitrofanoff technique. An unenhanced CT image is obtained in this patient who has had a cystectomy with creation of a pouch constructed from large bowel. This pouch is catheterized by the patient on a regular basis through the narrow port leading from the pouch to the abdominal wall (*arrow*). The appendix has been used as the port (Mitrofanoff technique).

catheterizing port. Kock pouch capacity can reach 800 to 1,000 mL, and reflux and incontinence are rare.

Large-bowel pouches are typically constructed from the cecum and an attached length of terminal ileum. Detubularization is typically accomplished by opening the cecum along its antimesenteric border and folding it into a pouch. Cecal pouches hold 500 mL or more of urine and provide satisfactory continence in more than 90% of patients. The continent catheterizing stoma may be a plicated segment of terminal ileum (Indiana pouch) or an intussuscepted ileocecal valve (King pouch). Alternatively, a

naturally narrow conduit, such as the appendix or a segment of ureter, may be attached between the skin and a closed cecal pouch (Mitrofanoff technique; Figs. 13.87D and 13.93). The antireflux mechanism in large bowel conduits is created by tunneling of the distal ureters into the taenia of the cecum. Reflux has not been a problem.

Use of continent cutaneous pouches has been facilitated by the proven safety of clean intermittent catheterization. Self-catheterization with a clean, but not sterile, catheter every 3 to 6 hours is acceptable to patients if continence is maintained during the intervening time. No external collecting device is needed.

Postoperative Complications after Continent Reservoir Surgery

Many postoperative complications are similar for both orthotopic and cutaneous pouches. Early problems that can be encountered include leakage of urine, pelvic abscess, obstruction at the point where bowel continuity has been reestablished after the ileal segments to be used have been isolated, and pyelonephritis. Late complications include incontinence, difficulty in catheterizing a stoma, strictures at the ureteroileal anastomoses (Fig. 13.94), stone formation (especially in those patients in whom staples are used for construction of the pouch), and, rarely, rupture of the pouch because of overdistention.

The postoperative radiographic evaluation of continent diversions requires that the radiologist be familiar with the bladder replacement procedure performed, as well as the location of any tubes, stents, or drains. For the first few postoperative days, it is not unusual to find ureteral stents and a catheter exiting the stoma of a cutaneous pouch. In an orthotopic pouch, the stents may exit the pouch anteriorly through a separate small incision in the lower abdominal wall. Bilateral stentograms may be performed to confirm that the upper urinary tracts are not dilated

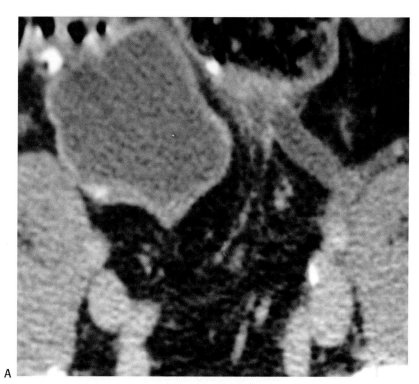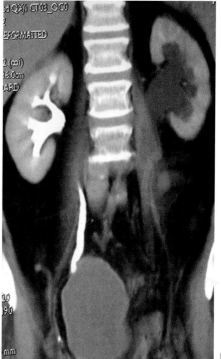

A   B

FIGURE 13.94. Fibrosis at a left ureteroileal anastomosis after creation of an orthotopic ileal neobladder. Axial **(A)** and coronal plane **(B)** excretory phase images from a CT urogram demonstrate marked left pelvocaliectasis and ureterectasis. The ureter is dilated to the level of its anastomosis with the afferent limb.

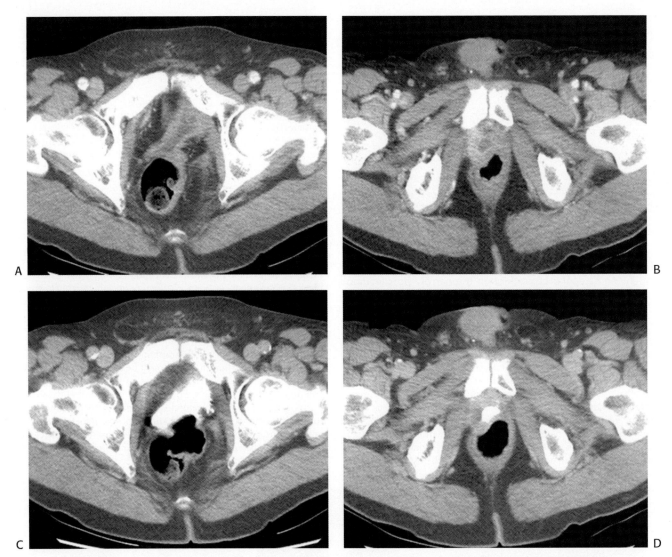

FIGURE 13.95. Bladder cancer recurrence at an ileourethral anastomosis in a patient with a neobladder. **A:** Early-enhanced axial image from a CT urogram demonstrates the caudal-most aspect of the reservoir of an orthotopic ileal neobladder. **B:** On a slightly more caudal image, an area of abnormally increased enhancement is noted along the right aspect of the anastomosis with the native urethra, corresponding to a region of tumor recurrence. **C:** The base of the neobladder reservoir fills with contrast material on a delayed enhanced image. **D:** On the more caudal excretory-phase image, the area of abnormal enhancement is no longer identified.

and that contrast medium passes freely down the ureters around the stents and through the anastomoses without leaking. If this study is satisfactory, the stents are removed. If desired, the pouch itself can be studied by dripping contrast medium through the pouch catheter. A relatively small amount of contrast material (250 mL), dripped, rather than injected, into the pouch is recommended to prevent stressing the fresh suture lines. This should occur under fluoroscopic control, and oblique views can be obtained as necessary to visualize all sides of the pouch for contrast medium extravasation. The presence or absence of reflux should be documented.

Follow-up studies after complete healing may be performed to document the capacity of the pouch, the postcatheterization residual urine, and whether reflux is present. Many patients with continent reservoirs have had surgery for bladder cancer, so that follow-up studies are also obtained to assess patients for locally recurrent or distant metastatic disease and for metachronous

upper tract neoplasms. Patients with ileal neobladders can develop local recurrences at the urethral anastomosis (Fig. 13.95) or pelvic lymph node metastases (Fig. 13.96). It is essential that the imager be aware of the normal appearance of continent reservoirs, so that normal and abnormal findings are not confused with one another.

BLADDER AUGMENTATION

Augmentation cystoplasty is a corollary of the continent orthotopic pouch in which various bowel segments are used to augment an existing small capacity bladder. A typical example would be to facilitate primary closure of an exstrophic bladder. It can also be used in patients who have interstitial cystitis. As with continent pouches, large or small bowel segments or a combination of both have proven effective. Radiographically, the appearance of the bladder in such cases will often reflect the specific method and bowel segment used for its augmentation.

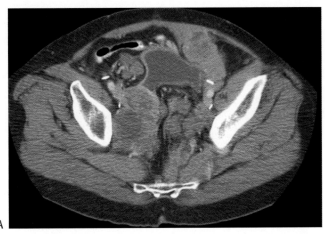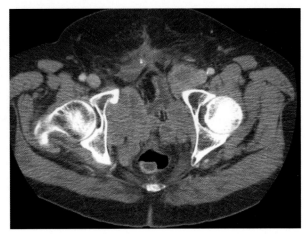

A   B

FIGURE 13.96. Recurrent bladder cancer after cystectomy and neobladder. Two contrast-enhanced axial CT images **(A, B)** through the pelvis in a patient who had a radical cystectomy for bladder cancer show multiple heterogeneous lobulated tumor masses throughout the pelvis, indicating the presence of extensive recurrent tumor.

NEUROGENIC BLADDER

The spectrum of neurogenic bladder disease is complex and often poorly understood. Evaluation of this condition is typically conducted by urologists in a laboratory specially equipped to perform video urodynamics, a highly sophisticated method for evaluating neurologic function of the bladder. However, the radiologist, by understanding the basics of bladder function, can play a role in detecting previously unsuspected neurologic abnormalities. When undiagnosed, the effects of neurogenic bladder on the upper urinary tract can be substantial, but when properly diagnosed and treated, renal function can almost always be preserved.

The following sections discuss various types of neurogenic bladder using a simplified classification (Table 13.1). It should be noted, however, that, on occasion, neurogenic bladders can be difficult to classify due to mixed features.

TABLE 13.1

Classification of Neurogenic Bladders

Uninhibited bladder (essentially normal urinary tract)
  Idiopathic
    Delayed maturation of cortical inhibitory center
    Delayed maturation of detrusor
  Acquired
    Stroke
    Brain tumor
    Normal pressure hydrocephalus
    Parkinson disease
Detrusor hyperreflexia
  Multiple sclerosis
  Myelodysplasia
  Spinal cord trauma
  Spinal cord tumors
  Spinal arteriovenous malformations
  Herniated intervertebral disc
Detrusor areflexia (large, atonic bladder)
  Herniated intervertebral disc (lower spine)
  Diabetic neuropathy
  Lower spinal cord tumors

Uninhibited Bladder

Uninhibited bladder may be idiopathic in origin, resembling a persistent infantile pattern of voiding. In such cases, there is usually incomplete or delayed maturation of the inhibitory mechanisms controlling the micturition reflex (Fig. 13.97). Whereas healthy individuals can allow their bladders to fill smoothly to capacity

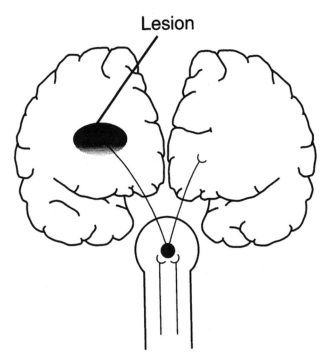

FIGURE 13.97. Schematic of an uninhibited bladder. The pontine micturition center and all pathways below it are intact in patients with uninhibited bladder. This protects the urinary tract, and it remains anatomically normal. The lesion in this case usually occurs in the cerebral cortex and may be a delayed maturation of its inhibitory mechanism or a result of acquired disease of the cerebral cortex such as stroke, brain tumor, normal pressure hydrocephalus, or Parkinson disease.

without thinking about it, patients with uninhibited bladder tend to suffer uninhibited (involuntary) bladder contractions. These contractions may occur spontaneously or be provoked by rapid filling of the bladder, a change in position, coughing, or other triggering mechanisms. These contractions are sensed by the patient as an urge to void that occasionally progresses to urge incontinence before the external urethral sphincter can be voluntarily contracted. This condition has been called nonneurogenic neurogenic bladder, or *Hinman syndrome*. In these patients, a functional bladder outlet obstruction is produced by voluntary contraction of the external sphincter during uninhibited voiding. The resulting pressure increase in the urethra results in dilation of the posterior urethra in male patients (typically young boys; Fig. 13.98) and of the entire urethra in females (Fig. 13.99). This has been termed the *spinning top* urethra in both males and females. The spinning top urethra in females has commonly been regarded as a normal variant. However, careful study of female patients with this configuration shows that a majority have uninhibited bladder. In boys, the dilated posterior urethra may occasionally resemble that seen with posterior urethral valves. In either case, the finding of a spinning top urethra in females or a wide posterior urethra in boys, especially when accompanied by urinary urgency, urge incontinence, daytime wetting, or enuresis, should prompt referral for urologic evaluation.

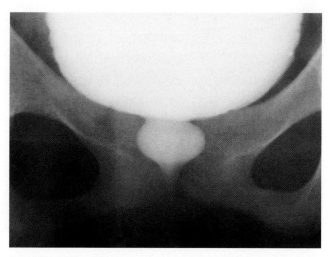

FIGURE 13.99. Spinning-top urethra in a woman. An anteroposterior radiograph obtained during a cystogram shows a dilated urethra. Although sometimes considered a normal variant, this appearance should suggest the possibility of uninhibited bladder.

Detrusor Hyperreflexia

Detrusor hyperreflexia is caused by lesions of the spinal cord above the sacral segments but below the pons (Fig. 13.100). Such patients have no perception of bladder filling or emptying and voluntary voiding is not possible. Voiding, when it does occur, is involuntary and uncoordinated, with simultaneous contractions of the detrusor and external sphincter muscles. This condition is known as detrusor–external sphincter dyssynergia (DESD) and occurs in up to 75% of patients with suprasacral spinal cord lesions. Contraction of the external sphincter occurs involuntarily at the same time a

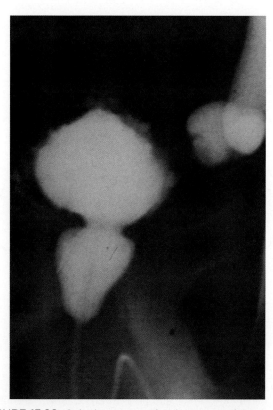

FIGURE 13.98. Spinning-top urethra in a young boy. A cystogram shows a dilated posterior urethra that resembles the pattern seen in posterior urethral valves. (From Saxton HM, Borzyskowski M, Robinson LB. Nonobstructive posterior urethral widening (spinning top urethra) in boys with bladder instability. *Radiology*. 1992;182:81, with permission.)

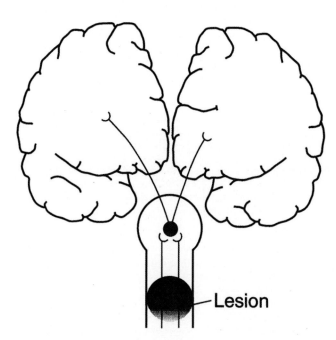

FIGURE 13.100. Schematic of detrusor hyperreflexia. Hyperreflexia occurs when a spinal cord lesion interrupts the neural pathways connecting the pontine micturition center to the sacral micturition center. Coordinated voiding is not possible in these patients. Common etiologies include trauma (most common), multiple sclerosis, myelodysplasia, spinal cord tumor, arteriovenous malformation of the spinal cord, and herniated intervertebral disks.

detrusor contraction occurs, impeding urine flow and resulting in bladder outlet obstruction. When this type of uncoordinated voiding occurs, intravesical pressure may become very high. This increased pressure ultimately can result in upper urinary tract deterioration. Although damage may occasionally be caused by vesicoureteral reflux, it is more common for a functional ureteral obstruction to occur because of the high intravesical pressure that must be overcome in the passage of a urine bolus from the kidney to the bladder. Common neurologic conditions resulting in DESD include multiple sclerosis, myelodysplasia, spinal cord trauma, spinal cord tumors, arteriovenous malformations of the spinal cord, and, occasionally, herniated intervertebral disks.

Radiographically, patients with long-term, untreated DESD have characteristic changes of the urinary tract (Fig. 13.101). The bladder is vertically oriented, with an irregular contour, consistent with trabeculation. There are frequently multiple diverticula. Such a bladder is referred to as a *Christmas tree* bladder. On voiding cystourethrography, there may or may not be vesicoureteral reflux. When the upper urinary tracts are studied by CT, generalized dilation and renal parenchymal thinning are frequently found.

If voiding can be induced during voiding cystourethrography, the posterior urethra is usually seen to be moderately dilated, and there can be reflux into the prostatic ducts in men. When such reflux is present, prostatic calculi on the plain film are a frequent accompaniment. The external sphincter at the level of the membranous urethra remains tightly contracted, with minimal passage of contrast medium into the anterior urethra and poor distention of the anterior urethra. If a 16- or 18-French catheter can be passed easily into the bladder to perform the cystography, significant stricturing in this area can be excluded and the diagnosis of DESD should be made.

When performing cystograms or other imaging studies on patients with suprasacral spinal cord lesions, the radiologist must be aware of the possibility of autonomic dysreflexia (Fig. 13.102). This is an acute syndrome of massive sympathetic hyperactivity that can be caused by stimuli such as urethral catheterization, pressure on the glans penis, bladder distention, manipulation of the renal pelvis (e.g., antegrade pyelography), and ileal conduit loopography. When so stimulated, these patients may exhibit severe paroxysmal hypertension, anxiety, sweating, piloerection, pounding headaches, and bradycardia.

More than half of all spinal cord injury patients undergoing urodynamic studies have been found to experience systolic blood pressure elevations during these procedures, with the likelihood of

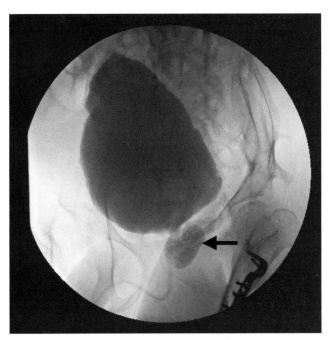

FIGURE 13.101. Detrusor–external sphincter dyssynergia (DESD). A voiding cystourethrogram demonstrates a vertically oriented bladder with an irregular contour due to trabeculation. The bladder is attempting to empty even with a catheter in place. Contrast material is seen in the prostatic urethra with extensive reflux into the prostatic glands (*arrow*).

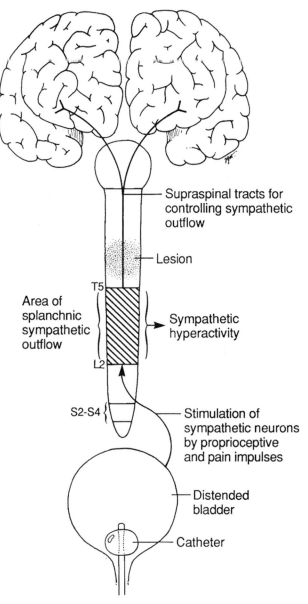

FIGURE 13.102. Schematic of autonomic dysreflexia. Autonomic dysreflexia can be seen in patients with detrusor hyperreflexia. Here, a spinal cord lesion blocks the moderating influence of the supraspinal tracts on sympathetic outflow. A distended bladder or other stimulus results in massive sympathetic hyperactivity.

this complication occurring being higher in patients with cervical spinal cord injuries, injuries that occurred more than 2 years prior to the procedure, and poor bladder compliance. Symptoms tend to be more severe in patients with complete spinal cord injuries and who are studied longer after their injury. In some patients, hypertension may be so profound as to result in stroke. If such symptoms occur during cystography, immediate draining of a full bladder and elevation of the head of the bed usually resolve the problem. Symptomatic treatment of the hypertension may also be required.

Detrusor Areflexia

Detrusor areflexia is caused by neurologic conditions affecting the sacral micturition center or pathways connecting this center with

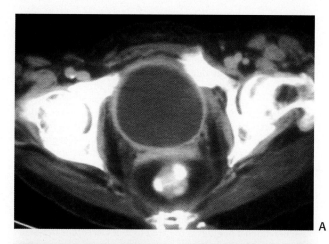

A

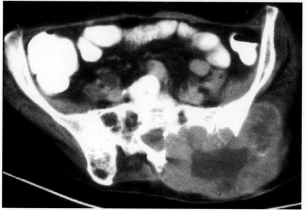

B

FIGURE 13.104. Detrusor areflexia. **A:** A contrast-enhanced axial CT image through the pelvis shows a distended bladder with only mild wall thickening. **B:** An axial image obtained slightly more cephalad shows a large sarcoma in the left hemipelvis invading the spinal canal.

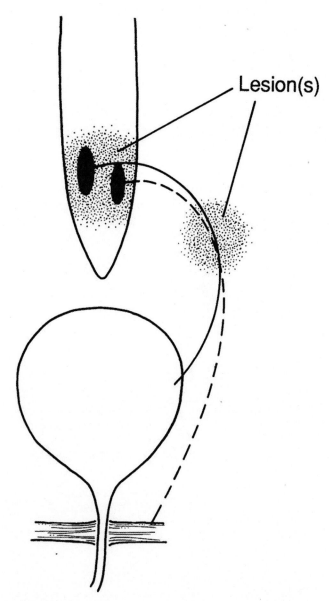

FIGURE 13.103. Schematic of detrusor areflexia. With detrusor areflexia, lesions of the sacral micturition center or sacral reflex arc result in a lack of perception of bladder filling. The bladder continues to fill until its ability to accommodate urine has been overcome and becomes grossly distended.

the bladder or both (Fig. 13.103). Conditions that can result in detrusor areflexia include herniated intervertebral discs in the lower spine, diabetic neuropathy, and lower spinal cord tumors. Because the sacral reflex arc is disrupted, there is no perception of bladder distention. Therefore, the bladder will continue to fill until the viscoelastic accommodating properties of the detrusor are overcome. Intravesical pressure increases rapidly at that point and eventually exceeds that exerted by the intact sphincter mechanisms. Overflow incontinence then occurs until the pressures in the bladder and urethra are equalized, at which point leakage ceases. The clinical pattern is that of a dribbling overflow incontinence that may or may not be constant.

Imaging studies in patients with detrusor areflexia reveal a smooth, thin-walled bladder with increased capacity, occasionally approaching several liters (Fig. 13.104). The grossly enlarged bladder may also be seen on plain film radiography (Fig. 13.105). During cystography, the patient is usually unable to void spontaneously on removal of a filling catheter. Intermittent or total dribbling incontinence may be seen. Even in patients with huge bladders, vesicoureteral reflux is rare because of the persistently relatively low intravesical pressures. If the patient is continent, he or she should be instructed to void by abdominal straining or by the Credé maneuver and the amount of residual urine should be documented by a postvoid radiograph.

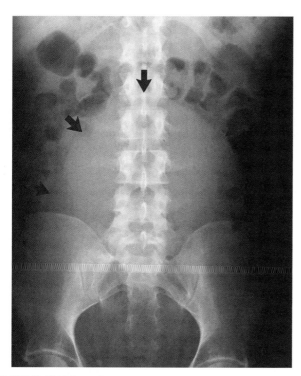

FIGURE 13.105. **Reflexive bladder.** Plain film radiograph of the abdomen reveals a soft tissue shadow from a hugely distended bladder (*arrows*) extending to the level of L2.

SUGGESTED READINGS

Benign Bladder Conditions

Amano M, Shimizu T. Emphysematous cystitis: a review of the literature. *Intern Med.* 2014;53:79–82.

Artibani W, Cerrruto MA. The role of imaging in urinary incontinence. *BJU Int.* 2005;95:699–703.

Chung AD, Schieda N, Flood TA, et al. Suburothelial and extrinsic lesions of the urinary bladder: radiologic and pathologic features with emphasis on MR imaging. *Abdom Imaging.* 2015;40:2753–2588.

Crew JP, Jephcott CR, Reynard JM. Radiation-induced haemorrhagic cystitis. *Eur Urol.* 2001;40:111–123.

Fall M, Peeker R. Classic interstitial cystitis: unrelated to BPS. *Curr Bladder Dysfunct Rep.* 2015;10:95–102.

Li G, Cai B, Song H, et al. Clinical and radiological character of eosinophilic cystitis. *Int J Clin Exp Med.* 2015;8:533–539.

Quint HJ, Drach GW, Rappaport WD, et al. Emphysematous cystitis: a review of the spectrum of disease. *J Urol.* 1992;147:134–137.

Shebel HM, Elsayes KM, About El Atta HM, et al. Genitourinary schistosomiasis: life cycle and radiologic-pathologic findings. *Radiographics.* 2012;32:1031–1046.

Yu J-S, Kim KW, Lee H-J, et al. Urachal remnant diseases: spectrum of CT and US findings. *Radiographics.* 2001;21:451–461.

Yu NC, Raman SS, Patel M, et al. Fistulas of the genitourinary tract: a radiologic review. *Radiographics.* 2004;24:1331–1352.

Zheng J, Wang G, He W, et al. Imaging characteristics of alkaline-encrusted cystitis. *Urol Int.* 2010;85:364–367.

Malignant Bladder Neoplasms

Abou-El-Gar ME, El-Assmy A, Refaie HF, et al. Bladder cancer: diagnosis with diffusion-weighted MR imaging in patients with gross hematuria. *Radiology.* 2009;251:415–421.

Aljabery F, Lindblom G, Skoog S, et al. PET/CT versus conventional CT for detection of lymph node metastases in patients with locally advanced bladder cancer. *BMC Urol.* 2015;15:87–92. doi:10.1186/s12894-015-0080-z.

Boyer AC, Jafri SZ, Jafri SM, Amin MB. Neuroendocrine carcinoma of the urinary bladder: a retrospective study of CT findings. *Abdom Imaging.* 2013;38:870–876.

Bretlau T, Hansen RH, Thomsen HS. CT urography and hematuria: a retrospective analysis of 771 patients undergoing CT urography over a 1-year period. *Acta Radiol.* 2015;56:890–896.

Ceci F, Bianchi L, Graiziani T, et al. 11-C-Choline PET/CT and bladder cancer: lymph node metastases assessment with pathological specimens as reference standard. *Clin Nucl Med.* 2015;40:e124–e128.

Cohan RH, Caoili EM, Cowan NC, et al. MDCT urography: exploring a new paradigm for imaging of bladder cancer. *AJR Am J Roentgenol.* 2009;293:1501–1508.

de Haas RJ, Steyvers MJ, Futterer JJ. Multiparametric MRI of the bladder: ready for clinical routine? *AJR Am J Roentgenol.* 2014;202:1187–1195.

Di Paulo PL, Vargas HA, Karlo CA, et al. Intradiverticular bladder cancer: CT imaging features and their association with clinical outcomes. *Clin Imaging.* 2015;39:94–98.

Donaldson SP, Bonington SC, Kershaw LE, et al. Dynamic contrast-enhanced MRI in patients with muscle-invasive transitional cell carcinoma of the bladder can distinguish between residual tumor and post-chemotherapy effect. *Eur J Radiol.* 2013;82:2161–2168.

Gautham K, Mallampati GK, Siegelman ES. MR imaging of the bladder. *Magn Reson Imaging Clin N Am.* 2004;12:545–555.

Helenius M, Dahlman P, Magnusson M, et al. Contrast enhancement in bladder tumors examined with CT urography using different scan phases. *Acta Radiol.* 2014;55:1129–1136.

Hitier-Berthault M, Ansquer C, Branchereau J, et al. 18-F-fluorodeoxyglucose positron emission tomography-computed tomography for preoperative lymph node staging in patients undergoing radical cystectomy for bladder cancer: a prospective study. *Int J Urol.* 2013;20:788–796.

Hoosein MM, Rajesh A. MR imaging of the urinary bladder. *Magn Reson Imaging Clin N Am.* 2014;22:129–134.

Jemal A, Siegel R, Ward E, et al. Cancer statistics, 2006. *CA Cancer J Clin.* 2006;56:106–130.

Kim JK, Park SY, Ahn HJ, et al. Bladder cancer: analysis of multi-detector row helical CT enhancement pattern and accuracy in tumor detection and perivesical staging. *Radiology.* 2004;231:725–731.

Kim JY, Kim SH, Hee JL, et al. MDCT urography for detecting recurrence after transurethral resection of bladder cancer: comparison of nephrographic with pyelographic phase. *AJR Am J Roentgenol.* 2014;203:1021–1027.

Ma W, Kang SK, Hricak H, et al. Imaging appearance of granulomatous disease after intravesical Bacille Calmette-Guerin (BCG) treatment of bladder carcinoma. *AJR Am J Roentgenol.* 2009;192:1494–1500.

Malayan AA, Pattanayak P, Apolo AB. Imaging muscle-invasive and metastatic urothelial carcinoma. *Curr Opin Urol.* 2015;25:441–448.

Maurer T, Horn T, Souvatzoglou M, et al. Prognostic value of 11C-Choline PET/CT and CT for predicting survival or bladder cancer patients treated with radical cystectomy. *Urol Int.* 2014;93:207–2013.

McKibben MJ, Woods ME. Preoperative imaging for staging bladder cancer. *Curr Urol Rep.* 2015;16:22. doi:10.1007/s11934-015-0496-8.

Patil VV, Wang ZJ, Sollitto RA, et al. 18-FDG PET/CT of transitional cell carcinoma. *AJR Am J Roentgenol.* 2009;193:W497–W504.

Rosenkrantz AB, Ego-Osuala IO, Khalef V, et al. Investigation of multi-sequence magnetic resonance imaging for detection of recurrent tumor after transurethral resection for bladder cancer. *J Comput Assist Tomogr.* 2016;40:201–205.

Rosenkrantz AB, Haghihi M, Horn H, et al. Utility of quantitative MRI metrics for assessment of stage and grade of urothelial carcinoma of the bladder: preliminary results. *AJR Am J Roentgenol.* 2013;201:1254–1259.

Rosenkrantz AB, Obele C, Rusinek H, et al. Whole lesion diffusion metrics for assessment of bladder cancer aggressiveness. *Abdom Imaging.* 2015;40:327–332.

Sadow CA, Silverman SG, O'Leary MP, et al. Bladder cancer detection with CT urography in an academic medical center. *Radiology.* 2008;249:195–202.

Sevcenko S, Ponhold L, Heinz-Peer G, et al. Prospective evaluation of diffusion-weighted MRI of the bladder as a biomarker for prediction of bladder cancer aggressiveness. *Urol Oncol.* 2014;32:1166–1171.

Shinagare AB, Ramaiua NH, Jagannathan JO, et al. Metastatic pattern of bladder cancer: correlation with the characteristics of the primary tumor. *AJR Am J Roentgenol.* 2011;196:117–122.

Sternberg IA, Keren Paz GE, Chen LY, et al. Upper tract imaging surveillance is not effective in diagnosing upper tract recurrence in patients followed for nonmuscle invasive bladder cancer. *J Urol.* 2013;190:1187–1191.

Takeuchi M, Sasaki S, Ito M, et al. Urinary bladder cancer: diffusion-weighted MR imaging—accuracy for diagnosing T stage and estimating histologic grade. *Radiology.* 2009;251:112–121.

Tekes A, Kamel I, Imam K, et al. Dynamic MRI of bladder cancer: evaluation of staging accuracy. *AJR Am J Roentgenol.* 2005;184:121–127.

Vikram R, Sandler CM, Ng CS. Imaging and staging of transitional cell carcinoma: part 1, lower urinary tract. *AJR Am J Roentgenol.* 2009;192:1481–1487.

Walker NF, Gan C, Olsburgh J, et al. Diagnosis and management of intradiverticular bladder tumors. *Urology.* 2014;11:383–390.

Witjes JA, Comperat E, Cowan NC, et al. EAU guidelines on muscle-invasive and metastatic bladder cancer: summary of the 2013 guidelines. *Eur Urol.* 2014;65:778–792.

Wu LM, Chen XX, Xu JR, et al. Clinical value of T2-weighted imaging combined with diffusion-weighted imaging in preoperative T staging of urinary bladder cancer. *Acad Radiol.* 2013;20:939–946.

Yoshita S, Koga F, Masude H, et al. Role of diffusion-weighted magnetic resonance imaging as an imaging biomarker or urothelial carcinoma. *Int J Urol.* 2014;21:1190–1200.

Yuan JB, Zu XB, Miao JG, et al. Laparoscopic pelvic lymph node dissection system based on preoperative primary tumour stage (T stage) by computed tomography in urothelial bladder cancer: results of a single institution prospective study. *BJU Int.* 2013;112:E87–E91.

Benign Bladder Neoplasms

Chen M, Lipson SA, Hricak H. MR imaging evaluation of benign mesenchymal tumors of the urinary bladder. *AJR Am J Roentgenol.* 1997;168:399–403.

Chung AD, Schieda N, Flood TA, et al. Suburothelial and extrinsic lesions of the urinary bladder: radiologic and pathologic features with emphasis on MR imaging. *Abdom Imaging.* 2015;40:2573–2588.

Takeuchi M, Sasaguri K, Naiki T, et al. MRI findings of inverted urothelial papilloma of the bladder. *AJR Am J Roentgenol.* 2015;205:311–316.

Zimmermann K, Amis ES Jr, Newhouse JH. Nephrogenic adenoma of the bladder: urographic spectrum. *Urol Radiol.* 1989;11:123–126.

Postoperative Bladder Changes

Catala V, Sola M, Smaniego J, et al. CT findings in urinary diversion after radical cystectomy: post-surgical anatomy and complications. *Radiographics.* 2009;29:461–476.

Heaney MD, Francis IR, Cohan RH, et al. Orthotopic neobladder reconstruction: findings on excretory urography and CT. *AJR Am J Roentgenol.* 1999;172:1213–1220.

Kawamoto S, Fishman EK. Role of CT in post-operative evaluation of patients undergoing urinary diversion. *AJR Am J Roentgenol.* 2010;194:690–696.

Keogan MT, Carr L, McDermott VG, et al. Continent urinary diversion procedures: radiographic appearances and potential complications. *AJR Am J Roentgenol.* 1997;169:173–178.

Ordorica R. The continent bladder: indications and techniques for the continent catheterizable segment. *Curr Opin Urol.* 2004;14:345–350.

Rink RC. Bladder augmentation: options, outcomes, future. *Urol Clin North Am.* 1999;26:111–123.

Sung DJ, Cho SB, Kim YH, et al. Imaging of the various continent urinary diversions after cystectomy. *J Comput Assist Tomogr.* 2004;28:299–310.

Neurogenic Bladder

Agrawal M, Joshi M. Urodynamic patterns after traumatic spinal cord injury. *J Spinal Cord Med.* 2013;38:128–133.

Amis ES Jr, Blaivas JG. The role of the radiologist in evaluating voiding dysfunction. *Radiology.* 1990;175:317–318.

Amis ES Jr, Blaivas JG. Neurogenic bladder simplified. *Radiol Clin North Am.* 1991;29:571–580.

Liu N, Zhou MW, Biering-Sorensen F, et al. Cardiovascular response during urodynamics in individuals with spinal cord injury. *Spinal Cord.* 2017;55:279–284. doi:10/1038/sc/2016/110.

Mahfouz W, Corcos J. Management of detrusor external sphincter dyssynergia in neurogenic bladder. *Eur J Phys Rehabil Med.* 2011;47:639–650.

14

Prostate and Seminal Vesicles

ANATOMY OF PROSTATE AND SEMINAL VESICLES

The prostate gland grows from epithelial buds of the male urogenital sinus in fetal life, from the same segment of the urogenital sinus that gives rise to a portion of the vagina in females. Male sexual differentiation requires that the müllerian duct structures regress under the influence of antimüllerian hormone, while the fetal testes provide an androgenic stimulus to support the development of both internal and external male genitourinary structures. In reproductively mature males, the prostate gland produces seminal fluid, which has important nutritive and enzymatic contributions to the function of spermatozoa produced in the testicles.

The prostate gland is shaped somewhat like a strawberry, with a rounded top, known as the "base," immediately below the bladder, and the mildly pointed tip directed inferiorly, known as the "apex" (Fig. 14.1). The prostatic urethra runs through the center of the gland. The anterior fibromuscular stroma is a midline component of the organ that contains no glandular tissue and no significant pathology. The glandular epithelium is organized into three areas that are distinguishable by MR imaging or dissection. These are (1) the transition zone (TZ), a rounded central mass of glandular tissue surrounding the upper prostatic urethra, superior to the verumontanum (Fig. 14.2); (2) the central zone (CZ), comprising much of the prostatic base and surrounding the paired ejaculatory ducts (Fig. 14.3); and (3) the peripheral zone (PZ), a pancake-shaped tissue component wrapping around the posterior and lateral aspects of the gland and containing up to 80% of the glandular tissue in a nonhypertrophied gland. A fibrous layer known as the "surgical capsule" separates the TZ from the PZ and is variable in diameter, becoming visible on MRI and occasionally mimicking cancer when it is thickened.

It is important to recognize that benign prostatic hyperplasia (BPH) predominantly involves the TZ, and enlargement of this area will both distort the glandular anatomy and change the relative proportions of glandular tissue in each area. About 75% of prostate adenocarcinoma occurs in the PZ, with the remaining 25% in the TZ and <3% of primary neoplasia in the CZ. The term "central gland" is sometimes used to refer to the combination of the TZ and the CZ, particularly when there is significant

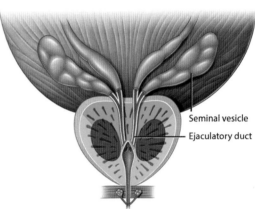

Seminal vesicle
Ejaculatory duct

Coronal section, posterior view

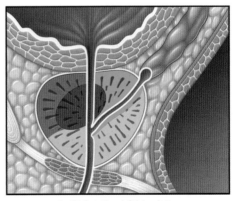

Sagittal section, left lateral view

■ Transition zone   ■ Peripheral zone
■ Central zone   ■ Anterior fibromuscular stroma

FIGURE 14.1. Prostatic zonal anatomy. The base is the broad top of the prostate gland and the apex is the pointed bottom. The majority of cancers occur in the peripheral zone (PZ), shown in lime green.

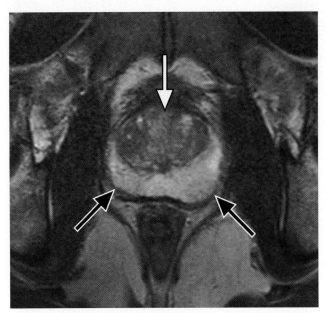

FIGURE 14.2. Axial T2WI showing high-signal C-shaped PZ (*black arrows*) wrapping around the lower-signal TZ (*white arrow*).

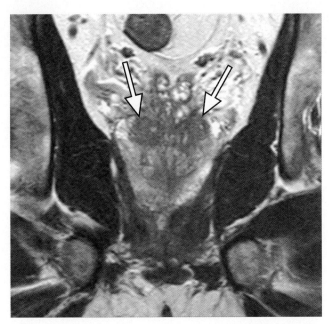

FIGURE 14.3. Coronal T2WI showing paired hypointense inverted teardrop shaped tissue components (*arrows*) surrounding the ejaculatory ducts. This is a physiologic appearance of CZ tissue but can be a mimic of malignancy on T2WI, especially if asymmetric.

distortion due to BPH, but is not anatomically precise. An alternative to zonal anatomy is lobar anatomy, which is less commonly used, with the exception of the "median lobe," a midline component of the central gland (Fig. 14.4) that is often enlarged in BPH.

The paired seminal vesicles extend superiorly and laterally from the base of the prostate, lying between the bladder and rectum (Figs. 14.1 and 14.5). The seminal vesicles have both secretory and reservoir functions for constituents of the ejaculatory fluid. Each seminal vesicle duct joins with the ipsilateral vas deferens conveying spermatozoa from the testis to form an ejaculatory duct. Each ejaculatory duct is about 2 cm in length and is surrounded by the prostatic parenchyma

of the CZ. The two ejaculatory ducts empty into the prostatic urethra at the verumontanum or prostatic colliculus.

IMAGING TECHNIQUES FOR THE PROSTATE AND SEMINAL VESICLES

Transrectal ultrasound (TRUS) enables the intracavitary probe to be in close proximity to the prostate and seminal vesicles, allowing for relatively high-resolution imaging and image-guided

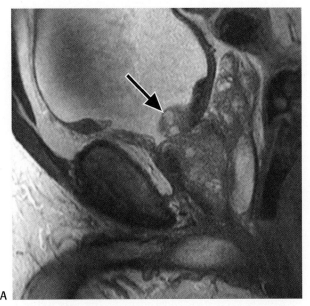

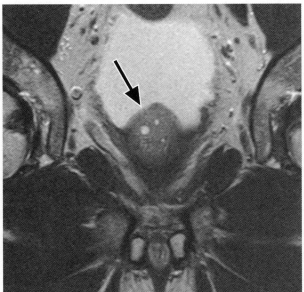

FIGURE 14.4. Nodular hypertrophy of the median lobe (*arrow*) on **(A)** sagittal and **(B)** coronal T2WI. This partially pedunculated tissue can prolapse into the urethral orifice and cause bladder outlet obstruction.

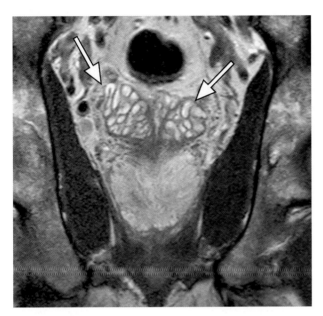

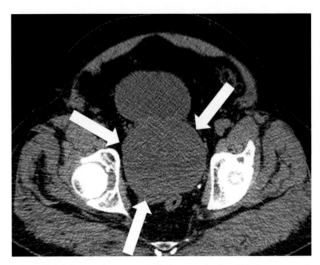

FIGURE 14.5. Normal seminal vesicles (*arrows*) on coronal T2WI. The seminal vesicles consist of curvilinear tubules whose volume varies physiologically.

FIGURE 14.6. Benign prostatic hyperplasia. CT shows markedly enlarged prostate (*arrows*); a portion of the bladder is seen anterior to the prostate.

interventions. However, both sensitivity and specificity of TRUS for prostate cancer remain low, and its use for primary diagnosis has waned. CT is not used for primary diagnosis of prostate cancer but may be the best and is often the most available choice when prostatic abscess is suspected. CT has an important role in staging and surveillance of prostate cancer. PET/CT, including both [18]FDG and prostate-directed novel radiotracers, has a recognized role in recurrent and metastatic disease.

In recent years, MRI has emerged as the primary imaging modality for the prostate gland. The term "multiparametric MRI" (mpMRI) is sometimes used to denote the importance of integrating information from multiple imaging sequences to improve diagnostic accuracy. There are three key sequences in prostate MRI: T2-weighted imaging (T2WI) with high spatial resolution and obtained in multiple planes if possible; diffusion-weighted imaging (DWI), with apparent diffusion coefficient (ADC) maps generated from the DWI data; and postcontrast T1WI, with a dynamic contrast-enhanced (DCE) acquisition allowing evaluation of enhancement kinetics. The utility of each of these sequences in distinguishing benign from malignant prostate disease will be detailed later in this chapter. The growing availability of 3T magnets and high-resolution surface coils—with their greater acceptability to both patients and operators—has driven the trend away from the use of endorectal MR coils, but either method can generate high-quality images.

BENIGN PROSTATIC DISEASE

Benign Prostatic Hyperplasia (BPH)

The term *BPH* refers to overgrowth of smooth muscle and epithelial cells of the prostate gland. This is the most common type of prostatic disease, affecting 50% to 75% of men over 50 years and as many as 80% of men over 70 years of age. Several factors increase the risk of developing BPH, including: age, diabetes mellitus, hypertension, obesity, and hypogonadism. Men who are more active, drink less alcohol, and eat more vegetables have a decreased risk of BPH. The prostate gland in adult males younger than 50 years is the size of a walnut (in its shell) and weighs 15 to 20 g; it enlarges gradually with age, even in men without BPH. The weight (g) and volume (cm³) of the prostate are considered roughly interchangeable.

When the histologic process of BPH increases the size or distorts the anatomy of the gland sufficiently to cause lower urinary tract symptoms (LUTS), men often seek medical attention. LUTS include sensations of diminished bladder capacity including frequent urination, urinary urgency, and nocturia and difficulties during urination itself including hesitancy, intermittent stream, and incomplete emptying. However, the correlation between the degree of prostatic enlargement and the presence or severity of symptoms is weak. Some men with very large glands are relatively asymptomatic, while many men with severe LUTS have only mildly to moderately enlarged glands (≤50 cm³). Understanding and quantification of the relationship between gland size and symptoms is further hampered by the fact that many men do not seek medical attention until BPH/LUTS have significantly impacted their quality of life. In the most advanced cases, BPH can result in urinary retention, recurrent stones and/or infection, obstructive uropathy, and renal failure.

Imaging may reveal enlargement and nodularity of the gland, as well as secondary findings of BPH. In young men, the prostate gland measures about 3 cm in diameter on axial images, whether by TRUS, CT, or MRI. The enlarged gland may be homogenous or heterogenous by CT (Fig. 14.6), but internal heterogeneity and nodularity are usually evident by US or MRI. BPH nodules on MRI tend to expand the TZ and may flatten and compress the PZ (Fig. 14.7). The signal characteristics of BPH nodules on T2WI are quite variable (Fig. 14.8), depending on the admixture of glandular and stromal elements. Glandular nodules often appear quite high in signal intensity on T2WI due to accumulated secretions, while stromal nodules tend to have lower signal on T2WI and are more challenging to distinguish from TZ carcinoma. Like TZ carcinomas, stromal nodules may have high signal on DWI and early hyperenhancement on DCE imaging. However, BPH nodules usually exhibit mixed (rather than homogenously hypointense) signal on T2WI, smooth well-defined margins and/or capsules, convex shapes, and ADC values somewhat higher than those of clinically significant carcinomas.

As the prostate enlarges, its mass effect on the bladder as well as morphologic changes of outlet obstruction may emerge. Findings include incomplete emptying of the bladder, varying degrees of thickening and trabeculation of the bladder wall, and indentation of the bladder base. The enlarged prostate elevates the interureteric ridge, producing a characteristic J shape or "hooking" of the distal ureters (Fig. 14.9). When detrusor hypertrophy can no longer compensate for

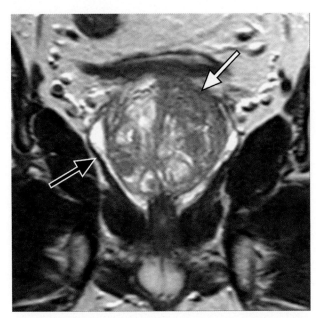

FIGURE 14.7. Benign prostatic hyperplasia. Coronal T2WI shows marked enlargement and heterogeneity in the TZ (*white arrow*) with compression and flattening of the PZ (*black arrow*).

bladder outlet obstruction, the bladder begins to dilate. Bladder diverticula result from long-standing outlet obstruction. Diverticula may grow larger than the bladder itself and may actually deviate the bladder. In such cases, the diverticulum is smooth walled, while the bladder has a thick, irregular (trabeculated) wall (Fig. 14.10). Associated urinary retention contributes to formation of bladder stones.

The median lobe of the prostate (Fig. 14.4) is particularly prone to enlargement in BPH, often taking on a pedunculated shape. Because it can prolapse into the bladder neck and produce obstruction during voiding, enlargement of this portion of the gland predicts risk of urinary retention better than overall prostate volume.

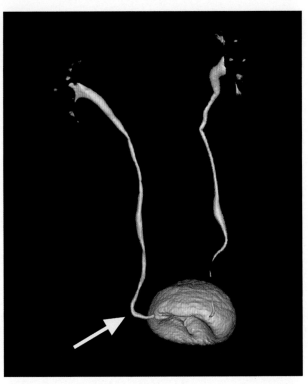

FIGURE 14.9. Benign prostatic hyperplasia. Coronal MIP from excretory phase CT demonstrates lobulated mass effect at bladder base and "fish hook" morphology (*arrow*) of distal ureter.

The median lobe can appear as a large, rounded filling defect in the center of the bladder on fluoroscopic studies, but ultrasound, CT, and MRI easily demonstrate the contiguity of the median lobe with the rest of the gland.

Moderate severity LUTS often respond well to oral medication, including alpha blockers such as doxazosin that reduce urinary tract smooth muscle tone and 5-*a*-reductase inhibitors like finasteride that reduce serum levels of dihydrotestosterone. However, persistent symptoms may require surgical intervention. For obstruction due to moderate enlargement of the prostate, transurethral resection of the prostate (TURP) is usually performed. This involves removal of the bladder neck and prostatic tissue surrounding the urethra through a resectoscope. With the internal sphincter at the bladder

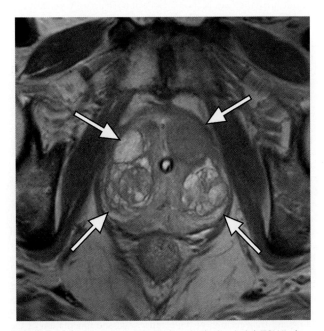

FIGURE 14.8. Benign prostatic hyperplasia. Axial T2WI demonstrates the pleomorphic nature and internal signal characteristic of BPH nodules (*arrows*). Note that despite their varying internal signal, all have well-circumscribed convex margins.

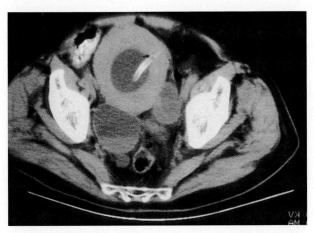

FIGURE 14.10. Bladder diverticula. The bladder is thick-walled due to chronic outlet obstruction and has an indwelling Foley catheter. There are two posterolateral diverticula, both with fluid–debris levels indicating stasis of urine.

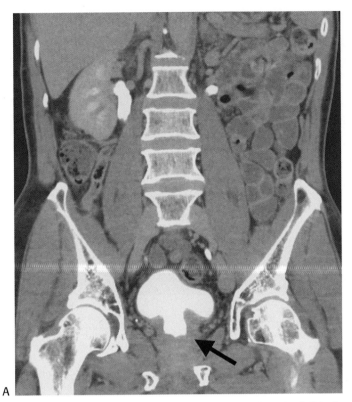 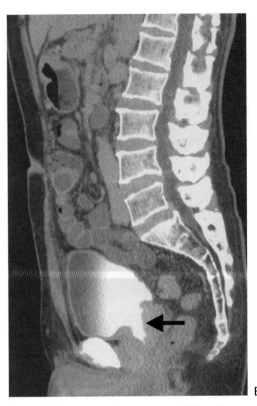

A   B

FIGURE 14.11. TURP defect. Coronal **(A)** and sagittal **(B)** views from a CT urogram show contrast filling the resected area of the prostate (*arrows*). The internal sphincter has been resected during the TURP, allowing passive filling of the cavity.

neck removed, urinary continence is maintained by the external sphincter surrounding the membranous urethra. During imaging of the bladder and urethra, the resected area of the prostate or "TURP defect" can be easily visualized because it is filled with urine (Fig. 14.11). Laser enucleation and high-frequency ultrasound (HIFU) ablation of the TZ are other alternatives for men with moderate to severe BPH. Men with very large glands (≥80 cm³) or contraindications to transurethral procedures are sometimes treated with simple prostatectomy.

Inflammation and Infection

The prostate may become infected by bacterial, viral, fungal, and mycobacterial agents and is occasionally inflamed by noninfectious processes. In contrast to prostate cancer, many of these conditions are quite symptomatic. Patients with prostatitis may complain of urinary frequency, urgency, nocturia, dysuria, fever, perineal pain, urethral discharge, and occasionally sexual dysfunction. In acute prostatitis, digital rectal exam reveals an exquisitely tender and swollen prostate gland that may be firm or fluctuant. In patients with chronic prostatitis, the prostate may be normal to the examining finger, asymmetrically hard, or diffusely enlarged and slightly tender.

Acute prostatitis is usually bacterial, most commonly due to retrograde infection by urinary tract pathogens. *Escherichia coli* infection accounts for more than 80% of bacterial prostatitis, and an additional 15% are caused by *Klebsiella*, *Proteus*, *Pseudomonas*, and *Enterobacter* or *Gonococcus* species. The etiology of chronic prostatitis, which commonly develops without an initial acute episode, can be infectious or inflammatory. Often, no pathologic organism is identified. Tuberculosis, fungi, interventions such as TURP or biopsy, and sarcoidosis may cause granulomatous prostatitis. Men with bladder cancer occasionally develop granulomatous prostatitis after intravesical treatment with bacillus Calmette–Guerin (BCG) (Fig. 14.12).

Clinical diagnosis rests on the digital rectal examination (DRE), culture of prostatic secretions expressed by digital transrectal massage, and biopsy of firm areas in the prostate gland that remain suspicious for tumor after appropriate antimicrobial therapy. A high index of suspicion for tumor is necessary, because both prostate cancer and prostatitis tend to occur in the PZ. TRUS does not reliably distinguish prostatitis from cancer, as both are hypoechoic masses in the PZ.

The distinction between inflammation and cancer remains challenging with MRI in some cases, but certain morphologic features are helpful. Prostatitis may be focal or diffuse and exhibits hypointense signal on T2WI compared to adjacent parenchyma. When focal, it is characteristically bandlike, triangular or geographic in morphology (Fig. 14.13), compared with the typical nodular or masslike configuration of cancer. When diffuse, the entire PZ may be "grayed out" or lower in signal than the very high signal expected in the PZ on T2WI (Fig. 14.14). Acute prostatitis may exhibit high signal on DWI but usually lacks the marked hypointensity of clinically significant cancers on ADC maps. Acute, chronic, and granulomatous prostatitis are all associated with hyperenhancement on arterial phase DCE. Granulomatous prostatitis can exhibit extracapsular extension (Fig. 14.12), making it very difficult to distinguish from locally advanced cancer and often requiring biopsy.

Bacterial, fungal, and granulomatous prostatitis may all be associated with abscess formation. Bacterial abscesses are most likely to be acutely symptomatic. At TRUS, prostatic abscesses are usually hypoechoic (Fig. 14.15) and avascular. Combined with the clinical presentation, a prostatic abscess may be suspected and proven by TRUS-guided aspiration. On CT, an abscess will manifest as a loculated, intraprostatic fluid collection, usually with enhancing walls (Fig. 14.16). Imaging should be extended through the urogenital diaphragm because prostatic abscesses can extend into the base

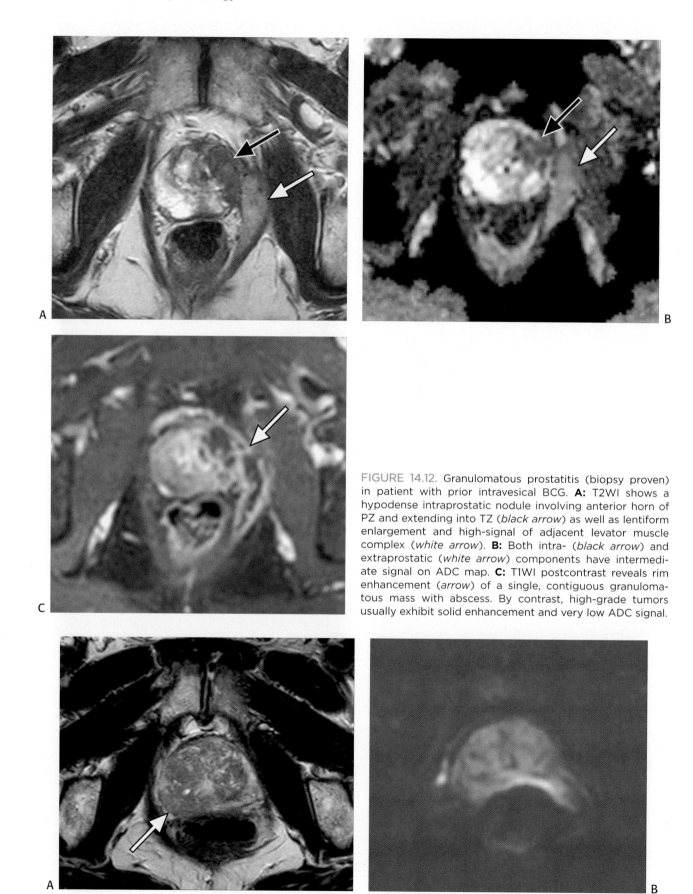

FIGURE 14.12. Granulomatous prostatitis (biopsy proven) in patient with prior intravesical BCG. **A:** T2WI shows a hypodense intraprostatic nodule involving anterior horn of PZ and extending into TZ (*black arrow*) as well as lentiform enlargement and high-signal of adjacent levator muscle complex (*white arrow*). **B:** Both intra- (*black arrow*) and extraprostatic (*white arrow*) components have intermediate signal on ADC map. **C:** T1WI postcontrast reveals rim enhancement (*arrow*) of a single, contiguous granulomatous mass with abscess. By contrast, high-grade tumors usually exhibit solid enhancement and very low ADC signal.

FIGURE 14.13. Focal prostatitis. Geographic low signal on T2WI **(A)** extends from surgical capsule to gland margin (*arrow*), with **(B)** no corresponding signal abnormality on DWI.

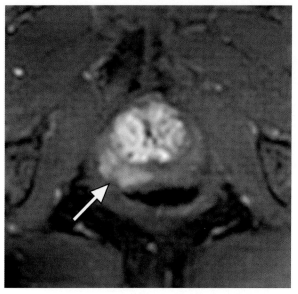

C

FIGURE 14.13. (continued) Focal prostatitis. **C:** T1WI post contrast illustrates focal early enhancement (*arrow*) equal to that of the TZ.

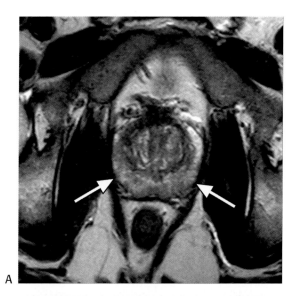

A

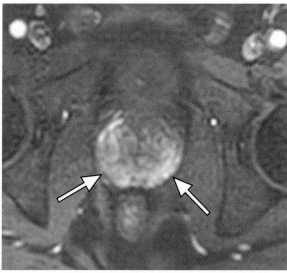

B

FIGURE 14.14. Diffuse prostatitis. **A:** T2WI demonstrates homogenous "grayed out" signal (*arrows*) in normally hyperintense PZ. **B:** T1WI postcontrast shows broad hyperenhancement in PZ (*arrows*). Normally, the PZ enhances later than the TZ.

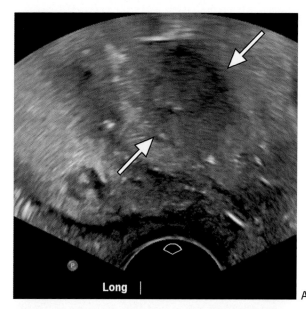

A

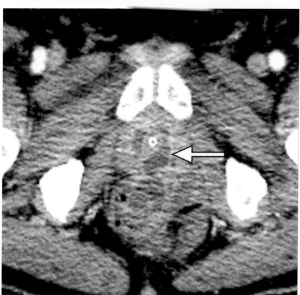

B

FIGURE 14.15. Prostatic abscess. **A:** TRUS sagittal image shows a hypoechoic collection (*arrows*) near prostatic apex. **B:** CT demonstrates an intraprostatic collection (*arrow*) extending posteriorly into rectal wall.

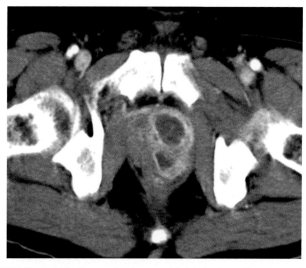

FIGURE 14.16. Prostatic abscess. Multiple rim enhancing collections are noted within the prostatic parenchyma.

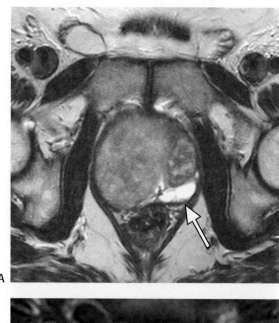

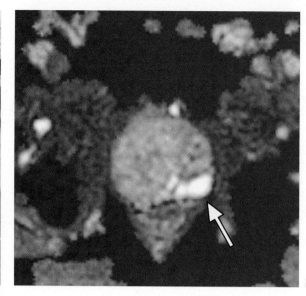

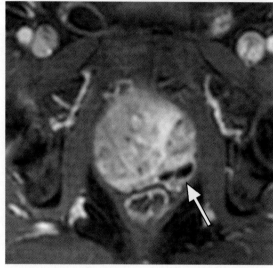

FIGURE 14.17. Prostatic abscess. **(A)** Small hyperintense collection in PZ on T2WI (*arrow*) shows **(B)** very high signal (*arrow*) on ADC map and **(C)** rim enhancement (*arrow*) on T1WI postcontrast.

of the penis. On MRI, fluid collections are generally hypointense on T1WI and hyperintense on T2WI and may exhibit peripheral enhancement (Fig. 14.17).

Prostatic inflammation, infection, and even necrosis can be associated with chronic adjacent infections such as perianal fistulas/abscesses or decubitus ulcers and prior therapeutic interventions such as pelvic surgeries and radiation (Fig. 14.18). In such cases, MRI is often helpful in evaluating the extent of organ involvement, using a combination of small and larger field of view images and T2WI and contrast-enhanced T1WI.

Prostatic Cysts

Developmental cysts within the prostate are not uncommon and can sometimes be symptomatic. However, with ongoing growth in prostate MRI, they are most often encountered incidentally. Midline prostatic cysts include prostatic utricle cysts, derived from the homologue of the vagina and uterus, and müllerian duct cysts, resulting from incomplete regression of the mesonephric duct. Prostatic utricular cysts are reported in slightly younger patients, are more commonly associated with other genitourinary tract malformations, and communicate with the prostatic urethra. They do not extend beyond the prostatic base (Fig. 14.19). Müllerian duct cysts extend above the prostatic base (Fig. 14.20) and do not communicate directly with

the urethra. Both can be associated with ejaculatory or urinary tract dysfunction, infection, or very rarely carcinoma and are sometimes surgically unroofed or resected. Paramidline and lateral prostatic cysts arise from the ejaculatory ducts and the prostate parenchyma respectively and are less common.

Prostatic Calcifications

The PZ of the prostate gland is the seat of the corpora amylacea, where calcifications with no known etiology and without pathologic effects tend to occur. These calcifications are discrete, vary in size from 1 to 5 mm, and are usually multiple. Calcification is also noted in some BPH nodules in the TZ. Prostatic calcifications have little clinical significance and are not useful in differentiating between benign and malignant diseases.

PROSTATE CANCER

Incidence

Prostate cancer is an important public health problem in the United States; there are expected to be nearly 200,000 new cases diagnosed in 2016, with over 25,000 deaths. Among American men, prostate cancer is the most common solid organ cancer, second only to lung

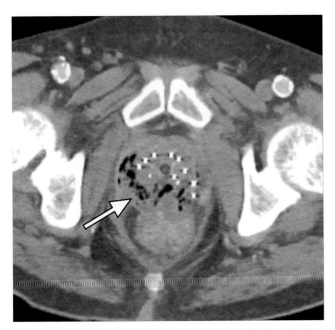

FIGURE 14.18. Prostatic necrosis. A gas and fluid collection replaces the posterior aspect of the gland (*arrow*) in this patient treated with radiation therapy for prostate cancer. Note radiopaque brachytherapy seeds anteriorly.

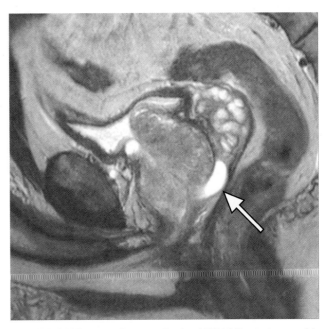

FIGURE 14.19. Utricular cyst. Sagittal T2WI illustrates a midline cyst (*arrow*) tapering toward the verumontanum, where it communicates with urethra. There is also marked BPH.

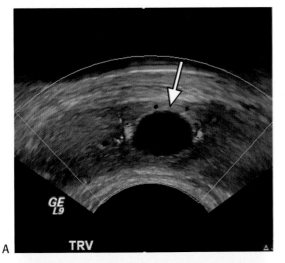

A   TRV

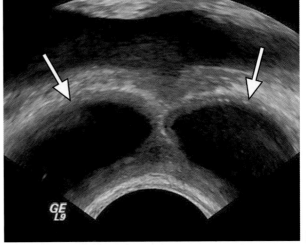

B

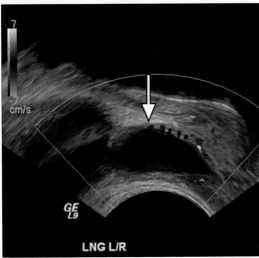

C   LNG L/R

FIGURE 14.20. Müllerian duct cyst. Axial TRUS shows a midline avascular cyst **(A)** (*arrow*) and dilated bilateral seminal vesicles **(B)** (*arrows*). **C:** Sagittal image illustrates this tear drop shaped cyst extending well above the prostatic base (*arrow*).

cancer as a cause of cancer death. However, early detection and advances in treatment have improved disease-specific mortality since the first few editions of this book.

Prostate cancer is rare in men younger than 50 years but risk increases with age thereafter. Significant geographic and racial differences in the incidence of prostate cancer are reported. The incidence of clinical prostate cancer is low in China, Japan, Israel, Latin and South America, and among Native Americans. The incidence is high in North America and Northern Europe. For reasons that remain incompletely understood, men of African ancestry living in the United States and the Caribbean have the highest risk of prostate cancer in the world. In the United States, African American men have a 70% higher risk of prostate cancer than non-Hispanic white men. Prostatic carcinoma, like prostatic hypertrophy, is androgen dependent. Positive family history and genetic mutations including Lynch syndrome are additional risk factors.

Pathology

More than 95% of prostatic neoplasms are adenocarcinomas, originating in the epithelium of prostatic acini in the PZ of the prostate. Other prostate tumors are rare but include squamous cell carcinomas, endometrioid carcinomas arising from the prostatic utricle, carcinosarcomas, melanomas and mesenchymal neoplasms such as rhabdomyosarcoma, leiomyosarcoma, or fibrosarcoma. The remainder of this discussion pertains to adenocarcinoma.

Originally established in the late 1960s, the Gleason pathologic system for grading prostate cancer involves a histologic evaluation of tissue for glandular pattern, size, and distribution; cells are examined for their degree of differentiation. Predominant and secondary patterns of tumor are identified; each of these is assigned a score of 1 through 5 and the two added to create an overall score ranging from 2 to 10. However, given that prostate cancer is not diagnosed unless the score is at least 3+3, the Gleason score for carcinoma in fact ranges from 6 to 10. Two cancers with the same total score but different predominant patterns may have contrasting prognoses, as a Gleason 7 (3+4) has at least 25% lower risk of progression than a Gleason 7 (4+3) at 10 years after surgery. In an effort to reflect these nuances and more closely tie pathologic grading to prognostic outcomes, a modified grading system with Grade Groups 1 to 5 has been proposed by the International Society of Urologic Pathology and accepted by the World Health Organization, though it is not yet in widespread use.

Screening

Detection of prostate cancer is performed by DRE and measurement of serum prostate-specific antigen (PSA). PSA is a serine protease that is normally secreted only into the ductal system of the prostate and is often elevated in patients with prostate cancer. Any derangement of the prostate architecture can cause PSA to leak from the acini into the stroma of the gland and enter the systemic circulation through lymphatics and capillaries. There are multiple benign causes for an elevated PSA level, including recent DRE or urinary intervention, prostatitis, prostatic infarct, acute urinary retention, advanced age, and benign hypertrophy of the prostate.

Interpretation of serum PSA in the clinical context improves its specificity. PSA levels below 4.0 ng/mL are considered "normal," but younger men with PSA as low as 2.5 ng/mL may have clinically significant cancers. The higher the PSA level, the higher the cancer risk, but inference is confounded by the factors detailed above. Dividing the serum PSA level by the volume of the prostate (usually determined by TRUS) yields "PSA density" and may be a more reliable screening value. Further, the rate of change of PSA over time (PSA velocity) is felt to be a better indicator of tumor likelihood than a single PSA determination. Finally, serum PSA is either free or bound to plasma proteins. A higher proportion of PSA is bound to proteins in patients with prostate cancer, resulting in a decrease in the ratio of free PSA to total (free plus protein bound) PSA in such patients.

Screening with DRE depends on the skill of the examiner and at best detects only about 40% of prostate cancers <1.5 cm. More than 50% of prostate cancers are clinically advanced at the time they are detected by DRE. Neither DRE nor PSA is highly sensitive, but their combined use improves screening performance. If both DRE and PSA are positive, 60% of those patients will have prostate cancer; if both DRE and PSA are normal, only 2% of those patients will have the disease.

Expansion of PSA screening has increased the diagnosis of small cancers, many of which are clinically undetectable and unlikely to impact the patient's long-term health. Treatments for localized cancer, including surgery, brachytherapy, external beam radiotherapy and ablation with cryotherapy or HIFU, confer a risk of side effects such as erectile dysfunction, urinary incontinence, fistula formation, and proctitis. The U.S. Preventive Services Task Force (USPSTF) recommends against PSA screening at all ages due to the risk of overdetection, overtreatment, and attendant morbidity, giving PSA screening a blanket grade of "D." However, the American Urological Association (AUA) recommends PSA screening for average risk men aged 55 to 69 who have discussed the test with their doctors and wish to proceed with an understanding of its limitations. In men ≤40 or ≥70 years with no special risk factors, there is consensus that PSA is not an appropriate screening test.

Currently, there is no evidence basis for the use of any imaging modality in prostate cancer screening. Broadly speaking, ultrasound, CT, magnetic resonance imaging (MRI), scintigraphy, and positron emission tomography (PET) are insufficiently accurate and/or too expensive to use for screening—though each has potential utility during the prostate cancer diagnosis and staging, treatment planning, and surveillance.

Diagnosis

When prostate cancer is suspected based on the DRE and/or PSA, "blind" (non–lesion-targeted) biopsy is usually performed by urologists. Because accurate prognosis incorporates histologic information, tissue diagnosis is pursued prior to treatment even when disease is obviously locally advanced or even metastatic on clinical grounds. Guided by TRUS, a spring-loaded biopsy gun obtains tissue cores from at least six representative portions of the gland. Multiple cores, sometimes as many as several dozen ("saturation" biopsy), may be obtained. Because the biopsy is transrectal, it is most effective in diagnosing cancers in the posterior PZ and more limited for diagnosis of anterior PZ and all TZ cancers.

TRUS is predominantly used to establish the location and borders of the prostate during biopsy, rather than for lesion detection or targeting. On TRUS, small carcinomas are typically hypoechoic relative to adjacent PZ parenchyma. However, margination and echogenicity are variable. Tumor is poorly distinguished from other processes such as prostatitis or BPH, with an overall positive predictive value for cancer remaining <50%. Color Doppler, ultrasound contrast enhancement, and elastography all improve diagnostic performance of TRUS for lesion detection and characterization.

When repeated TRUS-guided biopsy results are negative or equivocal but occult high-risk tumor is suspected, MRI has an important role in lesion localization and risk stratification. Suspicious areas can be biopsied under direct MRI guidance, although this is relatively involved technically and consumes substantial magnet time. Alternatively, real-time coregistration of MR images with TRUS guidance for biopsy can be performed in an outpatient setting. This method improves sampling of the most suspicious areas, increasing the accuracy of preoperative tumor grading and cancer staging compared with random biopsy, and has had a substantial impact on prostate cancer management. Research regarding its cost-effectiveness is ongoing.

Multiparametric MRI for evaluation of the prostate gland is an area of tremendous growth on both research and clinical fronts. The key sequences for prostate mpMRI are T2WI, DWI, and DCE (dynamic contrast enhanced T1WI with fat saturation). Maximum specificity is attained by integrating the level of risk conferred by signal abnormalities in each sequence, interpreted in the context of anatomic localization and known cancer mimics in that zone. Prostate MRI performed for cancer evaluation must be reported in a clear and actionable fashion, and there is a strong international trend toward standardized reporting. Two main approaches currently prevail, both rating lesions on a 1 to 5 scale, where 1 is highly unlikely and 5 is highly likely to represent clinically significant (Gleason 3+4 or greater) carcinoma. The first approach is an ordinal or Likert scale that does not formally assign categories based on specific features, but allows for a more global subjective assessment by the reader and summarizes the overall level of suspicion with a single number. This system performs well for experienced readers.

The second approach, Prostate Imaging and Reporting and Data System (PI-RADS), is more structured. PI-RADS was originally established by the European Society of Urogenital Radiology (ESUR) in 2012. The current Version 2 is intended to be more globally applicable and has been endorsed by a larger consortium including the American College of Radiology (ACR). PI-RADS v2 explicitly scores lesions according to their signal, morphology, and size on each sequence. It is important to recognize that the rating is governed primarily by DWI in the PZ and T2WI in the TZ. The details of this scoring system are somewhat beyond the scope of this chapter, and interested readers are referred to several PI-RADS references at the end.

Broadly speaking, in both systems, lesions are suspicious in any anatomic area when there is focal high signal on high B value DWI and associated markedly hypointense signal on ADC maps. On T2WI in the PZ, cancers are hypointense in signal and have a masslike (Fig. 14.21), nodular, or lentiform (Fig. 14.22) shape, while

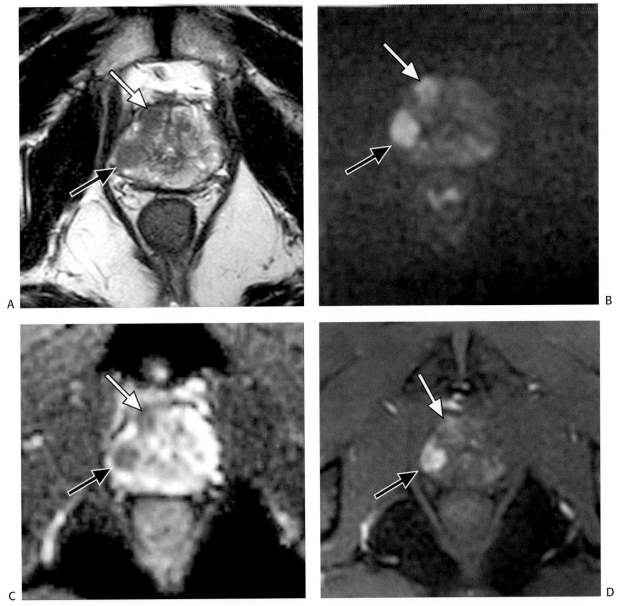

FIGURE 14.21. Multifocal carcinoma in the PZ with Gleason 7 (4+3) laterally (*black arrows*) and Gleason 6 (3+3) in the anterior horn (*white arrows*). Both lesions are **(A)** hypointense on T2WI, **(B)** markedly hyperintense on DWI, and **(C)** hypointense on ADC maps. **D:** The higher-grade carcinoma enhances more dramatically on DCE.

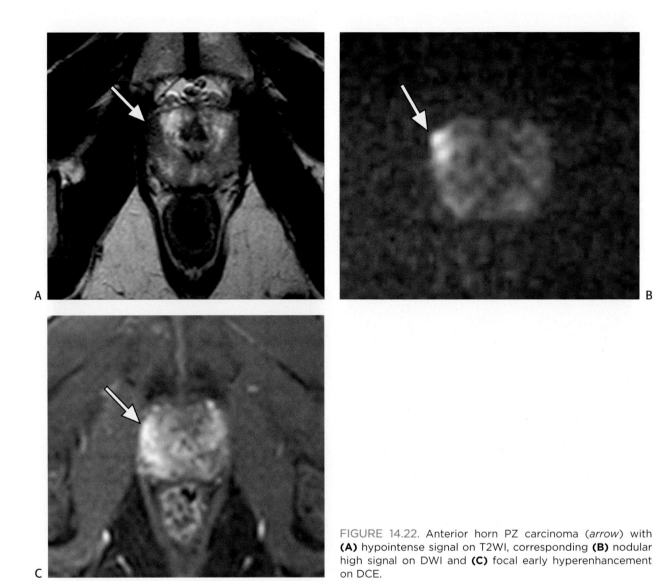

FIGURE 14.22. Anterior horn PZ carcinoma (*arrow*) with **(A)** hypointense signal on T2WI, corresponding **(B)** nodular high signal on DWI and **(C)** focal early hyperenhancement on DCE.

hypointense lesions that are geographic, nodular, or triangular are more likely prostatitis or hemorrhage. Both cancers and prostatitis (Figs. 14.13 and 14.14) may be hyperenhancing on DCE, and this sequence is generally third in importance. On T2WI in the TZ, cancers are poorly marginated (Fig. 14.23) or lenticular and often have intermediate "charcoal grey" signal, while BPH nodules are generally well circumscribed and often have very high (glandular nodule) or very low (stromal nodule) signal (Figs. 14.7 and 14.8). Just like carcinomas, BPH nodules may be hyperenhancing on DCE and hyperintense on DWI, underscoring the importance of lesion morphology on T2WI in the TZ. These cancer mimics and their appearances are discussed in more detail in their respective sections of the chapter.

The DCE sequence can provide several important pieces of diagnostic information. First, the precontrast T1WI should be scrutinized to evaluate for any hemorrhage from a prior TRUS biopsy. Hemorrhage is intrinsically hyperintense on T1WI (Fig. 14.24) and may persist for several months after a procedure. The citrate in the PZ glandular parenchyma is a natural anticoagulant and likely accounts for the relatively high prevalence of hemorrhage seen on postbiopsy imaging studies. A focal defect within a geographic area of high signal on pre contrast T1WI may reflect the presence of a tumor replacing normal PZ parenchyma, known as the "hemorrhage sparing" or "hemorrhage exclusion" sign. When

substantial hemorrhage is present on precontrast T1WI, subtracted images should be used for the postcontrast evaluation, if possible. It should also be noted that PZ hemorrhage usually creates a low-signal abnormality on T2WI and may act as another cancer mimic. Second, the presence or absence of enhancement within a lesion can be assessed in a binary fashion, which is helpful in characterization of nonmass lesions such as complex cysts, abscesses, and even calcifications. Third, the enhancement kinetics of a lesion or region of the prostate can be evaluated. This can be done formally using advanced postprocessing techniques to generate curves or visually by scrolling through multiple high temporal resolution images at the same level. Generally speaking, the TZ enhances prior to the PZ, and many BPH nodules are hyperenhancing in the early arterial images. If a lesion in the PZ enhances at the same time as the TZ, it is abnormal and may represent a cancer if it is nodular or lentiform (and has high signal on DWI) or an area of prostatitis if it is triangular, nodular, geographic, or diffuse.

Dissemination

Most carcinomas of the prostate arise in the PZ, closer to the prostatic capsule than to the urethra. Spread of prostatic carcinoma occurs by three methods: direct extension, lymphatic spread, and

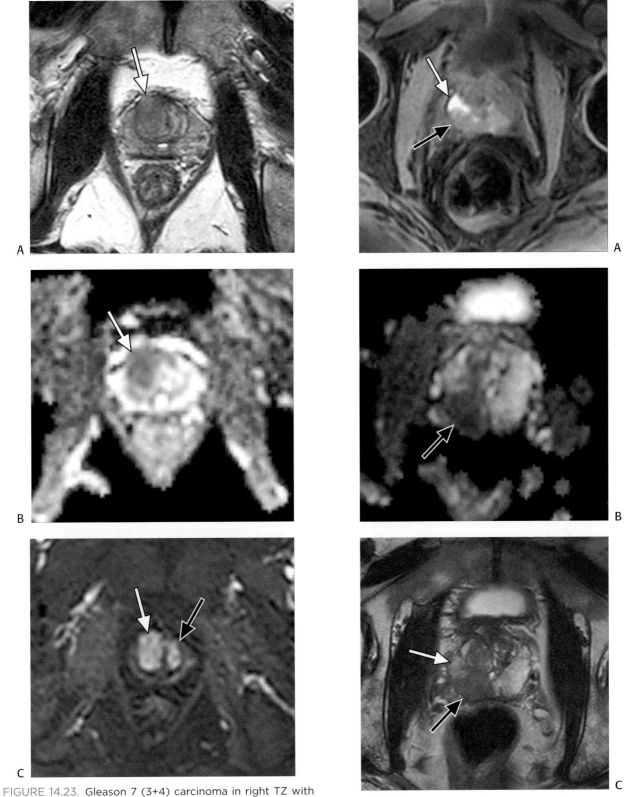

FIGURE 14.23. Gleason 7 (3+4) carcinoma in right TZ with (A) "smudged charcoal" appearance (*arrow*) and anterior capsular bulge on T2WI, (B) corresponding hypointensity on ADC (*arrow*), and (C) hyperenhancement on early DCE (*white arrow*). The lack of specificity of early enhancement in the TZ is apparent, with equally brisk enhancement of an adjacent benign BPH nodule (*black arrow*).

FIGURE 14.24. Hemorrhage exclusion sign. A: Precontrast T1WI shows hyperintense postbiopsy hemorrhage (*white arrow*) sparing an ovoid low-signal tumor (*black arrow*) in the right PZ. The tumor (B) has strikingly low signal on ADC map (*arrow*) and (C) is hypointense (*black arrow*) on T2WI compared to the more minimal loss of signal in the area of hemorrhage (*white arrow*).

hematogenous spread. Capsular invasion opens a route to perineural lymphatics and to the periprostatic venous plexus of Santorini, allowing distant metastases to the viscera and axial skeleton.

Local spread is to the seminal vesicles, the urethra, the bladder neck, the bladder base, and the interureteric ridge, sometimes with ureteral obstruction. Less commonly, prostatic cancer spreads posteriorly and superiorly, invading Denonvilliers fascia and the rectosigmoid colon. Rarely, rectal involvement produces an ulcerating lesion that is extremely difficult to distinguish from rectal carcinoma. Late local spread to the corpus cavernosa, corpus spongiosum, and scrotum has also been reported.

Lymphatic spread is from intraprostatic channels to the pelvic lymph nodes, initially the obturator, the external iliac, and the internal iliac nodes. The common iliac, para-aortic, mediastinal, and supraclavicular lymph nodes may be involved in advanced disease, but this is almost always after nodes become involved at the primary drainage sites.

Hematogenous spread is to the axial skeleton or viscera. Eighty-five percent of patients who die from prostatic carcinoma exhibit bony metastases in the axial skeleton. Sites of skeletal metastases are the lumbar spine, proximal femur, bony pelvis, thoracic spine, ribs, sternum, skull, and proximal humerus in order of decreasing frequency. The route of early hematogenous spread to the spine and pelvis is through the intervertebral venous plexus of Batson, which directly communicates with the periprostatic venous plexus of Santorini. More than 90% of prostatic metastatic lesions to bone are blastic. Spread to organs other than lymph nodes and bones is uncommon except in patients with widely disseminated disease.

Staging

Contemporary staging is performed using a tumor-node-metastasis (TNM) system (Fig. 14.25 and Table 14.1) with additional prognostic information derived from serum PSA level and Gleason score. Fundamentally, stages I to III indicate a tumor that does not involve adjacent structures and the absence of nodal or distant metastatic disease. The overall 5-year survival for men with prostate cancer is 95%. However, T4 tumors, N1, or M1 status denote stage IV disease and reduce the 5-year survival to about 28%. In an effort to incorporate the entire range of prognostic information including TNM staging, Gleason score, and PSA level, the National Comprehensive Cancer Network (NCCN) has designated five categories: very low risk, low risk, intermediate risk, high risk, and very high risk. This terminology is frequently used by clinicians and is relevant to prostate MRI interpretation because it is currently thought that MRI reliably detects high-risk and very high-risk cancers.

After prostate cancer is initially diagnosed, imaging plays an important role in staging. CT, like ultrasound, is relatively inaccurate in local staging. However, CT has an important role in systemic staging in patients with T3 or T4 disease, including assessment of lymph nodes and bones. MRI is by far the most accurate method for local anatomic staging of prostate cancer. Preoperative risk assessment may impact the surgical approach or direct patients toward nonoperative management. The suspicion or confirmation of extracapsular extension is the most important imaging distinction if a diagnosis of high-risk cancer has already been made by biopsy. Gross extension of tumor beyond the capsule (T3) or into adjacent structures (T4) may be readily apparent, but more subtle signs of capsular transgression include a bulge in the contour of the gland (Fig. 14.24) and discontinuity of the capsule in the region of the tumor. A smooth capsular bulge is predictive of capsular transgression in approximately 25% of cases, whereas an

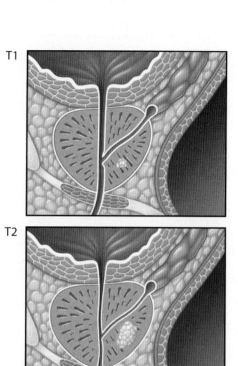
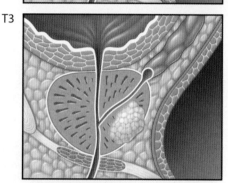
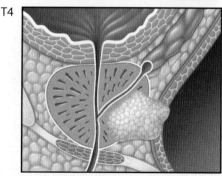

FIGURE 14.25. Schematic illustration of tumor (T) staging in prostate carcinoma.

irregular bulge is indicative of periprostatic spread in 75% of cases. Posterior tumors with capsular contact or extracapsular extension may involve the adjacent neurovascular bundle grossly or with more subtle signs such as loss of fat plane and adherence of the structures (Fig. 14.26).

The fluid in the lumina of normal seminal vesicles exhibits high signal on T2WI, while the thin walls are relatively low signal. Involvement by tumor may appear as obliteration of the normal anatomy and/or replacement of normally bright lumina

TABLE 14.1

Tumor (T) Staging for Prostate Cancer

T stage	Description
T0	**No evidence of tumor**
T1	**Tumor not clinically apparent**
T1a	Incidental finding at resection, ≤5% of gland
T1b	Incidental finding at resection, >5% of gland
T1c	Nonpalpable tumor detected on needle biopsy
T2	**Tumor confined to prostate**
T2a	Tumor involves ≤ half of one lobe
T2b	Tumor involves > half of one lobe, but not both lobes
T2c	Tumor involves both lobes
T3	**Tumor extends through prostate capsule**
T3a	Extracapsular extension (unilateral or bilateral)
T3b	Tumor invades seminal vesicles
T4	**Tumor is fixed in pelvis or invades extraprostatic structures other than seminal vesicles (rectum, levator complex, pelvic sidewall)**

with lower-signal intensity tumor (Fig. 14.27). Accuracy of MRI in detecting seminal vesicle involvement in patients with prostate cancer is reported as >90%. Finally, lymph nodes are hyperintense on both T2WI and DWI and can readily be detected and measured by MRI.

Treatment Planning

Treatment of patients with prostate carcinoma remains a complex subject, well beyond the scope of this chapter. But certain principles are useful in order to choose and interpret imaging studies correctly. Each patient's age, expected life span, tumor size and grade, PSA level, clinical and radiologic stage, and tolerance for risk from his tumor and from the potential complications of each of his potential treatments must be considered.

Very low-risk and low-risk tumors may not need treatment at all, but may be managed by active surveillance. Active surveillance may also be the preferred approach in patients with higher risk tumors but relatively short life expectancies. Active surveillance consists of periodic DRE and PSA, intermittent repeat biopsies, and MRI if suspicious findings emerge through other means of surveillance. Localized tumors that need therapy, and those which are felt to be curable because they have no demonstrable metastases and are relatively unlikely to recur after treatment, can be managed with surgery (usually radical prostatectomy), radiotherapy (brachytherapy or external beam irradiation) or occasionally with newer techniques such as cryotherapy or high-intensity focused ultrasound (HIFU). More detailed choices depend on the likelihood that the tumor is entirely contained within the prostatic capsule. None of these treatments is without risk, but these risks may be balanced by potential cure. Finally, tumors that are metastatic—or are felt to be very unlikely to be successfully treated by local therapy—usually require antiandrogen drugs, surgery, and/or chemotherapy.

Surveillance

The different treatments for prostate cancer may produce characteristic findings. Patients who have undergone prostate brachytherapy will have metallic seeds placed throughout the gland. During radical prostatectomy, the entire prostate gland with its contained segment of urethra and both seminal vesicles are removed en bloc. Continuity of the lower urinary tract must then

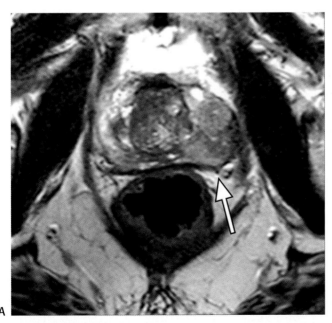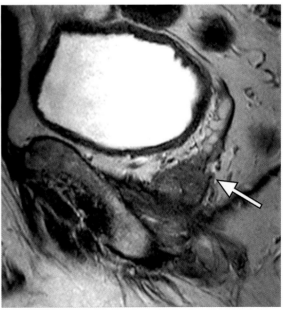

FIGURE 14.26. Gleason 9 (4+5) carcinoma in left PZ invades neurovascular bundle (*arrow*) on axial **(A)** and sagittal **(B)** T2WI.

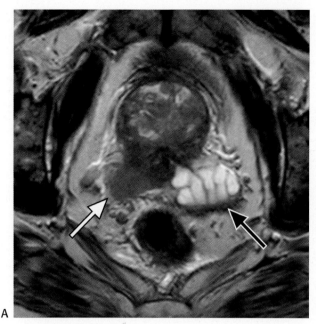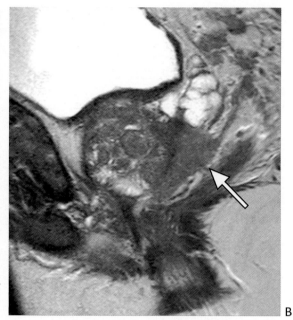

A B

FIGURE 14.27. Seminal vesicle (SV) invasion by prostate cancer. **A:** Axial T2WI shows tumor (*white arrow*) effacing the tubules on the right and causing obstruction on the left (*black arrow*). **B:** Sagittal T2WI shows extensive tumor extending posteriorly from the PZ (*arrow*) with obstructed SV superiorly.

be re-established by anastomosing the bladder neck to a stump of membranous urethra extending from the urogenital diaphragm. The end result is a funnel shape of the bladder base that extends well below the top of the pubic symphysis. Relevant complications include anastomotic leaks after radical prostatectomy, fistulae, and lymphoceles.

After treatment for localized prostate cancer, surveillance for recurrence is primarily performed by serial PSA determinations. If a continued rise in PSA above nadir is encountered, selection of treatment depends to a great degree upon whether the tumor has reappeared in the site of original treatment or has produced distant metastases. CT or MRI can demonstrate local recurrence,

usually evident as an enhancing soft tissue mass in the surgical bed (Fig. 14.28). If the original treatment was resection, salvage radiotherapy may be employed; if it was radiotherapy, salvage prostatectomy may be indicated. It is also crucial to exclude metastases; salvage therapy confers potential side effects and is ineffective if distant disease is present.

SEMINAL VESICLES

Due to the functional interrelationship and close proximity of the seminal vesicles and prostate gland, symptoms caused by seminal vesicle disease are often difficult to differentiate from primary prostatic disease. Relevant presenting symptoms include painful ejaculation, hematospermia, perineal or suprapubic pain, and infertility. Conditions affecting the seminal vesicles include calculi, cysts, inflammation, infection, and neoplasms.

The seminal vesicles can potentially be imaged by CT, TRUS, or MRI, listed with increasing degree of detail. The normal anteroposterior diameter of the seminal vesicles is ≤15 mm, and larger sizes may reflect engorgement due to obstruction. However, there is substantial physiological variation. Seminal vesicle obstruction may be unilateral or bilateral, arising from several potential causes, including stones, cysts, inflammation, or involvement by adjacent tumors.

Seminal vesicles may be obstructed by midline prostatic cysts (Fig. 14.20) or by seminal vesicle cysts. The latter are uncommon and are associated with ipsilateral renal agenesis in at least two-thirds of patients. Therefore, when a seminal vesicle cyst is identified, imaging of the kidneys is usually indicated. Seminal vesicle agenesis is also associated with ipsilateral renal agenesis. Acquired cysts can occur in the seminal vesicles secondary to obstruction or inflammation. Hemorrhage into the lumen of the cyst may result in a solid appearance on CT. Ultrasound will exhibit echoes or dependent debris in hemorrhagic cysts. MRI will typically

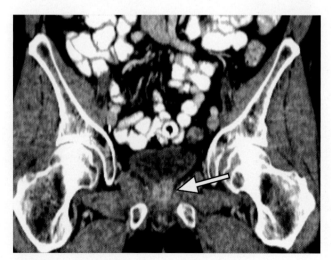

FIGURE 14.28. Prostate cancer recurrence (*arrow*) at bladder base after prostatectomy, on coronal CT reformat.

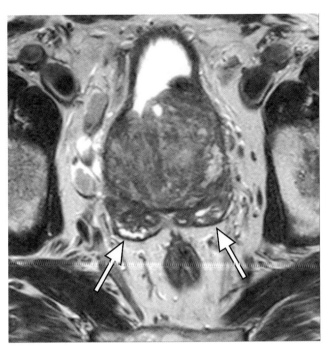

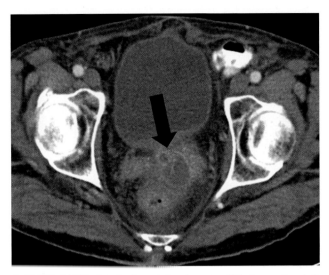

FIGURE 14.30. Seminal vesicle abscess. CT shows the left seminal vesicle to be enlarged; the abscess (*arrow*) has a fluid-filled center and faintly enhancing walls.

FIGURE 14.29. Seminal vesiculitis. Effacement of tubules and wall thickening (*arrows*) attributed to chronic vesiculitis in this patient with marked BPH.

show a high-signal intensity of a hemorrhagic cyst on both T1- and T2-weighted images.

Seminal vesicle inflammation (vesiculitis) may be associated with prostatitis or other urinary tract infection, causing wall thickening and hyperenhancement, which is increasingly recognized with prostate MRI (Fig. 14.29). Seminal vesicle abscesses have the characteristics of abscesses elsewhere (Fig. 14.30) and may be difficult to distinguish from infected cysts. Primary neoplasms of the seminal vesicles including cystadenomas and adenocarcinomas (Fig. 14.31) are extremely rare but can be quite aggressive. The most common cause of neoplastic involvement is direct invasion of the seminal vesicles by adjacent prostate or rectal carcinoma (Fig. 14.32).

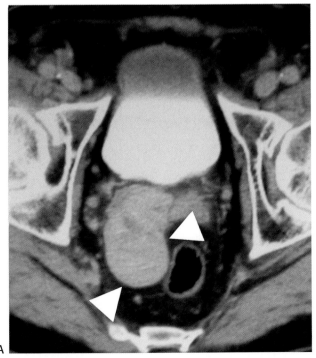

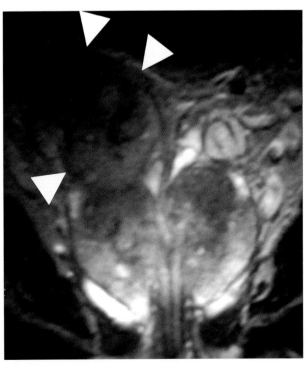

A

B

FIGURE 14.31. Seminal vesicle carcinoma. **A:** A large solid mass (*arrowheads*) arises from the right seminal vesicle on CT. **B:** Mass (*arrowheads*) replaces the normal high signal of the SV on coronal T2WI.

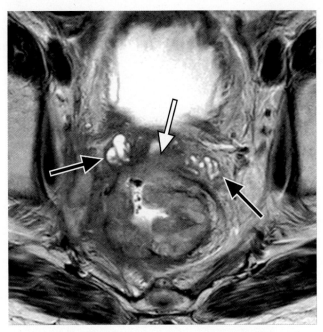

FIGURE 14.32. Midline seminal vesicle involvement (*white arrow*) by locally advanced anal cancer. The seminal vesicles (*black arrows*) are seen laterally, with some dilation of tubules on the right.

SUGGESTED READINGS

Aaron L, Franco OE, Wayward SW. Review of prostate anatomy and embryology and the etiology of benign prostatic hyperplasia. *Urol Clin North Am.* 2016;43(3):279–288.

American Joint Committee on Cancer (AJCC). *Prostate Cancer Staging.* 7th ed. https://cancerstaging.org/

American Cancer Society. *Cancer Facts & Figures 2016.* Atlanta, GA: American Cancer Society; 2016.

Barrett T, Vargas HA, Akin O, et al. Value of the hemorrhage exclusion sign on T1-weighted prostate MR images for the detection of prostate cancer. *Radiology.* 2012;263(3):751–757.

Carter HB, Albertsen PC, Barry MJ, et al. Early detection of prostate cancer: AUA guideline. *J Urol.* 2013;190(2):419–426.

Costa DN, Lotan Y, Rofsky NM, et al. Assessment of prospectively assigned Likert scores for targeted magnetic resonance imaging-transrectal ultrasound fusion biopsies in patients with suspected prostate cancer. *J Urol.* 2016;195(1):80–87.

Costa DN, Yuan Q, Xi Y, et al. Comparison of prostate cancer detection at 3-T MRI with and without an endorectal coil: a prospective, paired-patient study. *Urol Oncol.* 2016;34(6):255.

Dagur G, Warren K, Suh Y, et al. Detecting diseases of neglected seminal vesicles using imaging modalities: a review of current literature. *Int J Reprod Biomed (Yazd).* 2016;14(5):293–302.

Egan KB. The epidemiology of benign prostatic hyperplasia associated with lower urinary tract symptoms. *Urol Clin North Am.* 2016;43(3):289–297.

Epstein JI, Egevad L, Amin MB, et al.; Grading Committee. The 2014 International Society of Urological Pathology (ISUP) Consensus Conference on Gleason Grading of Prostatic Carcinoma: definition of grading patterns and proposal for a new grading system. *Am J Surg Pathol.* 2016;40(2):244–252.

Kim B, Kawashima A, Ryu JA, et al. Imaging of the seminal vesicle and vas deferens. *Radiographics.* 2009;29:1105–1121.

Kitzing YX, Prando A, Varol C, et al. Benign conditions that mimic prostate carcinoma: MR imaging features with histopathologic correlation. *Radiographics.* 2016;36:162–175.

Kongnyuy M, Sidana A, George AK, et al. Tumor contact with prostate capsule on magnetic resonance imaging: a potential biomarker for staging and prognosis. *Urol Oncol.* 2016;35(1):30.e1–30.e8. pii: S1078-1439.

Lee JY, Spratt DE, Liss AL, et al. Vessel-sparing radiation and functional anatomy-based preservation for erectile function after prostate radiotherapy. *Lancet Oncol.* 2016;17(5):e198–e208.

Macey MR, Raynor MC. Medical and surgical treatment modalities for lower urinary tract symptoms in the male patient secondary to benign prostatic hyperplasia: a review. *Semin Intervent Radiol.* 2016;33(3):217–223.

May EJ, Viers LD, Viers BR, et al. Prostate cancer post-treatment follow-up and recurrence evaluation. *Abdom Radiol (NY).* 2016;41(5):862–876.

Moyer VA; U.S. Preventive Services Task Force. Screening for prostate cancer: U.S. preventive services task force recommendation statement. *Ann Intern Med.* 2012;157(2):120–134.

NCCN. *Clinical Practice Guideline in Oncology: Prostate Cancer.* Version 3. 2016. http://www.nccn.org

Purysko AS, Rosenkrantz AB, Barentsz JO, et al. PI-RADS Version 2: a pictorial update. *Radiographics.* 2016;36(5):1354–1372.

Shebel HM, Frag HM, Kolokythas O, et al. Cysts of the lower male genitourinary tract: embryologic and anatomic considerations and differential diagnosis. *Radiographics.* 2013;33(4):1125–1143.

Siddiqui MM, Rais-Bahrami S, Truong H, et al. Magnetic resonance imaging/ultrasound–fusion biopsy significantly upgrades prostate cancer versus systematic 12-core transrectal ultrasound biopsy. *Eur Urol* 2013;64:713–719.

Weinreb JC, Barentsz JO, Choyke PL, et al. PI-RADS prostate imaging-reporting and data system: 2015, Version 2. *Eur Urol.* 2016;69(1):16–40.

Wong LM, Tang V, Peters J, et al. Feasibility for active surveillance in biopsy Gleason 3 + 4 prostate cancer: an Australian radical prostatectomy cohort. *BJU Int.* 2016;117(suppl 4):82–87.

15

Urethra and Penis

NORMAL MALE URETHRA

ACQUIRED URETHRAL
STRICTURES IN MEN
   Gonorrhea
   Tuberculosis
   Schistosomiasis

TRAUMA
   Instrument Strictures in Men
   Catheter Strictures

PERIURETHRAL ABSCESS

CONDYLOMA ACUMINATA

URETHRAL TUMORS IN MEN

URETHRAL TUMORS IN
WOMEN

FEMALE URETHRAL
DIVERTICULAE

URETHROVAGINAL
FISTULAE

URETHRAL CALCULI

POSTOPERATIVE URETHRAL
CHANGES
   Urethroplasty
   Prostatectomy

PENIS
   Penile Neoplasms
   Erectile Dysfunction
   Penile Prostheses
   Priapism
   Peyronie's Disease

NORMAL MALE URETHRA

A brief review of urethral anatomy as defined by radiographic landmarks is in order before discussing urethral strictures and tumors. During dynamic retrograde urethrography, the entire urethra can be visualized (Fig. 15.1A). If properly performed, contrast medium can be seen jetting through the bladder neck into the bladder. The verumontanum is seen as an ovoid filling defect in the prostatic urethra. The distal end of the verumontanum marks the proximal boundary of the membranous urethra. The distal boundary of the membranous urethra is the conical tip of the bulbar urethra. The membranous urethra is <1 cm in length and is that portion of the urethra that passes through the urogenital diaphragm. This is also the region of the external sphincter of the urethra. The anterior urethra extends from its junction with the membranous urethra to the urethral meatus. It is divided into the bulbar segment, which extends from the membranous urethra to the suspensory ligament at the penoscrotal junction, and the penile or pendulous segment. There is usually mild angulation of the urethra where these two segments join.

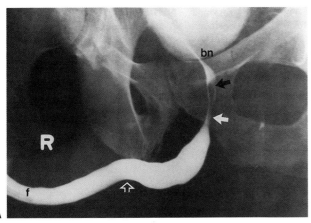
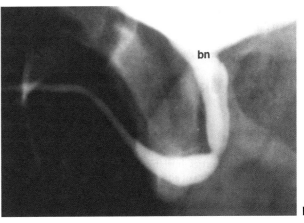

FIGURE 15.1. Normal male urethra. **A:** Dynamic retrograde urethrogram shows opacification of the entire urethra. Contrast can be seen jetting through the closed bladder neck (bn). The verumontanum (*black arrow*) is an ovoid filling defect in the prostatic urethra. The membranous urethra (*white arrow*) lies between the distal end of the verumontanum and the conical tip of the bulbous urethra. The mild angulation in the anterior urethra (*open arrow*) is the penoscrotal junction, dividing the bulbar and penile urethral segments. **B:** Voiding urethrogram shows funneling of the bladder neck (bn). The verumontanum is still clearly seen as a mound of tissue in the prostatic urethra. The membranous urethra is the narrow junction between the prostatic urethra and the bulbar urethra. The membranous urethra is significantly wider during voiding. (From Amis ES Jr, Newhouse JH. *Essentials of Uroradiology*. Boston, MA: Little, Brown and Company; 1991:336, with permission.)

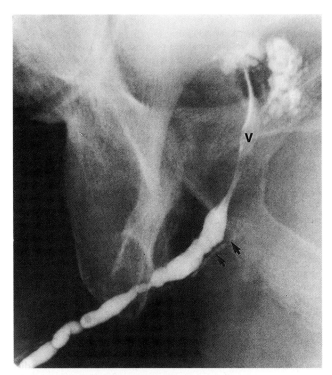

FIGURE 15.7. Gonococcal stricture. Retrograde urethrogram shows an irregular, beaded stricture involving the pendulous urethra and distal two-thirds of the bulbar urethra. The conical tip of the bulbar urethra is preserved and the verumontanum (v) is clearly seen, allowing easy identification of the membranous urethra. Cowper's duct is opacified (*arrows*) and reflux can be seen into the prostate.

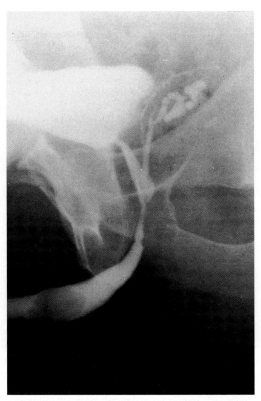

FIGURE 15.8. Dynamic retrograde urethrogram showing a bulbomembranous stricture and reflux into ejaculatory duct, seminal vesicle and vas deferens.

In the presence of a gonococcal stricture, the voiding study usually shows dilation of the proximal urethra (Fig. 15.3). The dilation may include the membranous urethra, even when the dynamic retrograde study indicates scarring extending into the membranous urethra.

The dynamic retrograde and voiding examinations may also indicate other complications of gonococcal urethral stricture. Reflux into prostatic ducts or bulbourethral (Cowper's) ducts are common findings. Reflux into the ejaculatory ducts, seminal vesicles, and vasa deferentia is uncommon (Fig. 15.8), as is reflux into the prostatic utricle, which may be dilated (Fig. 15.9).

Tuberculosis

Usually, genital tuberculosis is a descending infection, and renal tuberculosis is evident. However, in some patients with genital tuberculosis, the kidneys are normal, indicating the possibility of hematogenous spread directly to the urethra. The prostate is involved in most patients with genital tuberculosis. Prostatic abscesses may rupture into any surrounding structure, resulting in fistulae to the rectum or perineum and sinus tracts extending from the posterior urethra. Tuberculous epididymitis and scrotal abscess with fistulae may also be seen with genital tuberculosis, but few of these cases have urethral involvement. When urethral infection occurs, the development of one or more strictures may be followed by periurethral abscesses, producing numerous perineal and scrotal fistulae.

Dynamic retrograde urethrography and voiding cystourethrography typically show an anterior urethral stricture associated with multiple prostatocutaneous and urethrocutaneous fistulae, as well

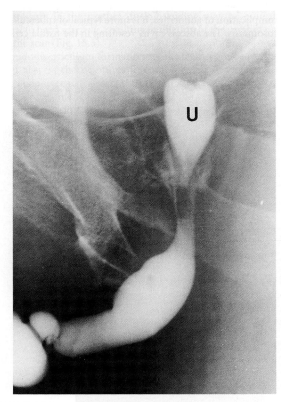

FIGURE 15.9. Dynamic retrograde urethrogram in a patient with multiple anterior urethral strictures. A dilated prostatic utricle (U) is arising from the verumontanum.

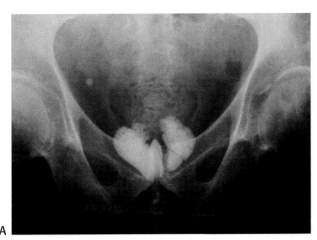 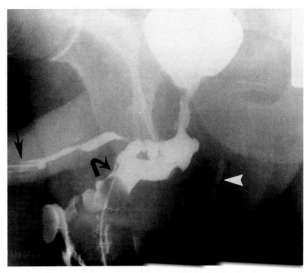

A   B

FIGURE 15.10. Tuberculosis. **A:** A plain film demonstrates an almost completely calcified prostate gland. **B:** A dynamic retrograde urethrogram with injection of contrast into the catheter (*arrow*) in the fossa navicularis shows a perineal fistula. A second catheter (*curved arrow*) is inserted into the perineal fistula orifice. Injection of both catheters simultaneously outlines a urethroperineal abscess cavity and a scarred urethra. Calcification is seen in the epididymis (*arrowhead*).

as blind-ending sinus tracts extending from the urethra. It may not be possible to visualize the entire urethra by standard means if most of the contrast medium exits the urethra through these perineal fistulae. It may be necessary to insert catheters into the fistulae and to inject the fistulae and urethra at the same time to obtain a satisfactory study (Fig. 15.10).

Schistosomiasis

Schistosoma haematobium often involves the bladder and ureters, but multiple fistulae may develop between the urethra and the suprapubic area, the perineum, and the scrotum. Radiographic features are similar to those described for tuberculous urethral disease.

TRAUMA

Most urethral trauma which leads to strictures is iatrogenic. Any penile injury sufficiently severe to affect the wall of the anterior urethra can cause strictures. Foreign bodies inserted into the urethra may produce traumatic strictures, and a straddle injury, in which a blow to the perineum crushes the bulbous urethra against the inferior surface of the pubic symphysis, may lead to a posttraumatic stricture.

Instrument Strictures in Men

The initial insult to the urethra resulting in an iatrogenic stricture is pressure necrosis from the passage of a straight rigid instrument through the curves of the urethra, which has points of relative fixation at the penoscrotal junction, which is attached to the symphysis pubis by the suspensory ligament of the penis, and the membranous urethra, which is fixed by the urogenital diaphragm. Most cystoscopies are currently performed via flexible instruments, but if a straight instrument—like a resectoscope used for transurethral prostatectomy—large diameter is left in the urethra for too long, or is moved in the urethra without appropriate lubrication, pressure necrosis can occur, resulting in scar formation and stricture formation. The incidence of urethral stricture after transurethral resection of the prostate (TURP) has been reported to be as high as 14%, and urethral contour irregularities or serrations are seen postoperatively in up to 30% of patients. However, meticulous technique results in a much lower complication rate.

Strictures arising from instrumentation tend to be short, while those due to inflammatory processes are longer and irregular, with less well-defined margins. Most instrument-related strictures occur in the bulbomembranous region (Fig. 15.11), and fewer than 20% occur at the penoscrotal junction (Fig. 15.12).

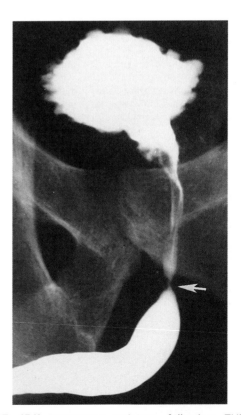

FIGURE 15.11. Instrument stricture following TURP. A dynamic retrograde urethrogram shows a short, tight stricture (*arrow*) in the bulbous urethra near the membranous urethra.

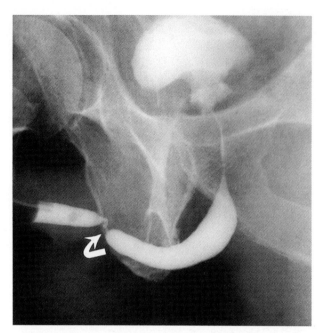

FIGURE 15.12. Instrument stricture following TURP. A dynamic retrograde urethrogram shows a short, tight instrument stricture (*curved arrow*) at the penoscrotal junction. The cone of the bulbous urethra is elongated and narrowed, suggesting bulbomembranous urethral scarring.

Catheter Strictures

Indwelling urethral catheters may also cause pressure necrosis at the fixed points of the urethra and almost invariably cause infection if the catheter is left in position for more than a few days. An indwelling catheter may evoke an inflammatory response and lead to a superimposed infection. With long-term indwelling catheters, diffuse urethritis is almost unavoidable. This infection spreads along the urethra involving the glands of Littré and extends into the submucosal tissues and corpus spongiosum. Urethrography typically reveals long and irregular strictures, often with visualiza-

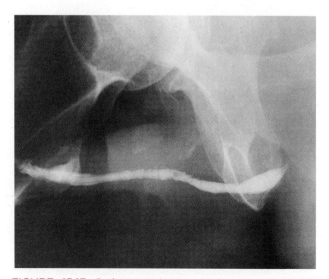

FIGURE 15.13. Catheter stricture. A dynamic retrograde urethrogram 1 year after 7 days of an indwelling bladder catheter. The penile and distal bulbous urethra are markedly narrowed and irregular, especially at the penoscrotal junction. Glands of Littré are visualized.

tion of the glands of Littré (Fig. 15.13). Catheter strictures affecting the bulbomembranous urethra cause irregularity and asymmetry of the cone of the proximal bulbous urethra.

PERIURETHRAL ABSCESS

Periurethral abscesses arise when a gland of Littré becomes obstructed by inspissated pus or fibrosis. Because the tunica albuginea resists the dorsal spread of infection, the abscess tracks ventrally into the corpus spongiosum, where it is confined by Buck fascia. If Buck fascia is perforated, the abscess may spread into the anterior abdominal wall, thighs, or buttocks.

Scrotal swelling and fever are the most common presenting complaints. Occasionally, an abscess may occlude the urethra, causing urinary retention. Most patients have a history of urethral strictures and many are associated with recent urethral instrumentation or catheterization. The most common infecting organisms are gram-negative rods, enterococci, and anaerobes.

If the abscess drains into the urethra, it may be demonstrated by urethrography. Edema and fluid collections may be recognized by MRI (Fig. 15.14) or ultrasound. Approximately 10% of periurethral abscesses drain spontaneously. Percutaneous aspiration and catheter drainage may be performed, usually through the perineal route.

CONDYLOMA ACUMINATA

Condylomata acuminata (venereal warts) are caused by a viral infection that usually produces sessile squamous papillomas on the glans and shaft of the penis and on the prepuce. Occasionally, these warts spread along the urethra (Fig. 15.15) and may even reach the bladder. Urethrography shows characteristic multiple frondlike papillary filling defects in the area of involvement. Occasionally, only isolated filling defects are seen in the penile urethra.

URETHRAL TUMORS IN MEN

Squamous cell and transitional cell carcinomas (TCCs) are the most common urethral malignancies in men. The incidence increases with age, peaking in the 75- to 84-year age cohort. TCC may extend into the urethra from the bladder or may arise in the prostatic urethra; adenocarcinoma occasionally arises in the glands of Littré and Cowper's glands. Benign urethral tumors are extremely rare.

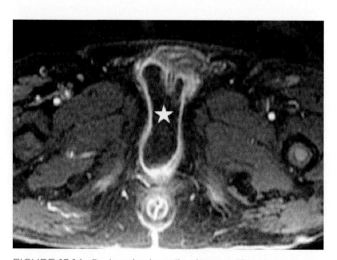

FIGURE 15.14. Periurethral penile abscess. The abscess cavity (*white star*) seen on this transverse gadolinium-enhanced fat-saturated MRI is surrounded by an enhancing wall; it has eroded into the corpora cavernosa and spongiosum.

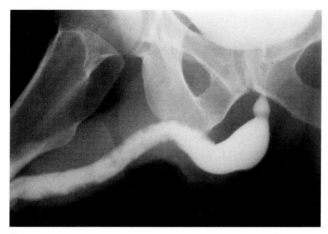

FIGURE 15.15. Condyloma acuminata. Multiple filling defects are seen in the anterior urethra.

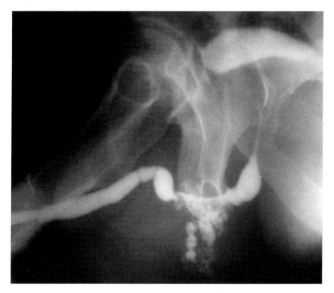

FIGURE 15.16. Squamous cell carcinoma. A spontaneous perineal fistula was the presenting complaint in this man with urethral carcinoma.

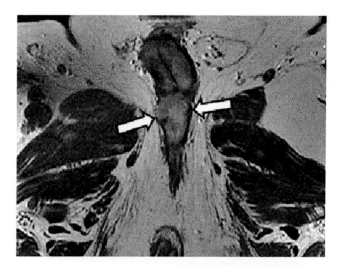

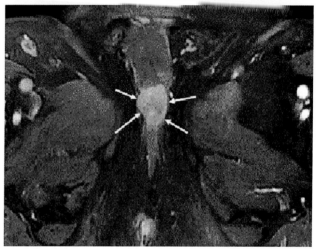

FIGURE 15.17. Squamous cell carcinoma of the urethra (*arrows*). T2-weighted image **(Top)** and T1-weighted gadolinium-enhanced fat-saturated image **(bottom)** reveals a mass in the shaft of the penis, invading the corpora cavernosa.

Squamous cell carcinoma is associated with previous urethral stricture in up to 75% of cases. Any condition that may result in urethral stricture should be considered a predisposing factor to squamous cell carcinoma. These include gonococcal urethritis, long-term urethral catheterization, and urethral trauma. Excess bleeding after stricture dilatation, the development of perineal fistula (Fig. 15.16), or a palpable hard mass in the bulbar region are all physical clues to the development of squamous cell carcinoma. Patients with urethral carcinoma may present with obstructive symptoms, serosanguinous discharge, perineal fistula, periurethral abscess, or a palpable mass in the perineum or along the shaft of the urethra.

Radiographically, urethral tumors have varied presentations. When associated with existing strictures, neoplastic change typically produces more narrowing and grossly irregular margins of the stricture. Such changes should lead to a high suspicion for tumor. In the absence of an existing stricture, urethral neoplasms may present as a de novo stricture or as a filling defect in the urethra; in either case, obstructive changes consisting of dilation and possibly extravasation into prostatic ducts may be seen proximal to the tumor. Early tumors may be detected as small mucosal nodules

without proximal urethral dilation. T1 and lower-stage tumors have not invaded beyond the subepithelial layer; T2 tumors have invaded the corpus spongiosum, prostate, or periurethral muscle; T3 tumors have invaded the corpora cavernosa or bladder neck; and T4 tumors have invaded further into adjacent organs. MRI is the modality of choice for local staging (Fig. 15.17).

Secondary tumors of the male urethra are uncommon. Bladder TCC may be spread to the anterior urethra by seeding during urethral instrumentation or at the time of cystectomy; these are usually seen as multiple small mucosal nodules during urethrography. Contiguous spread of carcinoma of the prostate (Fig. 15.18), rectum, spermatic cord, and testis may involve the corpus spongiosum, causing extensive urethral narrowing and irregularity. Erosion into the urethra from metastases to the corpus spongiosum may produce urethral irregularities, although hematogenous metastases to the corpora cavernosa and corpus spongiosum are exceedingly rare.

URETHRAL TUMORS IN WOMEN

Carcinoma of the female urethra is rare and accounts for <1% of genitourinary malignancies. Most female malignant urethral tumors are carcinomas. TCCs and adenocarcinomas involve the

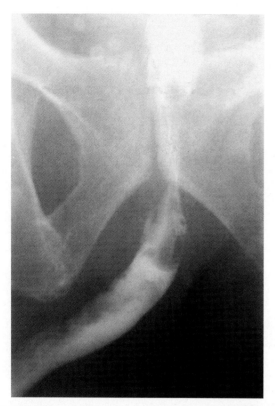

FIGURE 15.18. Contiguous spread of carcinoma of the prostate into the urethra. Multiple filling defects are appreciated in the bulbous and membranous portions of the urethra.

proximal urethra (Fig. 15.19), while squamous cell carcinomas arise in the distal two-thirds. Other histologic types are extremely rare.

The etiology of female urethral carcinomas remains controversial, but previous urethral infection, urethral trauma, and urethral caruncle may be predisposing factors. Female urethral diverticula may contain carcinomas as well as stones. Clinically, urethral tumors present with a mass projecting from the urethral orifice,

urethral bleeding, dysuria, and frequency. Sometimes they present only when urinary retention, urethral abscess, or urethrovaginal fistula have developed. Pain is a late and uncommon presentation.

The diagnosis of urethral tumor in a woman is usually clinical; urethrography is rarely useful. The local staging system is similar to that used for urethral cancer in males with the exception that a tumor may reach T3 status by invading the anterior bladder wall. MRI is useful in staging these tumors once the diagnosis has been established (Fig. 15.20).

FEMALE URETHRAL DIVERTICULAE

Urethral diverticulae in women are not uncommon. They should be sought in patients with chronic irritative voiding symptoms, postvoid dribbling, or dyspareunia. As pelvic imaging with CT and MRI becomes more common, they are often discovered as incidental findings. A diverticulum may cause irritative symptoms, including dyspareunia, by harboring chronic infection, and may produce postvoid dribbling if it fills during voiding and empties afterward. Although most diverticula lie posterior to the urethra, they can also be located laterally or anteriorly or even partially or completely surrounding the urethra.

A diverticulum may fill during the voiding phase of cystourethrography, presenting as a well-marginated fluid collection adjacent to the urethra (Fig. 15.21). Not all urethral diverticula fill during voiding, however, so that a normal voiding urethrogram does not exclude one. Direct-injection urethrography, using a "double bubble" catheter, which has two balloons which occlude the bladder neck and urethral meatus has largely been replaced by cross sectional imaging, especially MRI. A filling defect in a diverticulum is a rare finding but may be caused by stone, debris, or tumor. Adenocarcinoma is the most frequently diagnosed tumor in a diverticulum.

Transvaginal sonography, CT, and MRI are useful in detecting urethral diverticulae and may be more sensitive than urethrography. Ultrasound shows a relatively echo-free cavity adjacent to the urethra (Fig. 15.21); it may also demonstrate inflammatory debris and/or surrounding inflammatory edema. T2-weighted MR images reveal the diverticulum as a high-signal structure and can easily define the full extent and configuration of the diverticulum (Fig. 15.22).

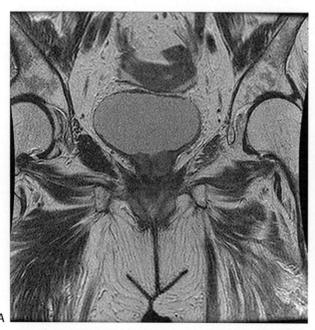
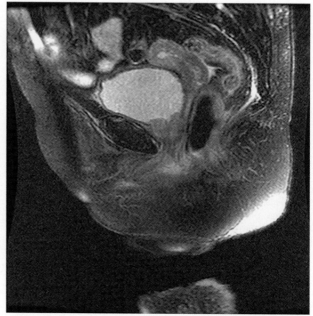

FIGURE 15.19. Transitional cell carcinoma invading the bladder neck and proximal urethra is seen on **(A)** coronal and **(B)** sagittal T2-weighted MR images. (Case courtesy of Akira Kawashima, M.D.)

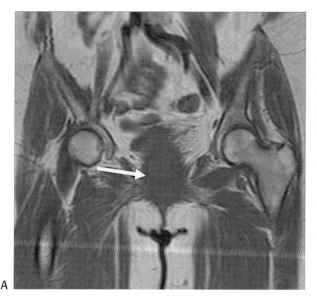
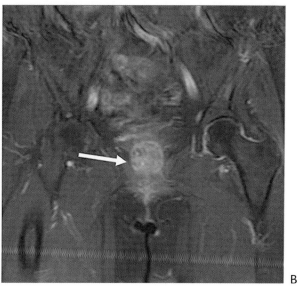

A   B

FIGURE 15.20. Squamous cell carcinoma of the female urethra. Precontrast T1-weighted coronal image **(A)** (*arrow*) below the bladder and postcontrast T1-weighted image **(B)** with fat suppression showing an enhancing mass (*arrow*).

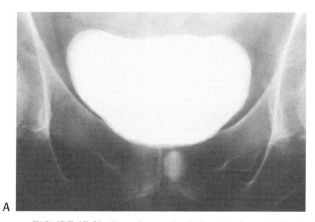
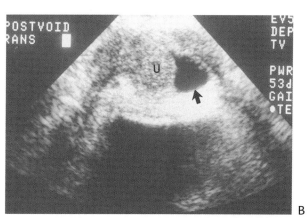

A   B

FIGURE 15.21. Female urethral diverticulum. **A:** Postvoid film from a voiding cystourethrogram reveals a collection of contrast below the bladder base slightly to the left of midline. **B:** Transvaginal sonography reveals a cystic mass (*arrow*) adjacent to the urethra (U).

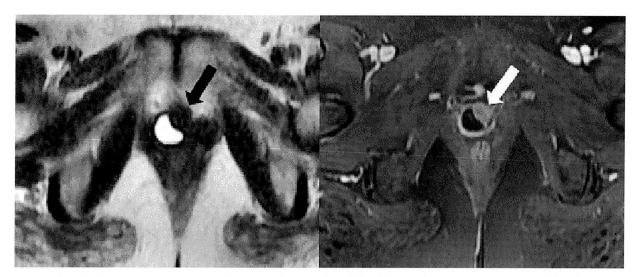

FIGURE 15.22. MRI of periurethral diverticulum. **Left:** T2-weighted image. The urine in the lumen of the diverticulum is bright. **Right:** T1-weighted gadolinium-enhanced fat-saturated image. The urine is dark; the wall of the diverticulum is enhanced. The *arrow* indicates the urethra.

URETHROVAGINAL FISTULAE

Urethrovaginal fistulae are much less common than vesicovaginal fistulae. In the Western world, they are most frequently caused by iatrogenic trauma and may appear as complications after procedures such as urethral diverticulectomy, urethral sling procedures, traumatic catheterizations, and hysterectomy. In undeveloped parts of the world, they occur more often after traumatic childbirth. Fluoroscopic urethrography, either voiding or via a double bubble direct urethrography catheter, is most effective to demonstrate them (Fig. 15.23).

URETHRAL CALCULI

Calculi from the upper urinary tract or bladder that are small enough to pass through the bladder neck into the urethra are usually small enough to pass through the urethra during voiding. Occasionally, however, a stone may be large enough to become lodged at a point of urethral narrowing such as the membranous urethra or a urethral stricture (Fig. 15.24). Primary formation of stones in the urethra may be seen within a congenital or acquired diverticulum (Fig. 15.25). Symptoms of a urethral stone include a weak stream, dysuria, and hematuria. The stones are usually easily visible on radiographs and CT; retrograde urethrography usually will identify a rounded filling defect in the urethra.

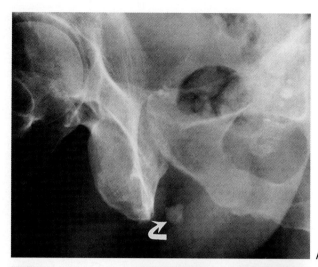

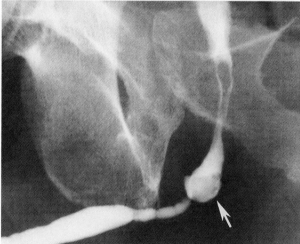

FIGURE 15.24. Urethral stone. **A:** A small stone is seen (*curved arrow*) in the expected location of the urethra. **B:** A dynamic retrograde urethrogram shows severe scarring in the bulbous urethra. The filling defect (*arrow*) in the dilated urethra proximal to the scarring is a urethral stone.

POSTOPERATIVE URETHRAL CHANGES

Urethroplasty

Urethroplasty, particularly two-stage procedures performed as definitive therapy for anterior urethral strictures, may result in saccular dilations of the urethra, particularly near the proximal and distal ends of the repair (Fig. 15.26). These sacculations may be so large as to resemble urethral diverticulae. Because of their size, they may collect urine during voiding and cause postvoid dribbling. Retrograde urethrography easily demonstrates sacculations or acquired diverticulae.

Prostatectomy

In rare instances, nodules of benign prostatic hyperplasia can reform in the resected urethra following a TURP procedure; these are most commonly found near the distal end of the resection, because the urologist may be less vigorous in resecting this area in an effort not

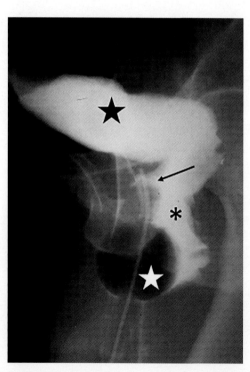

FIGURE 15.23. Urethrovaginal fistula after surgery for urethral diverticulum. A double balloon catheter is in the urethra. An air-filled balloon (*white star*) occludes the urethral meatus; the other balloon is obscured by contrast in the bladder (*black star*). Contrast has been injected into the urethra via a side hole in the catheter; the contrast has leaked into the vagina (*asterisk*) which has filled via the fistula (*arrow*).

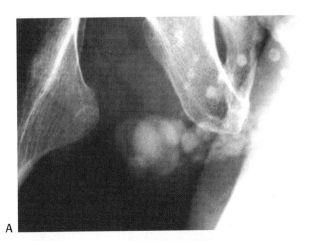

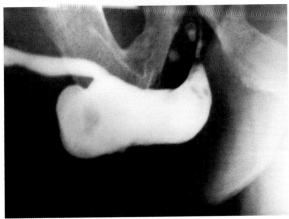

FIGURE 15.25. Calculi in a urethral diverticulum. **A:** Multiple calculi are appreciated on the scout film. **B:** Filling defects are seen in the contrast-filled urethral diverticulum.

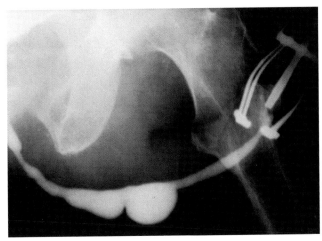

FIGURE 15.26. Urethral sacculations after urethroplasty. Retrograde urethrogram using a Brodney clamp shows two saccular dilations of the midurethra after urethroplasty for urethral stricture. (From Taveras JM, Ferrucci J. *Radiology: Diagnosis-Imaging-Intervention.* Philadelphia, PA: JB Lippincott Co.; 1986:6, chapter 114, with permission.)

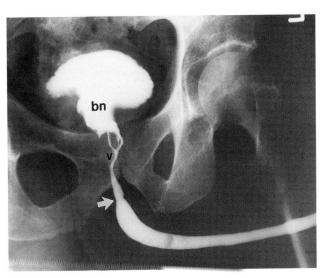

FIGURE 15.27. Recurrent prostatic nodule after TURP. Retrograde urethrogram shows a widely resected prostatic urethra and bladder neck (bn). Immediately above the verumontanum (V) is a nodule protruding into the lumen. The narrowing of the proximal bulbar urethra (*arrow*) is the musculus compressor nuda.

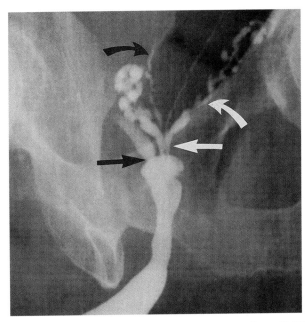

FIGURE 15.28. Bladder neck contracture after TURP. Retrograde urethrogram shows a narrow bladder neck (*straight black arrow*). Contrast is taking the path of least resistance and opacifying the ejaculatory ducts (*straight white arrow*) and the convoluted portion of the vasa (*curved black arrow*) and the seminal vesicles (*curved white arrow*). (From Amis ES Jr, Newhouse JH, Cronan JJ. Radiology of the male periurethral structures. *AJR Am J Roentgenol.* 1988;151:321.)

to compromise the external sphincter. These nodules typically are smooth and round or ovoid and are best demonstrated by retrograde urethrography (Fig. 15.27). Another, although fortunately rare, complication of TURP or other interventions is bladder neck contracture (Fig. 15.28). These are being seen less frequently given the declining use of TURP for obstructive voiding problems. After open prostatectomy for benign disease, the proximal prostatic urethra may appear patulous and irregular when imaged by urethrography, CT, MRI, or transrectal ultrasound.

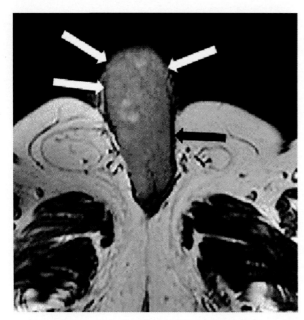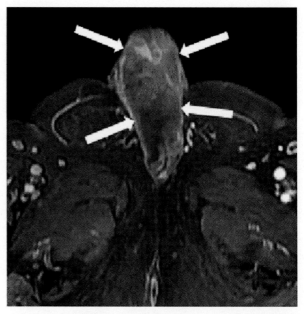

FIGURE 15.29. Squamous cell carcinoma of the penis. The tumor (*arrows*) is seen invading the corpora and urethra in T2-weighted **(left)** and T1-weighted gadolinium-enhanced fat-saturated images **(right)**.

PENIS

Penile Neoplasms

Primary penile cancer is a rare entity, accounting for only 0.4% of all malignancies in males in the United States. Squamous cell carcinoma accounts for nearly all penile tumors and usually occurs in the sixth and seventh decades. Penile cancers are most commonly located on the glans penis and usually occur in uncircumcised men. Survival is dependent on the depth of invasion of the primary tumor and the status of the draining inguinal lymph nodes. Tumors which do not invade the corpora are considered stage T1, stage T2 tumors invade either the corpora cavernosa or corpus spongiosum, stage T3 lesions invade the urethra, and stage T4 lesions extend to other adjacent structures. MRI is the most sensitive method for making these assessments. T2-weighted and gadolinium-enhanced T1-weighted sequences accurately define the extent of the primary lesion. The tumor is typically hypointense relative to the corpora on both T1- and T2-weighted images and enhances following gadolinium (Fig. 15.29), although less than the corpora cavernosa. As might be expected, higher local stages are associated with higher metastatic likelihood and lower survival. Metastatic nodes occur first in the inguinal and then in the iliac regions (Fig. 15.30).

Secondary tumors of the penis can occur, and in most cases, the primary tumor is found in the urogenital system. These typically manifest on MRI as multiple discrete masses in the corpora cavernosa and corpus spongiosum which have low-signal relative to normal corporal tissue on both T1- and T2-weighted sequences.

Erectile Dysfunction

Erectile dysfunction (ED) is the most common male sexual complaint, affecting up to 30 million men in the United States. The etiologies of the condition are numerous and include vascular, neurologic, traumatic, endocrine, psychologic, and drug-related factors, as well as Peyronie's disease (see below). In most cases, imaging workup is not necessary: history and physical examination may reveal the cause, and if the dysfunction responds to oral pharmacologic agents, specific diagnostic tests are only infrequently performed.

Nevertheless, in circumstances in which optimal therapy is not immediately evident, Doppler ultrasound may be of value to distinguish some of the pathophysiologic causes of ED. Stenoses of the arteries supplying the corpora, including the internal pudendal, penile, dorsal penile, and cavernosal arteries (Fig. 15.31) may be amenable to direct intervention, and diminished cavernosal flow velocity in the flaccid penis often indicates these conditions. CT arteriography or catheter arteriography may then demonstrate specific lesions to guide therapy. Alternatively, the resistance to venous outflow from the sinusoids, which is normally high enough to reduce venous flow almost to zero and produce erections by increasing the volume of the corpora and elevating the blood pressure within the corpora, may be abnormally low. When Doppler studies demonstrate high venous flow after intracorporal injections of papaverine, correctible arterial lesions are unlikely to be responsible.

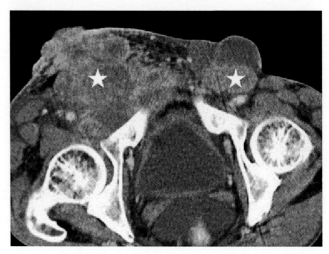

FIGURE 15.30. Metastatic squamous cell carcinoma of the penis. Matted enlarged lymph nodes (*stars*) are seen in both the inguinal and femoral regions.

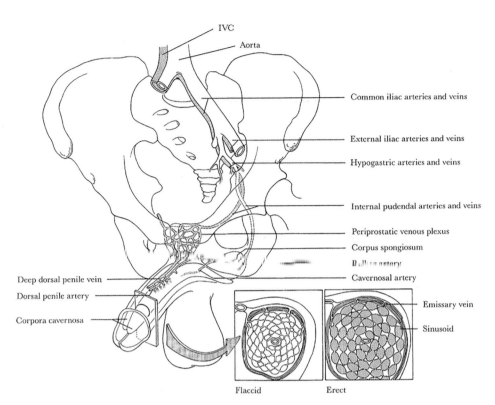

FIGURE 15.31. Simplified diagram of erectile function. During erection, the sinusoids in the corpora cavernosa distend and compress the emissary veins against the rigid tunica albuginea, thus occluding venous outflow. Leakage via these veins is the cause of venogenic impotence. Obstruction of the arterial supply to the penis from atherosclerosis causes arteriogenic impotence. (IVC, inferior vena cava.) (From Amis ES Jr, Newhouse JH. *Essentials of Uroradiology*. Boston, MA: Little, Brown and Company; 1991:382, with permission.)

Penile Prostheses

When standard therapies prove unsuccessful or are not well tolerated, the implantation of a penile prosthesis may be considered. This option is feasible for nearly every man with ED, and current device survival rates and patient/partner satisfaction rates are high. Contemporary implantable penile prostheses are either solid or hydraulic. The solid types may be malleable or mechanically positionable. The hydraulic types are much more commonly used; each consists of a pair of inflatable cylinders with a reservoir (Fig. 15.32) in the abdomen and a pump in the scrotum or both reservoir and pump in the scrotum. New products and variations on existing devices are continually introduced, although the basic function and radiographic appearance of these implants are relatively constant.

Radiographic evaluation is usually requested to evaluate these devices when they fail to function properly. For the inflatable prosthesis, radiographs will indicate if the reservoir, which may be filled with radiopaque fluid, is intact or leaking (Fig. 15.33) and if the tubing connecting the various parts is kinked (Fig. 15.34) or disconnected. MRI and CT can easily display the various components of various types of prostheses (Fig. 15.35).

Priapism

Priapism is a condition characterized by a prolonged erection, with 4 hours as a commonly accepted threshold. So-called low-flow priapism is the more common variety; it is usually painful, is due to pathologic obstruction to blood flow at the sinusoidal level and, if not promptly treated, may cause chronic ED. Priapism may be idiopathic and may also occur with conditions, like sickle cell disease, which lead to small vessel occlusive crises. High-flow priapism is caused by low-resistance shunts between cavernosal or dorsal penile arteries and cavernosal sinusoids; it is usually the result of trauma. It is seldom painful, may resolve spontaneously

or with angioembolic therapy, and is less likely to have long-term consequences.

Doppler ultrasound reveals extremely low or absent flow in cavernosal arteries and in the corpora cavernosa in low-flow priapism and rapid flow, often with characteristics of arteriovenous shunts, in the arteries and cavernosal sinusoids in high-flow priapism. CT and MR arteriography have been used to demonstrate

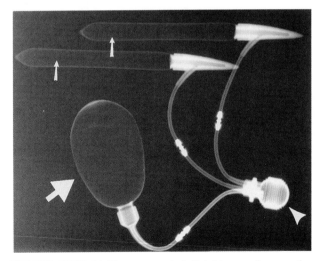

FIGURE 15.32. Multicomponent inflatable penile prosthesis (IPP). This radiograph of a Mentor IPP demonstrates the reservoir (*large arrow*), valve mechanism (*arrowhead*), and penile cylinders (*small arrows*). (From Cohan RH. Radiology of penile prostheses: normal appearance and evaluation of malfunctions. In: *Uroradiology Syllabus*. Leesburg, VA: American Roentgen Ray Society; 1989:169, with permission.)

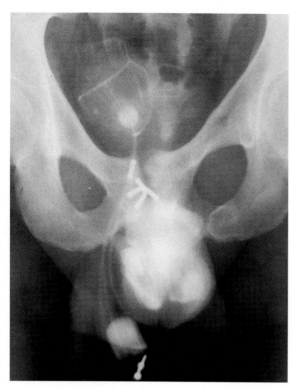

FIGURE 15.33. Fluid leak from an IPP. Only a minimal amount of fluid remains within the reservoir and penile cylinders, indicating fluid leak.

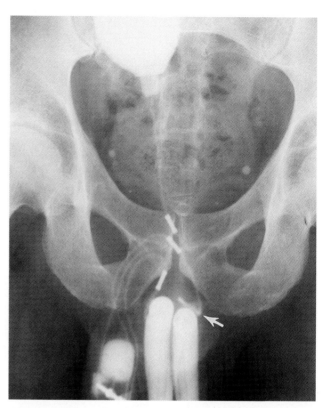

FIGURE 15.34. Kink in connecting tubing. The abrupt angulation (*arrow*) indicates a kink in the connecting tubing. (From Cohan RH. Radiology of penile prostheses: normal appearance and evaluation of malfunctions. In: *Uroradiology Syllabus*. Leesburg, VA: American Roentgen Ray Society; 1989:170, with permission.)

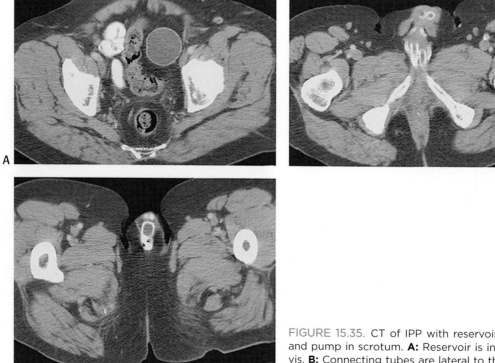

FIGURE 15.35. CT of IPP with reservoir in abdomen and pump in scrotum. **A:** Reservoir is in the true pelvis. **B:** Connecting tubes are lateral to the implants in the corpora cavernosa. **C:** The pump is in the scrotum.

the vascular anatomy of the shunt, as has catheter arteriography; the last has the advantage of enabling direct progression to embolic therapy.

Peyronie's Disease

Peyronie's disease is an uncommon, idiopathic condition in which parts of the tunica albuginea become inflamed and then thickened and fibrotic. During the inflammatory phase, pain is a common symptom; the subsequent fibrosis leads to focal limitation of expansion during erections, which can lead to penile deformity and pain during erections. MRI is the most effective imaging method to demonstrate the condition; it reveals thickening of regions of the tunica with fibrous tissue which is of low intensity on both T1- and T2-weighted images (Fig. 15.36). In some cases, the abnormal regions of the tunica calcify (Fig. 15.37).

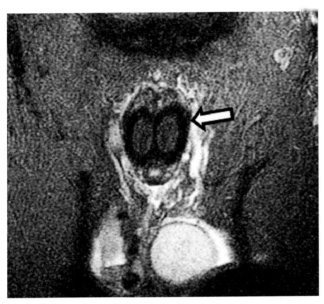

FIGURE 15.36. Peyronie's disease. Coronal MRI reveals circumferential thickening of the tunica albuginea around the corpora cavernosa; the tunica is thickest at the site indicated by the *arrow.*

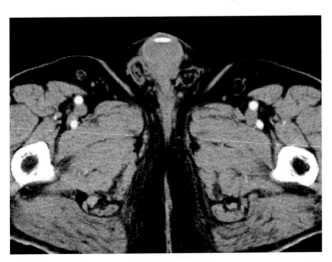

FIGURE 15.37. Peyronie's disease. A calcified plaque in the tunica albuginea is visible in the ventral portion of the penis.

SUGGESTED READINGS

Urethra

Amis ES Jr, Newhouse JH, Cronan JJ. Radiology of male periurethral structures. *AJR Am J Roentgenol.* 1988;151:321.

Chaudhari VV, Patel MK, Douek M, et al. MR Imaging and US of female urethral and periurethral disease. *Radiographics.* 2010;30:1857–1874.

Chou C-P, Levenson RB, Elsayes KM, et al. Imaging of female urethral diverticulum: an update. *Radiographics.* 2008;28:1917.

Crescenze IM, Goldman HB. Female urethral diverticulum: current diagnosis and management. *Curr Urol Rep.* 2015;16(10):71.

Fernbach SK, Feinstein KA, Schmidt MB. Pediatric voiding cystourethrography: a pictorial guide. *Radiographics.* 2000;20:155.

Gallentine ML, Morey AF. Imaging of the male urethra for stricture disease. *Urol Clin North Am.* 2002;29:361.

Hosseinzadeh K, Furlan A, Torabi M. Pre- and postoperative evaluation of urethral diverticulum. *AJR Am J Roentgenol.* 2008;190:165–172.

Kawashima A, Sandler CM, Wasserman NF, et al. Imaging of urethral disease: a pictorial review. *Radiographics.* 2004;24:S195.

Pavlica P, Barozzi L, Menchi I. Imaging of male urethra. *Eur Radiol.* 2003;13:1583.

Pollack HM, DeBenedictis TJ, Marmar JL, et al. Urethrographic manifestations of venereal warts (condyloma acuminata). *Radiology.* 1978;126:643.

Prasad SR, Menias CO, Narra VR, et al. Cross-sectional imaging of the female urethra: technique and results. *Radiographics.* 2005;25:749.

Ryu J, Kim B. MR imaging of the male and female urethra. *Radiographics.* 2001;21:1169.

Shebel HM, Fag HM, Kolokythas O, et al. Cysts of the lower male genitourinary tract: embryologic and anatomic considerations and differential diagnosis. *Radiographics.* 2013;33:1125.

Singla P, Long SS, Long CM, et al. Imaging of the female urethral diverticulum. *Clin Radiol.* 2013;68(7):e418–e425.

Swartz MA, Porter MP, Lin DW, et al. Incidence of primary urethral carcinoma in the United States. *Urology.* 2006;68:1164–1168.

Symes JM, Blandy JP. Tuberculosis of the male urethra. *Br J Urol.* 1973;5:432.

Penis

Andipa E, Liberopoulos K, Asvestis C. Magnetic resonance imaging and ultrasound evaluation of penile and testicular masses. *World J Urol.* 2004;22:382.

Avery LL, Scheinfeld MH. Imaging of penile and scrotal emergencies. *Radiographics.* 2013;33:721.

Bertolotto M, Pavlica P, Serafini G, et al. Painful penile induration: imaging findings and management. *Radiographics.* 2009;29:477.

Halls J, Bydawell G, Patel U. Erectile dysfunction: the role of penile Doppler ultrasound in diagnosis. *Abdom Imaging.* 2009;34:712.

Hanchanale V, Lehana Y, Subedi N, et al. The accuracy of magnetic resonance imaging (MRI) in predicting the invasion of the tunica albuginea and the urethra during the primary staging of penile cancer. *Br J Urol Int.* 2016;117(3):439–443.

Huang Y-C, Harraz AM, Shindel AW, et al. Evaluation and management of priapism: 2009 update. *Nat Rev Urol.* 2009;6(5):262–271.

Kirkham APS, Illing RO, Minhas S, et al. MR Imaging of nonmalignant penile lesions. *Radiographics.* 2008;28:837.

Kirkham APS. MRI of the penis. *Br J Radiol.* 2012;85(Spec No 1):586–593.

Moncada I, Jara J, Cabello JJ, et al. Radiological assessment of penile prosthesis: the role of magnetic resonance imaging. *World J Urol.* 2004;22:371.

Parker RA, Menias CO, Quazi R, et al. MR imaging of the penis and scrotum. *Radiographics.* 2015;35:1033.

Patel DV, Halls J, Patel U. Investigation of erectile dysfunction. *Br J Radiol.* 2012;85(Spec Iss 1):S69–S78.

Pretorius ES, Siegelman ES, Ramchandani P, et al. MR imaging of the penis. *Radiographics.* 2001;21:S283.

Shenoy-Bhangle A, Perez-Johnston R, Singh A. Penile imaging. *Radiol Clin North Am.* 2012;50(6):1167–1181.

Singh AK, Saokar A, Hahn PF, et al. Imaging of penile neoplasms. *Radiographics.* 2005;25:1629.

Wang AC, Wang CR. Radiologic diagnosis and surgical treatment of urethral diverticulum in women. A reappraisal of voiding cystourethrography and positive pressure urethrography. *J Reprod Med.* 2000;45(5):377–382.

White C, Gulati M, Gomes A, et al. Pre-embolization evaluation of high-flow priapism: magnetic resonance angiography of the penis. *Abdom Imaging.* 2013;38(3):588–597.

16

Scrotum and Contents

The major indications for scrotal imaging include pain, palpable mass or asymmetry, male infertility, and cryptorchidism. Ultrasound—which is widely available, relatively inexpensive, and free of ionizing radiation—is the dominant modality in contemporary imaging of the scrotum and its contents. The exam can be targeted to areas of patient or physician clinical concern such as focal pain or nodule. Dynamic imaging with changes in patient position and/or Valsalva maneuver can be particularly helpful to distinguish intratesticular from extratesticular processes and for specialized applications including evaluation of inguinal hernias and varicoceles. Doppler imaging helps to distinguish vascularized solid masses from complex cysts and can demonstrate hyperemia in an inflamed testis or epididymis or diminished vascularity in a torsed testis.

CT is rarely used for primary evaluation of the scrotum, though it is important for retroperitoneal staging in testicular cancer and may contribute to evaluation of inguinal hernias, scrotal abscesses, and soft tissue gas in necrotizing fasciitis. More often, scrotal pathologies are incidentally detected on CT and further characterized by ultrasound. MRI using high-resolution surface coils can be helpful for characterization of sonographically indeterminate processes in the scrotum due to its excellent soft tissue contrast.

ANATOMY AND EMBRYOLOGY

The testes form within the abdominal cavity in embryonic life and descend into the inguinal region by the end of the first trimester. Each testis is tethered inferiorly by a gubernaculum testis, which persists as a fibrous band in adult life, and each is encased within a peritoneal extrusion known as a processus vaginalis, which later becomes the tunica vaginalis, or lining of the scrotal sac (Fig. 16.1). Incomplete testicular descent and persistent patency of the processus vaginalis are each associated with specific clinical manifestations.

Undescended Testes

Final descent from the internal inguinal ring into the scrotum occurs late in gestation, between the 34th and the 36th week of fetal life. Thus, the prevalence of undescended testes is much higher in premature (30%) than full-term (3%) newborns. Although 75% of undescended testes are found in the inguinal canal, the descent may be arrested at any level, and the testicle may lie anywhere in the abdominal cavity from the kidneys to the pelvis. Spontaneous descent after birth reduces the overall prevalence of undescended testis to only about 1% at the age of 1 year.

Many undescended testes are palpable within the inguinal canal or retractile within the upper scrotum. Imaging may be helpful for precise localization and for evaluation of size,

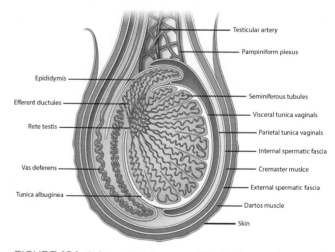

FIGURE 16.1. Schematic diagram of testicular anatomy and scrotal layers.

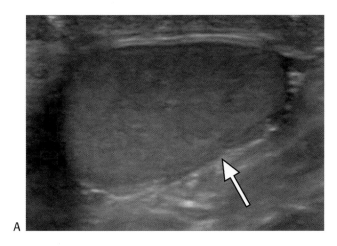
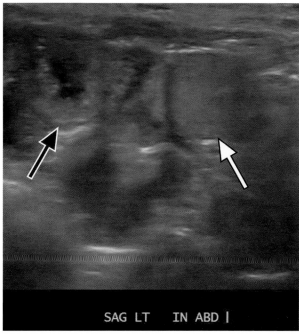

FIGURE 16.2. Undescended testis in a 10-month-old boy. **A:** Normally positioned right testis (*arrow*). **B:** Left testis (*white arrow*) at apex of inguinal canal, surrounded by peristalsing bowel (*black arrow*).

vascularity, and parenchymal characteristics. Ultrasound accurately localizes undescended testes in more than 90% of cases when the organ is in or near the inguinal canal (Fig. 16.2). The examination should begin with the scrotum to identify the normal descended testis. The undescended testis is usually smaller and more elongated than the normal testis, with similar or slightly diminished echogenicity. The bulbous end of the gubernaculum (*pars infravaginalis gubernaculi*) may be of similar size and echogenicity as an undescended testis; therefore, identification of the mediastinum testis is needed in order to confirm the structure is a testicle.

When ultrasound fails to locate the undescended testis, CT, MRI, or rarely arteriography or venography may be employed. The reported sensitivity of CT in the detection of undescended testes in or near the inguinal canal is excellent. An ovoid mass of soft tissue density is seen along the line of testicular descent, with absent ipsilateral spermatic cord structures. On MR images (Fig. 16.3), cryptorchid testes have similar signal to normal testes (intermediate to hypointense on T1WI; hyperintense on T2WI). Ultrasound, CT, and MRI may all fail to identify an undescended testis, sometimes necessitating further hormonal and karyotypic evaluation, particularly when neither testis is identified.

Since normal testicular development occurs only if the testicle is in the typical vascular, hormonal, and thermal milieu of the scrotum, undescended testes are associated with subfertility and an increased risk of neoplasia, the latter about five times greater than that of the normal population. (Notably both risks are higher when the condition is bilateral and lower than reported in older literature.) Orchiopexy is usually performed at about 1 year of age if the testis has not spontaneously descended, with the intent to preserve function and prevent malignancy. In patients who are beyond the age of puberty, an undescended testis is often resected to avoid malignancy. In older men with incidental detection of predominantly fibrous testicular remnants, observation may be reasonable.

Patent Processus Vaginalis

The processus vaginalis is patent in many newborns and closes over the first few years of life in most boys. When the processus vaginalis maintains a small aperture of communication with the peritoneal space, fluid may become entrapped within this space and present as a congenital communicating hydrocele. When the opening is larger, it may accommodate herniation of bowel loops into the scrotum.

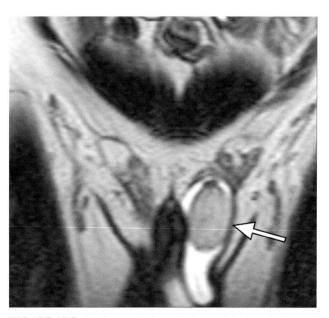

FIGURE 16.3. Undescended testis (*arrow*) in inguinal canal on coronal T2WI.

TESTICULAR AND SCROTAL EMERGENCIES

For the radiologist in training, or the seasoned radiologist with a specialty outside of the genitourinary tract, the following four conditions are highlighted as essentials of on-call scrotal sonography. Neoplasia is a very important diagnosis and will be addressed subsequently in the chapter, but these four conditions are truly urgent, and timely diagnosis will impact management and patient outcomes.

Testicular Torsion

Testicular torsion is abnormal twisting of the testis on its vascular pedicle, the spermatic cord. When the testis twists, the testicular artery may become occluded. Vascular engorgement and edema tend to worsen the occlusion. If torsion is unrelieved, acute ischemia of the testis can result. Pain is usually severe and acute in onset and only rarely associated with trauma. Most patients are infants, boys, or young men. Intrascrotal twists associated with congenital incomplete fixation of the testis by leaves of the tunica vaginalis—so-called "bell-clapper deformity"—are known as "intravaginal torsion." When the twist of the spermatic cord is superior to the scrotum, it is known as "extravaginal torsion."

Immediately after symptom onset, gray-scale ultrasound images of a torsed testis may be normal. Within a few hours, the torsed testis will usually become asymmetrically enlarged, hypoechoic, and mottled in its parenchymal echogenicity (Fig. 16.4). Asymmetrically diminished vascular flow is usually evident on color or power Doppler images including both testes (Fig. 16.5). However, this may be technically challenging due to patient size or discomfort, and it is important to ensure that settings—including gain and pulse repetition frequency—are optimized to detect slow flow if present.

Incomplete or intermittent torsion can pose a diagnostic challenge. Spectral Doppler images may demonstrate a patent testicular

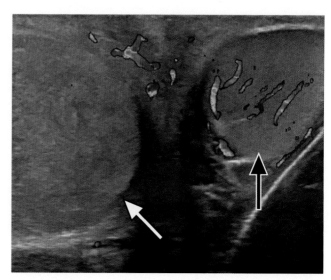

FIGURE 16.5. Acute testicular torsion. Enlarged, hypoechoic, and avascular torsed right testis (*white arrow*) compared to the normal contralateral side (*black arrow*) on color Doppler.

artery, with diminished diastolic flow due to edema and venous outflow obstruction. Rarely, if there has been no infarction, spontaneous detorsion can result in transient testicular hyperemia demonstrable by Doppler ultrasound. Extratesticular findings of torsion include enlargement of the epididymis, thickening of the scrotal skin, hydrocele, and a visible twist of the spermatic cord; occasionally, a torsed testis may be accompanied by an extratesticular hematoma.

Dynamic testicular scintigraphy has been entirely supplanted by ultrasound in most centers. Due to cost, availability, and prolonged examination times, MRI is rarely used in the setting of acute suspected torsion. However, MRI does have characteristic findings including asymmetric enlargement, knotted appearance or "whirl-pool" pattern in the spermatic cord. MRI with gadolinium enhancement and dynamic imaging is highly accurate for demonstrating testicular ischemia (Fig. 16.6), but there are no specific findings for intermittent torsion.

Acute severe testicular ischemia from torsion requires immediate surgery. The testicular salvage rate in the first few hours of symptoms approaches 100% but decreases rapidly to approximately 20% by 12 to 24 hours. Complete testicular ischemia lasting longer than 24 hours virtually always causes irreversible infarction and is known as a *missed torsion*. When the testis can be salvaged, surgical orchiopexy fixes it to the scrotum. Because the bell-clapper deformity tends to be bilateral, orchiopexy is often performed bilaterally and may be indicated even for the normal testis in patients who have had missed torsion.

Rarely, either the appendix testis or the appendix epididymis may undergo torsion. On ultrasound, the appendix testis may appear as an enlarged echogenic structure adjacent to the superior pole of the testis near the pole of the epididymal head. Doppler ultrasound reveals the appendix as an avascular mass. Torsion of an appendage is self-limited, and surgery is unnecessary.

Scrotal Trauma

Scrotal hematomas are fairly common and rarely require intervention. By contrast, intrinsic testicular trauma is unusual and may need urgent surgical attention. Testicular rupture results

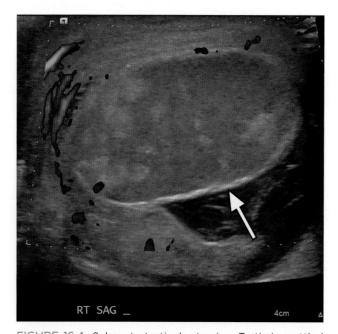

FIGURE 16.4. Subacute testicular torsion. Testis is mottled and avascular (*arrow*) on power Doppler.

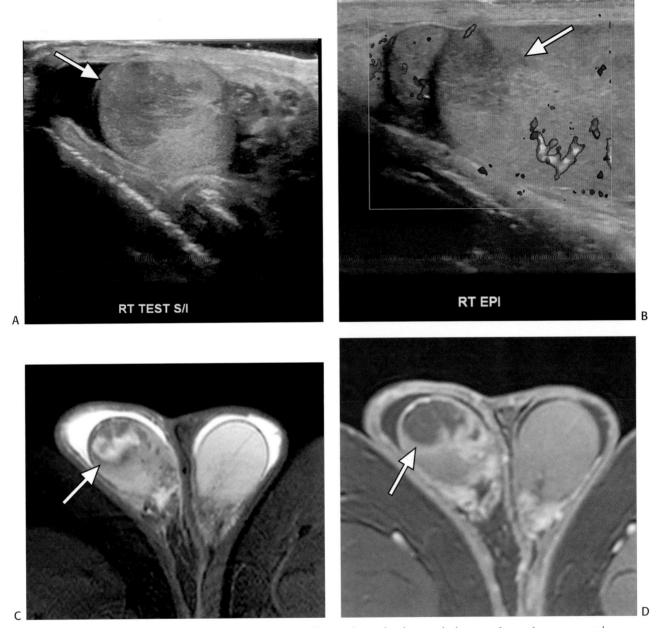

FIGURE 16.6. Testicular infarct demonstrating **(A)** an irregular hypoechoic area (*arrow*) on grayscale US, **(B)** with no internal vascularity (*arrow*) on color Doppler, helping to distinguish it from neoplasm. MR was performed given the indeterminate appearance, with **(C)** a geographic area of altered signal (*arrow*) on axial T2WI and **(D)** a focal enhancement defect (*arrow*) on postcontrast imaging, confirming the diagnosis.

most commonly from athletic injuries, vehicular accidents, and assaults, often when the testis is compressed between the osseous pelvis and an external object. The tunica albuginea ruptures, and hemorrhage occurs into the scrotum and/or testis itself. If surgical intervention occurs within 72 hours, the testis can be saved in approximately 90% of cases, whereas later surgery is associated with a salvage rate of only 55%. Therefore, testicular trauma is an indication for emergency ultrasound examination, which is extremely accurate in diagnosing or excluding testicular hematomas and lacerations.

The diagnosis depends upon careful evaluation of the integrity of the tunica albuginea, parenchymal homogeneity, and altered vascularity. Both testicular laceration and intratesticular hematoma produce focal, often linear or ovoid, alterations of the normal testicular echogenicity; the lesions may be heterogeneous, hypoechoic, or hyperechoic with diminished vascularity (Figs. 16.7 and 16.8). Focal testicular infarction may also accompany trauma and may produce alterations in echogenicity. With testicular rupture, it may be impossible to detect even a portion of the normal testicular outline or tissue, and only a large heterogenous mass

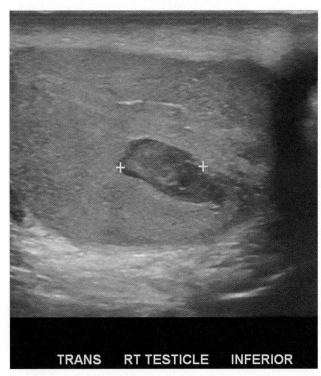

TRANS   RT TESTICLE   INFERIOR

FIGURE 16.7. Small hypoechoic testicular hematoma (*calipers*) in patient kicked by a horse.

comprising hematoma and portions of remaining testis may be seen. If evident, a focal discontinuity of the tunica is a key sign of parenchymal injury (Fig. 16.9). A hydrocele or hematocele may accompany testicular injury; hematoceles may sometimes demonstrate low-level mobile echoes.

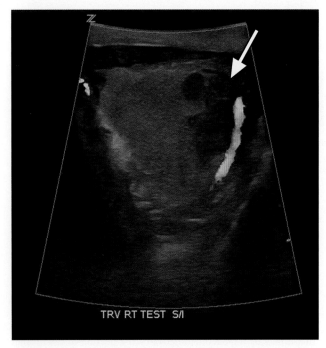

TRV RT TEST S/I

FIGURE 16.8. Large testicular hematoma (*arrow*) is hypoechoic and avascular compared to surrounding parenchyma.

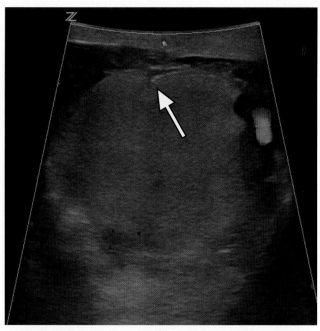

FIGURE 16.9. Testicular rupture with focal defect in tunica albuginea (*arrow*).

Of note, a focal region of testicular injury may not be distinguishable from an intratesticular neoplasm on ultrasonographic grounds alone; the history is necessary. If clinical ambiguity persists, short-term follow-up may be helpful because contusions and hematomas tend to resolve rapidly, whereas tumors change very slowly. Finally, MRI may be helpful when ultrasound findings are unclear in patients with testicular trauma. MRI is particularly effective at demonstrating the testicular tunica albuginea, which appears as a circumferential dark line when intact, making testicular rupture or major laceration unlikely. Like hematomas elsewhere in the abdomen and pelvis, scrotal hematomas exhibit variable signal on T1WI and T2WI, depending upon the age of blood products.

Epididymitis and Orchitis

Epididymitis is the most common inflammatory process in the scrotum, affecting young, often sexually active men, and older men, who may have risk factors such as urinary stasis or indwelling bladder catheters. The condition is rare in children. Although urinary tract pathogens such as *Escherichia coli*, *Pseudomonas*, and *Aerobacter* are most commonly implicated, only a minority of men report associated dysuria. Sexually transmitted organisms including *chlamydia* and *gonococcus* are also associated with epididymitis, and there are occasional cases of mycobacterial or viral epididymitis. Epididymitis can spread to the testis, then termed "epididymo-orchitis," in a minority of cases. Isolated orchitis may be caused by the mumps virus or syphilis but is otherwise a secondary process.

Patients with acute epididymitis present with acute pain and tenderness in the scrotum. Fever, dysuria, or pyuria with urethral discharge may be present. The onset tends to be more subacute than torsion, but the clinical distinction of epididymitis from acute torsion is sometimes difficult. Fortunately, the sonographic findings are quite different.

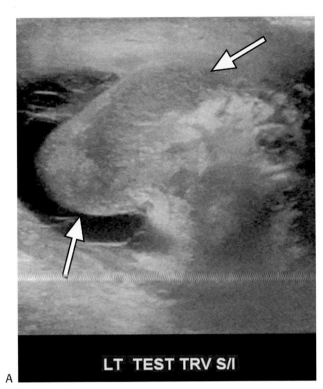
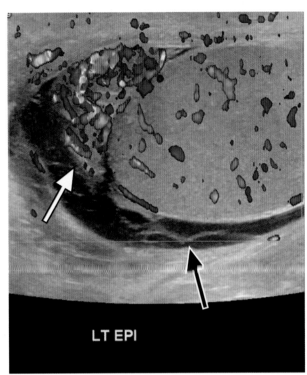

FIGURE 16.10. Acute epididymitis with **(A)** enlarged featureless epididymis (*arrows*) and **(B)** marked hypervascularity (*white arrow*) on color Doppler. Note also complex reactive hydrocele (*black arrow*).

Ultrasound examination reveals that some or all of the head and body of the inflamed epididymis is enlarged and of altered echogenicity (Fig. 16.10). The echogenicity is usually decreased, but epididymitis may also present with hyperechoic regions in the epididymal head. On color or power Doppler images, the inflamed epididymis appears much more vascular than the ipsilateral testis if there is no orchitis; alternatively, in the setting of epididymo-orchitis, both the testis and epididymis are more highly

vascularized than the contralateral side. Associated findings may include a reactive hydrocele or pyocele or occasionally an epididymal abscess.

When orchitis coexists with epididymitis, the testicle is enlarged and of reduced echogenicity and may resemble a torsed testis at gray-scale imaging but is striking in its hypervascularity (Fig. 16.11). Focal orchitis is less common than involvement of the entire testis, but it may occur immediately adjacent to the inflamed epididymis and occasionally may resemble a testicular tumor. An abscess generally manifests as a hypoechoic nonperfused region on ultrasound (Fig. 16.12) or a rim-enhancing collection on MRI. After acute orchitis has resolved, the affected testis may atrophy. A complication of severe acute epididymitis is ischemia of the testis, sometimes followed by infarction, presumably caused by compression of the testicular vessels from epididymal swelling. Chronic epididymitis, which may present clinically as a painless nodular mass on palpation, may appear relatively hypoechoic on ultrasound examination.

Fournier Gangrene

This rare but fulminant necrotizing fasciitis of the penis, scrotum, and perineum was described by Fournier in 1883 and remains a much-feared and frequently litigated diagnosis. Approximately one-half of patients have diabetes mellitus, which both predisposes patients to infection and may limit patient awareness of cellulitis due to neuropathy. Other risk factors include malignancy, paraplegia, alcohol abuse, and prolonged hospitalization. Most patients have had an underlying urinary tract infection, recent urologic instrumentation, or perirectal or colonic disease. Localized cellulitis leads to a diffuse inflammatory reaction within the deep fascial

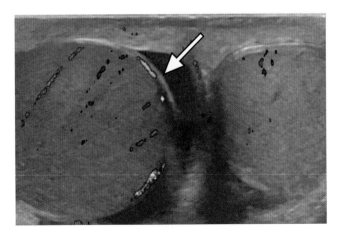

FIGURE 16.11. Acute epididymo-orchitis demonstrating an enlarged hypoechoic right testis (*arrow*) with asymmetric hypervascularity. The contralateral testis provides a helpful internal control in evaluation of torsion or orchitis.

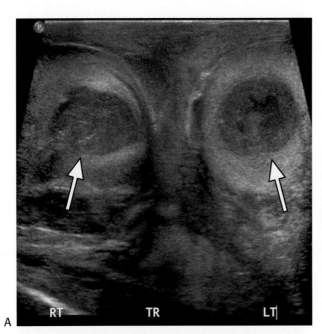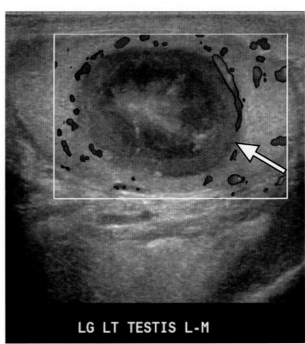

FIGURE 16.12. Bilateral testicular abscesses demonstrating **(A)** hypoechoic intratesticular collections (*arrows*) with **(B)** no internal vascularity (*arrow*).

planes, which notoriously is not as symptomatic as it is potentially deadly. The condition may progress rapidly to extensive gangrene. The diagnosis of subcutaneous emphysema may be made by physical exam, with plain radiographs, ultrasound (Fig. 16.13), or CT (Fig. 16.14). Important distinctions include the involvement of deep spaces of the pelvis and presence of any drainable collections. Treatment includes intravenous antibiotic therapy and surgical debridement.

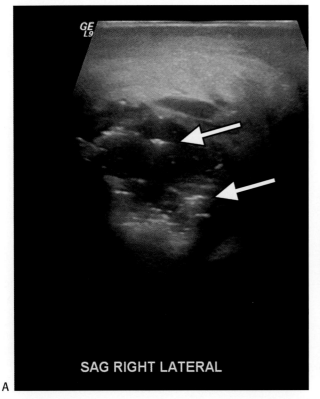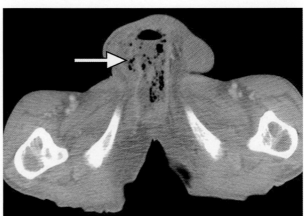

FIGURE 16.13. Fournier gangrene with **(A)** small echogenic foci of gas (*arrows*) with posterior "ring-down" artifact within the scrotum on ultrasound and **(B)** scrotal abscess (*arrow*) on CT.

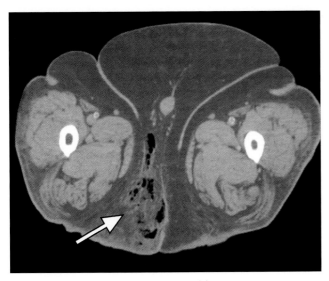

FIGURE 16.14. Fournier gangrene with multifocal gas in the right gluteal region (*arrow*). The presence of ischiorectal fossa or supralevator extension should be commented upon in CT reports for surgical planning.

INTRATESTICULAR LESIONS

Testicular Tumors

Testicular cancer accounts for approximately 1% of all cancers in men. Testicular tumors include primary germ cell and stromal neoplasms, metastases (including lymphoma), and adrenal rest tumors. Germ cell tumors (GCTs) account for up to 95% of primary testicular neoplasms, and about half of these are pure seminoma (*see schematic below*). Some seminomas are intermixed with other germ cell types and are considered nonseminomatous germ cell tumors (NSGCTs), including components of embryonal cell carcinoma, choriocarcinoma, teratoma, and/or yolk sac tumor. NSGCTs including yolk sac tumors and teratomas are more common in children than in adults. The remaining 5% of primary testicular neoplasms arise from stromal cells and are often benign.

There is an association between testis tumors and cryptorchidism. However, the contemporary understanding of the attributable risk of cryptorchidism is lower than was reported in older literature, due to conflation of increased risk conferred by underlying hormonal and genetic syndromes in those studies. The relative risk of testicular cancer is about double that of the normal population in men who underwent orchiopexy prior to puberty and about five times that of the normal population in those with later orchiopexy. Overall, about 10% of testis tumors occur in cryptorchid testes. As in normally positioned testes, seminoma is the most common cell type.

Testicular tumors are usually painless but often palpable. Acute scrotal pain generally favors another process such as torsion or epididymo-orchitis. Occasionally, an asymptomatic, intratesticular, nonpalpable mass may be encountered in a scrotal ultrasound performed for other reasons. In patients with advanced disease, metastatic signs and symptoms such as supraclavicular lymphadenopathy, dyspnea, and back pain may lead to the diagnosis.

Occasionally, testicular tumors may present with upper retroperitoneal metastases but without a palpable tumor in the scrotum (Fig. 16.15). In such cases, ultrasound is particularly important in searching for the primary tumor. Ultrasound of a testis tumor usually reveals the primary lesion to be an intratesticular mass; deciding on the relative location of a mass may be the most important step toward diagnosis of malignancy because so few extratesticular scrotal lesions are neoplasms.

Histologic subtypes cannot be distinguished accurately by ultrasound, but most seminomas are homogeneous, and most nonseminomatous tumors are not. Small tumors tend to be hypovascular by color Doppler, while flow may be more conspicuous in larger tumors. Compared with normal parenchyma on MRI, tumors are generally hypointense in T2WI though often isointense on precontrast T1WI. Gadolinium-enhanced MRI is highly accurate in local tumor depiction and can detect local stage (breach of the tunica albuginea, invasion of the epididymis, invasion of the scrotal wall, etc.) in greater detail than other modalities. However, local tumor staging is almost always performed surgically rather than preoperatively by imaging.

Testicular cancer is staged using a tumor–node–metastasis (TNM) system. Tumors confined to the scrotum are defined as stage I. Stage II involves regional lymph nodes, and stage III indicates various combinations of distant lymph nodes, extranodal metastasis, or markedly elevated postorchiectomy serum tumor markers. Tumor markers, including lactate dehydrogenase (LDH), α-fetoprotein

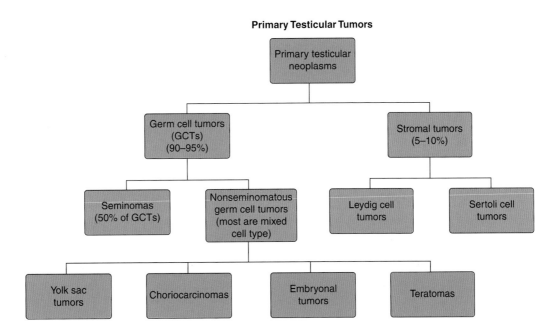

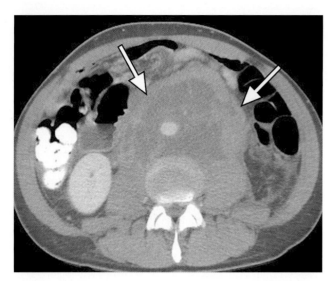

FIGURE 16.15. Retroperitoneal metastasis with abdominal pain as initial presentation of seminoma. Contrast-enhanced CT shows centrally necrotic mass (*arrows*) at the level of the kidneys.

(αFP), and human chorionic gonadotropin (hCG), are used for both primary staging and surveillance. Imaging studies include a chest radiograph and CT of the abdomen and pelvis. Chest CT is performed in the setting of abdominal masses, an abnormal radiograph, or associated symptoms. Current NCCN guidelines do not recommend [18]fluorodeoxyglucose positron emission tomography ([18]FDG-PET) for initial staging, but it is useful in restaging to assess the viability of any measurable disease persisting after chemotherapy.

Testis tumors may spread by direct invasion of the epididymis or spermatic cord, through the lymphatics to upper retroperitoneal nodes, or hematogenously. Hematogenous spread is most common in choriocarcinoma. Retroperitoneal lymph node involvement often appears first at the level of the renal hilum on the left and slightly lower on the right, near the sites of insertion of the gonadal veins into the left renal vein and IVC, respectively. Right-sided tumors are known to cross into the left retroperitoneum via lymphatics, presenting initially in the para-aortic space, for example, but left-sided tumors rarely present with initial metastasis in the right retroperitoneum. Inguinal and external iliac nodes are usually spared unless there is involvement of scrotal skin. Continued lymphatic spread may occur through the thoracic duct and to supraclavicular lymph nodes. Hematogenous metastases usually appear in the lungs, where they form multiple pulmonary nodules or masses.

Imaging diagnosis of nodal metastases remains focused on size. We assume that the larger the lymph node, the more likely it is to contain metastatic disease, while recognizing the possibility that small nodes may contain neoplastic cells and large nodes may reflect benign reactive changes. A measurement of 10 mm in short-axis diameter is typically used, although other features such as craniocaudal length, cortical irregularity, globular shape, internal necrosis, clustering of nodes, and asymmetry in number or size should also be considered.

Radical inguinal orchiectomy remains the primary diagnostic and therapeutic intervention in evaluation of testicular neoplasia. Percutaneous biopsy is almost never performed, due to the risk of tumor seeding in the scrotal skin or lymphatics.

Seminoma

Seminoma is the most common testicular neoplasm, making up about half of GCTs. Seminoma occurs in slightly older men than do other types of testicular tumors; patients are often 30 to 45 years of age. The majority of these men present with highly curable stage I disease, conferring a 10-year disease-specific survival rate of 99.6%. The prognosis in stage II disease remains excellent, with a 98% cure rate. In the last half century, combination chemotherapies including platinum-based agents have dramatically improved survival even in metastatic and/or recurrent disease, with complete cure rates up to 80%.

Masses may be detected by palpation or imaging. On ultrasound images, seminomas are usually hypoechoic compared to adjacent parenchyma and are variable in size. Doppler ultrasound with appropriate settings virtually always demonstrates internal vascularity (Fig. 16.16). Testicular seminomas are often well

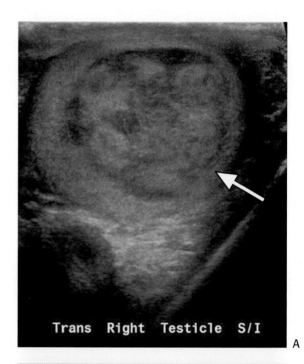

Trans Right Testicle S/I

A

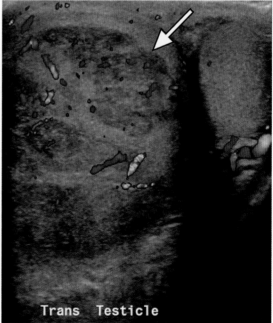

Trans Testicle

B

FIGURE 16.16. Seminoma with **(A)** mixed echogenicity, well-circumscribed mass (*arrow*) and **(B)** brisk internal vascularity (*arrow*).

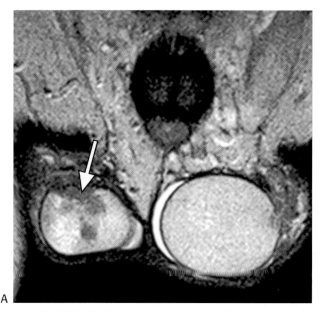
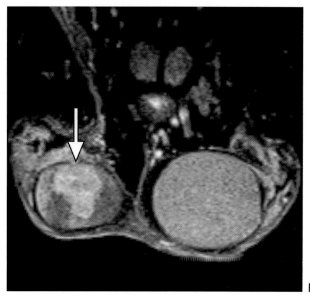

FIGURE 16.17. Pure seminoma manifesting as **(A)** low-signal mass (*arrow*) on T2WI with **(B)** hyperenhancement (*arrow*) compared to surrounding parenchyma.

circumscribed and rarely involve the tunica albuginea, though satellite nodules can be seen at tumor margins. Unlike NSGCTs, seminomas tend to be homogenous and rarely become necrotic, cystic, or hemorrhagic. On MRI, the background signal intensity of the testis is high on T2WI due to fluid within seminiferous tubules. Seminomas replace normal parenchyma and have comparatively low signal intensity on T2WI (Fig. 16.17), with enhancement postcontrast.

In the absence of high-risk histologic features or extrascrotal disease, there are three potential pathways after orchiectomy for stage I seminoma. Active surveillance, postoperative radiotherapy, and postoperative chemotherapy are all associated with >99% long-term survival. The strategy of active surveillance—physical exam, tumor markers, and CT of the abdomen and pelvis—is associated with no immediate side effects, but an approximately 20% rate of relapse. Such patients are then treated with salvage chemotherapy with no detriment to long-term survival. Postoperative radiotherapy and chemotherapy have short-term side effects but reduce the chance of relapse to 4%. Low-volume stage II seminoma is treated with radiation to the para-aortic and ipsilateral iliac nodes, while larger volume and higher-stage disease requires combination chemotherapy.

Nonseminomatous Germ Cell Tumors

NSGCTs are defined as any GCT containing nonseminomatous components. Seminoma is often admixed with these. Pure NSGCTs are relatively rare, and treatment guidelines largely consider these as a group of mixed cellularity tumors. NSGCTs occur in slightly younger patients than do seminomas, with a peak age in the late teens to midtwenties. The serum αFP is often elevated. Although NSGCTs tend to be slightly more aggressive than seminomas histologically, and more frequently invade the tunica albuginea, most patients with NSGCT present with stage I disease.

Embryonal cell carcinoma, teratoma (Fig. 16.18), yolk sac carcinoma, and choriocarcinoma are fairly rare in their pure forms and are poorly distinguished from one another by imaging. Cystic components, coarse calcifications (Fig. 16.19), internal heterogeneity, marginal irregularity, and tunica invasion are more common

than in pure seminoma. Such internal heterogeneity is also reflected in MR imaging, but there are no specific features enabling histologic diagnosis by imaging.

After orchiectomy, stage I NSGCTs are separated into risk categories based on the presence of lymphovascular invasion at histologic examination. High-risk patients have up to 50% risk of relapse in active surveillance, while only 15% of low-risk patients

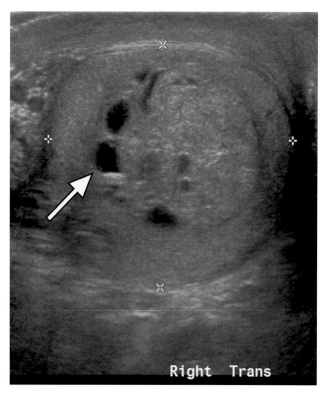

FIGURE 16.18. Mixed-type NSGCT comprised of 60% teratoma, demonstrating heterogenous intratesticular mass with cystic elements (*arrow*).

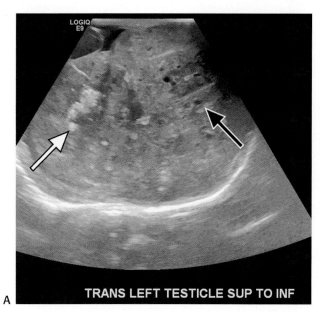

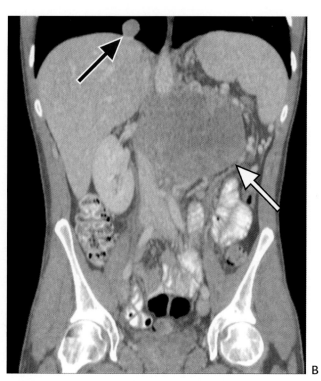

FIGURE 16.19. Mixed-type NSGCT with **(A)** large tumor containing coarse calcifications (*white arrow*) and cysts (*black arrow*) on US and **(B)** coronal CT reformat illustrating retroperitoneal mass (*white arrow*) at level of left renal vein with sparing of more caudal nodes and lung metastasis (*black arrow*) at presentation.

will recur without adjuvant therapy. Other initial options include nerve sparing retroperitoneal lymph node dissection (RPLND) and short-course chemotherapy. As in seminoma, there is a 99% long-term cure rate in stage I NSGCT. Stage II NSGCT can be treated with chemotherapy with or without RPLND. Stage III disease is further stratified into risk categories based on tumor type, sites of involvement, and serum tumor marker levels. The overall cure rate declines with increasing risk level, with an approximately 50% to 60% overall cure rate in the highest risk group.

Nongerminal Testis Tumors

Primary tumors arising from the gonadal sex cord and stroma include Leydig, Sertoli or granulosa cell tumors. The most common are Leydig cell tumors, which develop in the interstitial cells of the fibrovascular stroma. They may present with excessive virilization and increased muscle mass due to their production of testosterone. Leydig cell hyperplasia has also been described in the presence of seminoma. Sertoli cell tumors develop from the basement membranes of seminiferous tubules and produce estrogen and occasionally gynecomastia. About 90% of these tumors are indolent, but 10% will behave like GCTs and metastasize to the retroperitoneum. Unfortunately, testicular sex cord–stromal tumors are less sensitive to chemotherapy and radiation than are GCTs, so retroperitoneal metastasis often confers a fatal prognosis.

Imaging features of sex cord–stromal tumors are not specific (Fig. 16.20) and the radiologist's task is to identify an intratesticular mass, confirm internal vascularity, assess disease extent, and evaluate retroperitoneal lymph nodes if possible. As in GCTs,

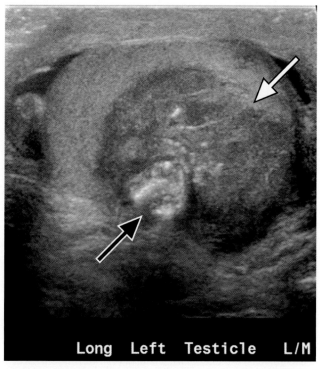

FIGURE 16.20. Sex cord–stromal tumor presenting as hypoechoic mass (*white arrow*) with coarse calcification (*black arrow*). Internal vascularity was present, not shown.

orchiectomy is essential for tissue diagnosis and prognosis. The role and timing of retroperitoneal node dissection is controversial in these rare tumors, but it is often considered earlier in the course of treatment than in otherwise comparable patients with GCT, due to the absence of effective salvage treatments.

Other rare primary testicular tumors do not arise from germ cells. These include gonadoblastoma, adenocarcinoma of the rete testes, and mesenchymal neoplasms such as fibromas and leiomyomas. Adenomatoid tumors, which are small and benign, may occur in the testis but are more commonly found in the epididymis.

Testicular Metastases, Lymphoma, and Leukemia

Metastatic disease to the testis is more common than primary testicular tumors in men older than 50 years. Metastases have been reported from a variety of primary tumors arising in the prostate, kidney, lung, gastrointestinal tract, skin, and other sites. Testicular metastases are usually bilateral, multiple, and often hypoechoic.

Testicular lymphoma is usually of the non-Hodgkin type and most common in the setting of systemic disease. Lymphoma accounts for 25% of testicular tumors in men older than 50 years. Lymphoma tends to be hypoechoic, poorly marginated, hypervascular, and bilateral (Fig. 16.21) but sometimes presents as a diffusely enlarged testis. It is not uncommon for testicular lymphoma to infiltrate the epididymis. Lymphoma has low signal intensity on both T1- and T2-weighted MR sequences and shows less enhancement than normal testicular tissue. Testicular leukemia is similar in appearance to lymphoma. The testis is a characteristic initial site of relapse in boys treated for systemic leukemia, due to limited perfusion of chemotherapy into the testis, allowing persistence of leukemic cells.

Benign Intratesticular Processes

Cysts

Cysts of varying sizes may be centered in the testis, tunica albuginea, or tunica vaginalis. Intratesticular simple cysts are rare. They are usually idiopathic but may be postinflammatory or posttraumatic. They arise from efferent ductules of the rete testes, are lined by cuboidal or low columnar epithelium, and are located peripherally within or adjacent to the mediastinum testis. Their average size is 5 to 7 mm, and they are not palpable. Ultrasound examination reveals peripheral, well-defined anechoic lesions with normal surrounding testicular echogenicity (Fig. 16.22). Septations are occasionally seen. No intervention is generally needed.

Epidermoid cysts arise from epithelial rests within the testis and are probably a very low-grade germ cell neoplasm consisting of ectodermal products including squamous cells and keratin debris. Ultrasound shows them to be avascular solitary structures with concentric hyperechoic and hypoechoic rings; they have been described as having a "bull's eye" or "onion skin" appearance (Fig. 16.23). Unlike most tumors, epidermoid cysts are usually of high signal intensity on T2-weighted MRI (Fig. 16.24). Also in contrast to other intratesticular neoplasms, epidermoid cysts can be treated with enucleation of the mass from the testis, rather than orchiectomy. Although true epidermoid cysts are benign, histologic examination is needed to exclude the presence of premalignant components given their germ cell origin.

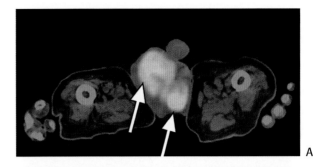

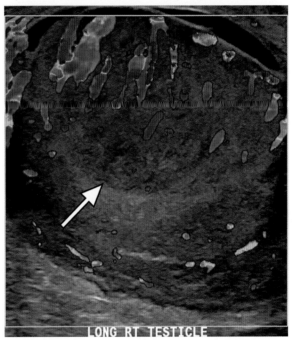

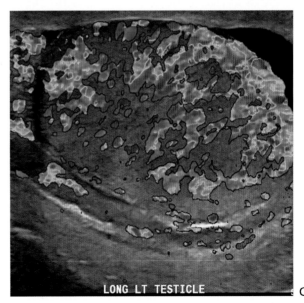

FIGURE 16.21. Testicular lymphoma with **(A)** bilateral avid masses (*arrows*) on ¹⁸FDG-PET, and **(B, C)** multifocal, hypervascular masses (*arrow*) on Doppler US. Ultrasound vascularity of lymphoma is often even greater than that of primary testicular neoplasms.

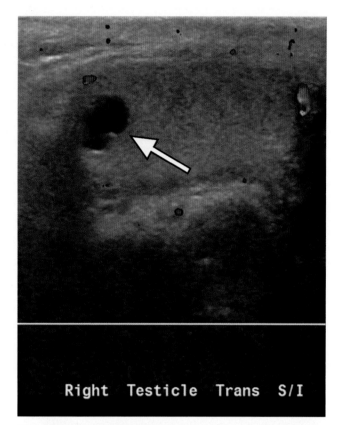

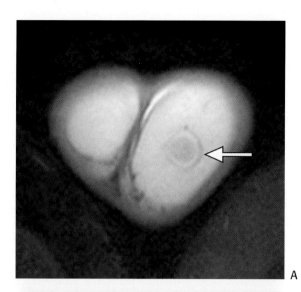

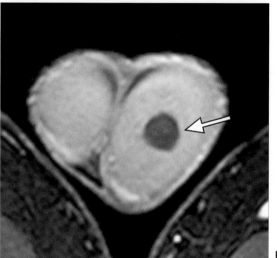

FIGURE 16.22. Testicular cyst (*arrow*) is anechoic, well circumscribed, and avascular.

Tunica albuginea cysts are palpable due to their superficial location on the testis and are usually small (2- to 5-mm), smooth, and painless. Palpation does not permit distinction of cyst from tumor, but ultrasound examination reveals tiny anechoic lesions with no solid elements (Fig. 16.25).

Ectasia of the Rete Testis

Obstruction of epididymal outflow due to trauma, inflammation, cysts, or vasectomy may lead to cystic dilation of the rete testis. This

FIGURE 16.24. Epidermoid cyst with **(A)** concentric high-signal rings surrounding a high-signal round lesion (*arrow*) on T2WI and **(B)** no enhancement (*arrow*) postcontrast.

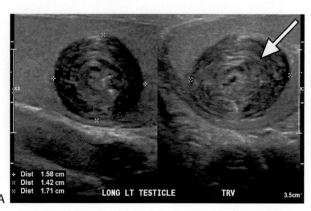

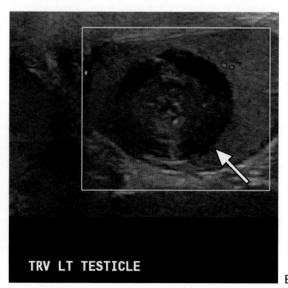

FIGURE 16.23. Epidermoid cyst showing **(A)** lamellated, "onion skin" appearance (*arrow*) and **(B)** no internal vascularity (*arrow*).

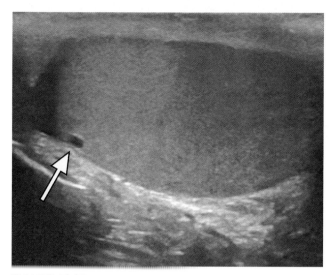

FIGURE 16.25. Tunica albuginea cyst manifesting as a tiny peripheral anechoic lesion (*arrow*).

condition is often bilateral and more common in men over 50 year of age. Ectasia of the rete testis manifests as numerous ovoid and/ or tubular lesions clustered along one side of the testis (Fig. 16.26). These cysts converge on the mediastinum testis and do not alter the external contour. There may be an associated spermatocele. This is a benign process that may visually mimic a tumor but can be distinguished by its morphology and lack of internal vascularity. It requires no intervention.

Microlithiasis

The presence of multiple tiny (<1 mm) calcifications or hematoxylin bodies interspersed within the testicular parenchyma is termed microlithiasis. The process is usually diffuse and bilateral but can be unilateral or focal. Ultrasound demonstrates multiple tiny echogenic foci (Fig. 16.27), without posterior acoustic shadowing or associated vascularity.

Approximately 5% of asymptomatic men and 2% of asymptomatic boys have microlithiasis. Men with other testicular disorders including subfertility, cryptorchidism, Klinefelter syndrome, and testicular cancer—particularly seminoma (Fig. 16.28)—are more likely to have microlithiasis. These statistical associations have led to speculation regarding causal and temporal relationships between microlithiasis and other conditions, particularly neoplasia. Concern that microlithiasis is a precursor lesion for cancer has led to a variety of recommendations in the literature, from surveillance with self- or physician exam to evaluation with tumor markers, ultrasound, and even testicular biopsy. However, current evidence does not support these aggressive approaches. In the absence of other risk factors for testicular neoplasia, microlithiasis should be considered a benign finding that does not warrant imaging surveillance or intervention.

Testicular Adrenal Rest Tumors

Adrenal tissue remnants persist in the testes of up to 15% of neonates but normally regress during infancy. In patients with increased levels of adrenocorticotropic hormone (ACTH), usually due to impaired adrenal steroid synthesis in the setting of 21-hydroxylase deficiency, both the adrenal glands and intratesticular adrenal remnants undergo hyperplasia. The hyperplastic adrenal rests can become quite large, distorting and obstructing normal seminiferous tubules and causing infertility. Tumors

usually, though not always, regress with hydrocortisone replacement therapy, because the ACTH stimulus is removed.

Testicular adrenal rest tumors (TARTs) are usually bilateral, multiple (Fig. 16.29), and may produce testicular enlargement. They tend to be eccentrically located in the testes. Sonographic features are variable; small tumors are hypoechoic (Fig. 16.30) but TARTs may become hyperechoic with posterior acoustic shadowing when large. Internal vascularity is minimal or absent. Like other intratesticular masses, TARTs are hypointense to normal testis on T2WI and may be multiple.

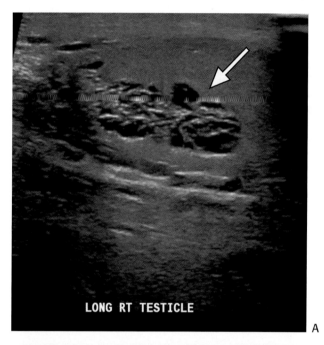

LONG RT TESTICLE

A

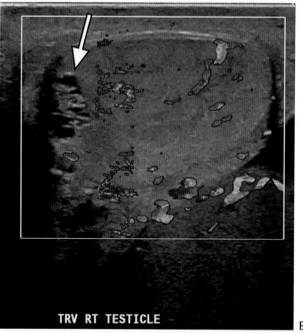

TRV RT TESTICLE

B

FIGURE 16.26. Rete testis ectasia shows **(A)** clustered cysts or tubules in an eccentric linear configuration (*arrow*) with **(B)** no internal vascularity (*arrow*).

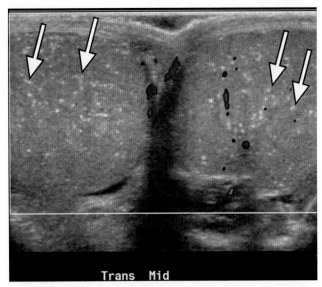

FIGURE 16.27. Microlithiasis with innumerable tiny echogenic foci (*arrows*) in otherwise normal testes.

Testicular Miscellany

Other benign intratesticular lesions include abscesses, hamartomas, intraparenchymal varicoceles, pseudoaneurysms, arteriovenous malformations, and granulomas due to tuberculosis or sarcoidosis. Some of these are detailed elsewhere in the chapter and others are quite rare and beyond the present scope.

EXTRATESTICULAR SCROTAL PATHOLOGY

Hernia

Hernias containing structures normally found within the abdomen may extend through the inguinal canal into the scrotum.

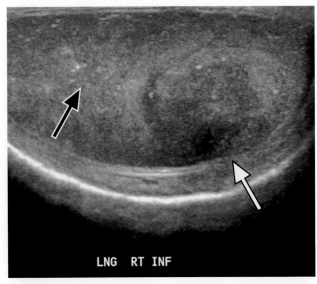

FIGURE 16.28. Seminoma and testicular microlithiasis with hypoechoic mass (*white arrow*) and tiny echogenic foci (*black arrow*) in background parenchyma.

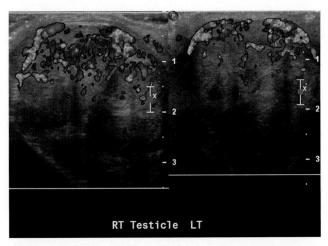

FIGURE 16.29. Bilateral testicular adrenal rest tumors (TARTs) with shadowing posterior masses exhibiting minimal vascularity compared to the preserved normal parenchyma anteriorly.

Contents may include fat, bowel, ascitic fluid, or occasionally bladder. Ultrasound or CT examination with Valsalva maneuver can provide dynamic information about structures traversing the inguinal canal. Ultrasound may demonstrate a characteristic gut signature or peristalsing bowel, while CT may demonstrate enteric or excreted contrast in a bowel loop or herniated bladder, respectively. Management depends on size, location, symptoms, and reducibility.

Hydrocele

A hydrocele is an abnormal collection of fluid between the visceral and the parietal layers of the tunica vaginalis. Congenital

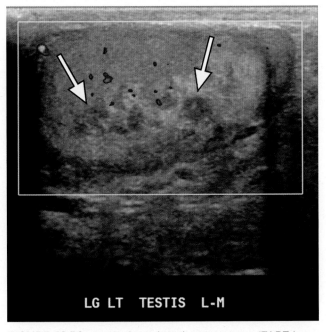

FIGURE 16.30. Testicular adrenal rest tumors (TARTs) are small, hypoechoic (*arrows*), and hypovascular in this patient.

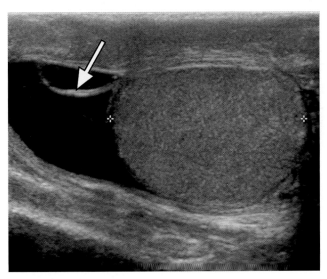

FIGURE 16.31. Hydrocele with single thin septation (*arrow*) and normal testis.

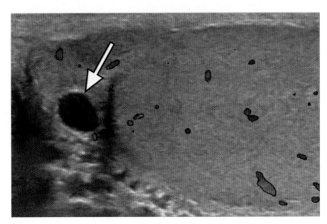

FIGURE 16.32. Epididymal cyst with small, anechoic avascular structure (*arrow*) in epididymal head.

(communicating) hydroceles arise from incomplete closure of the processus vaginalis, as discussed above. In adults, small (noncommunicating) idiopathic hydroceles are common and usually asymptomatic. In fact, small hydroceles are noted sonographically in more than half of normal men. Hydroceles are less frequently secondary to inflammatory disease, tumor, or trauma. Traumatic hydroceles may contain blood and are termed hematoceles, while pyoceles contain pus.

The common small, simple, idiopathic hydrocele usually involves only a fraction of the testicular circumference (Fig. 16.31). A large hydrocele may surround the entire testis but is usually posterolateral, where the tunica vaginalis invests the testis and epididymis. Thin septations can be demonstrated within a sterile hydrocele, while thick septations raise suspicion for infection. Low-level echoes may indicate blood, pus, or debris.

Epididymal Cyst and Spermatocele

Epididymal cysts are caused by dilation of the tubules in the epididymis. They are often small and multiple but may range up to several centimeters in diameter. Epididymal cysts contain serous fluid and may occur anywhere within the epididymis. Spermatoceles usually represent retention cysts of the small tubules in the epididymal head and may be loculated. They contain sperm-filled fluid, thicker and sometimes more echogenic than that found in serous epididymal cysts. They may be idiopathic or be associated with vas deferens obstruction from surgery; they may also follow epididymitis and are thus more common among older men. Spermatoceles and epididymal cysts are usually indistinguishable from each other, but occasionally a spermatocele demonstrates internal echoes as a result of the presence of spermatozoa.

Both types of cysts may be unilateral or bilateral and are usually palpated as extratesticular masses posterior to the testes. Ultrasound demonstrates thin walled, anechoic structures with posterior acoustic enhancement (Fig. 16.32). Even when large, they can usually be distinguished from hydroceles by their position. A hydrocele surrounds the testis, usually anteriorly, whereas epididymal cysts and spermatoceles lie in the epididymis superior or posterior to the testis.

Varicocele

The pampiniform plexus is the main venous drainage of the testis, while the cremasteric plexus drains the epididymis and the scrotal wall. When these veins become dilated >3 mm in diameter, the resulting tangle of vessels is termed a varicocele. Primary varicoceles are idiopathic and more common on the left—perhaps due to the more acute angle of the gonadal vein entry into the left renal vein, compared to the oblique entry of the right gonadal vein into the inferior vena cava. Secondary varicoceles result from incompetent valves in the left gonadal vein or rarely from left gonadal or renal vein occlusion. Ten percent to 20% of healthy men have a varicocele, and up to 50% of men evaluated for infertility have varicoceles—often bilateral. Varicoceles may diminish fertility due to increased scrotal temperature, preferential drainage of renal or adrenal metabolites to the testis, testicular hypoxemia, and/or insufficient testicular hormone production. Surgical varicocelectomy or endovascular occlusion is often followed by an improvement in sperm quality and increased fertility.

High-resolution, real-time Doppler ultrasound is an excellent method for demonstrating a varicocele. Small varicoceles may be made more visible by examining the patient in the upright position or by the Valsalva maneuver in the supine position. Small varicoceles may be demonstrated as serpentine, tubular, elongated anechoic fluid collections in the spermatic cord adjacent to the testis (Fig. 16.33). These veins usually measure >3 mm in diameter and should increase in caliber and demonstrate a Doppler "flash" with a Valsalva maneuver. Doppler ultrasound may reveal antegrade flow, stasis, or retrograde flow at rest.

Tumors and Pseudotumors

Primary extratesticular neoplasms are unusual; in fact, a commonly cited principle of scrotal ultrasound is that intratesticular lesions are very likely to be malignant tumors, whereas extratesticular abnormalities are almost always benign. The most common among rare extratesticular neoplasms is the benign adenomatoid tumor, which appears as a small solid echogenic mass (Fig. 16.34). Adenomatoid tumors most commonly involve the epididymal head or tunica albuginea. Rare spermatic cord neoplasms, including lipoma, liposarcoma (Fig. 16.35), and lymphoma, can occasionally present with both intra-abdominal and intrascrotal components.

Other benign extratesticular scrotal masses include mobile calcifications, sometimes called scrotal pearls (Fig. 16.36), and fibrous

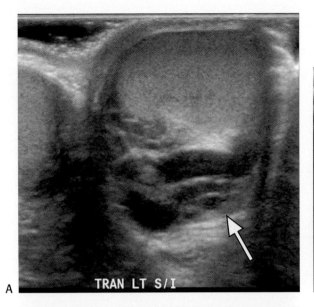

A

TRAN LT S/I

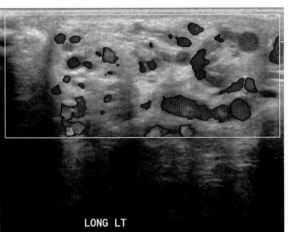

LONG LT

B

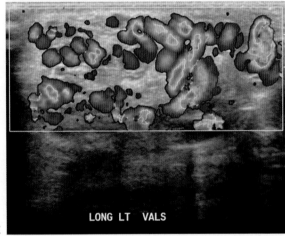

C

LONG LT VALS

FIGURE 16.33. Varicocele with **(A)** dilated tubular veins (*arrow*), **(B)** modest flow on initial color Doppler, and **(C)** greatly augmented flow with aliasing after Valsalva maneuver.

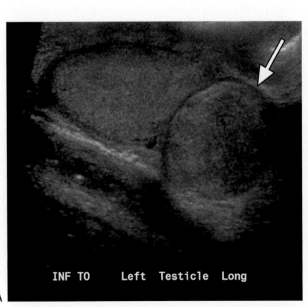

A

INF TO   Left Testicle Long

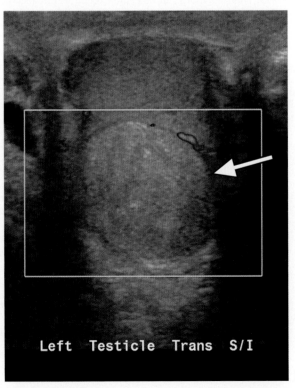

B

Left Testicle Trans S/I

FIGURE 16.34. Adenomatoid tumor of epididymis with **(A)** hypoechoic, well-circumscribed extratesticular mass (*arrow*), **(B)** without conspicuous internal vascularity (*arrow*).

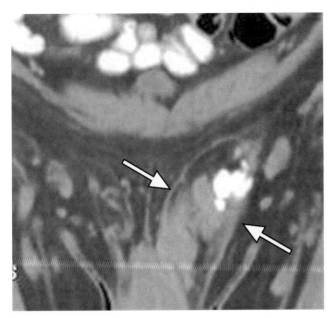

FIGURE 16.35. Liposarcoma exhibits soft tissue masses, calcifications, and fat expanding the left inguinal canal (*arrows*) on coronal CT reformat.

pseudotumors. Pseudotumors probably reflect scarring after a prior traumatic or inflammatory insult, may be variable in echogenicity, and are usually mobile and avascular.

Scrotal Edema

Diffuse scrotal edema is caused by anasarca (due to organ failure or hypoproteinemia) or lymphatic obstruction (due to filariasis, lymph node dissection or metastasis, pelvic tumor, or retroperitoneal fibrosis). Scrotal edema, a mural process, should be distinguished from hydroceles. Ultrasound reveals thickened subcutaneous tissue (Fig. 16.37) with echogenicity greater than normal fat, CT shows infiltration and skin thickening, and MRI will

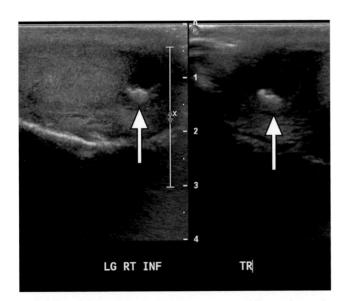

FIGURE 16.36. Scrotal "pearls" are mobile echogenic (*arrows*) extratesticular calcifications.

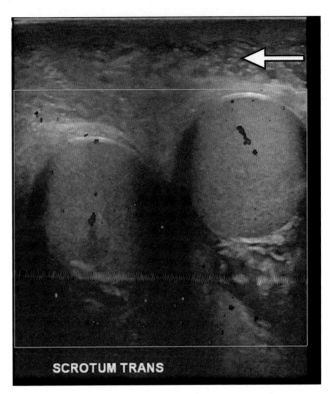

FIGURE 16.37. Scrotal edema manifests as thickening (*arrow*) and increased echogenicity of subcutaneous tissues.

reveal edematous subcutaneous fat with correspondingly altered signal on all sequences. This process can be very uncomfortable for patients; clinical management depends upon the underlying condition.

CONCLUSION

Ultrasound is the primary imaging modality for evaluation of the scrotum and its contents. Urgent diagnoses include torsion, trauma, epididymo-orchitis, and necrotizing fasciitis (Fournier gangrene). Seminoma is by far the most common testicular neoplasm and is usually diagnosed at stage I with an excellent long-term prognosis. Most extratesticular processes are benign and many require no further intervention.

SUGGESTED READINGS

Alleman WG, Gorman B, King BF, et al. Benign and malignant epididymal masses evaluated with scrotal sonography: clinical and pathologic review of 85 patients. *J Ultrasound Med.* 2008;27(8):1195–1202.

Avery LL, Scheinfeld MH. Imaging of penile and scrotal emergencies. *RadioGraphics.* 2013;33(3):721–740.

Barrisford GW, Kreydin EI, Preston MA, et al. Role of imaging in testicular cancer: current and future practice. *Future Oncol.* 2015;11(18):2575–2586.

Bernard B, Sweeney CJ. Diagnosis and treatment of testicular cancer: a clinician's perspective. *Surg Pathol Clin.* 2015;8(4):717–723.

Bhatt S, Rubens DJ, Dogra VS. Sonography of benign intrascrotal lesions. *Ultrasound Q.* 2006;22(2):121–136.

Buckley JC, McAninch JW. Use of ultrasonography for the diagnosis of testicular injuries in blunt scrotal trauma. *J Urol.* 2006;175(1):175–178.

Cassidy FH, Ishioka KM, McMahon CJ, et al. MR imaging of scrotal tumors and pseudotumors. *RadioGraphics.* 2010;30(3):665–683.

Cooper ML, Kaefer M, Fan R, et al. Testicular microlithiasis in children and associated testicular cancer. *Radiology.* 2014;270(3):857–863.

Hedgire SS, Pargaonkar VK, Elmi A, et al. Pelvic nodal imaging. *Radiol Clin North Am.* 2012;50(6):1111–1125.

Heller HT, Oliff MC, Doubilet PM, et al. Testicular microlithiasis: prevalence and association with primary testicular neoplasm. *J Clin Ultrasound.* 2014;42:423–426.

Howard SA, Gray KP, O'Donnell EK, et al. Craniocaudal retroperitoneal node length as a risk factor for relapse from clinical stage I testicular germ cell tumor. *AJR Am J Roentgenol.* 2014;203(4):W415–W420.

Kim W, Rosen MA, Langer JE, et al. US MR imaging correlation in pathologic conditions of the scrotum. *Radiographics.* 2007;27:1239–1253.

National Cancer Care Network (NCCN). *Guidelines in Oncology: Testicular Cancer.* Version 2.2016. Accessed August 2016, NCCN.org.

Parker RA III, Menias CO, Quazi R, et al. MR imaging of the penis and scrotum. *RadioGraphics.* 2015;35(4):1033–1050.

Pedersen MR, Rafaelsen SR, Moller H, et al. Testicular microlithiasis and testicular cancer: review of the literature. *Int Urol Nephrol.* 2016;48(7):1079–1086.

Philips S, Nagar A, Dighe M, et al. Benign non-cystic scrotal tumors and pseudotumors. *Acta Radiol.* 2012;53(1):102–111.

Qublan HS, Al-Okoor K, Al-Ghoweri AS, et al. Sonographic spectrum of scrotal abnormalities in infertile men. *J Clin Ultrasound.* 2007;35(8):437–441.

Shetty D, Bailey AG, Freeman SJ. Testicular microlithiasis an ultrasound dilemma: survey of opinions regarding significance and management amongst UK ultrasound practitioners. *Br J Radiol.* 2014;87(1034):20130603.

Sielberstein JL, Bazzi WM, Vertosick E, et al. Clinical outcomes of local and metastatic testicular sex cord-stromal tumors. *J Urol.* 2014;192(2):415–419.

Tsili AC, Argyropoulou MI, Giannakis D, et al. MRI in the characterization and local staging of testicular neoplasms. *AJR Am J Roentgenol.* 2010;194(3):682–689.

Vasdev N, Chadwick D, Thomas D. The acute pediatric scrotum: presentation, differential diagnosis and management. *Curr Urol.* 2012;6(2):57–61.

Walsh TJ, Dall'Era MA, Croughan MS, et al. Prepubertal orchiopexy for cryptorchidism may be associated with lower risk of testicular cancer. *J Urol.* 2007;178(4 Pt 1):1440–1446.

Wasnik AP, Maturen KE, Shah S, et al. Scrotal pearls and pitfalls: ultrasound findings of benign scrotal lesions. *Ultrasound Q.* 2012;28(4):281–291.

Winter TC, Kim B, Lowrance WT, et al. Testicular microlithiasis: what should you recommend? *AJR Am J Roentgenol.* 2016;206(6):1164–1169.

Wood HM, Elder JS. Cryptorchidism and testicular cancer: separating fact from fiction. *J Urol.* 2009;181(2):452–461.

Yu MK, Jung MK, Kim KE, et al. Clinical manifestations of testicular adrenal rest tumor in males with congenital adrenal hyperplasia. *Ann Pediatr Endocrinol Metab.* 2015;20(3):155–161.

Ovaries and Adnexa

NORMAL ANATOMY

The term "adnexa" refers to the connective tissue and other structures adjacent to or associated with any organ. Each uterine adnexa includes the respective ovary, fallopian tube, ligaments, and other connective tissue, as well as neurovascular structures lateral to the uterus. At physical examination, these individual structures are difficult to distinguish, and the entire area lateral to the uterus on each side is described as the "adnexal region."

Each ovary is only about 1 to 3 mL in volume in neonates, growing slowly throughout childhood and more rapidly during puberty to reach normal volumes of 4 to 16 mL in the reproductive years. The ovarian volume is usually calculated with the prolate ellipse formula, length × width × height × 0.52, and a simple way to remember normal ovarian size during reproductive life is roughly 2 × 3 × 4 cm. It is normal and physiologic to see multiple unilocular follicles bilaterally with any imaging modality, commonly up to 2.5 cm but sometimes up to 7 cm, discussed in more detail below (Fig. 17.1). Zonal anatomy of the ovary is evident at MR imaging, with hypointense central stroma and hyperintense peripheral follicles on T2-weighted images (T2WI). After menopause, the size and conspicuity of the ovaries decrease with all imaging modalities, and the normal ovarian volume decreases to 1 to 6 mL.

FOLLICLES AND CYSTS

Normal, physiologic follicles form multiple "cysts" in reproductive-age women every month, and benign simple cysts remain relatively common after menopause. It is important to recognize that the vast majority of ovarian cysts diagnosed by imaging are incidental and benign and do not require monitoring with imaging. However, given the aggressiveness and morbidity of some types of ovarian cancer, it is equally important to distinguish sonographically indeterminate lesions requiring further workup from these common, benign, simple cysts.

Approximately once a month during reproductive life, one or more dominant follicles will grow to about 2 to 3 cm in size and eventually release an oocyte. These simple follicular cysts are unilocular and anechoic at ultrasound and exhibit fluid density at CT

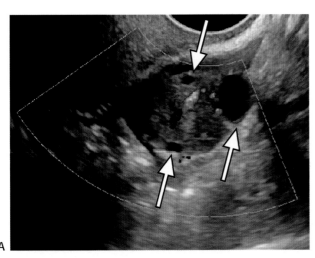
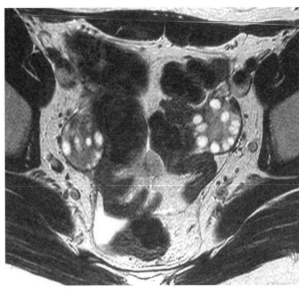

FIGURE 17.1. Normal follicles of varying sizes on **(A)** TVUS (*arrows*) and **(B)** T2WI.

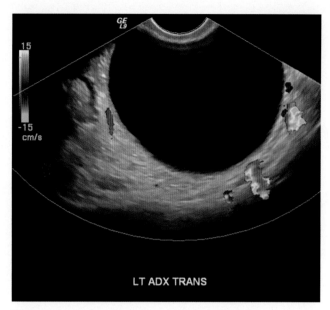

FIGURE 17.2. Simple cyst is anechoic, sharply marginated, and avascular on TVUS with color Doppler.

and fluid signal at MRI. They have a thin, sharply defined wall and no internal soft tissue features (Fig. 17.2). Sometimes, there are 1 or 2 thin (≤2 mm) septations, but no demonstrable vascularity. After ovulation, a corpus luteum may be evident as an annular, vascularized soft tissue stricture (Fig. 17.3) at US, sometimes as a round or irregular crenulated hypervascular stricture at CT or MR or an area of hyperintense ¹⁸FDG uptake at PET/CT. These are physiologic findings and do not require imaging follow-up in most cases. The 2010 Society of Radiologists in Ultrasound (SRU) consensus guidelines for asymptomatic adnexal cysts suggest that annual US monitoring be performed for simple cysts 5 to 7 cm in diameter in

reproductive age women and 1 to 7 cm in postmenopausal women, while cysts >7 cm should be evaluated by a gynecologic surgeon in all age groups.

Hemorrhagic cysts are also physiologic but are sometimes symptomatic, particularly when ruptured. On US, hemorrhagic cysts may be hyperechoic acutely, later developing hematocrit levels, an avascular "cobweb" or reticular pattern due to fibrin strands, and finally a characteristic pattern of triangular or convex retractile clot (Fig. 17.4). Hemorrhagic cysts are hyperdense at CT, usually between 30 and 100 HU, and may be accompanied by simple or hemorrhagic free fluid in the pelvis (Fig. 17.5). On T1-weighted images, hemorrhagic cysts are hyperintense and do not exhibit enhancement after contrast administration. Hemorrhagic cysts are more commonly acutely symptomatic than endometriomas, which may have similar imaging appearances. (Endometriosis is discussed in more detail in a separate section below.) Sometimes, the only way to distinguish these entities is with follow-up imaging: hemorrhagic cysts resolve and endometriomas do not.

Since luteal cysts are the most likely to bleed, hemorrhagic cysts are usually physiologic in reproductive age women. Hemorrhagic cysts are not physiologic in postmenopausal women, and gynecologic consultation is suggested when they are detected. In reproductive-age women, the SRU guidelines suggest that no follow-up is needed for hemorrhagic cysts ≤5 cm in diameter. For larger hemorrhagic cysts (>5 cm) in premenopausal women, or hemorrhagic cysts of any size in perimenopausal women (<5 years after menopause), US follow-up in 6 to 12 weeks is suggested to ensure resolution. In late postmenopausal women, all hemorrhagic cysts should be surgically evaluated.

A few other types of nonneoplastic cysts deserve mention. Theca lutein cysts appear in response to high levels of human chorionic gonadotropin (β-hCG) in women with gestational trophoblastic disease including molar pregnancy (Fig. 17.6) and multiple gestations and in women undergoing pharmacologic ovulation induction. They are usually large, unilocular, and multiple. Ovarian hyperstimulation is characterized by marked enlargement of the ovaries, sometimes with associated ascites and pleural effusions. Paraovarian cysts are adnexal cysts that arise in the broad ligament instead of the ovary; they can be diagnosed by demonstrating that the lesion is separate from the ovary. SRU guidelines suggest that these may be managed just as ovarian cysts—that is, little imaging follow-up is needed unless soft tissue elements or vascularity are present. Peritoneal inclusion cysts are another ovarian cyst mimic. They form as a result of adhesions, sometimes resulting from pelvic surgery or inflammation. These adhesions entrap ovulatory fluid and normal serous peritoneal fluid, forming collections that characteristically invaginate around existing structures (Fig. 17.7). MRI is often helpful as peritoneal inclusions may be hard to diagnose sonographically.

Polycystic ovary syndrome, or Stein–Leventhal syndrome, consists of oligomenorrhea or amenorrhea, obesity, infertility, and hirsutism. Similar "polycystic" ovaries may also be seen in other hormonal disorders. The imaging findings are not dramatic. The ovaries are slightly enlarged, may be hyperechoic, and exhibit an increased number of tiny—usually <5 mm—follicular cysts, distributed at the periphery of the ovary (Fig. 17.8).

Ectopic pregnancy is an important differential diagnosis whenever adnexal cysts are encountered. Every pelvic ultrasound should be interpreted with the following three questions in mind: "How old is she? Is she pregnant? What's the serum β-hCG level?" Full consideration of obstetric ultrasound and complications is beyond the scope of this text, but ectopic pregnancy is an important and highly morbid condition that must always be considered in reproductive age women. Tubal ectopic pregnancy is the most common and the most likely to mimic an ovarian cyst. Unlike physiologic cysts, ectopic pregnancy is usually symptomatic, any

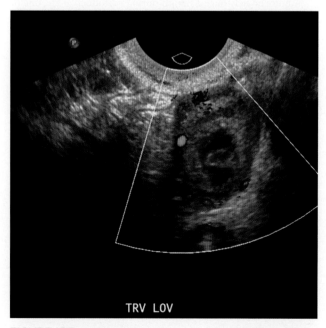

FIGURE 17.3. Corpus luteal cyst has a thick wall and appears "collapsed" but lacks internal vascularity on TVUS with power Doppler.

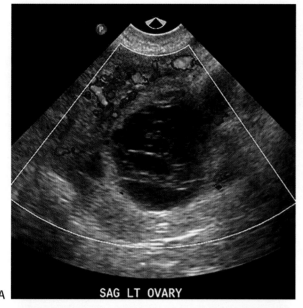

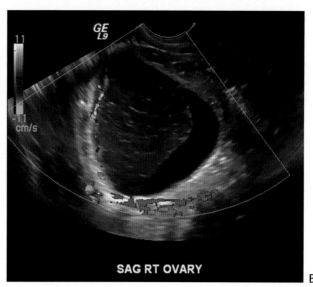

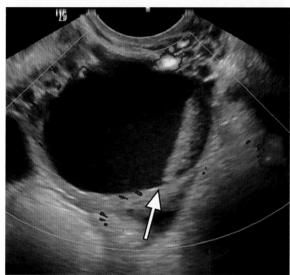

FIGURE 17.4. Hemorrhagic cysts on TVUS demonstrating **(A)** characteristic reticular pattern due to fibrin strands, **(B)** retractile clot appearance, and **(C)** layering blood products (*arrow*).

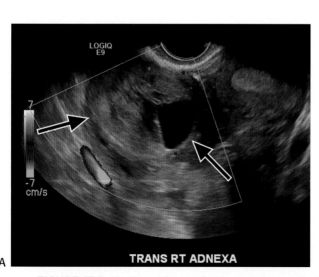

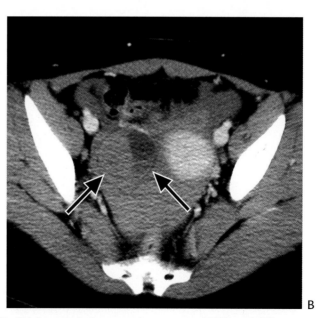

FIGURE 17.5. Ruptured hemorrhagic cyst (*arrows*) with **(A)** hyperechoic avascular mass on TVUS and **(B)** mixed density mass and hemoperitoneum on CECT. Pelvic fluid measured >70 HU.

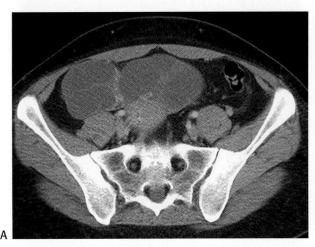 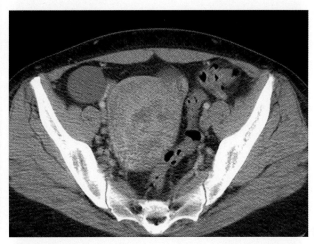

FIGURE 17.6. Multiple theca lutein cysts due to elevated β-hCG in invasive gestational trophoblastic disease. CECT images show **(A)** enlarged, multicystic ovaries and **(B)** enlarged, heterogenous uterus.

"cyst" is complex and thick walled, and is often associated with complex pelvic free fluid, particularly if ruptured (Fig. 17.9). When a pregnant woman has no demonstrable intrauterine pregnancy by TVUS and a serum β-hCG >3,000 mIU/mL, the likelihood of a viable intrauterine pregnancy is approximately 0.5%. In this setting, all apparent "cysts" must be carefully scrutinized for imaging features that would favor ectopic pregnancy and expedite appropriate treatment.

TORSION

Torsion is pathologic rotation of the ovary on its vascular pedicle. This process may impede ovarian perfusion and is often acutely symptomatic. Ovarian torsion is more likely to occur in young women and girls than in older women; it has even been reported in utero. Ovarian masses, especially cystic teratomas (dermoids) predispose to torsion, although torsion may also occur with a morphologically normal ovary or in association with physiologic follicles or a corpus luteum.

Ovarian torsion produces acute lower abdominal or pelvic pain, which is often severe and abrupt in onset. The clinical differential diagnosis includes appendicitis, hemorrhagic cyst, ruptured ectopic pregnancy, and ureteral stone. The degree of ovarian ischemia depends on the duration and severity of the torsion. The ovary has a dual blood supply via uterine and ovarian arteries, and partial or intermittent torsion may occur, so the extent of vascular compromise is variable. In some cases, torsion resolves spontaneously. Transient or partial ischemia may be reversed by surgical detorsion, with maintenance of a viable ovary. However, complete ischemia of more than several hours'

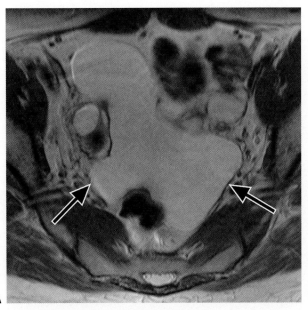 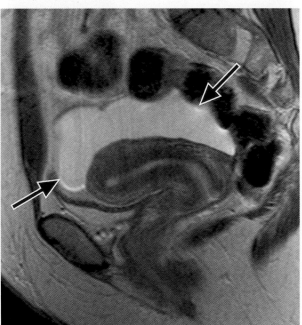

FIGURE 17.7. Peritoneal inclusion cyst (*arrows*) on **(A)** axial and **(B)** sagittal T2WI, with unilocular collection in central pelvis taking the shape of adjacent structures. This patient had chronic pelvic fullness and later underwent successful sclerotherapy.

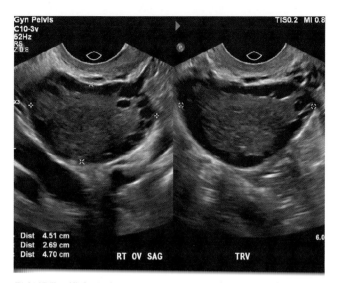

FIGURE 17.8. Polycystic ovary syndrome with mildly enlarged ovary exhibiting multiple tiny peripheral follicles. This is a clinical rather than an imaging diagnosis.

duration usually leads to irreversible necrosis of the ovary, which must be resected.

Torsion occludes flexible, low-pressure venous structures before thick-walled, high-pressure arteries, so that venous drainage is impaired before the arterial supply. As a result, the torsed ovary becomes edematous, congested, and sometimes hemorrhagic. On US, a torsed ovary is asymmetrically enlarged, usually with altered or mottled echogenicity, and peripheralized follicles (Fig. 17.10). Color Doppler ultrasound may show absent or diminished vascularity, even with low pulse repetition frequency (PRF) settings to optimize detection of slow flow. Power Doppler ultrasound further augments the sensitivity. Spectral Doppler images may show impaired diastolic flow or reduced venous flow (Fig. 17.11). Near normal Doppler vascularity can be seen in ovaries with partial or intermittent torsion, so the presence of flow does not exclude the diagnosis. However, the absence of flow is highly predictive of torsion, assuming that the study has been technically optimized. Ultrasound may also reveal a twist, or "whirlpool" sign, in the ovarian pedicle at the site of torsion and/or free fluid in the pelvis.

Torsion can be more difficult to diagnose if the torsed ovary contains a mass, particularly if it is an avascular or hypovascular mass such as an endometrioma, mature teratoma, or cyst

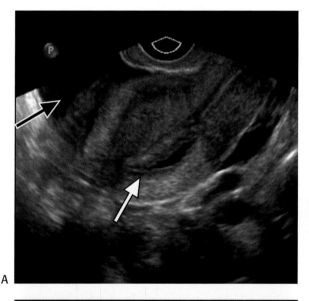

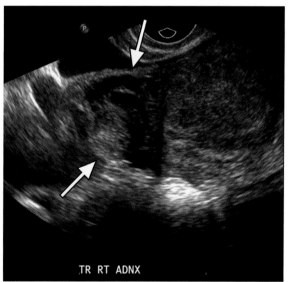

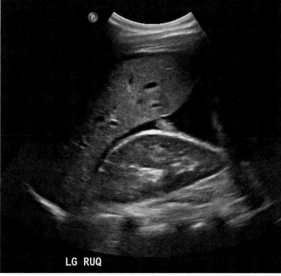

FIGURE 17.9. Ruptured ectopic pregnancy with TVUS showing **(A)** intrauterine "pseudosac" (*white arrow*) and complex pelvic fluid (*black arrow*), **(B)** mass representing gestational sac and hemorrhage (*white arrows*) in the right adnexa, and **(C)** transabdominal US image showing free fluid.

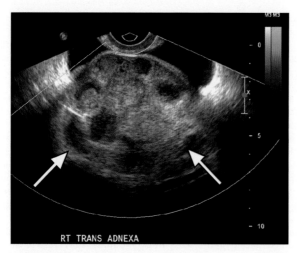

FIGURE 17.10. Torsed right ovary (*arrows*) in a woman undergoing pharmacologic ovulation stimulation is enlarged and edematous, with no demonstrable flow even with power Doppler on TVUS.

(Fig. 17.12). The ovarian tissue at the periphery of the mass can be evaluated with Doppler, but it may be stretched and distorted by the mass or other process. Fallopian tube torsion is less common than ovarian torsion, manifesting as an edematous and twisted tubular structure on all modalities, but often with a normal ovary.

Although CT is not usually performed to evaluate ovarian torsion, the diagnosis may be made incidentally by CT when other entities like appendicitis are suspected. When both ovaries are visualized and normal in size on CT, torsion is no longer in the differential diagnosis. On CT imaging, a torsed ovary is typically enlarged; has a low density, with peripheral and sometimes hemorrhagic follicles; and is often "flipped" into an unusually high or medial position (Fig. 17.13). Pelvic edema and free fluid are common.

On MRI, the diagnosis of ovarian torsion is readily made with multiplanar T2-weighted imaging, demonstrating an enlarged ovary with a high signal in the acute setting (Fig. 17.14), sometimes with an evident beak, twist, or knot in the fallopian tube. MRI is highly sensitive for edema and a small amount of fluid almost always surrounds the torsed ovary. Regions of ovarian or tubal hemorrhage may show high signal on precontrast T1-weighted images; the affected ovary will often have differential

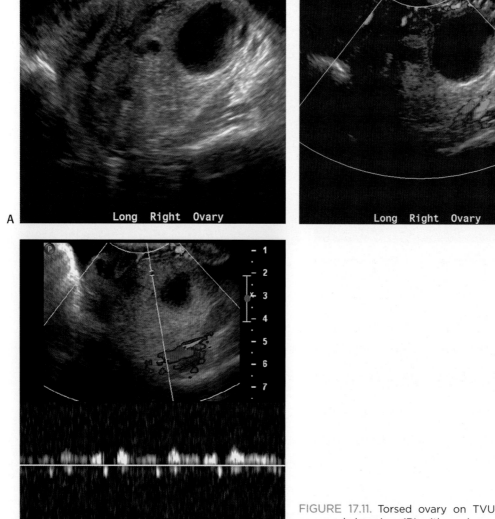

FIGURE 17.11. Torsed ovary on TVUS is **(A)** enlarged on gray-scale imaging, **(B)** with no demonstrable flow on power Doppler, and **(C)** equivocal arterial pulsatility on spectral Doppler.

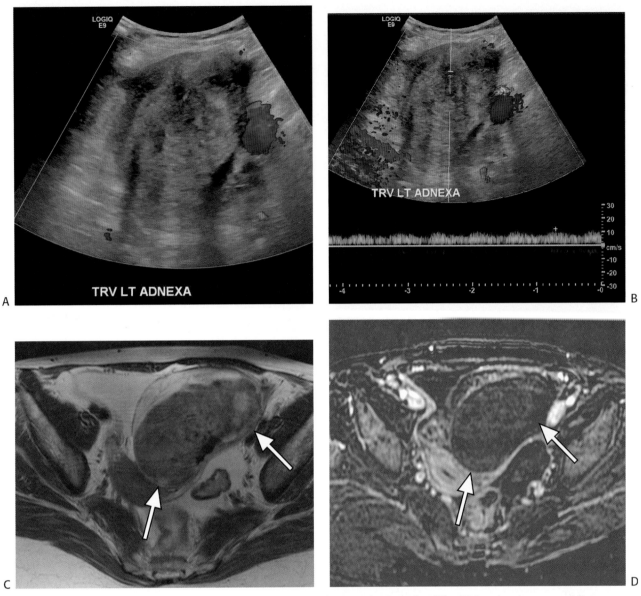

FIGURE 17.12. Torsed ovarian fibroma is **(A)** hypovascular on color Doppler, **(B)** with low-level preserved flow on spectral Doppler. The expected low signal of fibromas is obscured by edema **(C)** (*arrows*) on T2WI and the mass exhibits no enhancement **(D)** (*arrows*) on subtracted T1WI postcontrast.

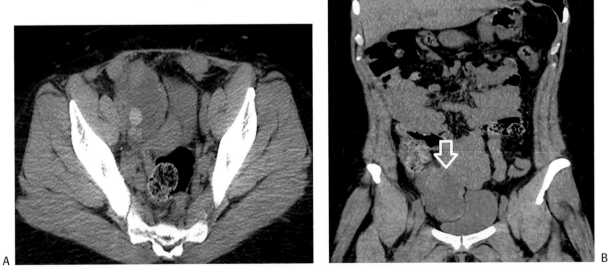

FIGURE 17.13. Right ovarian torsion on **(A)** axial and **(B)** coronal noncontrast CT. The ovary is enlarged with an unusual vertical orientation (*arrow*, **B**), showing multiple peripheral hemorrhagic follicles.

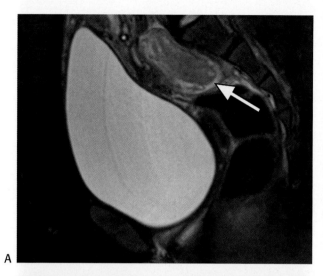

A

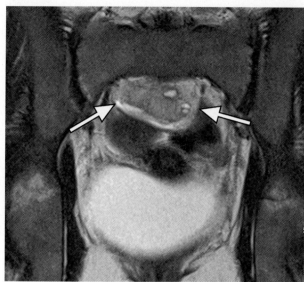

B

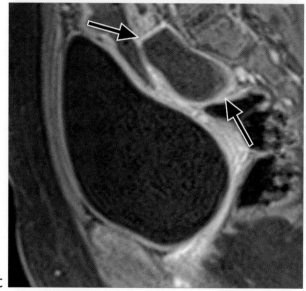

C

FIGURE 17.14. Ovarian torsion with **(A)** sagittal and **(B)** coronal T2WI showing an enlarged, very edematous ovary (*arrows*) with peripheral displacement of follicles, and **(C)** complete lack of enhancement (*arrows*) on sagittal postcontrast T1WI.

enhancement from the contralateral normal ovary after contrast administration.

ENDOMETRIOSIS

Endometriosis is proliferation of endometrial tissue outside the uterus. The most commonly recognized finding is an endometrioma, or cystic adnexal collection of blood products. Endometriosis may also form small solid deposits of endometrial tissue along peritoneal surfaces, sometimes deeply infiltrating the peritoneal lining or serosal surfaces of pelvic organs. The sites of implantation may include the uterus itself, the uterosacral ligament, the pouch of Douglas, the fallopian tubes, the rectum, bladder, and rectovaginal septum and any parietal or visceral peritoneal surface in the pelvis or lower abdomen. Etiologic hypotheses include endometrial differentiation of müllerian rests and retrograde spread of endometrial cells through the fallopian tube into the peritoneal cavity. Endometriosis occasionally appears in caesarian section or other surgical scars (Fig. 17.15), presumably having seeded the incision during pelvic surgery.

Endometriosis most frequently affects women 30 to 40 years of age. Endometriosis may cause dysmenorrhea, infertility, pelvic pain, and dyspareunia; rarely, endometriosis or adhesions may obstruct the bowel or ureter. Like adenomyosis, endometriosis is estrogen dependent, may resolve spontaneously with menopause, and has some response to hormonally directed pharmacologic therapies. Serum CA-125, a circulating substance often used to diagnose or follow ovarian cancer, may be elevated in patients with endometriosis. Laparoscopy is used frequently for the diagnosis of endometriosis and its adhesions, while TVUS and MRI are frequently used for surveillance. TVUS has the advantages of availability and low cost, with performance augmented by technical innovations such as 3D and contrast-enhanced imaging. However, considerable expertise is needed to detect the more subtle findings of endometriosis, and this approach is more common outside the United States. MRI has very high sensitivity for the range of endometriotic disease but remains costly and time consuming.

Endometriomas tend to grow gradually due to repeated cycles of hormonally dependent hemorrhage, akin to the normal endometrium, and often reach 5 to 10 cm or larger. On US,

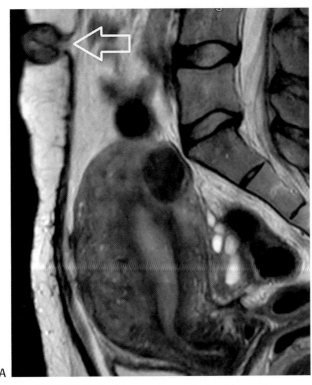

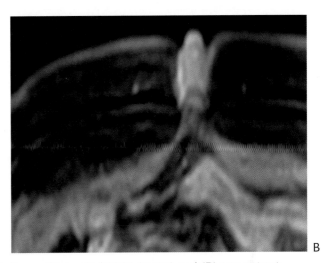

FIGURE 17.15. Scar endometriosis at laparotomy port site on **(A)** sagittal T2WI (*arrow*) and **(B)** precontrast T1WI. Deposits of endometriotic tissue may have signal characteristics of soft tissue without significant accumulations of blood products.

endometriomas usually have a homogenous "ground-glass" appearance of numerous fine, punctate internal echoes, which may be mobile (Fig. 17.16). The classic MR imaging features are marked hyperintensity on pre contrast T1-weighted images, both with and without fat saturation (Fig. 17.17) and intermediate signal known as "shading," with a layered or annular gradient of

signal intensity, on T2WI. When hemosiderin accumulates at the margin of an endometrioma, it may form small echogenic crystals with ring-down artifact on US and blooming at T2WI and in phase GRE (Fig. 17.18). Endometriomas should not have internal vascularity. Long-standing and large endometriomas are associated with the development of clear cell and endometrioid ovarian adenocarcinomas (Fig. 17.19). Thus, annual TVUS surveillance is recommended for unresected endometriomas, and the development of any vascularized soft tissue is a highly concerning feature supporting surgical intervention.

In contrast to cystic endometriomas, solid deposits of endometriosis are usually numerous but very small. They may be difficult to evaluate with TVUS, especially in larger patients, and are more conspicuous with MRI, which demonstrates small high-signal locules on precontrast T1-weighted images (Fig. 17.20). Endometriosis incites a local inflammatory response and is associated with adhesions, which range in size and distribution from tiny filaments to densely packed regions of fibrotic tissue. Endometriosis and associated fibrosis may be infiltrative and masslike, with hypoechoic stellate soft tissue on US and low-signal masses with spiculated margins at T2-weighted sequences (Fig. 17.21). Deeply infiltrative endometriosis often involves the rectouterine pouch, with characteristic elevation of the peritoneal reflection due to chronic adhesions. Other sequelae include hydrosalpinx, adhesions involving and sometimes obstructing small or large bowel, and mural invasion of the bladder (Fig. 17.22).

FIGURE 17.16. Large endometrioma on TVUS, showing characteristic fine, homogenous "ground-glass" pattern of low-level internal echoes, with no demonstrable color Doppler vascularity.

PELVIC INFLAMMATORY DISEASE

Pelvic inflammatory disease (PID) is a general term referring to gynecologic infection. In North America, sexually transmitted *Neisseria gonorrhoeae* or *Chlamydia trachomatis* are common

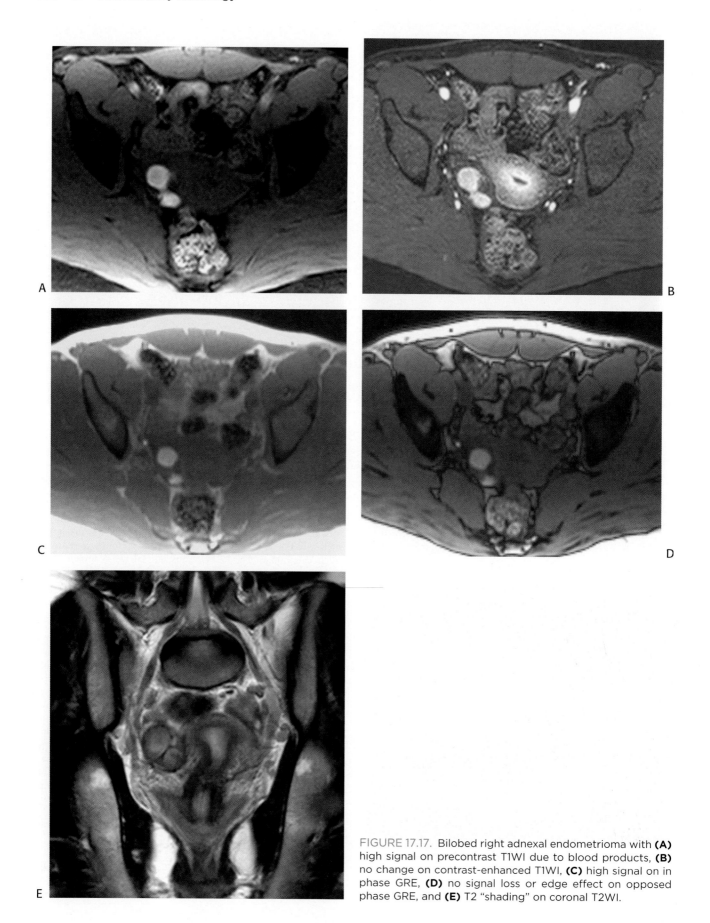

FIGURE 17.17. Bilobed right adnexal endometrioma with **(A)** high signal on precontrast T1WI due to blood products, **(B)** no change on contrast-enhanced T1WI, **(C)** high signal on in phase GRE, **(D)** no signal loss or edge effect on opposed phase GRE, and **(E)** T2 "shading" on coronal T2WI.

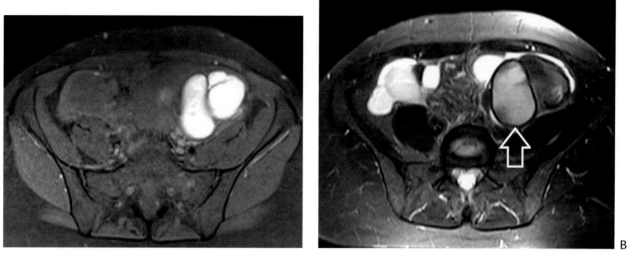

FIGURE 17.18. Left adnexal endometrioma with **(A)** very high signal on precontrast T1WI with fat saturation and **(B)** a hemosiderin ring with very low signal (*arrow*) on T2WI.

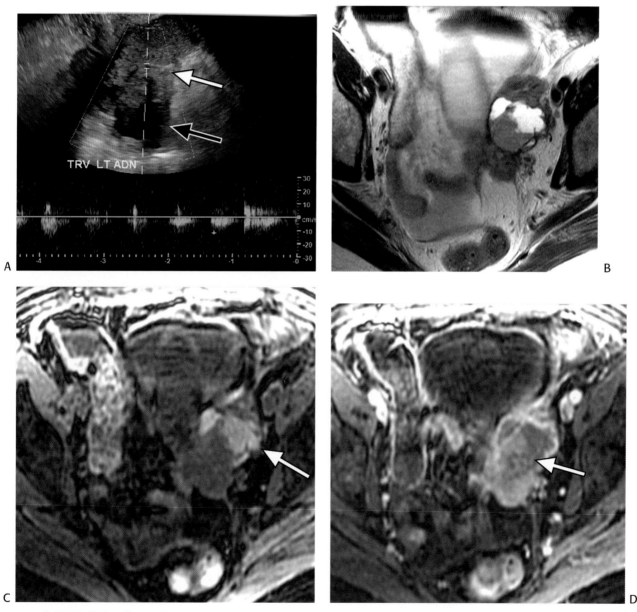

FIGURE 17.19. Clear cell carcinoma arising in endometriosis with **(A)** hemorrhagic (*black arrow*) and vascularized solid components (*white arrow*) on TVUS, **(B)** similar bimodal appearance on T2WI, **(C)** high-signal blood products (*arrow*) on precontrast T1WI, and **(D)** enhancement of solid component (*arrow*) on postcontrast T1WI.

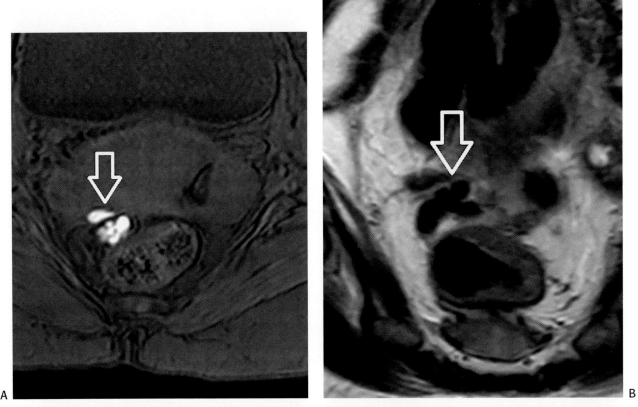

FIGURE 17.20. Small solid endometrial deposits (*arrows*) in the rectouterine pouch with **(A)** very high signal on axial precontrast T1WI with fat saturation and **(B)** low signal on oblique uterine short-axis T2WI.

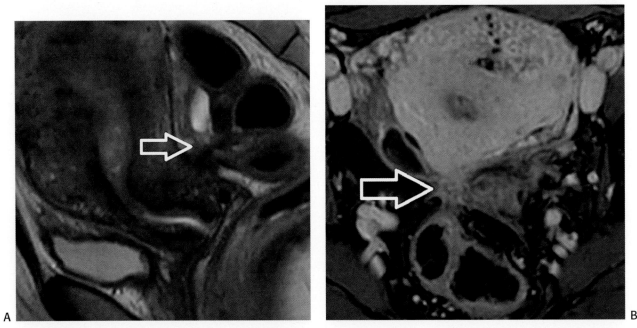

FIGURE 17.21. Infiltrative rectocervical endometriosis with **(A)** stellate low-signal mass (*arrow*) elevating the posterior cul-de-sac on sagittal T2WI and **(B)** enhancing soft tissue tethering pelvic structures (*arrow*) on axial T1WI postcontrast.

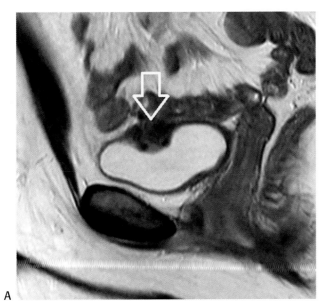
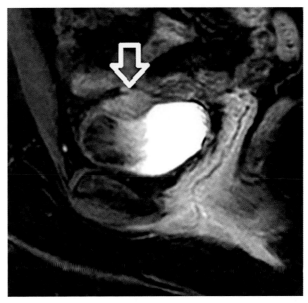

A
B

FIGURE 17.22. Infiltrative endometriosis involving bladder dome (*arrows*) with **(A)** low-signal mass on sagittal T2WI and **(B)** enhancement on postcontrast T1WI in a woman with prior hysterectomy.

causes, with typical risk factors of multiple sexual partners and lack of barrier contraception. Although this is most commonly a disease of young women, there has been a surge in sexually transmitted disease among sexually active elderly men and women in the last two decades.

PID is often asymptomatic. However, characteristic symptoms prompting patients to seek medical attention may include pelvic pain, fever, dyspareunia, and vaginal discharge. Sequelae of PID include endometritis, salpingitis, oophoritis, pyosalpinx, tuboovarian abscesses, and local peritonitis, sometimes with subsequent development of hydrosalpinx, salpingitis isthmica nodosa (SIN), pelvic adhesions, and, especially if there has been intrauterine instrumentation, endometrial synechiae (Asherman syndrome). Occasional long-term complications include infertility and ectopic pregnancy. Rarely, acute inflammation may spread to the right upper quadrant (Fitz–Hugh–Curtis syndrome), with associated peritonitis and adhesions.

Most PID is diagnosed clinically, but imaging can provide important information about disease extent and complications. Ultrasound is the mainstay of imaging diagnosis. Women with active PID often experience discomfort from the TVUS probe, giving a clue to the diagnosis prior to image review. As with other pelvic pathologies, CT is rarely used for the primary evaluation of PID, but may contribute to management. MRI provides excellent soft tissue detail and is more sensitive for findings of early infection. Most women with PID are treated successfully with antibiotics. A minority require image-guided interventional procedures for abscess drainage. Occasionally, surgery is required to resect a chronically inflamed tuboovarian abscess with pyosalpinx.

Imaging findings are quite variable in extent and severity. Free fluid is often present, sometimes complex. Inflamed and edematous fat is more hyperechoic than normal fat, and the lack of normal mobility of pelvic structures on TVUS may be notable. Cervicitis and endometritis are the earliest manifestations of this ascending infectious process, but are hard to diagnose by TVUS. The cervix and uterus may be edematous, sometimes with fluid in the endometrial canal. MRI can demonstrate loss of normal zonal anatomy due to high-signal edema on T2WI. Inflamed fallopian tubes may

exhibit wall thickening or hyperenhancement or may be distended with complex fluid or pus, known as pyosalpinx (Fig. 17.23). One or both ovaries may be enlarged by edema initially or involved by a tuboovarian abscess (Fig. 17.24) at later stages. Tuboovarian abscesses vary widely in size and complexity. When the appearance is masslike rather than predominantly cystic, the term tuboovarian complex may be used. Due to surrounding inflammation and patient discomfort, TVUS is sometimes limited for the diagnosis of tuboovarian abscess or complex, and CT and MR are particularly helpful. Bubbles of gas in tuboovarian abscesses are extremely rare; when they are encountered, strong consideration should be given to an abscess of enteric origin.

Chronic inflammation of the fallopian tubes is associated with SIN. This condition is diagnosed laparoscopically or with fluoroscopic hysterosalpingography (HSG). HSG is contraindicated in acute PID due to the risk of ascending spread of an existing infection by retrograde contrast injection, but it may be used in the subacute or chronic setting as part of an infertility workup. SIN is characterized by multiple tiny diverticula or cavities within small nodules of postinflammatory tissue involving the isthmic portions of the tubes. These nodules are visible and palpable at surgery, whereas the diverticula are demonstrated at HSG, with filling of clustered linear and flask-shaped outpouchings from the tubal lumens (Fig. 17.25). SIN frequently appears along with other hysterosalpingographic evidence of prior inflammatory disease, such as tubal occlusion and hydrosalpinx.

Treated salpingitis is associated with the subsequent development of sterile hydrosalpinx resulting from tubal scarring and obstruction of the fallopian tubes. The fallopian tubes are not normally visible at imaging, but when distended by fluid, they are tubular and usually form "C" or "S" shapes in the adnexal regions. Simple hydrosalpinx has luminal contents that are anechoic on TVUS (Fig. 17.26), fluid density on CT, low signal on T1-weighted images, and high signal on T2-weighted sequences. The linear longitudinal folds of the normal tube may be seen in cross section on TVUS or MR images, helping to make the diagnosis of hydrosalpinx and distinguish it from a cystic mass. Unlike pyosalpinx, hydrosalpinx is unlikely to be acutely symptomatic and does not

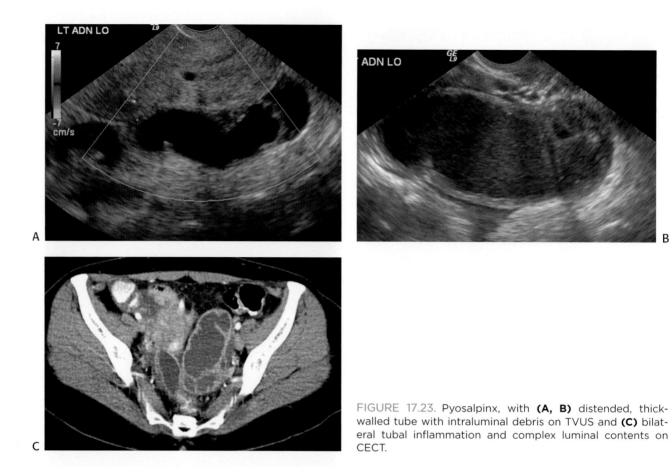

FIGURE 17.23. Pyosalpinx, with **(A, B)** distended, thick-walled tube with intraluminal debris on TVUS and **(C)** bilateral tubal inflammation and complex luminal contents on CECT.

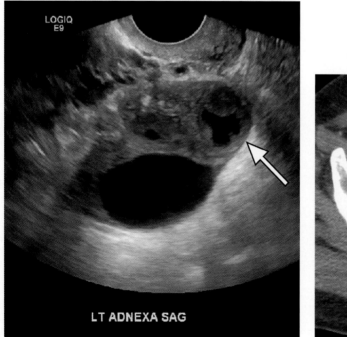

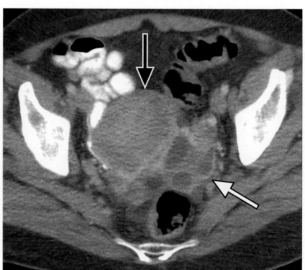

FIGURE 17.24. Tuboovarian abscess with **(A)** cystic mass incorporating thick-walled tube (*arrow*) on TVUS and **(B)** multilocular inflammatory left pelvic mass (*white arrow*) on CT. Note also the edematous and hypoenhancing uterus (*black arrow*), a finding of endometritis.

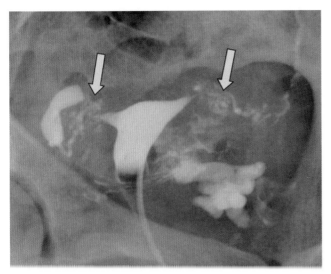

FIGURE 17.25. Salpingitis isthmica nodosa (SIN). HSG reveals multiple small diverticula (*arrows*) arising from the isthmic portions of the tubes. Pelvic adhesions prevent free intraperitoneal spill.

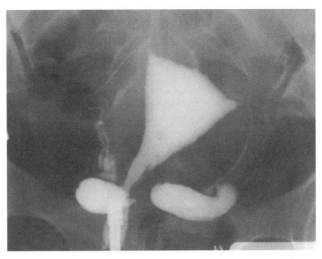

FIGURE 17.27. Bilateral hydrosalpinges on HSG. The ampullary portions of the fallopian tubes are dilated, and there is no peritoneal spill.

require antibiotic therapy, but hydrosalpinx is associated with sub-fertility and may be an indication for salpingectomy or tubal aspiration (paired with assisted reproductive technologies) in women desiring pregnancy. HSG may reveal various abnormalities. The tubes may be occluded and fail to opacify. Alternatively, the distal ends of the tubes may be occluded, so that the tubes fill and distend during injection, but do not spill contrast into the peritoneum (Fig. 17.27). Not infrequently, there is a discrepancy in the degree of hydrosalpinx demonstrated by HSG and by other techniques. A fallopian tube that is occluded at two points, and that is distended

in between, may appear as a hydrosalpinx on US, CT, or MR, but fail to opacify on HSG. Alternatively, a distally occluded tube may be transiently distended by active injection during HSG, but have a normal diameter when other techniques are used.

NEOPLASIA

Primary ovarian neoplasms may be benign or malignant, arising from epithelial, germ cell, or sex cord–stromal origins. Metastatic disease, most often from gastrointestinal or endometrial primary cancers, may also involve the ovaries. The radiologist's task is rarely to make a histologic diagnosis, but more often to identify the typical

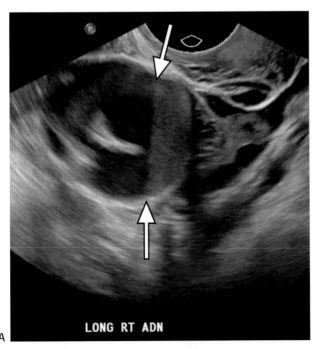

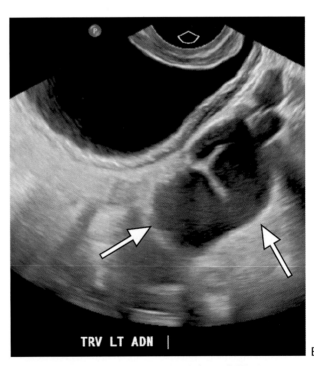

FIGURE 17.26. Bilateral hydrosalpinges on TVUS (*arrows*) with **(A)** layering debris on the right and **(B)** more simple fluid contents on the left.

TABLE **17.1**	
2014 FIGO Staging of Ovarian Carcinoma	
Stage	Description
Stage I	Tumor confined to ovaries A. One ovary, capsule intact B. Both ovaries C. One or both ovaries, with ruptured capsule and/or malignant cells in ascites or peritoneal washings
Stage II	Pelvic extension A. Extension and/or implant on surface of uterus and/or tubes B. Extension to other intraperitoneal pelvic tissues
Stage III	Ovarian tumor with extrapelvic peritoneal tumor and/or retroperitoneal nodes A. Positive nodes and/or microscopic abdominal peritoneal implants B. Macroscopic, extrapelvic, peritoneal implants ≤2 cm in diameter ± positive retroperitoneal nodes (includes surface deposits on liver and spleen) C. Macroscopic, extrapelvic, peritoneal implants >2 cm in diameter ± positive retroperitoneal nodes (includes surface deposits on liver and spleen)
Stage IV	Distant metastases excluding peritoneal metastases A. Pleural effusion with positive cytology B. Abdominal or extra-abdominal parenchymal metastases, inguinal or distant nodes

imaging features of characteristic benign and physiologic lesions in order to avoid unnecessary workup while remaining alert to imaging features concerning for aggressive or malignant neoplasms. Ovarian cancer is the most deadly gynecologic malignancy, but most ovarian lesions are not cancer. When ovarian cancer is diagnosed, imaging can provide important information relevant to staging (Table 17.1) and surveillance, to be discussed in more detail below.

Imaging Features of Tumors

When adequately visualized with any imaging modality, unilocular cysts containing simple fluid with no internal soft tissue elements can be considered benign at any age. Simple cysts span a range of diagnoses from functional cysts and follicles to cystadenomas. It is important for radiologists to recognize and confidently diagnose simple cysts, to avoid unnecessary diagnostic workup and even surgery, with associated patient anxiety, cost, and related complications.

It is equally important for radiologists to identify imaging features associated with neoplasia and recommend appropriate management. Relevant ultrasound guidelines for adnexal cyst evaluation include the International Ovarian Tumor Analysis (IOTA) model and the SRU guidelines. These and other consensus recommendations vary in their emphasis and specifics but share certain

fundamental concepts. Simple cysts, hemorrhagic cysts, endometriomas, and mature teratomas (dermoids) often have pathognomonic sonographic features and should be managed according to the specific diagnosis, to be detailed below. When a lesion is poorly or incompletely visualized, or sonographically indeterminate, further characterization with MR is recommended.

In general, the risk of ovarian malignancy increases with cyst size, number and size of soft tissue elements including mural nodules and thick (>2 mm) septations, vascular flow within soft tissue elements, bilaterality, and ascites. Although low-resistance spectral Doppler arterial waveforms are associated with malignancy, this sign has poor sensitivity and specificity. Clinical features associated with ovarian malignancy include postmenopausal status and elevated tumor markers, particularly CA-125 but also HE-4, inhibins A and B, CEA (carcinoembryonic antigen), β-hCG (human chorionic gonadotropin), and α-FP (fetoprotein).

When an ovarian cyst has very suspicious imaging features by US, such as large, vascularized mural nodules and ascites, further imaging characterization may not be needed and the patient may be referred directly to a gynecologist or gynecologic oncologist. However, many benign and malignant lesions are sonographically indeterminate, and further characterization with MRI may be needed to guide management and prevent unnecessary surgery. Pelvic MRI for adnexal mass characterization may be performed on a 1.5T or 3T magnet. Intravenous or intramuscular administration of glucagon or another antiperistaltic agent is very helpful to reduce artifact from bowel motion, especially for large masses extending superiorly out of the pelvis. Important sequences include multiplanar T2WI, DWI, and pre- and postcontrast T1WI with fat saturation. High temporal resolution true dynamic postcontrast imaging is performed in some centers, allowing evaluation of enhancement curves that help to delineate benign from malignant neoplasms. Multiphasic postcontrast imaging is more commonly performed, with 3 to 5 whole pelvis postcontrast acquisitions that can be performed in any plane preferred by the interpreting radiologist. In- and opposed-phase GRE is also helpful for evaluation of fat within dermoids and blooming of blood products.

As with US imaging, certain broad concepts govern MR characterization of pelvic masses. Macroscopic lipid within a mass is characteristic of benign dermoids. Low or very low signal within a solid mass on T2-weighted imaging is a benign prognostic sign associated with exophytic leiomyomas, fibromas, fibrothecomas, and Brenner tumors. Most primary ovarian malignancies have a mixture of cystic and solid elements, so a purely solid mass is relatively reassuring unless there is a known extraovarian primary malignancy. Unilocular cysts are benign, and if mural nodules or papillations are present, the risk of malignancy increases with their number and size. Enhancement of any solid components including thick septations or mural nodules should be carefully evaluated on postcontrast images, using image subtraction to separate true enhancement from intrinsic hyperintensity of blood products as needed. Almost all aggressive neoplasms have high signal on DWI within their solid components, but the presence of high DWI signal is not specific as it is may also be present in a variety of benign lesions. However, very low apparent diffusion coefficient (ADC) values are predictive of malignancy. These concepts will be illustrated below, in the context of specific tumor histologies.

Epithelial Tumors

Epithelial histologies constitute the majority of ovarian neoplasms overall and the majority of cancers. Serous and mucinous subtypes are the most common and the most important to understand, with less common types including endometrioid and clear cell ovarian cancer and Brenner tumors. Epithelial ovarian cancer is the leading cause of gynecologic cancer death in the United States, with risk factors including early menarche and delayed menopause, nulliparity, obesity, hormone replacement therapy, and BRCA gene mutations. Associations with endometriosis and PID are less well established. Protective factors include oral contraceptive use, pregnancy, and breastfeeding.

As in endometrial cancer, epithelial ovarian cancers are currently understood to arise from two distinct lineages, known as type I and type II cancers. Type I epithelial tumors are low grade and slow growing and probably develop stepwise from benign precursors such as cystadenomas. This type of orderly progression or spectrum from dysplasia to neoplasia is analogous to tumors in many other body sites, such as the colonic adenoma to carcinoma pathway. By contrast, type II tumors are high grade and usually in an advanced stage at presentation. Despite the "ovarian cancer" appellation, many type II epithelial tumors such as high-grade

serous cancer (HGSC) are thought to arise from a tubal epithelial precursor known as serous tubal intraepithelial carcinoma (STIC).

Serous Tumors

Serous histology is the most common epithelial cell type in ovarian neoplasia. Type I serous tumors include benign serous cystadenomas—which are sometimes completely simple—and cystadenofibromas (Fig. 17.28), characterized by one or a few small mural nodules within an otherwise simple, unilocular cyst. The presence of demonstrable Doppler vascularity is variable, but these mural papillations almost always show enhancement at MRI. Small psammomatous calcifications may be seen in the nodule, with occasional thin mural calcifications. Cystadenomas and cystadenofibromas never become high-grade, type II cancers, so they may be safely

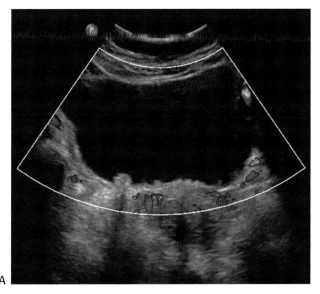
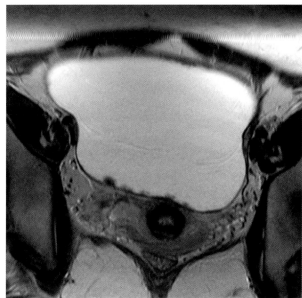
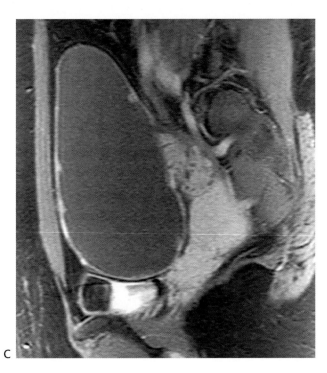

FIGURE 17.28. Benign serous cystadenofibroma is predominantly cystic with tiny mural papillations on **(A)** transabdominal US, **(B)** axial oblique T2WI, and **(C)** sagittal T1WI postcontrast.

managed with imaging and tumor marker surveillance. However, they do predispose to torsion and have the long-term capacity to develop into borderline or low-grade tumors and are usually resected in young and middle-aged women. These benign lesions may be resected with cystectomy or oophorectomy.

Malignant type I serous tumors include borderline and low-grade serous cancers, which are distinguished histologically, rather than imaging. "Borderline" is a specific histologic designation indicating serous epithelial neoplasia that does not invade the ovarian stroma, though it is considered malignant. Borderline tumors may have superficial peritoneal deposits strongly resembling carcinomatosis by imaging, but they do not exhibit true peritoneal invasion under the microscope. By imaging, both borderline and low-grade serous tumors exhibit papillary and frondlike soft tissue elements (Fig. 17.29), with more and larger mural nodules than their benign counterparts. Image-based staging should include evaluation of both ovaries, uterus, peritoneal surfaces, and pelvic

and retroperitoneal lymph nodes. Low-grade serous tumors are true invasive cancers, though slow growing. Some subtypes exhibit extensive psammomatous calcifications with linear coating of peritoneal surfaces (Fig. 17.30). Intraoperative frozen section is often used to determine the degree of surgical intervention that is needed; current National Comprehensive Cancer Network (NCCN) guidelines favor complete surgical staging.

HGSC is the "classic" and the most common ovarian cancer cell type. This is a rapidly growing type II cancer with marked cytologic atypia and frequent p53 gene mutations. HGSC does not arise from benign precursors such as cysts and cystadenomas, but most likely from tiny STIC. HGSC has a single imaging and histologic appearance, treatment pathway, and prognosis whether it is known as ovarian carcinoma, fallopian tubal carcinoma, or primary peritoneal carcinoma. HGSC is most commonly a mixed cystic and solid mass at imaging (Fig. 17.31), often with a substantial and poorly marginated solid component. HGSC invades

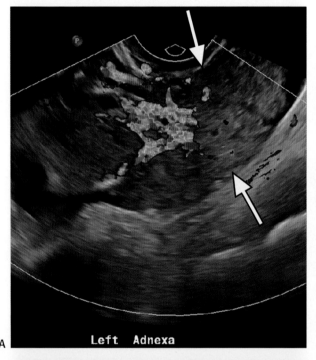

A — Left Adnexa

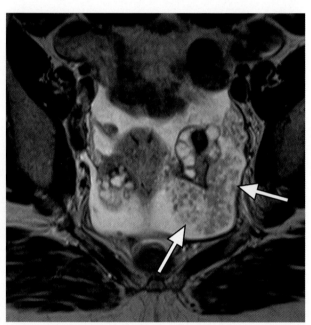

B

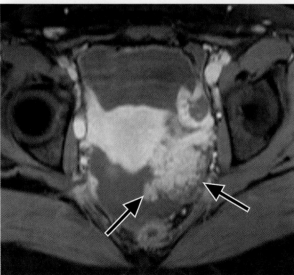

C

FIGURE 17.29. Serous borderline tumor with exophytic frondlike tissue (*arrows*) extending posterior to left ovary on **(A)** TVUS with color Doppler showing vascular pedicle, **(B)** papillary tissue surrounded by ascites on T2WI, and **(C)** enhancement on postcontrast T1WI. This cannot be reliably distinguished from HGSC by imaging, and complete surgical staging is indicated.

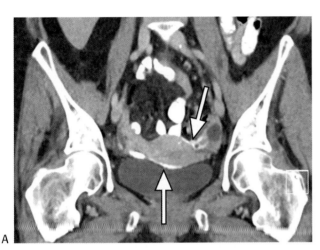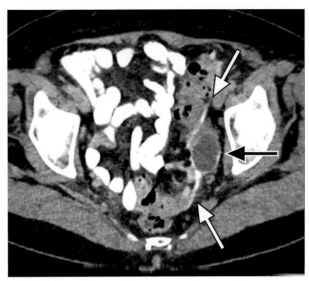

FIGURE 17.30. Psammomatous calcifications (*white arrows*) coating peritoneal surfaces **(A)** on coronal and **(B)** axial CECT images, with associated left ovarian cystic lesion (*black arrow*) containing papillations not visible by CT. Psammomatous calcifications are classically associated with low-grade serous carcinomas but can be seen microscopically with any serous tumor.

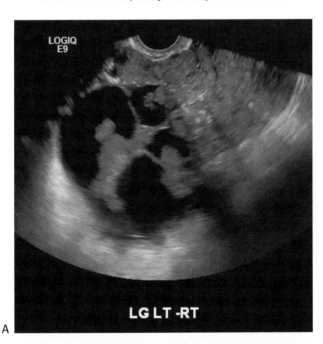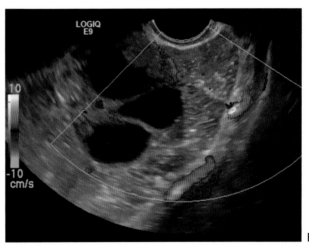

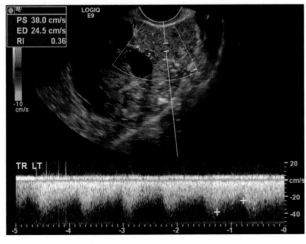

FIGURE 17.31. High-grade serous ovarian carcinoma with **(A)** many papillary nodules studding thin septations, **(B)** color Doppler vascularity in solid elements, and **(C)** a low-resistance (high diastolic flow) waveform associated with, but not specific or sensitive for, disrupted vasoregulation in tumor vessels.

the ovarian stroma and spreads directly into adjacent organs and into the peritoneal cavity, blanketing coelomic surfaces and obscuring margins between organs (Fig. 17.32). HGSC is most commonly stage III or IV at diagnosis and 5-year survival rates of approximately 39% and 17%, respectively. STIC and HGSC are associated with the BRCA gene mutations and are the basis of currently recommended prophylactic bilateral salpingo-oophorectomy for these women, but interestingly, patients with BRCA mutations have more chemoresponsive tumors than the general population.

CT of the abdomen and pelvis is often performed prior to surgery. Comprehensive surgical staging and debulking, performed via open laparotomy, includes evacuation of any ascites and/or peritoneal lavage for cytology, hysterectomy, bilateral salpingo-oophorectomy, omentectomy, complete visualization of peritoneal surface with excision of any nodules, and pelvic and retroperitoneal lymph node dissection. Thus, the presence of peritoneal carcinomatosis is not a contraindication to surgery in HGSC, as it is in many other abdominal and pelvic malignancies, nor is the presence of carcinomatosis a binary assessment. Very extensive intraperitoneal disease may be a contraindication to primary debulking and require neoadjuvant chemotherapy prior to definitive surgery (Fig. 17.33). The presence and extent of soft tissue nodules on the peritoneal surfaces, within the omental fat and along leaflets of the mesentery

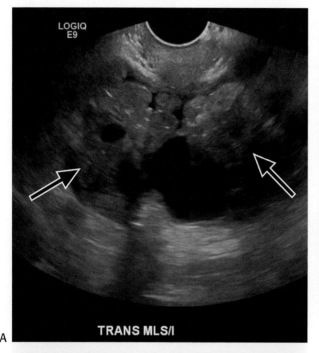

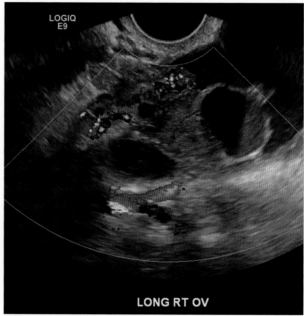

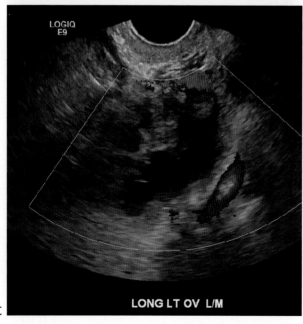

FIGURE 17.32. High-grade serous ovarian carcinoma with **(A)** diffuse papillary soft tissue (*arrows*) obscuring organ margins in deep pelvis and **(B, C)** bilateral adnexal masses.

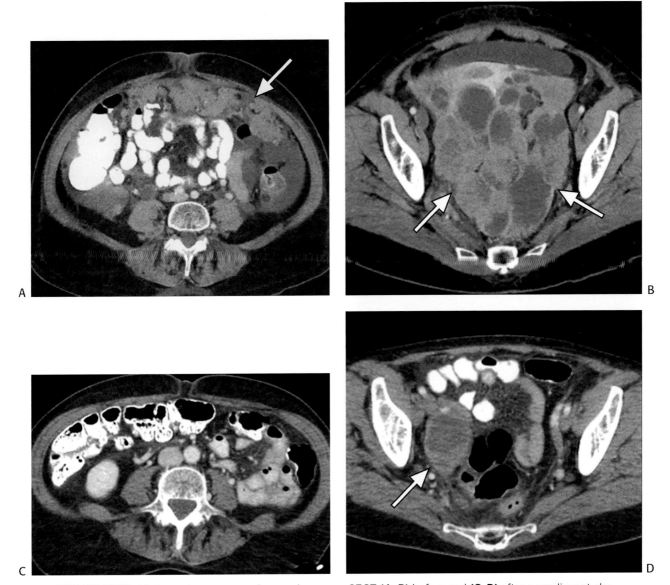

FIGURE 17.33. High-grade serous ovarian carcinoma on CECT **(A, B)** before and **(C, D)** after neoadjuvant che-motherapy. Note **(A, C)** near-complete resolution of omental cake (*arrows*) and **(B, D)** substantial decrease in size of pelvic mass (*arrows*). Surgical staging with optimal debulking was then performed, demonstrating no viable tumor histologically.

should be separately described. In particular, bulky disease under the right hemidiaphragm, retroperitoneal nodes at or above the renal hila, and mesenteric (as distinct from omental) nodules >1 cm are predictive of suboptimal debulking (Fig. 17.34) and should be specifically described.

PET/CT is usually not used during initial diagnosis and staging but may be helpful in the recurrent setting, particularly when there is a new elevation in serum CA-125. PET/CT augments the sensitivity of other modalities for detecting small areas of intraperitoneal recurrence. Most series have shown PET/CT (Fig. 17.35) to be more sensitive than CT for detecting all foci of metastatic disease and for localizing recurrences after major therapy; changes in SUV may permit earlier evaluation of treatment efficacy than imaging that relies on tumor size. PET/CT may even detect recurrent disease in some cases in which the CA-125 is normal.

Mucinous Tumors

Most mucinous tumors are benign or low grade. Mucinous ovarian carcinoma is less common than previously thought, due to increasing recognition that many ovarian mucinous carcinomas are actually metastatic from gastrointestinal primary sites. Primary mucinous ovarian carcinomas are type I tumors, meaning that they develop in a stepwise fashion from benign mucinous cystadenoma, to mucinous borderline tumor, to mucinous carcinoma. Mucinous cystadenomas are unilocular or multilocular, often with smooth vascularized septations (Fig. 17.36) but no dominant solid component. The cystic components of mucinous tumors accumulate large amounts of mucin produced by a relatively modest amount of epithelium, so mucinous tumors may reach a large size while remaining benign. Mucinous cystadenomas may be treated with cystectomy or unilateral oophorectomy. Mucinous borderline

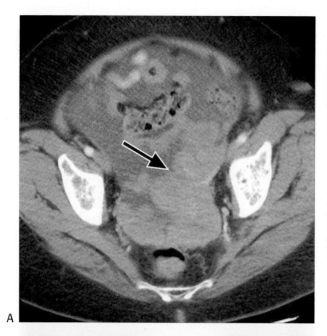

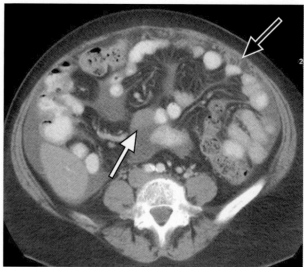

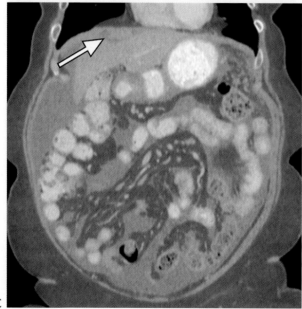

FIGURE 17.34. High-grade serous ovarian carcinoma with **(A)** confluent pelvic masses (*arrow*) on CECT. Factors that may preclude primary surgical debulking include **(B)** mesenteric masses (*white arrow*), which should be distinguished from omental implants (*black arrow*), and **(C)** subdiaphragmatic nodules at liver dome (*arrow*).

tumors and carcinomas have a larger solid component and/or thick, nodular septations (Fig. 17.37). The solid elements are not usually papillary or frondlike as in serous tumors. Coarse or septal calcifications may be seen. They are treated with complete surgical staging as described above in the discussion of serous tumors.

Only 20% of mucinous ovarian tumors are malignant, and only 20% of those are of primary ovarian origin. The remaining 80% are metastatic deposits from gastrointestinal, often appendiceal, mucinous neoplasms. Despite the low-grade histology of these neoplasms, they are often associated with disseminated peritoneal adenomucinosis (DPAM), also known as pseudomyxoma peritonei, where the peritoneal space is filled with hypocellular mucinous material (Fig. 17.38). This can be a clinically aggressive process, causing abdominal enlargement, bloating, pain, and even bowel obstruction. Although pseudomyxoma peritonei is associated with ovarian cancer, it more often arises from appendiceal mucinous

tumors. Thus, the appendix is usually also resected when a mucinous tumor is identified at oophorectomy.

Other Epithelial Tumors

Endometrioid and clear cell ovarian neoplasms are much less common than serous or mucinous epithelial tumors and most commonly present as overt carcinomas. Both are associated with long-standing endometriosis, which may enable a correct prospective diagnosis by imaging. The presence of a vascularized nodule within an otherwise typical endometrioma on US or MR (Fig. 17.19) is highly suspicious for endometrioid or clear cell carcinoma. Endometrioid ovarian carcinoma is also associated with synchronous intrauterine endometrial proliferation, either carcinoma or hyperplasia, in up to 40% of women (Fig. 17.39).

Brenner tumors are benign epithelial ovarian neoplasms that histologically resemble urothelium. They tend to be predominantly

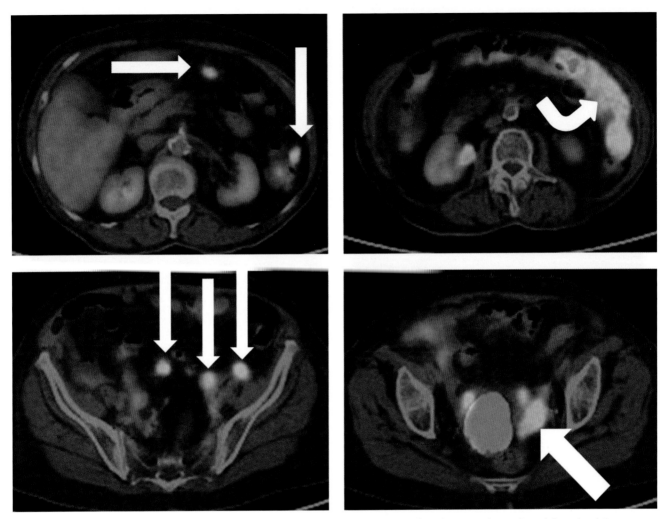

FIGURE 17.35. Metastatic serous ovarian carcinoma. Fused ¹⁸FDG PET/CT shows peritoneal, nodal, and pelvic deposits (*arrows*) and omental disease (*curved arrow*). The patient also has a densely calcified uterine fibroid.

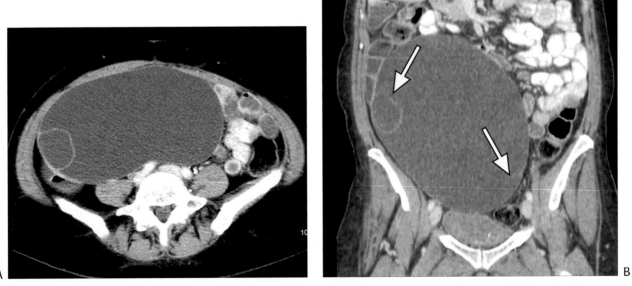

FIGURE 17.36. Mucinous cystadenoma on CECT is a **(A)** large predominantly cystic mass with **(B)** only a few scattered thin septations (*arrows*). This was an incidental finding.

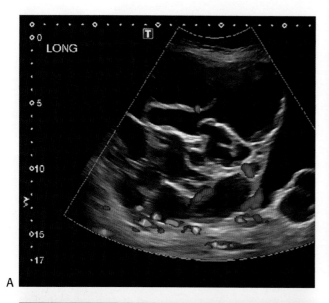

A

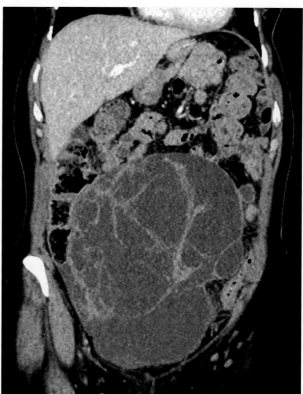

B

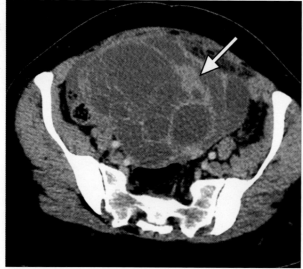

C

FIGURE 17.37. Mucinous borderline tumor presenting as a large mass **(A)** with thick vascular septations on transabdominal US, **(B)** extension into the abdomen on coronal CECT, and **(C)** nodular soft tissue components (*arrow*) on axial CECT. The number, thickness, and nodularity of the septations and overall size of the mass increase the likelihood of malignancy; this borderline tumor cannot be distinguished from cystadenocarcinoma by imaging.

solid with a significant fibrous stromal component, resulting in their typical sonographic appearance of a hypoechoic vascularized mass and low-signal homogenous mass on T2WI (Fig. 17.40).

Other epithelial carcinomas include mixed epithelial tumor, which is usually treated in accordance with the most aggressive cell type and carcinosarcoma (also called malignant mixed mesodermal/müllerian tumor or MMMT). MMMT has a blend of epithelial and sarcomatoid elements and tends to be more solid than the typically mixed cystic/solid pure epithelial tumors. However, a specific preoperative diagnosis cannot be made by imaging, and these tumors are surgically staged just like other epithelial tumors.

Germ Cell Tumors

Germ cell tumors (GCTs) affect younger women more often than do epithelial ovarian cancer, and they are most commonly benign. Mature teratoma (dermoid) is the most common GCT and probably the most common ovarian neoplasm overall. It is a well-differentiated benign neoplasm with elements of two or more of the three embryonic layers: ectoderm, mesoderm, and endoderm. As such, dermoids contain a variety of tissue types including teeth, hair, and oily, sebaceous, or fatty material and neural tissue. The presence of intralesional lipid is a major feature enabling their identification on imaging studies. Depending on whether it is solid or

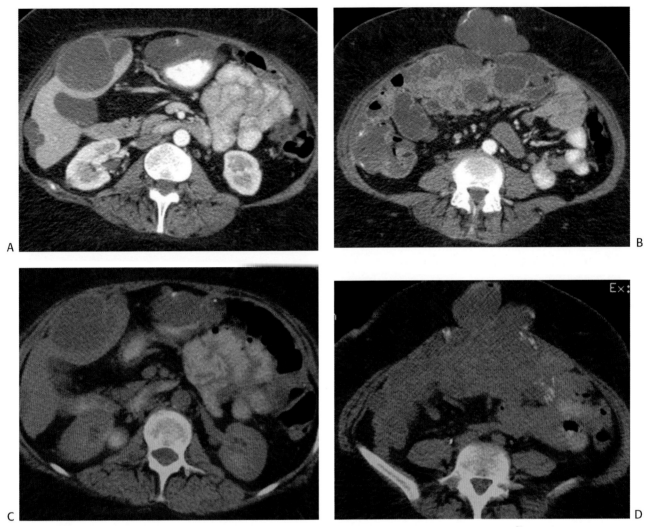

FIGURE 17.38. Pseudomyxoma peritonei on CECT **(A, B)** with gelatinous mucinous material anterior to liver and stomach, coating bowel loops, and extending through the umbilicus. This material is hypocellular, accounting both for the lack of uptake on fused ¹⁸FDG PET/CT images **(C, D)** and its poor responsiveness to chemotherapy.

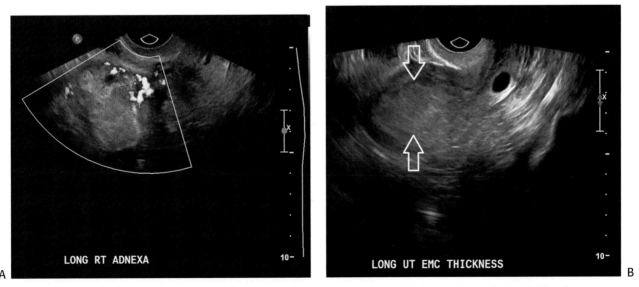

FIGURE 17.39. Synchronous **(A)** right ovarian endometrioid adenocarcinoma and **(B)** endometrioid endometrial carcinoma with markedly thickened stripe (*arrow*) on TVUS.

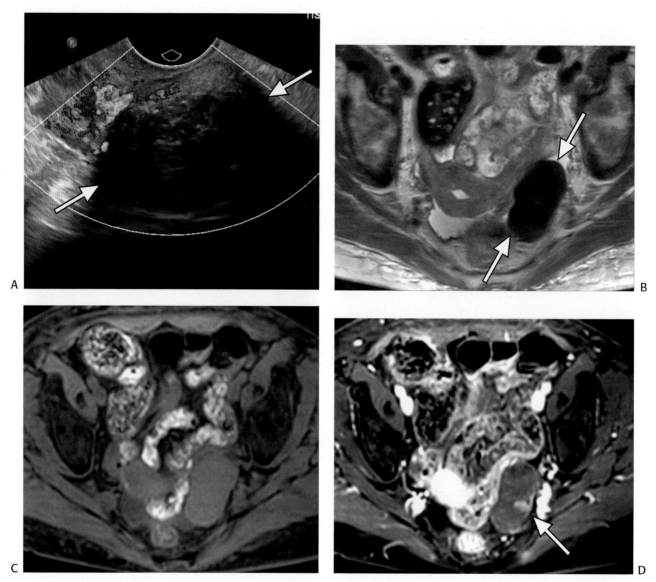

FIGURE 17.40. Brenner tumor (*arrows*) with **(A)** hypoechoic shadowing mass strongly resembling a fibroid on TVUS, **(B)** very low signal on axial T2WI, **(C)** signal similar to skeletal muscle on precontrast T1WI, and **(D)** low-level enhancement on postcontrast T1WI.

liquid, lipid content in a dermoid may manifest as an echogenic mass, a fat–fluid level, or even floating mobile fat lobules on TVUS (Fig. 17.41). Hair often forms an echogenic nest, sometimes with a "dot–dash" sign and posterior acoustic shadowing. Coarse calcifications of teeth are also highly echogenic, with posterior acoustic shadowing. Lipid and calcifications are readily apparent at CT (Fig. 17.42). Depending on the admixture of fat and other elements, the signal within lipid components of dermoids is variably suppressed with fat-saturated MR sequences and may exhibit diffuse signal loss or a surrounding chemical shift artifact on opposed phase GRE (Figs. 17.41 and 17.43). Dermoids may have enhancing soft tissue elements and remain benign.

Immature teratomas are rare solid masses without specific imaging features and are most often seen in teenagers. Malignant degeneration of mature teratomas is also rare, usually squamous cell degeneration in older women, and manifests as growth of an internal solid nodule or direct invasion of adjacent structures. The vanishingly small risk of malignant degeneration of mature teratomas is much smaller than the risk of torsion. Some patients elect annual ultrasound surveillance, though most undergo cystectomy.

Among overt cancers, malignant GCTs are more common than epithelial ovarian carcinomas in young women and girls. Among malignant GCTs, the most common is dysgerminoma, the female equivalent of seminoma. It is a small solid mass, sometimes bilateral and sometimes with central necrosis or hemorrhage. Yolk sac tumors grow rapidly, are often large and necrotic at presentation, and are associated with elevated α–FP levels. Embryonal tumor is also unilateral and large, presenting in children and adolescents, with elevated α–FP and/or β-hCG. Choriocarcinoma is characteristically highly vascular and hemorrhagic, with elevated β-hCG levels.

Sex Cord–Stromal Tumors

The least frequently encountered group of primary ovarian tumors is the sex cord–stromal tumors (SCSTs), which arise from the intraovarian matrix supporting the germ cells. SCSTs include

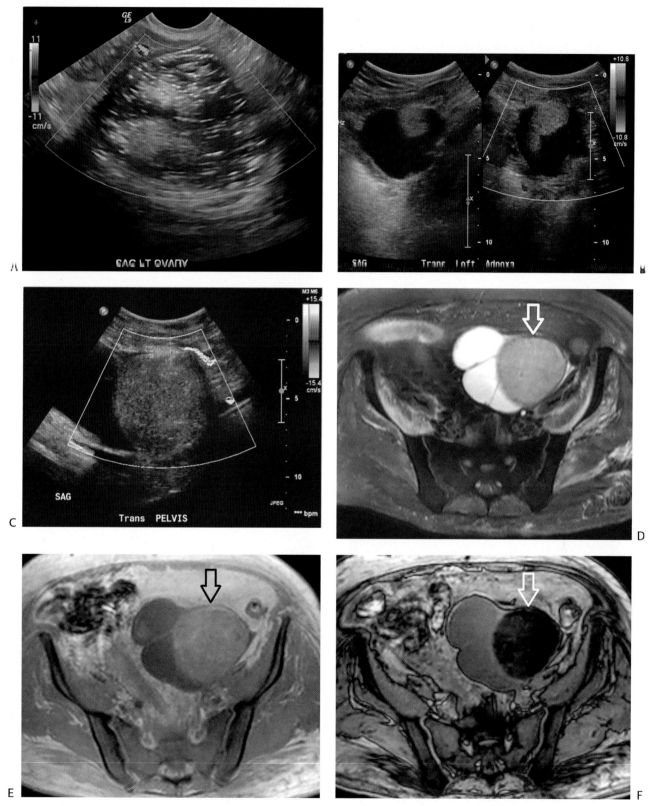

FIGURE 17.41. Dermoids may have a variety of sonographic appearances including **(A)** echogenic fat nodules within a mesh of hair, **(B)** echogenic mural nodules (usually without vascularity), or **(C)** a dominant solid mass requiring further characterization by MRI. In this case the mixed lipid content (*arrows*) causes **(D)** incomplete fat saturation on axial T2WI, **(E)** intermediate signal on in phase GRE, and **(F)** diffuse signal dropout on opposed phase GRE.

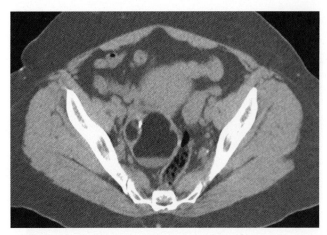

FIGURE 17.42. Small ovarian dermoid. Noncontrast CT shows a septated fat density mass containing a small focus of calcium. A dependent layer of denser fluid is seen in the larger chamber.

fibroma, thecoma, and fibrothecoma, granulosa cell tumor, and Sertoli–Leydig cell tumor. These tumors are diagnosed in women of all ages and are usually benign or of low malignant potential. However, their tendency to elaborate steroid hormones creates characteristic clinical presentations usually related to excess estrogen, but sometimes including virilization.

Fibroma is the most common SCST and is usually an incidental finding at imaging. Like fibroids and Brenner tumors, fibromas are hypoechoic with internal vascularity on TVUS and low signal on T2WI (Fig. 17.44). They are not hormonally active, but are often admixed with thecoma elements, which produce estrogen. Thus, the most common clinical presentation of thecomas and fibrothecomas is vaginal bleeding due to endometrial hyperplasia.

Granulosa cell tumor is the most common malignant SCST. It is usually low grade but has the tendency to recur after many years or even decades. Granulosa cell tumors produce estrogen, resulting in precocious puberty in girls, menometrorrhagia in reproductive age women, and postmenopausal bleeding in older women. They are characteristically large, contain multiple blood filled cysts

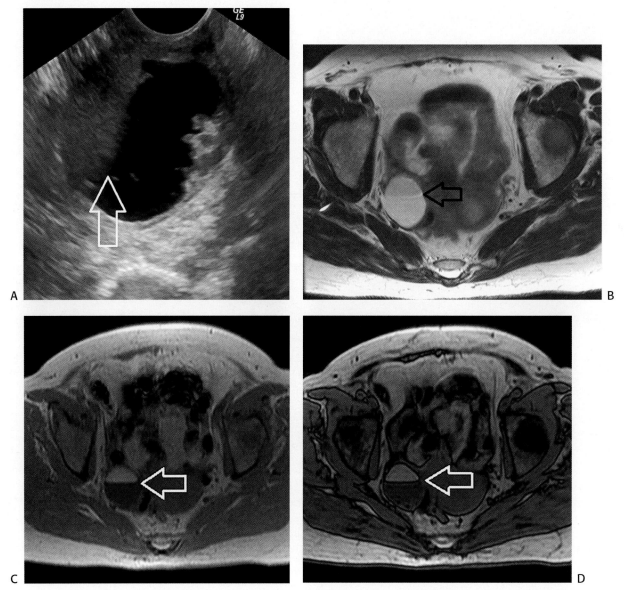

FIGURE 17.43. Dermoid with fat–fluid level (*arrows*) on **(A)** TVUS, where echogenic fat is nondependent in the supine patient, **(B)** T2WI, **(C)** in phase GRE, and **(D)** opposed-phase GRE, where a chemical shift artifact occurs in the mixed voxels at the interface between dependent fluid and floating fat.

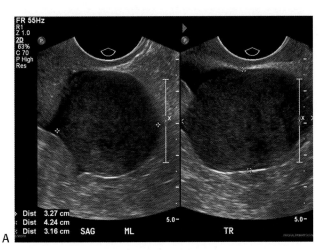
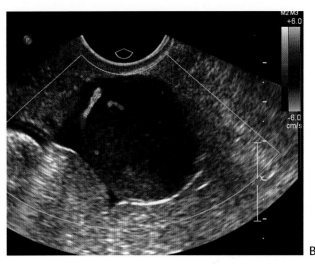

FIGURE 17.44. Ovarian fibrothecoma with **(A)** homogeneous, hypoechoic mass on TVUS and **(B)** internal vascularity distinguishing it from an endometrioma or other cyst with complex contents.

(Fig. 7.45), and are associated with endometrial stripe thickening, uterine enlargement, and/or adenomyosis.

Sertoli cells produce estrogen and Leydig cells produce androgens but the two cell types are often mixed. Sertoli–Leydig tumors are usually solid and enhancing, with somewhat higher tissue signal on T2WI than fibromas (Fig. 17.46). They have low malignant potential and favorable long-term outcomes.

CONCLUSION

Ovarian and adnexal abnormalities, including cysts, masses, and inflammation, are common and frequently incidental findings on a variety of imaging studies. Pelvic imaging is appropriately performed and interpreted with awareness of the patient's menstrual and pregnancy status. Radiologists should be familiar with the normal appearance of the ovaries and adnexa throughout the life cycle, understand contemporary recommendations for follow-up

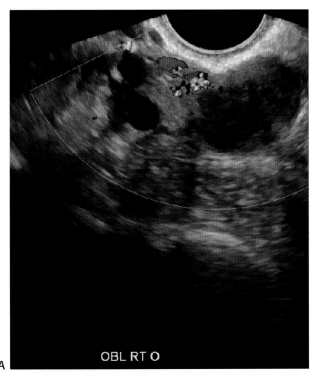
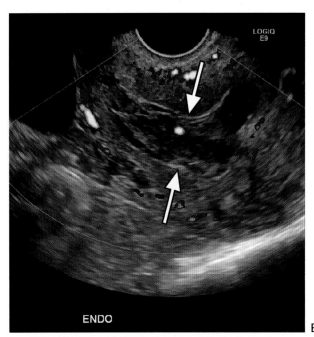

FIGURE 17.45. Granulosa tumor presenting with **(A)** small mixed echogenicity right ovarian mass on TVUS and **(B)** complex atypical endometrial hyperplasia (*arrows*) due to estrogen production by the tumor.

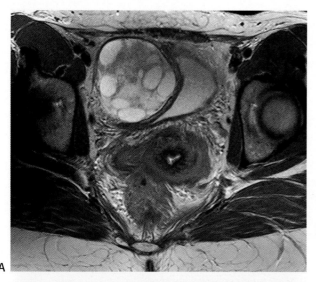

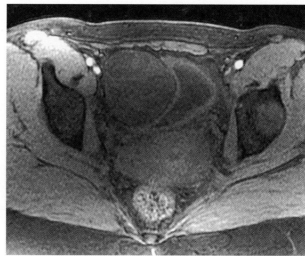

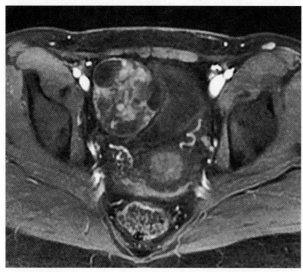

FIGURE 17.46. Sertoli–Leydig cell tumor in the right ovary with **(A)** central solid stroma and peripheral cysts on T2WI, **(B)** low signal on precontrast T1WI, and **(C)** enhancement of the solid elements on postcontrast T1WI.

of incidental lesions, and recognize specific imaging features that heighten suspicion for malignancy. High-quality imaging, interpreted within a context of understanding of ovarian physiology and disease, has tremendous capacity to influence and improve patient care.

SUGGESTED READINGS

Chang HC, Bhatt S, Dogra VS. Pearls and pitfalls in diagnosis of ovarian torsion. *Radiographics*. 2008;28(5):1355–1368.

Coutinho A Jr, Bittencourt LK, Pires CE, et al. MR imaging in deep pelvic endometriosis: a pictorial essay. *Radiographics*. 2011;31(2):549–567.

Czeyda-Pommersheim F, Kalb B, Costello J, et al. MRI in pelvic inflammatory disease: a pictorial review. *Abdom Radiol (NY)*. 2017;42(3):935–950.

Davarpanah AH, Kambadakone A, Holalkere ME, et al. Diffusion MRI of uterine and ovarian masses: identifying the benign lesions. *Abdom Radiol (NY)*. 2016;41(12):2466–2475.

Doubilet PM, Benson CB, Bourne T, et al. Diagnostic criteria for non-viable pregnancy early in the first trimester. *N Engl J Med*. 2013;369(15):1443–1451.

Forstner R, Thomassin-Naggara I, Cunha TM, et al. ESUR recommendations for imaging of the sonographically indeterminate adnexal mass: an update. *Eur Radiol*. 2017;27(6):2248–2257.

Histed SN, Desmukh M, Masamed R, et al. Ectopic pregnancy: a trainee's guide to making the right call: women's imaging. *Radiographics*. 2016;36(7):2236–2237.

Horta M, Cunha TM. Sex cord-stromal tumors of the ovary: a comprehensive review and update for radiologists. *Diagn Interv Radiol*. 2015;21(4):277–286.

Iyer VR, Lee SI. MRI, CT, and PET/CT for ovarian cancer detection and adnexal lesion characterization. *AJR Am J Roentgenol*. 2010;194(2):311–321.

Kaijser J, Bourne T, Valentin L, et al. Improving strategies for diagnosing ovarian cancer: a summary of the International Ovarian Tumor Analysis (IOTA) studies. *Ultrasound Obstet Gynecol*. 2013;41(1):9–20.

Langer JE, Oliver EO, Lev-Toaff AS, et al. Imaging of the female pelvis through the life cycle. *Radiographics*. 2012;32:1575–1597.

Levine D, Brown DL, Andreotti RF, et al. Management of asymptomatic ovarian and other adnexal cysts imaged at US: Society of Radiologists in Ultrasound Consensus Conference Statement. *Radiology*. 2010;256(3):943–954

Masch WR, Kamaya A, Wasnik AP, et al. Ovarian cancer mimics: how to avoid being fooled by extraovarian pelvic masses. *Abdom Radiol*. 2016;41(4):783–793.

Moyle P, Addley HC, Sala E. Radiological staging of ovarian carcinoma. *Semin Ultrasound CT MR*. 2010;31(5):388–398.

National Comprehensive Cancer Network (NCCN). *Guidelines: Ovarian Cancer, Including Fallopian Tube Cancer and Primary Peritoneal Cancer, Version 1.2016*. www.nccn.org.

Patel MD, Ascher SM, Paspulati RM, et al. Managing incidental findings on abdominal and pelvic CT and MRI, part 1: white paper of the ACR incidental findings committee II on adnexal findings. *J Am Coll Radiol*. 2013;10:675–681.

Prakash P, Cronin CG, Blake MA. Role of PET/CT in ovarian cancer. *AJR Am J Roentgenol.* 2010;194(6):W464–W470.

Revsin MV, Mathur M, Dave HB, et al. Pelvic inflammatory disease: multimodality imaging approach with clinical-pathologic correlation. *Radiographics.* 2016;36(5):1579–1596.

Rezvani M, Shaaban AM. Fallopian tube disease in the nonpregnant patient. *Radiographics.* 2011;31:527–548.

Shaaban AM, Rezvani M, Elsayes KM, et al. Ovarian malignant germ cell tumors: cellular classification and clinical and imaging features. *Radiographics.* 2014;34(3):777–801.

Stein EB, Wasnik AP, Sciallis AP, et al. MRI-Pathologic correlation in ovarian cancer. *MR Clin North Am.* 2017, in press.

Timmerman D, Testa AC, Bourne T, et al. Simple ultrasound-based rules for the diagnosis of ovarian cancer. *Ultrasound Obstet Gynecol.* 2008;31(6):681–690.

Thomassin-Naggara I, Aubert E, Rockall A, et al. Adnexal masses: development and preliminary validation of an MR imaging scoring system. *Radiology.* 2013;267(2):432–443.

Thomassin-Naggara I, Toussaint I, Perrot N, et al. Characterization of complex adnexal masses: value of adding perfusion- and diffusion-weighted MR imaging to conventional MR imaging. *Radiology.* 2011;258(3):793–803.

Young SW, Saphier NB, Dahiya N, et al. Sonographic evaluation of deep endometriosis: protocol for a US radiology practice. *Abdom Radiol (NY).* 2016;41(12):2364–2379.

Uterus and Cervix

UTERINE ZONAL ANATOMY
MYOMETRIUM
    Leiomyoma (Fibroid)
    Adenomyosis
    Sarcoma

ENDOMETRIUM
Hyperplasia
Polyps
Carcinoma

CERVIX
Carcinoma

This chapter provides an overview of imaging for common non-obstetric gynecologic conditions. Ultrasound is the most important initial imaging modality in female pelvic imaging, and many conditions can be definitively diagnosed sonographically. MRI provides the next level of detail, with exquisite soft tissue contrast and emerging methods for functional assessment, including diffusion-weighted images (DWI) and dynamic contrast-enhanced (DCE) imaging enabling accurate lesion characterization and tumor staging. Obstetrical imaging is beyond the scope of this text, and congenital uterine anomalies are discussed in Chapter 1.

UTERINE ZONAL ANATOMY

The uterine lining, or endometrial epithelium, is separated from the myometrium by an embryologically distinct layer of myometrium called the junctional zone. Zonal anatomy of the uterus can be appreciated on MRI (Fig. 18.1) and is most conspicuous in reproductive-age women. The junctional zone, which is müllerian in origin, is more hormonally responsive than the remainder of the myometrium and is responsible for physiologic uterine peristalsis during reproductive life. Real-time cine MR or US imaging can be used to observe peristalsis, which is cephalad during the first half of the menstrual cycle, facilitating sperm transport, and most active in the periovulatory period. By contrast, normal uterine peristalsis is caudad in the second half of the menstrual cycle. Disruption in the direction, amplitude, and/or frequency of normal peristaltic waves has been implicated as a cause of both pain symptoms and infertility in women with leiomyomas and adenomyosis (discussed below).

MYOMETRIUM

Leiomyoma (Fibroid)

Uterine leiomyomas are benign, monoclonal smooth muscle tumors of the myometrium. They are very common, as they are diagnosed in as many as 30% of women seen in clinical practice and 50% in autopsy series. They are most prevalent in African American women. Because they are responsive to estrogen, leiomyomas are rare in premenarchal girls, enlarge with pregnancy, and tend to involute after menopause.

Leiomyomas are masses of smooth muscle cells. Despite their colloquial name "fibroid," and their tough and rubbery quality at gross pathologic examination (Fig. 18.2), they are not composed of

fibroblasts. Leiomyomas are often multiple and vary in size from sub-centimeter nodules to huge masses filling the abdomen. Leiomyomas may be entirely contained within the uterine wall (mural), distort or protrude into the uterine cavity (submucosal), extend beyond the peritoneal surface of the uterus (subserosal) in an exophytic or pedunculated fashion, or a combination. Pedunculated leiomyomas may become adherent to adjacent structures such as the broad ligament and develop collateral circulation, while the primary supply from the uterus involutes. These are known as parasitic leiomyomas.

Leiomyomas may exhibit several types of internal degeneration, including necrosis, hemorrhage, hyalinization, and rarely infection. These phenomena tend to alter the imaging appearance of the masses on all modalities, detailed below, and in some cases can cause

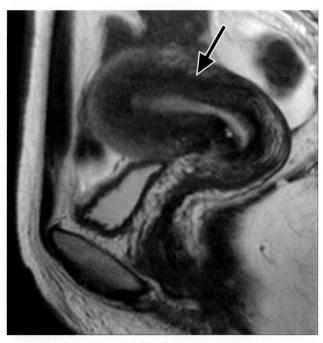

FIGURE 18.1. Normal zonal anatomy of the uterus on sagittal T2WI. Note high-signal endometrium, lower-signal junctional zone (*arrow*), and intermediate-signal outer myometrium.

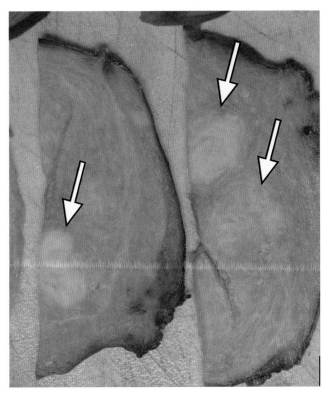

FIGURE 18.2. Gross pathologic image of uterine leiomyomas (*arrows*), which are pale and bulge outward from the cut surface of the adjacent normal myometrium.

acute symptoms. Leiomyomas are benign and do not metastasize, but the clinical entities of parasitic leiomyoma and peritoneal leiomyomatosis reflect varying degrees of superficial implantation of leiomyomas on extrauterine surfaces. There are reports of dedifferentiation of cellular leiomyomas into leiomyosarcomas, but the most recent literature suggests that this is extremely rare.

Leiomyomas are often asymptomatic and detected only incidentally. However, they may produce a variety of symptoms depending on their size and location, including abnormal bleeding, pelvic pain, dyspareunia, infertility, urinary frequency, and abdominal enlargement. Most uterine leiomyomas require no treatment, but symptoms may have a significant impact on quality of life for some women. Treatment options include pharmacologic agents including oral contraceptives and gonadotropin-releasing hormone analogs, levonorgestrel intrauterine devices, myomectomy, hysterectomy, and ablative techniques including uterine artery embolization and high intensity focused ultrasound. Treatment selection incorporates the dominant symptoms (bleeding versus bulk versus pain), leiomyoma size and location, and patient goals with respect to fertility. Localization is important in therapeutic planning and is most accurately assessed with MRI.

Imaging

Ultrasound is the primary imaging modality for the diagnosis and surveillance of uterine leiomyomas, with additional information regarding precise location, internal degeneration, vascular supply, and presence of concomitant adenomyosis provided by MRI when desired for treatment planning purposes. Leiomyomas are occasionally seen incidentally on plain radiographs as "popcorn" calcifications in the pelvis and are evident on fluoroscopic hysterosalpingograms (HSG) when they are submucosal and distort the endometrial cavity. Leiomyomas are evident as uterine masses with varying degrees of internal enhancement and calcification on CT (Fig. 18.3), but this is usually an incidental observation rather than an exam ordered for the specific evaluation of leiomyomas.

Leiomyomas are usually hypoechoic compared to adjacent myometrium on ultrasound imaging. Because of their complex internal architecture of crossing bands of smooth muscle fibers, leiomyomas attenuate the ultrasound beam and are often associated with posterior acoustic shadowing (Fig. 18.4). Linear shadows at the margins between leiomyomas and adjacent myometrium are also commonly seen. Leiomyomas may exhibit central or peripheral calcifications (Fig. 18.5), with internal heterogeneity that tends to be more hypoechoic in the setting of cystic degeneration and

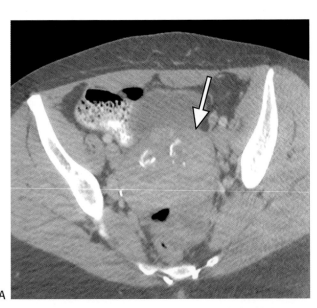

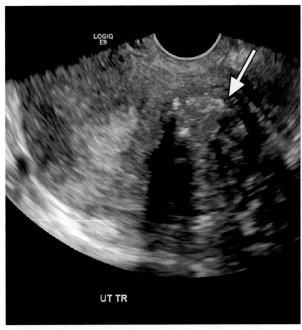

FIGURE 18.3. Calcified leiomyoma (*arrows*) on **(A)** CT and **(B)** TVUS.

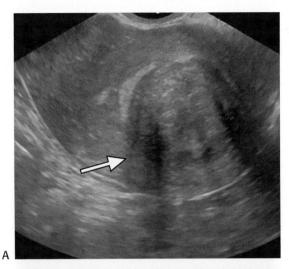

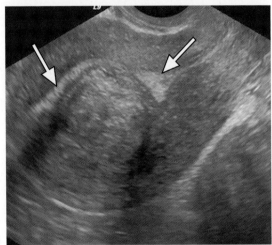

FIGURE 18.4. Large submucosal leiomyoma on TVUS shows typical features of **(A)** posterior acoustic shadowing (*arrow*) and **(B)** distortion of the normal echogenic endometrial stripe (*arrows*).

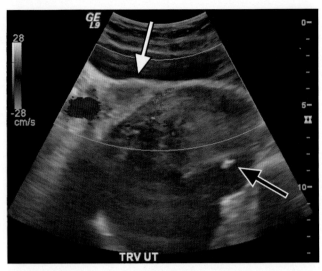

FIGURE 18.5. Large exophytic leiomyoma with coarse calcification (*black arrow*) dwarfs the uterus (*white arrow*) on transabdominal US.

hyperechoic in the context of internal hemorrhage or fat (lipoleiomyoma) (Fig. 18.6). Pedunculated submucosal leiomyomas may prolapse into the uterine cavity or vagina and are usually more hypoechoic than endometrial polyps owing to their muscular rather than epithelial content. Exophytic or pedunculated subserosal leiomyomas can often be distinguished from adnexal or other intraperitoneal masses by the presence of vessels crossing from the uterus into the mass (Fig. 18.7). Acoustic shadowing may obscure the posterior margins of the uterus itself as well as the adnexa, particularly on transvaginal imaging, and a combination of transvaginal and transabdominal images is generally needed for diagnostic assessment. Color and power Doppler vascularity is demonstrable within most leiomyomas, but they are rarely hypervascular on ultrasound.

Leiomyomas are usually well-circumscribed, low-signal masses on T2WI (Fig. 18.8). However, highly cellular leiomyomas or those containing myxoid degeneration may have intermediate to high signal on T2WI. The superior tissue differentiation

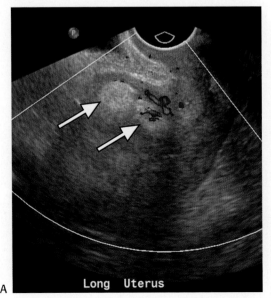

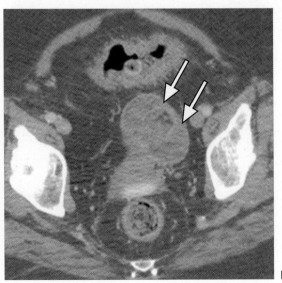

FIGURE 18.6. Lipoleiomyomas manifest as **(A)** echogenic masses (*arrows*) within an enlarged uterus on TVUS and **(B)** areas of very low (<0 HU) attenuation (*arrows*) in the uterus on CT.

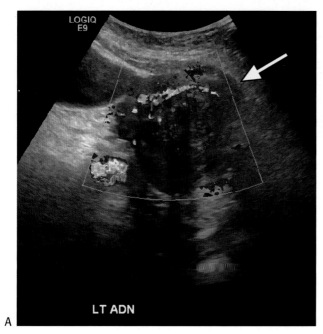
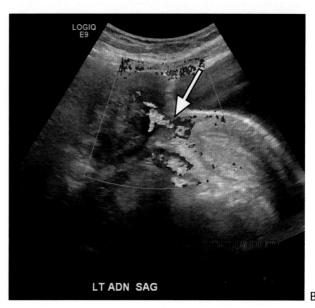

FIGURE 18.7. **A:** Pedunculated leiomyoma (*arrow*) mimics left ovarian mass on transabdominal US, transverse orientation. **B:** The mass, now at the left side of the sagittal image, is connected to the uterus at the right side of the image by a vascular stalk (*arrow*).

of MRI allows precise localization of subserosal, intramural, and submucosal masses (Fig. 18.9). Vessels bridging myometrium and mass are often evident on MRI, improving anatomic localization and diagnostic accuracy for sonographically indeterminate masses. Progressive enhancement is observed in dynamic postcontrast T1WI (Fig. 18.10), while signal characteristics on DWI are rather variable, depending on the degree of cellularity or degeneration within the mass. During preoperative

assessment for uterine artery embolization, specific diagnostic considerations include: any pedunculated lesions that could necrose and drop off into the peritoneal cavity or be delivered vaginally; collateral vascularity from ovarian artery, requiring additional embolization; and the presence of enhancement—an important predictor of response to endovascular treatment—within individual leiomyomas.

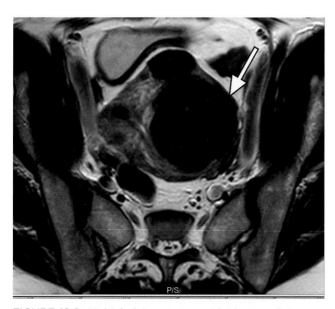

FIGURE 18.8. Multiple leiomyomas, with characteristic very low signal intensity on axial T2WI. The largest (*arrow*) is intramural in location but extends to both the mucosal and serosal surfaces.

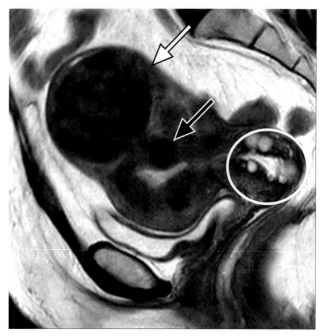

FIGURE 18.9. Large subserosal leiomyoma (*white arrow*) and smaller submucosal leiomyoma (*black arrow*) on sagittal T2WI. Note also benign Nabothian cysts (*circle*) in the cervix.

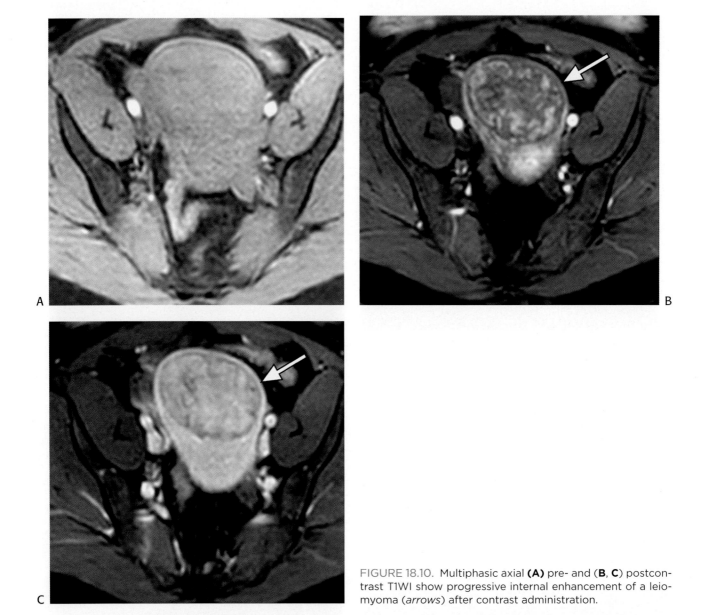

FIGURE 18.10. Multiphasic axial **(A)** pre- and **(B, C)** postcontrast T1WI show progressive internal enhancement of a leiomyoma (*arrows*) after contrast administration.

Treated, degenerated (Figs. 18.11 and 18.12), or devascularized masses have less predictable internal signal intensity and enhancement. Gas bubbles within a recently treated mass are a normal postprocedural finding and do not necessarily indicate infection. Uterine necrosis due to ischemia is a rare complication of embolization (Fig. 18.13). Transient hypoperfusion of the myometrium surrounding devascularized leiomyomas is an expected postprocedural finding for days to weeks, but normal uterine enhancement should be restored on follow-up imaging over the course of weeks to months, while the completely embolized and nonenhancing leiomyomas will gradually decrease in size.

Adenomyosis

Adenomyosis is the abnormal proliferation of endometrial glands within the myometrium. It is believed to result from invagination of normal endometrial tissue into the myometrium or possibly from endometrial differentiation of müllerian rest tissue. Adenomyosis may be focal or diffuse. Each nidus of ectopic endometrial tissue

causes local smooth muscle proliferation (Fig. 18.14), eventually leading to uterine enlargement. Adenomyosis is associated with multiparity and uterine interventions, suggesting that disruption of the uterine lining has a role in its pathophysiology. Adenomyosis is also strongly associated with other estrogen-sensitive conditions including uterine leiomyomas and endometriosis. Adenomyosis is diagnosed histologically in more than half of women who undergo hysterectomy for pelvic pain or bleeding, but is diagnosed preoperatively in <25% of cases. This disease is underdiagnosed both clinically and by imaging at present.

Adenomyosis is associated with symptoms of dysmenorrhea, menorrhagia, and subfertility. Ectopic glands involve the uterine junctional zone and disrupt normal uterine peristalsis, which may be an underlying driver of all three symptom types. Pharmacologic treatments of adenomyosis include oral aromatase inhibitors or gonadotropin-releasing hormone agonists and the levonorgestrel-releasing intrauterine device. Although there is increasing evidence supporting the efficacy of uterine artery embolization and high-frequency ultrasound ablation for

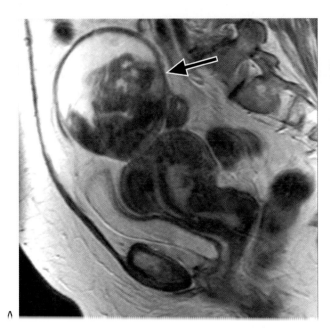

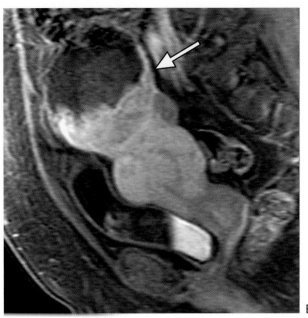

FIGURE 18.11. **A:** Sagittal T2WI shows mixed signal intensity of a subserosal leiomyoma (*arrow*) with cystic degeneration. **B:** Postcontrast sagittal T1WI demonstrates enhancement only at the inferior aspect of the mass (*arrow*), the solid area that was low signal on T2WI.

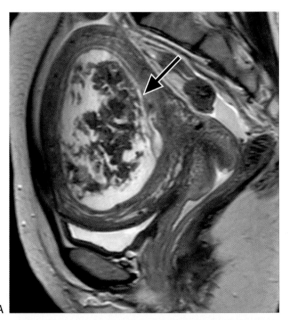

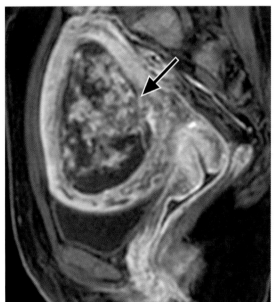

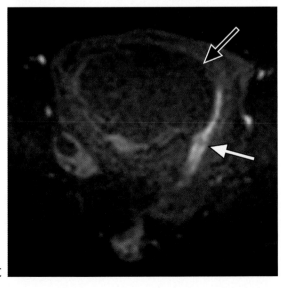

FIGURE 18.12. Necrosis and cystic degeneration of submucosal leiomyoma with **(A)** mixed low and very high signal intensity (*arrow*) on sagittal T2WI and **(B)** heterogenous enhancement (*arrow*) on postcontrast T1WI. **C:** DWI shows very low signal within the mass (*black arrow*), which distorts the normally high-signal endometrial stripe (*white arrow*).

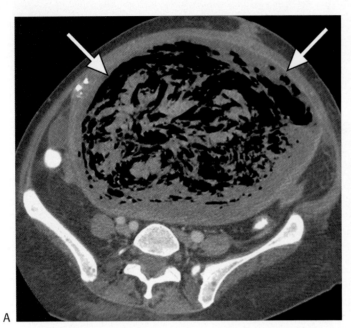
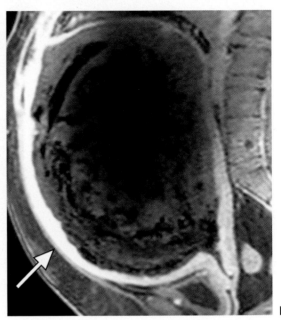

A

B

FIGURE 18.13. Uterine necrosis after emergent embolization for hemorrhage. **A:** Axial CT image shows extensive gas (*arrows*) within the uterine corpus, beyond the normally expected low volume gas after embolization. **B:** There is little or no enhancement within the fundus on sagittal postcontrast T1WI, with some preserved myometrial enhancement (*arrow*) in the lower uterine segment and cervix. A frankly necrotic uterus was found at surgery.

adenomyosis, hysterectomy remains the definitive therapy for women with severe symptoms.

Imaging

Adenomyosis has characteristic imaging features in transvaginal ultrasound (TVUS) imaging, fluoroscopic HSG, and MRI. The positive predictive value for the diagnosis of adenomyosis with TVUS

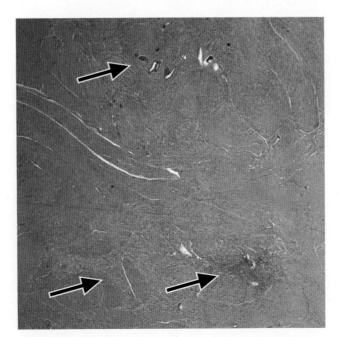

FIGURE 18.14. Microscopic image of adenomyosis showing clumps of glandular tissue (*arrows*) surrounded by bands of uterine smooth muscle.

interpreted by expert readers is approximately 68%, compared to about 76% with MRI. However, about 50% of women with adenomyosis have concomitant leiomyomas, decreasing the sensitivity of TVUS to only 33%. MRI is better able to distinguish between and localize the two conditions, and remains the preferred diagnostic modality for adenomyosis. HSG can sometimes demonstrate filling of the "flasklike" subendometrial outpouchings, but it is an invasive test whose true sensitivity for diagnosis of adenomyosis is unknown.

Sonographic features of adenomyosis include an asymmetrically thickened and globular uterus (Fig. 18.15), heterogeneity of the myometrium, loss of definition or thickening of the uterine junctional zone, subendometrial cysts (Fig. 18.16), and linear myometrial striations. On hysterosonography, patent channels connecting the endometrium to the myometrium may become distended during saline infusion, appearing as myometrial "cracks" (Fig. 18.17). Tiny bubbles of infused air may also travel into the myometrium, resulting in hyperechoic myometrial foci. However, the sensitivity of these unique features is reported as <30%, and hysterosonography is not widely employed for the diagnosis of adenomyosis.

Sagittal T2WI is the single most useful MR sequence for assessment of adenomyosis. T2WI reveals focal or diffuse thickening (>12 mm) (Fig. 18.18) of the uterine junctional zone (JZ) due to smooth muscle proliferation around microscopic deposits of endometrial tissue. Other metrics expressing JZ proliferation have been proposed and can be used in equivocal cases, including a JZ-to-myometrial thickness ratio of >40% and JZ difference (maximum–minimum JZ thickness) > 5 mm. It is important to recognize that transient uterine contractions can mimic JZ thickening, and findings should be confirmed on T2WI in another plane (Fig. 18.19). Focal adenomyomas are also difficult to distinguish from leiomyomas but are generally less hypointense on T2WI and have small cystic inclusions (Fig. 18.20). Subendometrial cysts, hyperintense on T2WI and usually nested within the thickened JZ, are the single most specific (>98%) MRI sign of adenomyosis

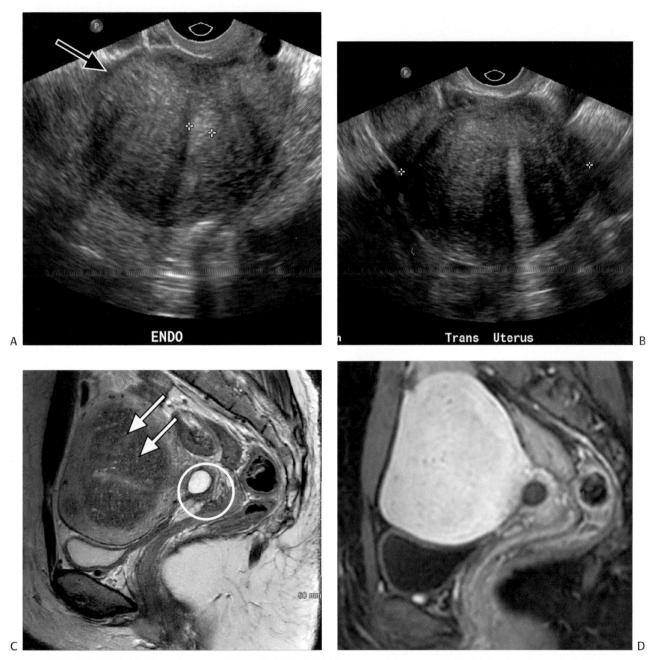

FIGURE 18.15. Uterine adenomyosis on TVUS with **(A)** asymmetric myometrial thickening (*arrow*) distorting the normal endometrium (*calipers*) on sagittal image and **(B)** striated pattern of shadowing resembling leiomyoma on transverse image. **C:** Sagittal T2WI shows marked thickening of the uterine junctional zone with multiple tiny cysts (*arrows*) in areas of endometrial inclusion. Note benign Nabothian cysts in the cervix (*circle*). **D:** Areas of adenomyosis are isointense to normal myometrium on postcontrast T1WI.

(Fig. 18.21) but are seen in fewer than 50% of cases. Occasional hemorrhage within these cysts manifests as areas of high signal on precontrast T1WI. The entire affected area usually enhances on postcontrast T1WI, and this sequence does not add major diagnostic information.

Sarcoma

Mesenchymal tumors of the uterus account for <10% of uterine malignancies. More than half of uterine sarcomas are leiomyo-

sarcomas, with less common subtypes including endometrial stromal sarcomas, carcinosarcomas, and adenosarcomas. Most leiomyosarcomas are believed to arise *de novo*, rather than from a benign leiomyoma precursor. Uterine sarcomas occur in pre-, peri-, and postmenopausal women, although carcinosarcomas in particular are more common in postmenopausal women. The most common presenting symptom is vaginal bleeding. Other presentations include abdominal pain, enlargement of the uterus, and systemic symptoms such as weight loss. Occasionally, sarcoma is detected incidentally during pathologic examination of

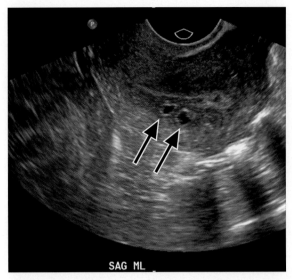

FIGURE 18.16. Adenomyosis with subendometrial inclusion cysts (*arrows*) on TVUS.

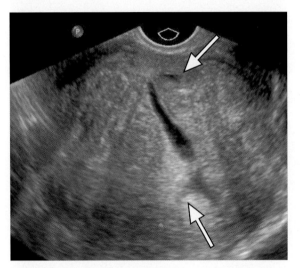

FIGURE 18.17. Adenomyosis with myometrial "cracks" (*arrows*) during saline-infused hysterosonography.

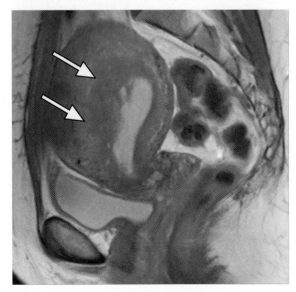

FIGURE 18.18. Adenomyosis with marked thickening of the anterior JZ (*arrows*) on sagittal T2WI. Note normal JZ posteriorly.

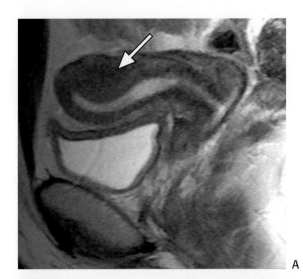

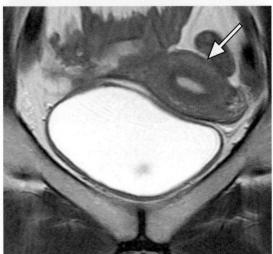

FIGURE 18.19. Focal uterine contraction **(A)** mimics leiomyoma or adenomyosis on sagittal T2WI (*arrow*) but **(B)** has completely resolved (*arrow*) by the time coronal T2WI was acquired.

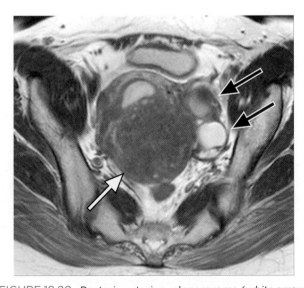

FIGURE 18.20. Posterior uterine adenomyoma (*white arrow*) with intermediate hypointensity and multiple small high-signal inclusions on axial T2WI. Note endometriomas (*black arrows*) with "T2 shading" in left adnexa—many women with adenomyosis also have endometriosis.

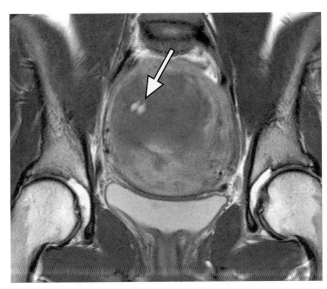

FIGURE 18.21. Adenomyosis in the posterior myometrium with conspicuous subendometrial cysts (*arrow*) on coronal T2WI.

hysterectomy specimens after surgery performed for presumed leiomyomas. The risk of intraperitoneal dissemination that is posed by inadvertent morcellation of a sarcoma has sparked considerable controversy about surgical technique in the gynecologic literature in recent years.

Imaging

Imaging studies do not reliably differentiate uterine sarcomas from other tumors, particularly leiomyomas. Unusual and bizarre leiomyomas remain much more common than leiomyomas, and benign leiomyomas can grow rather rapidly during the reproductive years. However, ongoing or rapid growth of a presumed leiomyoma in a postmenopausal woman remains a concerning clinical sign. Broadly speaking, sarcomas may exhibit internal necrosis (Fig. 18.22), disordered vascularity, indistinct margins (Fig. 18.23), and invasion or obstruction of adjacent structures on all imaging studies. Findings of high signal on T2WI and DWI, very low signal on apparent diffusion coefficient (ADC) maps, and marked hypervascularity have all been described in uterine sarcomas, but all of these features are occasionally seen in highly cellular or degenerated leiomyomas. The presence of nodal metastases is specific for malignancy but is relatively insensitive as it indicates International Federation of Gynecology and Obstetrics (FIGO) stage IIIc disease.

ENDOMETRIUM

The endometrium undergoes substantial change throughout each menstrual cycle and over the course of a woman's life—both histologically and by imaging. During reproductive life, the endometrial stripe undergoes substantial cyclic change every month. It is very thin at the beginning of each cycle and is thickest just before menstruation. It starts in the menstrual phase as a thin echogenic line at the interface of endometrial surfaces and reaches a maximum of 10 to 14 mm during the secretory phase, or second half of the cycle, when it may have a trilaminar appearance (Fig. 18.24). After menopause, the maximum normal stripe thickness is 8 mm, but a stripe > 5 mm is usually considered sufficient basis for endometrial biopsy if there is postmenopausal bleeding.

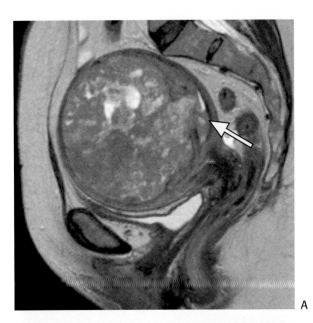

A

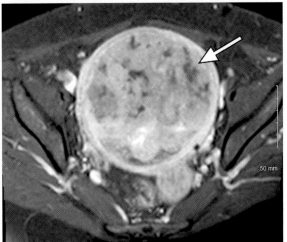

B

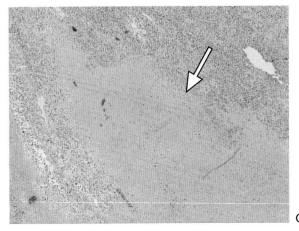

C

FIGURE 18.22. Leiomyosarcoma with **(A)** heterogenous internal signal on T2WI and extrusion of myometrial tumor into the endometrial canal (*arrow*). **B:** Postcontrast T1WI illustrates marked heterogeneity of enhancement (*arrow*), poorly distinguished from a degenerating leiomyoma by imaging. **C:** Microscopic image with abrupt transition (*arrow*) between viable **(top)** and necrotic **(bottom)** tissue, which is a distinctive histologic feature of leiomyosarcoma absent in infarcted leiomyomas.

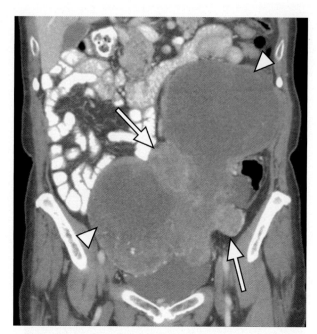

FIGURE 18.23. Leiomyosarcoma with cystic (*arrowheads*) and solid (*arrows*) components on coronal CT image.

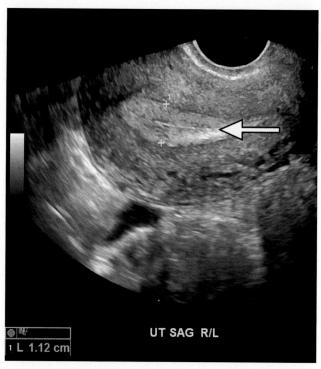

FIGURE 18.24. Normal secretory phase trilaminar endometrial stripe (*calipers*) with echogenic interface (*arrow*) between opposing endometrial surfaces on TVUS.

Hyperplasia

Driven by hyperestrogenism, endometrial hyperplasia may occur in premenopausal or postmenopausal women. The underlying estrogen excess may be a result of anovulatory states, estrogen-producing tumors, exogenous administration of estrogen or tamoxifen, or, perhaps most commonly, the peripheral conversion of androstenedione to estrone in adipose tissue of obese women. Pathologically, the hyperplastic endometrium may exist as a smoothly thickened layer, a micronodular surface, or macroscopic polyps. Endometrial hyperplasia may produce menometrorrhagia or postmenopausal bleeding. Most cases of endometrial hyperplasia do not progress to endometrial carcinoma, but those that reveal severe cytologic atypia may do so.

Imaging

TVUS provides accurate measurement of the endometrial stripe in most patients. Measurements should include the sum of both sides of the endometrial lining, even when separated by endogenous or infused fluid within the canal. In premenopausal women, a full-thickness stripe > 14 mm may indicate endometrial hyperplasia or other pathology; in asymptomatic postmenopausal women, the stripe should be considered abnormal if it is >8 mm in thickness. The stripe may range from homogenous and hyperechoic (Fig. 18.25)

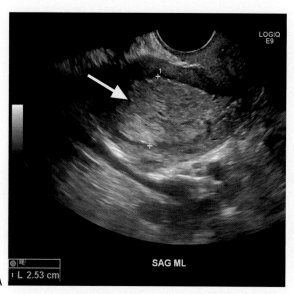

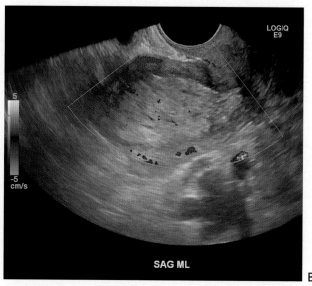

FIGURE 18.25. Benign endometrial hyperplasia in a 60-year-old woman, with **(A)** markedly thickened endometrial stripe (calipers, *arrow*) on gray scale and **(B)** scattered internal vascularity without a dominant vascular stalk on color Doppler TVUS images.

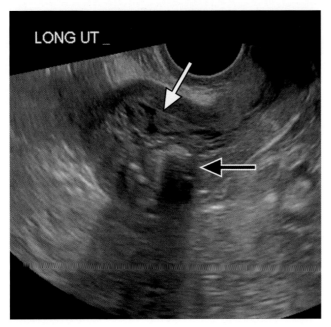

FIGURE 18.26. Benign endometrial hyperplasia in a 56-year-old woman, with cystic appearance (*white arrow*) of the thickened endometrial stripe and a posterior submucosal leiomyoma (*black arrow*) slightly indenting the canal.

to complex and cystic (Fig. 18.26) in appearance. In a woman with postmenopausal bleeding, a more stringent standard of 5 mm is used as a cutoff for recommendation of further evaluation by blind, in-office endometrial pipelle biopsy. Hysterosalpingography

and saline infusion hysterosonography (Fig. 18.27) may reveal a hyperplastic endometrium to be irregular, nodular, or polypoid.

CT is not normally used to evaluate the endometrial stripe. It should be noted however that low-density material in the endometrial canal of a premenopausal women is usually the endometrial epithelium itself, rather than fluid within the canal. Thus, a conspicuous endometrial stripe on CT can be a completely normal finding in women of reproductive age. MRI can readily distinguish zonal anatomy of the uterus and enables detailed evaluation of the endometrial stripe in patients with anatomic or other limitations to high-quality ultrasound imaging. The normal endometrial lining (Fig. 18.1) has very high signal on T2WI due to fluid content within glandular epithelium, high signal on DWI due to its dense cellularity, and exhibits diffuse enhancement after contrast administration. The hyperplastic endometrium appears similar but is thicker. The normal junctional anatomy is preserved and there is no myometrial invasion.

Polyps

Polypoid masses within the endometrial canal may be pedunculated submucosal leiomyomas, benign epithelial polyps, endometrial polyps with cellular atypia, or pedunculated cancers. These filling defects cannot be distinguished from one another on fluoroscopic HSGs. Leiomyomas tend to follow the appearance of myometrium on all other modalities, meaning that they are relatively hypoechoic on US and have a low signal on T2WI compared to the endometrium. Endometrial polyps are hyperechoic and have a higher signal on T2WI, reflecting their epithelial origin. In the absence of frankly invasive behavior, imaging is insensitive for distinguishing benign and malignant epithelial polyps. As discussed below in the section on endometrial cancer, malignancies tend to have slightly lower signal intensity than normal endometrium on T2WI and are less enhancing in the delayed

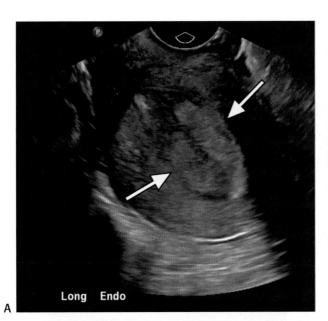
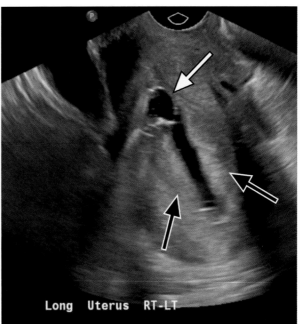

FIGURE 18.27. Benign endometrial hyperplasia in a morbidly obese 28-year-old woman with **(A)** marked thickening of the stripe (*arrows*) on TVUS. **B:** Smooth, symmetric thickening of both sides of the endometrium (*black arrows*) revealed by saline-infused hysterosonogram, which distends the canal (*white arrow*) and enables exclusion of a focal polyp that would have required hysteroscopic biopsy.

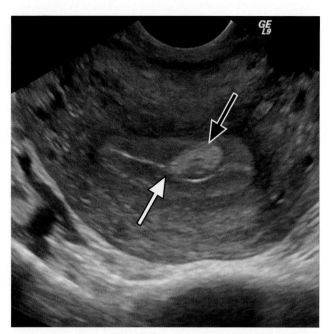

FIGURE 18.28. Endometrial polyp on TVUS with a distinct hyperechoic nodule (*black arrow*) within the endometrial lining, focally interrupting the normal hyperechoic interface (*white arrow*) between the two sides.

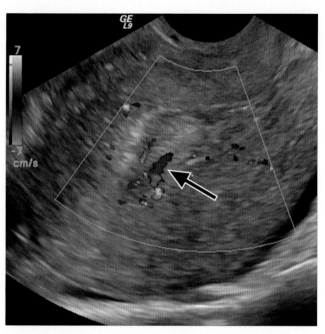

FIGURE 18.29. Endometrial polyp on TVUS with color Doppler, with vascular stalk (*arrow*).

hysterosonography (Fig. 18.30) may be helpful to separate and distinguish polyps.

Carcinoma

Endometrial carcinoma is the most common primary gynecologic malignancy. Emerging evidence supports the concept of two distinct clinical groups (Table 18.1): type I, low-grade, predominantly endometrioid adenocarcinomas, arising in a stepwise and estrogen-dependent fashion from hyperplastic precursors, and type II, high-grade endometrioid, serous, and clear cell adenocarcinomas and carcinosarcomas presenting at more advanced initial stages, without estrogen dependency. Type I cancers are much more common

phase. However, such features are less conspicuous in low-grade and small cancers.

At TVUS, endometrial polyps are hyperechoic and characteristically interrupt the endometrial line (Fig. 18.28) or interface between the two surfaces, because they are intracavitary. A conspicuous vascular stalk (feeding or draining vessel) (Fig. 18.29) is frequently identified. When these features are seen in a woman with abnormal bleeding, additional imaging workup is unlikely to provide additional information, and hysteroscopic biopsy is a reasonable next step. However, if there is endometrial thickening and a discrete polyp is not identified, saline-infused

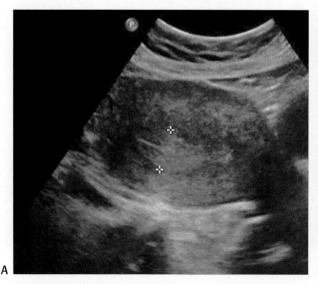

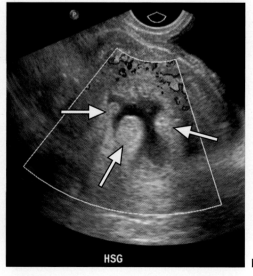

FIGURE 18.30. Endometrial polyps with **(A)** thickened endometrial stripe but no discrete lesion on transabdominal ultrasound, but **(B)** at least three distinct polyps (*arrows*) on saline-infused hysterosonogram.

TABLE 18.1

Characteristics of Type I and Type II Endometrial Carcinoma

	Type I	Type II
Proportion of cases	85%	15%
Primary risk factor	Unopposed estrogen	Older age
Primary histologic subtypes	Endometrioid	Other (serous, clear cell, etc.)
Tumor grade	Low	High
Stage at presentation	I–II	III–IV
5-year survival	>80%	<50%

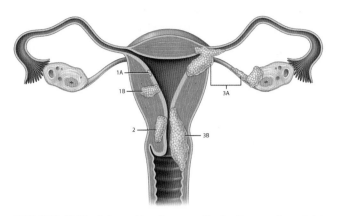

FIGURE 18.31. Schematic diagram illustrating endometrial cancer staging.

(about 85% of all endometrial cancer), present at early initial disease stage, and are associated with >80% five year survival. Type II cancers are less common and have an aggressive growth pattern, with <50% five-year disease-related survival. Type I cancers largely arise in pre- and perimenopausal women and are associated with the same factors as hyperplasia, including hyperestrogenic states arising from obesity, prolonged menses (early menarche, late menopause, and/or nulliparity), hormone-secreting tumors, and exogenous hormone administration. Endometrioid adenocarcinoma is also associated with Lynch syndrome. Type II cancers usually arise in postmenopausal women but do not have other known risk factors. Like high-grade ovarian cancers with similar natural histories, type II endometrial cancers frequently exhibit p53 mutations.

Women with endometrial carcinoma most commonly present with abnormal uterine bleeding. The diagnosis of endometrial cancer is pathologic; endometrial tissue is obtained by pipelle biopsy or by dilation and curettage. Histologic grading (FIGO grades 1 to 3, with increasing aggressiveness) and subtyping of tumors impact surgical planning and prognosis. As with other gynecologic cancers, staging is performed according to the surgically based FIGO system (Table 18.2, Fig. 18.31). Because most endometrial cancers are type I (slow growing) and commonly cause abnormal uterine bleeding, most endometrial cancer presents at stage I (limited to the uterine

TABLE 18.2

FIGO Staging of Endometrial Carcinoma

Stage I	Tumor confined to uterus
	A. No or less than half myometrial invasion
	B. >50% myometrial invasion
Stage II	Invasion of cervical stroma
Stage III	Locoregional disease
	A. Tumor invades uterine serosa or adnexae
	B. Vaginal and/or parametrial involvement
	C. Metastases to pelvic and/or paraortic lymph nodes
Stage IV	Local organ invasion and/or distant metastases
	A. Bladder and/or bowel mucosal invasion
	B. Distant metastasis, including intra-abdominal metastasis and/or inguinal nodes

corpus) and II (involving the cervical stroma). Cancers with extra-serosal extension, and/or pelvic or para aortic nodal involvement are stage III, while distant metastases to nonregional lymph nodes, liver, lung, or brain are classified as stage IV.

Hysterectomy and bilateral salpingo-oophorectomy are the standard surgical treatments for endometrial cancer. Lymph node staging is a topic of ongoing debate, with varied practice patterns ranging from routine pelvic lymph node dissection to a sentinel node approach or limitation of node dissection to women with high-risk disease (FIGO grade 2 or 3 endometrioid or more aggressive types such as clear cell and serous) according to preoperative histology. Para-aortic node dissection is also usually performed in women with aggressive histologies or known lymph node enlargement. This is an important question because lymphadenectomy is associated with increased operative time and associated costs, perioperative complications, and lymphedema, yet the vast majority of women with endometrial cancer do not have lymph node involvement.

About a third of women with endometrial cancer are considered to be completely cured after surgery and are simply followed clinically. The remaining women receive adjuvant therapy with one of several possible combinations of vaginal cylinder brachytherapy (to reduce vaginal cuff recurrence), external beam radiation to the whole pelvis (to minimize nodal recurrence), and/or chemotherapy (to reduce the risk of distant metastasis). Adjuvant therapy decisions are based upon final tumor histology, depth of myometrial invasion, presence of lymphovascular space invasion, nodal involvement, and patient age.

Imaging

Ultrasound is the initial imaging modality of choice in the setting of abnormal uterine bleeding. As discussed above in the context of hyperplasia, a thickened endometrial stripe may reflect carcinoma, hyperplasia, or a polyp. 5 mm is the usual threshold for postmenopausal women, with thicker stripes prompting biopsy. Early carcinoma cannot be distinguished from hyperplasia by imaging (Fig. 18.32). Features that may increase suspicion for carcinoma include deep myometrial invasion (Fig. 18.33), with interruption of the thin hypoechoic line along the inner myometrium, and hematometra (Fig. 18.34), though this can also be seen in benign cervical stenosis. Ultrasound is insufficiently sensitive for primary tumor staging in endometrial cancer, though myometrial invasion is often evident when extensive.

Endometrial cancer may be incidentally detected at CT, or CT may be ordered for preoperative systemic staging. CT is not sensitive for local tumor staging in endometrial cancer. A thickened endometrial stripe may be evident even in stage I or II disease

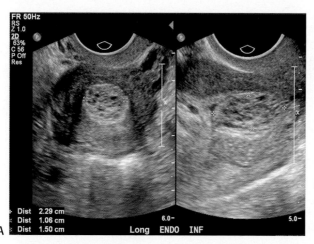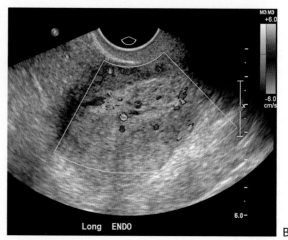

FIGURE 18.32. Endometrioid adenocarcinoma, nonmyoinvasive (stage IA), with **(A)** cystic-appearing endometrial thickening and **(B)** scattered vascularity on TVUS.

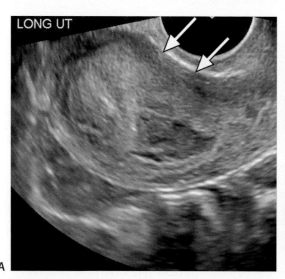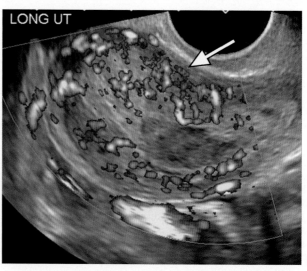

FIGURE 18.33. Endometrioid adenocarcinoma with deep myoinvasion (stage IB) showing **(A)** loss of delineation of tumor and myometrial thinning (*arrows*) and **(B)** deep extension of tumor vascularity (*arrow*) into myometrium on TVUS. The avascular material in the canal is likely clot.

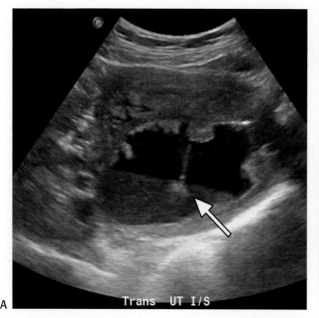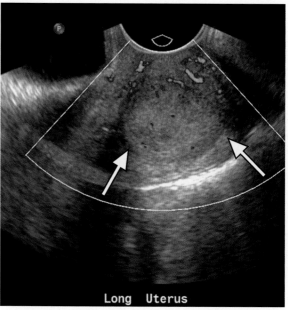

FIGURE 18.34. Stage II endometrioid adenocarcinoma with **(A)** hematometra and dangling strands of clot (*arrow*) on transabdominal image and **(B)** vascularized tumor (*arrows*) involving the cervix.

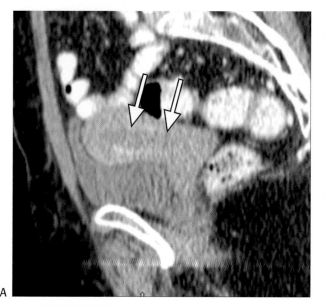 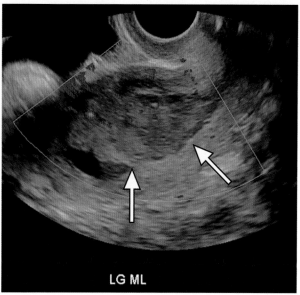

FIGURE 18.35. Stage IA endometrioid adenocarcinoma with **(A)** endometrial stripe thickening (*arrows*) on CT sagittal reformat, much more obvious on **(B)** TVUS, with a thickened vascularized stripe but preserved myometrial margin (*arrows*).

(Fig. 18.35), while extrauterine and nodal involvement in stage III and IV disease is more conspicuous (Fig. 18.36). Nodal involvement usually follows a stepwise pathway in endometrial cancer, with mid- and lower uterine masses draining to parametrial, paracervical, and obturator lymph nodes, while upper uterine and fundal tumors drain to common iliac and para-aortic nodes. Although sensitivity is imperfect, nodes that are >1 cm in short axis, globular, clustered, or asymmetric are suspicious and should be reported. Inguinal lymph nodes are not regional nodes in endometrial cancer, and their involvement indicates stage IV disease. Finally, in the surveillance setting, it is important for radiologists to be aware that the vaginal cuff is the most common site of recurrence for early-stage disease (Fig. 18.37), and it should be specifically included in the search pattern.

MRI has excellent diagnostic performance for preoperative tumor staging in endometrial cancer and is an optional part of

the National Comprehensive Cancer Network (NCCN) guidelines for patients with high-grade or clinically suspected high-stage endometrioid cancers as well as the higher-risk histologies including serous, clear cell, and carcinosarcoma. The three essential sequences for tumor staging are high-resolution multiplanar T2WI, multiphase or DCE T1WI with fat saturation, and DWI. Off-axial short-axis T2WI and DWI acquisitions orthogonal to the endometrial canal are particularly helpful for assessing the depth of myometrial invasion. Pretreatment with an antiperistaltic agent such as glucagon is helpful to minimize bowel motion artifact.

Endometrial carcinoma has intermediate signal intensity on T2WI—lower than the normal high-signal endometrium and higher than the normal myometrium (Fig. 18.38). Short-axis T2WI is the essential sequence for evaluating the depth of

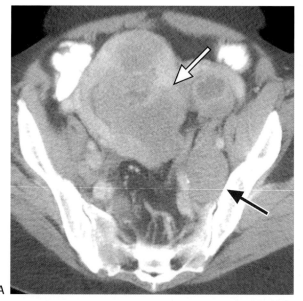 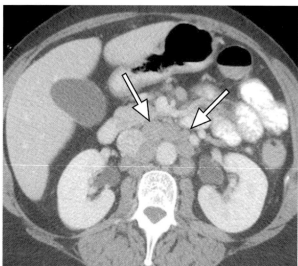

FIGURE 18.36. Stage IV mixed-type endometrial adenocarcinoma with **(A)** obvious myometrial invasion (*white arrow*), involvement of adjacent left ovary, enlarged obturator lymph node (*black arrow*), and **(B)** enlarged upper retroperitoneal nodes (*white arrows*).

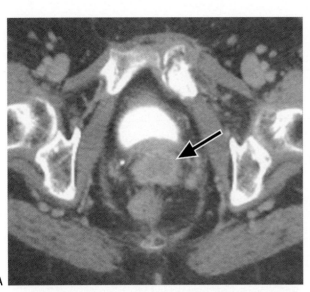

A

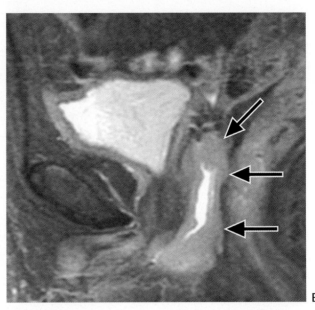

B

FIGURE 18.37. Endometrioid adenocarcinoma with vaginal cuff recurrence after hysterectomy. **A:** CECT shows a vaginal mass (*arrow*). **B:** Sagittal T2WI confirms extensive involvement of the apex and posterior wall (*arrows*) of the vaginal cuff.

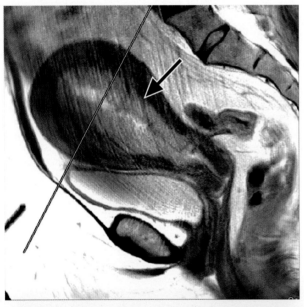

A

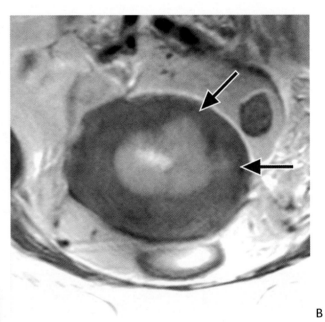

B

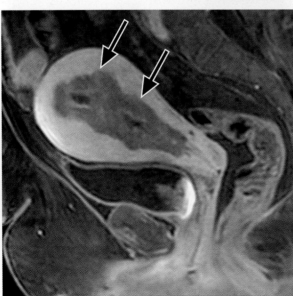

C

FIGURE 18.38. Endometrioid adenocarcinoma, stage IB, involving outer myometrium. **A:** Tumor (*arrow*) has an intermediate "gray" signal on sagittal T2WI. Orthogonal short-axis plane is indicated by yellow line. **B:** Short-axis T2WI demonstrates nodular growth of tumor (*arrows*) into the outer 50% of the myometrium. **C:** Maximum tumor to myometrial contrast (*arrows*) is attained in the portal venous to delayed phases on T1WI with fat saturation.

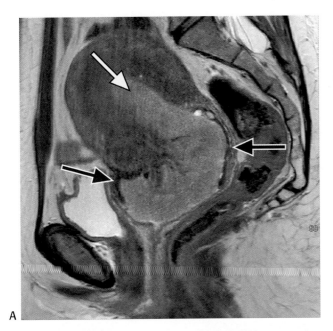

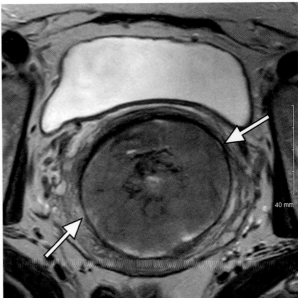

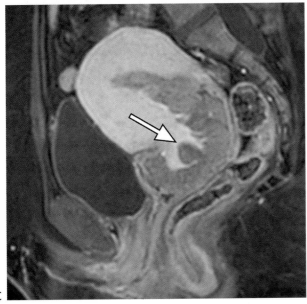

FIGURE 18.39. Endometrioid adenocarcinoma, stage II, arising from lower uterine segment and prolapsing into the cervical canal. **A:** Sagittal T2WI shows intermediate-signal tumor (*white arrow*) expanding the endometrial canal and stretching the cervix, whose intact outer stroma is evident as thin low-signal bands (*black arrows*) anteriorly and posteriorly. **B:** Short-axis T2WI demonstrates markedly thin but intact cervical stroma (*arrows*). Absence of transserosal/parametrial extension keeps this from being a stage III tumor. **C:** Delayed postcontrast sagittal T1WI shows nodular hypoenhancing tumor (*arrow*) extending into, but not through, cervical stroma.

myometrial invasion, which is an important prognostic indicator and will change the surgical approach—deeply invasive tumors should be fully staged with pelvic lymphadenectomy. On contrast-enhanced imaging, maximum contrast between tumor and normal endometrium occurs in the latter postcontrast phases, when tumor is hypointense to adjacent normal parenchyma (Fig. 18.39). Small tumors may be hard to distinguish from normal endometrium on anatomically based imaging sequences, and staging is augmented by functional imaging sequences such as DWI. The highly cellular endometrial epithelium has high signal on DWI normally, but tumors, especially if high grade, tend to have even higher signal on DWI and low signal on corresponding ADC maps (Fig. 18.40). Known pitfalls in tumor staging include inaccurate measurement of the myometrial depth of invasion in cancers involving the (normally thin) cornual portions of the uterus or areas of myometrium distorted by adenomyosis or leiomyomas.

CERVIX

The cervix is the "neck" of the uterus, starting at the internal os and extending distally into the vaginal apex, where it is surrounded by a potential space called the vaginal fornix. The cervical stroma is more fibrous and contains less water than the myometrium and is more hypoechoic on TVUS and has lower signal intensity on T2WI. The endocervix is the lining of the cervical canal, lined by a single layer of columnar mucus-secreting epithelium. The ectocervix is the portion of the cervix that extends into the vaginal canal and is covered by a multilayered squamous epithelium, like the rest of the vagina. The squamocolumnar junction is usually at the level of the external os.

Sometimes, the squamous epithelium overlaps portions of the columnar epithelium and entraps mucus, forming Nabothian cysts. These benign cysts are frequently identified incidentally on ultrasound, where they are usually anechoic unless complicated by prior infection, and MRI, where they are evident as very high-signal

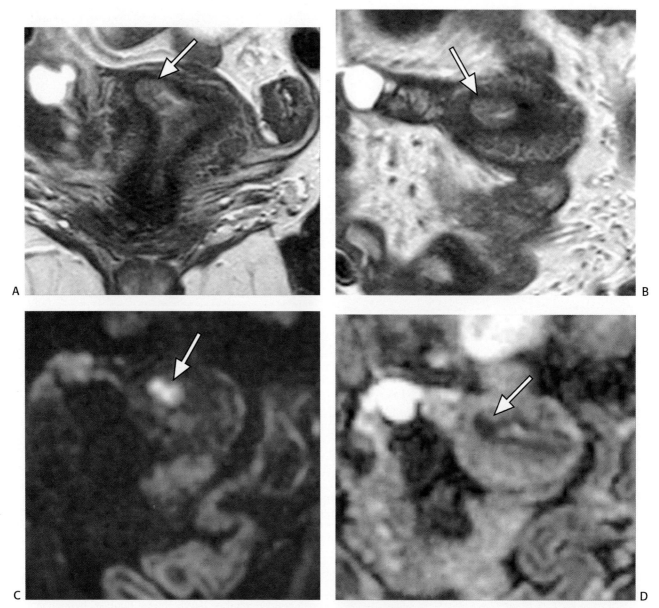

FIGURE 18.40. Small endometrioid adenocarcinoma, stage IA, involving the right cornua (*arrows*), has intermediate signal on **(A)** long-axis and **(B)** axial T2WI. There is corresponding discrete, focal high signal on **(C)** DWI and **(D)** low signal on ADC map.

ovoid structures on T2WI (Figs. 18.9 and 18.15), sometimes large or multiloculated. Another benign variant can be seen in women with cystic fibrosis, who have unusually viscous cervical mucus. Their enlarged endocervical glands may be manifest on pelvic exam and imaging as an exophytic mass (Fig. 18.41).

When the external os is obstructed by scar tissue or a mass, hematometra may result. Benign cervical stenosis may be idiopathic, related to prior inflammation or intervention, or associated with pelvic irradiation. Endometrial and cervical carcinomas, discussed in detail below, may cause malignant cervical stenosis.

Carcinoma

Cervical cancer is the third most common cancer in women worldwide. 85% of cervical cancer is squamous cell type, and the majority of these are associated with human papilloma (HPV) virus,

particularly the high-risk subtypes HPV-16 and HPV-18. Cervical cancer is less common in the United States than in developing countries because of widespread Pap smear screening and increasing HPV vaccination in girls and young women. Despite these advances, cervical cancer remains highly morbid and represents the leading cause of cancer death in younger women.

Cervical epithelial dysplasia, known as cervical intraepithelial neoplasia (CIN), progresses to invasive squamous cell carcinoma in <1% of women. The risk of progression is higher in treatment-resistant or high-grade dysplasia and in association with highly oncogenic HPV subtypes. Early-stage disease is often asymptomatic but sometimes causes vaginal discharge and/or postcoital bleeding. Advanced disease may cause pelvic pain, obstructive uropathy, and systemic symptoms.

Staging is performed using the FIGO system, which maintains primacy as a globally available staging method despite its lack of

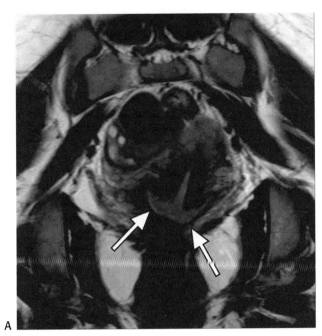 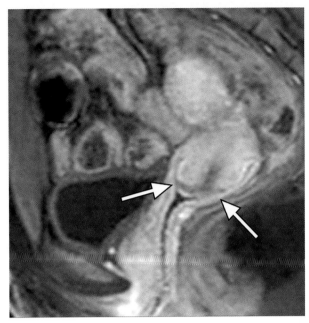

FIGURE 18.41. Cystic fibrosis with benign ectatic cervical mucus glands manifesting as a mass on physical exam. **A:** Long-axis T2WI through the cervix shows a cap of high signal (*arrows*) extending from the endocervix and covering the ectocervix. **B:** Corresponding hypoenhancement (*arrows*) on sagittal postcontrast T1WI.

incorporation of advanced imaging and thus subclinical nodal disease. FIGO staging, summarized in Table 18.3 and Figure 18.42, is based on physical exam augmented by cystoscopy and/or sigmoidoscopy, chest and/or skeletal radiography, IV urography, and open surgical staging. CT and MRI are suggested as adjuncts where available. By contrast, information from advanced imaging studies including CT, MRI, PET/CT, and image-guided biopsies can be formally expressed in the tumor–node–metastasis (TNM) system and is incorporated in the NCCN guidelines and in treatment decision making at most centers in industrialized countries.

The fundamental staging distinction governing treatment and prognosis in cervical cancer is between early-stage and locally advanced disease. Depending on the size of the tumor and the patient's desire for fertility sparing, early-stage tumors may be treated with surgical removal of the cervix (trachelectomy) or simple or radical hysterectomy. Traditionally, the division was made between IIA and IIB disease, but women with IB2 and higher disease are now considered to be locally advanced. Locally advanced disease involves the parametrium by definition and is treated with primary chemoradiation using a combination of intracavitary

TABLE 18.3

TNM + FIGO Staging Summary for Cervical Carcinoma

TNM Staging	FIGO Staging	Description
TX	None	Primary tumor cannot be assessed.
T0	0	No evidence of primary tumor
Tis		Carcinoma in situ
T1	I	Disease confined to the cervix and uterine corpus
T1a	IA	Microscopic invasive tumor
T1b	IB	Clinically visible tumor ≤4.0 cm (IB1) or >4.0 cm (IB2)
T2	II	Carcinoma extends outside of the uterus but not to pelvic sidewall or lower 1/3 of vagina.
T2a	IIA	Tumor without parametrial invasion ≤4.0 cm (IIA1) or >4.0 cm (IIA2)
T2b	IIB	Tumor with parametrial invasion
T3	III	Tumor involves lower 1/3 of the vagina (IIIA), pelvic wall (IIIB), and/or obstructs ureter (IIIB).
T4	IV	Tumor invades mucosa of the bladder or rectum (IVA) or extends beyond the true pelvis (IVB).
NX	Defer to local stage	Regional nodes cannot be assessed.
N0		No regional node metastasis
N1	IIIB	Positive regional node metastasis
M0	Defer to local stage	No distant metastasis
M1	IVB	Positive distant metastasis (includes para-aortic nodes)

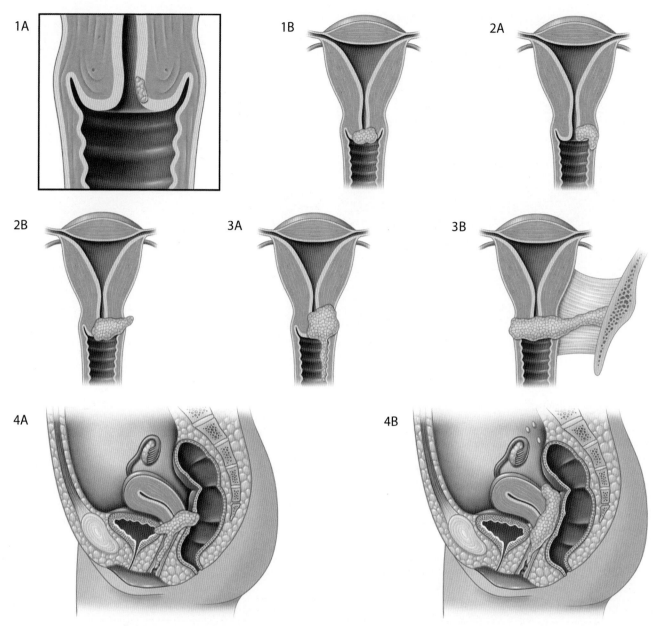

FIGURE 18.42. Schematic diagram of FIGO cervical cancer staging.

(tandem-based) brachytherapy and external beam radiotherapy. The intention is definitive treatment, not debulking prior to surgery.

Early-stage cervical cancer is highly treatable, with 93% five-year survival for stage IA and 80% for stage IB disease. However, long-term survival declines rather precipitously with more locally advanced and distant disease, with only about 15% five-year survival of women with stage IV disease. When advanced disease is suspected clinically, a combination of MRI for local tumor staging and PET/CT for systemic staging is often used. MRI is more accurate than physical exam for measuring tumor size, assessing the presence and extent of parametrial extension and/or pelvic sidewall involvement, and pelvic nodal staging. PET/CT can demonstrate metabolic activity even in normal-sized nodes and detect more distant disease. MRI is also used in image-based planning of radiation therapy for cervical cancer, particularly brachytherapy, and for evaluation of suspected pelvic recurrence. Thus, there is ongoing expansion of

the role of imaging in the management of locally advanced cervical carcinoma and an opportunity for radiologists to contribute to the care of these patients.

Imaging

Ultrasound is the appropriate initial imaging modality for women with pelvic masses or bleeding and may sometimes be the first imaging study demonstrating a cervical mass. Cervical carcinoma is usually hypoechoic, irregularly marginated, and hypervascular (Fig. 18.43). More advanced tumors may be associated with obstruction and dilatation of the endometrial canal or ureters (Fig. 18.44). When other imaging modalities are available, ultrasound should not be used for primary tumor staging in endometrial cancer.

CT has poor tissue contrast for pelvic organs and is unlikely to detect small tumors. Larger tumors, particularly those involving the pelvic sidewalls, bladder, or rectum, are usually evident as poorly

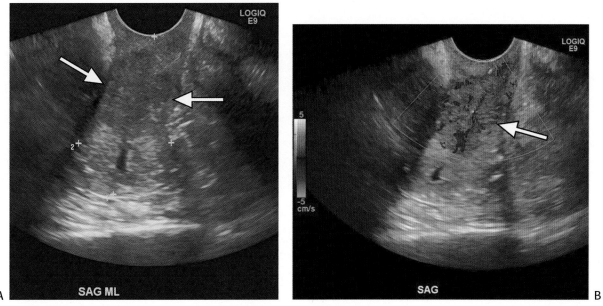

FIGURE 18.43. Squamous cell carcinoma of the cervix with **(A)** hypoechoic mass (*arrows*) on gray scale and **(B)** hypervascularity (*arrow*) on color Doppler TVUS.

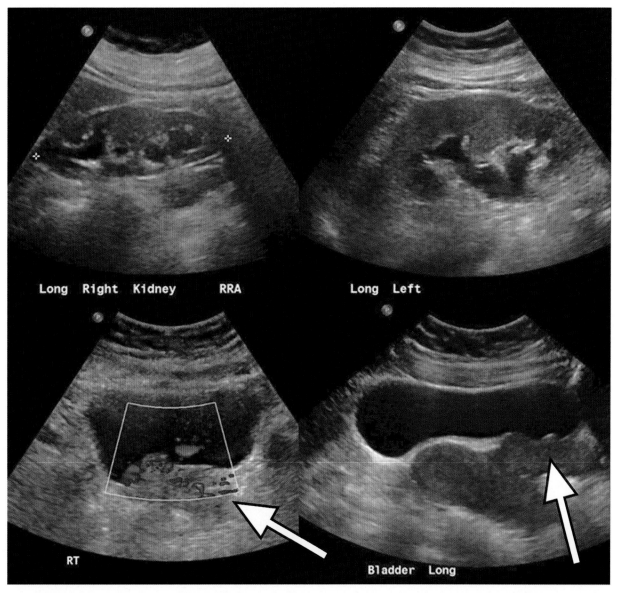

FIGURE 18.44. Squamous cell carcinoma of the cervix with transabdominal ultrasound images showing bilateral hydronephrosis due to a locally advanced tumor (*arrows*) involving the posterior bladder wall and distal ureters.

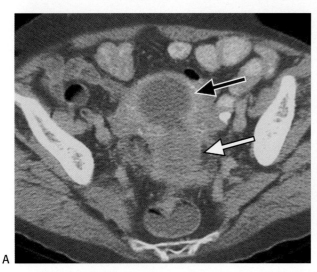
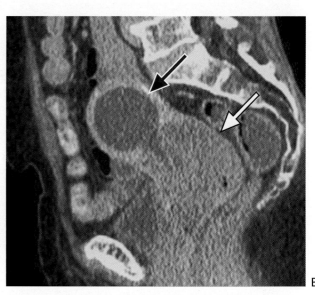

FIGURE 18.45. Squamous cell carcinoma of the cervix on **(A)** axial and **(B)** sagittal reformatted CT images showing hematometra (*black arrows*) due to obstructing cervical mass (*white arrows*).

marginated masses (Fig. 18.45). Enhancement depends upon prior treatment and central necrosis. CT is very helpful for evaluation of pelvic and para-aortic lymph node enlargement, which will alter staging and radiation treatment planning if present.

MRI is the most accurate imaging modality for local tumor staging. The protocol is similar to endometrial cancer, relying on multiplanar small field of view T2WI with short-axis images obtained orthogonal to the cervical canal, multiphasic contrast-enhanced T1WI with fat saturation, and DWI. Imaging with a high-field strength magnet (3.0T) improves spatial resolution, while images obtained with low-field strength (<1.0T) open magnets are rarely diagnostic. An IV or IM peristaltic agent also improves image quality, and intravaginal gel is very helpful to delineate tumor and evaluate forniceal involvement (Fig. 18.46).

Very small tumors and those with minimal stromal invasion are usually staged clinically. Although this is an epithelial neoplasm, all of the important information governing treatment and prognosis pertains to the degree of tumor invasion into or through the cervical stroma. Cervical carcinoma exhibits intermediate "gray" signal on T2WI, which is much higher in signal intensity than the normal hypointense cervical stroma. As in endometrial cancer, short-axis T2WI is essential for determining the depth of invasion (Fig. 18.47). Inflammation and architectural distortion after conization or other biopsy may increase the signal of an uninvolved cervix. DWI is helpful to distinguish tumor from benign edema in this setting.

Cervical cancer enhancement is somewhat variable, but is usually distinct from normal background tissue in all phases.

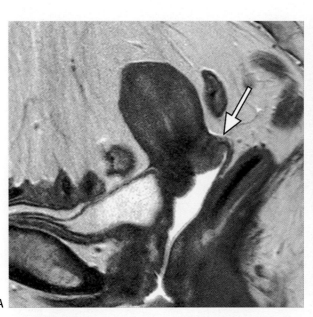
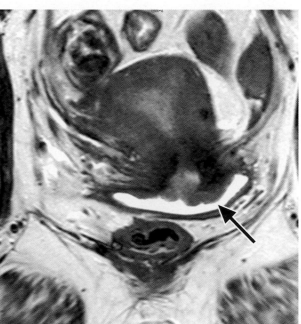

FIGURE 18.46. Squamous cell carcinoma of the cervix arising in a condyloma. **A:** High-signal gel distends the vagina and helps to delineate involvement of the posterior fornix (*arrow*) on sagittal T2WI. **B:** Long-axis T2WI shows tumor (*arrow*) outlined by gel.

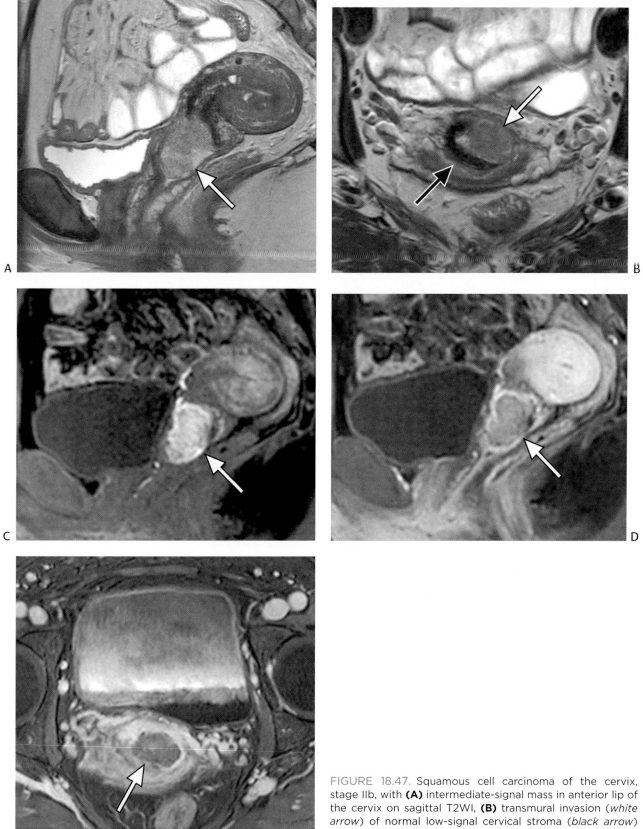

FIGURE 18.47. Squamous cell carcinoma of the cervix, stage IIb, with **(A)** intermediate-signal mass in anterior lip of the cervix on sagittal T2WI, **(B)** transmural invasion (*white arrow*) of normal low-signal cervical stroma (*black arrow*) on short-axis T2WI, and **(C)** hyperenhancement (*arrow*) in the arterial phase and relative hypoenhancement (*arrows*) in later phases on **(D)** sagittal and **(E)** axial postcontrast T1WI.

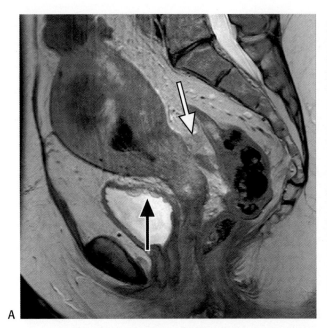
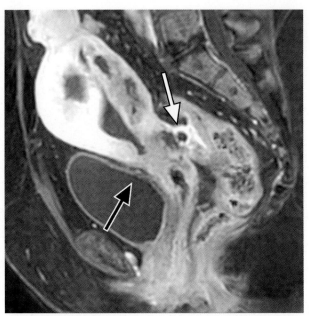

FIGURE 18.48. Squamous cell carcinoma of the cervix, stage III, with **(A)** bulky cervical mass extending posteriorly to involve rectal serosa (*white arrow*) and bullous edema (*black arrow*) of the bladder wall due to impaired lymphatic drainage. **B:** Sagittal postcontrast T1WI shows brisk enhancement of the tumor in the posterior cul-de-sac (*white arrow*) but sparing of rectal and bladder (*black arrow*) mucosal surfaces. Transmural enhancement would indicate stage IV disease.

Cervical carcinomas are often hypervascular in the arterial phase, may exhibit central necrosis, and tend to enhance less than normal stroma in later phases. Contrast-enhanced imaging is particularly useful for evaluation of transmural bladder or bowel invasion. Submucosal bladder wall involvement obstructs lymphatic drainage and causes bullous edema of the bladder mucosa (Fig. 18.48), which must be distinguished from transmural bladder wall invasion with enhancing intraluminal soft tissue, indicating stage IV disease. Viable tumors have high signal on DWI and low signal on

ADC maps, and these sequences are also useful for monitoring response to therapy.

Other cervical neoplasms include adenosquamous, mucinous, and small cell cancers and occasionally lymphoma. Adenoma malignum is a rare type of very well-differentiated mucinous adenocarcinoma of the cervix with an unusual and characteristic appearance; on T2-weighted MRI, it appears as a cluster of cystic lesions, usually in the endocervical canal (Fig. 18.49) and may even mimic Nabothian cysts. Radiologists should also be aware of this

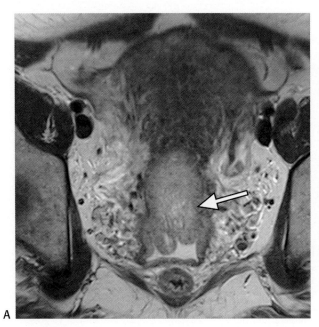
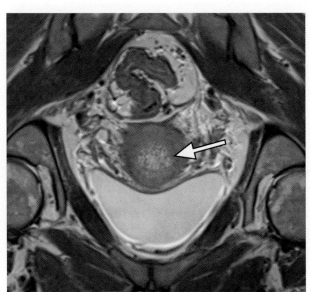

FIGURE 18.49. Adenoma malignum of the cervix with tiny intratumoral cysts (*arrows*) on **(A)** long- and **(B)** short-axis T2WI. In some patients, this mucinous tumor can appear almost entirely cystic and may be mistaken for Nabothian cysts.

rare diagnosis, also known as "minimal deviation adenocarcinoma," when asked to stage cervical carcinoma.

Preoperative staging of cervical cancer on MRI should include three-dimensional measurements of tumor size; the presence and location of parametrial involvement; presence and extent of invasion of the vagina, bladder, urethra, ureters, rectum, or sidewall strictures; and nodal assessment. Overall staging accuracy of MRI has been quoted as ranging from 76% to 94%. Armed with an understanding of the technical aspects of high-quality imaging and the clinical significance of the findings, radiologists have the opportunity to make substantial contributions to the care of women with gynecologic cancers.

SUGGESTED READINGS

Adelman MR. The morcellation debate: the history and the science. *Clin Obstet Gynecol.* 2015;58(4):710–717.

Bazot M, Cortez A, Darai E, et al. Ultrasonography compared with magnetic resonance imaging for the diagnosis of adenomyosis: correlation with histopathology. *Hum Reprod.* 2001;16(11):2427–2433.

Chuang LT, Temin S, Camacho R, et al. Management and care of women with invasive cervical cancer: American Society of Clinical Oncology Resource-Stratified Clinical Practice Guideline. *J Global Oncol.* 2016;2(5):311–339.

Choi HJ, Ju W, Myung SK, et al. Diagnostic performance of computer tomography, magnetic resonance imaging, and positron emission tomography or positron emission tomography/computer tomography for detection of metastatic lymph nodes in patients with cervical cancer: meta-analysis. *Cancer Sci.* 2010;101(6):1471–1479.

Deng L, Wang QP, Chen X, et al. The combination of diffusion- and T2-weighted imaging in predicting deep myometrial invasion of endometrial cancer: a systematic review and meta-analysis. *J Comput Assist Tomogr.* 2015;39(5):661–673.

Deshmukh SP, Gonsalves CF, Guglielmo FF, et al. Role of MR imaging of uterine leiomyomas before and after embolization. *Radiographics.* 2012;32(6):E251–E281.

Dueholm M, Lundorf E. Transvaginal ultrasound or MRI for diagnosis of adenomyosis. *Curr Opin Obstet Gynecol.* 2007;19:505–512.

Early HM, McGahan JP, Scoutt LM, et al. Pitfalls of sonographic imaging of uterine leiomyoma. *Ultrasound Q.* 2016;32:164–174.

Freeman SJ, Aly AM, Kataoka MY, et al. The revised FIGO staging system for uterine malignancies: implications for MR imaging. *Radiographics.* 2012;32:1805–1827.

Gaetke-Udager K, McLean K, Sciallis AP, et al. Diagnostic accuracy of ultrasound, contrast-enhanced CT, and conventional MRI for differentiating leiomyoma from leiomyosarcoma. *Acad Radiol.* 2016;23(10):1290–1297.

Kamaya A, Yu PC, Lloyd CR, et al. Sonographic evaluation for endometrial polyps: the interrupted mucosa sign. *J Ultrasound Med.* 2016;35(11):2381–2387. pii: 15.09007.

Langer JE, Oliver ER, Lev-Toaff AS, et al. Imaging of the female pelvis through the life cycle. *Radiographics.* 2012;32:1575–1597.

Levy G, Dehaene A, Laurent N, et al. An update on adenomyosis. *Diagn Interv Imaging.* 2013;94:3–25.

Munro MG, Critchley HOD, Broder MS, et al. FIGO classification system for causes of abnormal uterine bleeding in nongravid women of reproductive age. *Int J Gynaecol Obstet.* 2011;113:3–13.

Nakai A, Reinhold C, Noel P, et al. Optimizing cine MRI for uterine peristalsis: a comparison of three different single shot fast spin echo techniques. *J Magn Reson Imaging.* 2013;38:161–167.

National Comprehensive Cancer Network (NCCN). *Clinical Practice Guidelines in Oncology: Uterine Neoplasms (Version 2.2016) and Cervical Cancer (Version 1.2016).* National Comprehensive Cancer Network. www.nccn.org

Novellas S, Chassang M, Delotte J, et al. MRI characteristics of the uterine junctional zone: from normal to the diagnosis of adenomyosis. *AJR Am J Roentgenol* 2011;196:1206–1213.

Rauch GM, Kaur H, Choi H, et al. Optimization of MR imaging for pretreatment evaluation of patients with endometrial and cervical cancer. *Radiographics.* 2014;34(4):1082–1098.

Sala E, Rockall AG, Freeman SJ, et al. The added role of MR imaging in treatment stratification of patients with gynecologic malignancies: what the radiologist needs to know. *Radiology.* 2013;266(3):717–740.

Siddiqui N, Nikolaidis P, Hammond N, et al. Uterine artery embolization: pre- and postprocedural evaluation using magnetic resonance imaging. *Abdom Imaging.* 2013;38:1161–1177.

Son H, Kositwattanarerk A, Hayes MP, et al. PET/CT evaluation of cervical cancer: spectrum of disease. *Radiographics.* 2010;30(5):1251–1268.

Timmermans A, Opmeer BC, Khan KS, et al. Endometrial thickness measurement for detecting endometrial cancer in women with postmenopausal bleeding: a systematic review and meta-analysis. *Obstet Gynecol.* 2010;116(1):160–167.

Verma SK, Lev-Toaff AS, Baltarowich OH, et al. Adenomyosis: sonohysterography with MRI correlation. *AJR Am J Roentgenol.* 2009;192:1112–1116.

Wildenberg JC, Yam BL, Langer JE, et al. US of the nongravid cervix with multimodality imaging correlation: normal appearance, pathologic conditions, and diagnostic pitfalls. *Radiographics.* 2016;36:596–617.

Female Perineum and Vagina

The urinary, reproductive, and gastrointestinal systems converge in a small space at the female perineum. The anatomy is complex and many different types of pathology are possible. Because the perineum is readily accessible to physical examination, clinicians often make these diagnoses without the use of imaging. However, in many cases, imaging provides important anatomic and functional information that can guide management. Perineal conditions are occasionally diagnosed incidentally on CT examinations, though CT is usually not appropriate for primary assessment of the vagina or perineum. Translabial or transvaginal ultrasound and high-resolution MRI provide the most useful information about these small structures, with PET/CT offering additional staging information in the setting of malignancy.

ANATOMY

The perineum is a diamond-shaped space (Fig. 19.1) bounded by the pubic symphysis anteriorly, ischial tuberosities laterally, and coccyx posteriorly. The relevant anatomy is briefly reviewed, proceeding from superficial to deep. Unlike many other anatomic locations, this also means from caudal to cranial, because the perineum is a horizontally oriented "upside down" surface in a standing woman.

The mons pubis is the subcutaneous tissue overlying the symphysis, and the labia majora are the exterior skin folds evident on superficial physical exam. The labia are homologous to the scrotum in men, which is fused in the midline raphe. The labia minora are paired mucosal folds medial to the labia majora, parting to reveal the vaginal opening, or introitus. Anterior to the vaginal opening is the urethral meatus, with its paired periurethral glands, or Skene glands. These glands drain the paired vestibular bulbs (Fig. 19.2), pear shaped mounds of erectile tissue that are the bifurcated homologue of the single male corpus spongiosum. The vestibular bulbs are surrounded by the superficial bulbospongiosus muscles. The vestibular bulbs lie in close apposition to the clitoral crura (corpora cavernosa), which converge in the midline clitoral body and glans (Fig. 19.3). The clitoral crura are covered by the ischiocavernosus

muscles, paralleling the inferior pubic rami. Female erectile tissue may be well depicted by several imaging modalities, including translabial ultrasound or MR images. The term vulva incorporates all of the above structures: the labia, openings of urethra and vagina, and erectile tissue.

The perineal membrane or urogenital diaphragm is the most superficial muscular layer of the pelvic floor, stretching between the inferior rami to form a triangle anteriorly (Fig. 19.1). The deep and superficial transverse perineal muscles are the major elements of the perineal membrane, which coalesces posteriorly

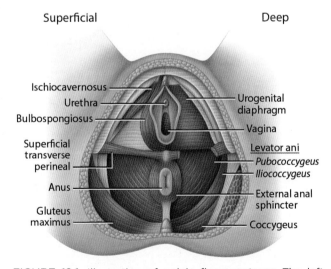

FIGURE 19.1. Illustration of pelvic floor anatomy. The left side (patient's right) shows the superficial musculature and the right side shows the deep musculature. Posteriorly, the ischiorectal fat has been removed, revealing the levator ani complex and other musculature.

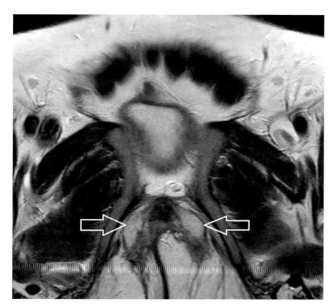

FIGURE 19.2. Vestibular bulbs are paired mounds of erectile tissue (*arrows*) converging at the urethra, showing intermediate signal on T2WI. On contrast-enhanced CT or MRI, the vestibular bulbs often exhibit transient hypervascularity, analogous to the common incidental finding in male erectile tissue.

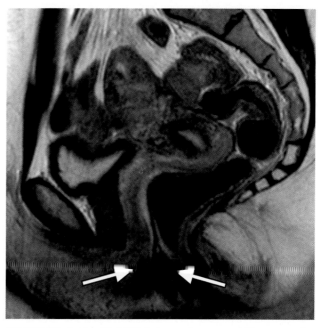

FIGURE 19.4. Sagittal T2WI shows the normal fibromuscular perineal body (*arrows*) posterior to the vaginal introitus and anterior to the anus.

to form the perineal body (Fig. 19.4), between the vagina and anus. The perineal membrane has midline openings for the urethra and vagina.

The vagina is a muscular tube of 8 to 12 cm in length, lined by squamous epithelium with conspicuous transverse folds, or rugae. At rest (Fig. 19.5), the mucosal surfaces are apposed and the vagina is flat, with a typical H-shape on axial images. The upper portion of the vagina fuses with the cervix in the vaginal fornix or arch, a circular potential space surrounding the cervix. When a hysterectomy has been performed, the vaginal cuff is closed in a linear fashion with suture material at its apex.

The funnel-shaped levator ani complex (Fig. 19.6) provides primary muscular support of the pelvic organs. The levator complex has several distinct components: the iliococcygeus and pubococcygeus muscles extend from the pelvic sidewalls to the coccyx and anococcygeal raphe, while the puborectalis muscle is a U-shaped sling suspending the anorectal junction, with insertions near the symphysis pubis. The levator complex merges caudally with the external anal sphincter complex.

The endopelvic fascia is a network of thin fascial sheets that invest and support the pelvic organs and tether them to the osseous pelvis. The endopelvic fascial structures are largely invisible by imaging, but damage can be inferred from abnormal descent of pelvic organs.

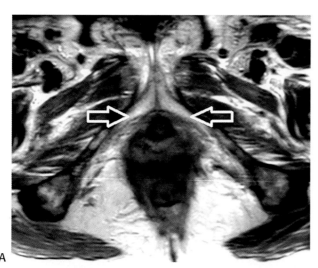

A

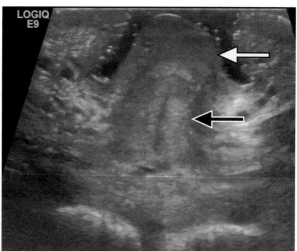

B

FIGURE 19.3. Clitoral structures include the paired clitoral crura on **(A)** T2WI, showing crura as intermediate signal tubular structures (*arrows*) paralleling inferior rami and converging anteriorly, and **(B)** translabial ultrasound, demonstrating midline clitoral body (*black arrow*) and head (*white arrow*).

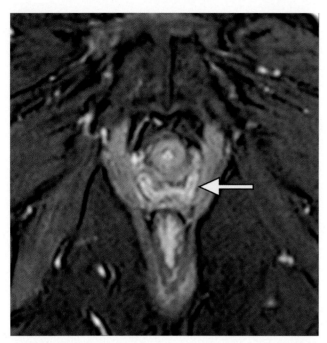

FIGURE 19.5. Axial T1WI postcontrast shows the normal H- or W-shaped collapsed vagina (*arrow*) posterior to the urethra and anterior to the anus.

CYSTIC LESIONS OF THE PERINEUM

Benign perineal cysts may be incidentally detected, or they may cause symptoms due to mass effect or infection. The most common types are readily distinguished by location and are summarized in Table 19.1. The primary reason to distinguish among these benign lesions is to guide clinical management by appropriate anatomic localization. Finally, these lesions should be

TABLE 19.1	
Benign Perineal Cysts	
Cyst	Location
Urethral diverticulum	Posterolateral or encircling midurethra, above meatus, luminal communication
Skene gland (periurethral) cysts	At urethral meatus, 4 and 8 o'clock positions
Bartholin gland cysts	Posterior vaginal introitus
Gartner duct cysts	Anterolateral upper vagina, above inferior margin of pubic symphysis
Canal of Nuck cyst	Intralabial, may extend to inguinal canal

meticulously distinguished from perineal solid masses by Doppler US imaging or IV contrast-enhanced CT or MR examinations whenever possible.

Urethral Diverticulum

Infection or inflammation of periurethral glands may lead to abscess formation and secondary communication with the urethral lumen. These epithelialized outpouchings, or diverticula, are usually tear drop shaped (Fig. 19.7) and involve the midurethra. When large, they may dissect throughout the urethral–vaginal space and become horseshoe shaped. Urethral diverticula have imaging characteristics of simple fluid on all imaging studies, with additional findings of wall thickening, debris, and/or septa when inflamed. Symptoms include urinary dribbling or recurrent infection; symptomatic diverticula are usually excised or marsupialized. Diverticular adenocarcinoma is a rare long-term complication.

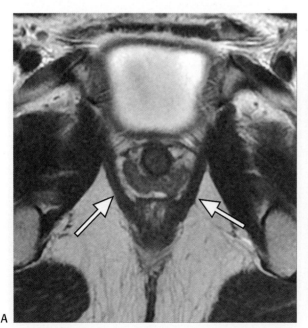

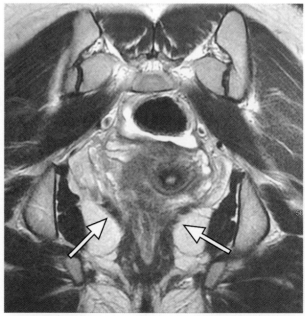

A   B

FIGURE 19.6. Pelvic floor muscular structures. **A:** Axial T2WI shows the puborectalis sling (*arrows*) suspending the anorectal junction from the posterior aspect of the pubic symphysis. **B:** Coronal T2WI shows the funnel-shaped levator ani muscular complex (*arrows*) separating the mesorectal space from ischiorectal fat. The perineal membrane is also seen at the inferior aspect of the image.

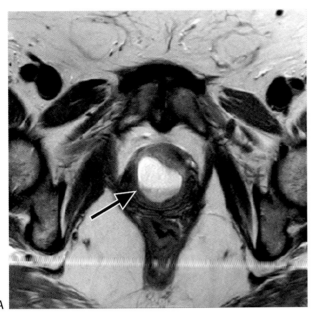
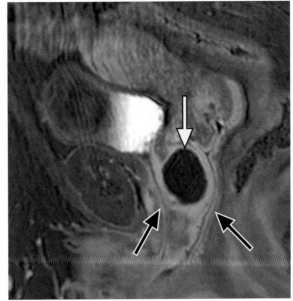

FIGURE 19.7. Large urethral diverticulum **(A)** with layering debris (*arrow*) on T2WI and **(B)** with lack of internal enhancement on sagittal T1WI postcontrast imaging. Note splaying of collapsed urethral and vaginal lumens (*black arrows*) by this large diverticulum (*white arrow*).

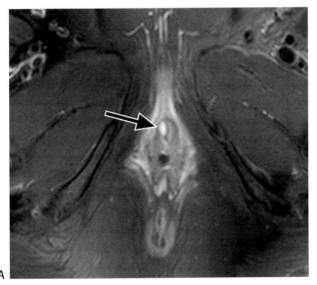
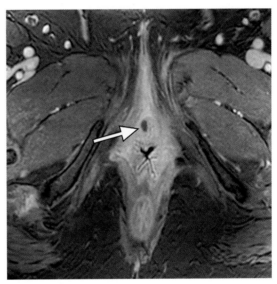

FIGURE 19.8. Tiny Skene gland cyst (*arrows*) at posterolateral urethral meatus on axial **(A)** T2WI and **(B)** T1WI postcontrast.

Skene Gland Cyst

Unlike diverticula, Skene gland cysts (Fig. 19.8) do not directly communicate with the urethral lumen and are located at the meatus. They also arise from duct obstruction but without abscess or formation of a secondary communication. Skene gland cysts are often asymptomatic, though occasionally cause problems due to mass effect or difficulty in differentiation from a diverticulum.

Bartholin Gland Cyst

Paired Bartholin glands lie at the posterior aspect of the vaginal introitus and may form cysts when obstructed (Fig. 19.9). Like the

other cysts, they are well circumscribed, with imaging features of simple fluid except when inflamed.

Gartner Duct Cyst

Gartner ducts involve the upper two-thirds of the vagina and are usually anterolateral. Gartner duct cysts (Fig. 19.10) are intramural and may be difficult to distinguish from vaginal inclusion cysts resulting from trauma or surgery. Because they arise from mesonephric duct remnants, these cysts are occasionally associated with other anomalies such as renal agenesis or cross-fused ectopia.

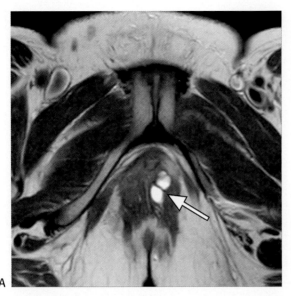 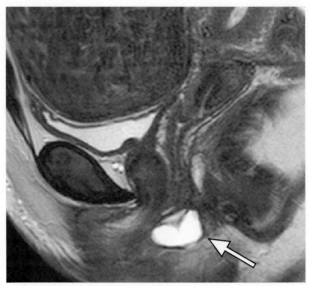

FIGURE 19.9. Bartholin gland cyst at the left introitus (*arrows*) on axial **(A)** and sagittal **(B)** T2WI. This patient also has a large uterine leiomyoma.

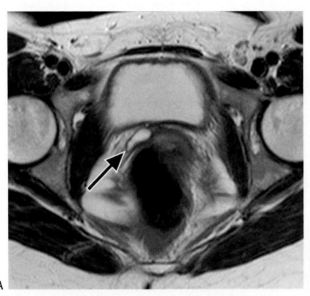 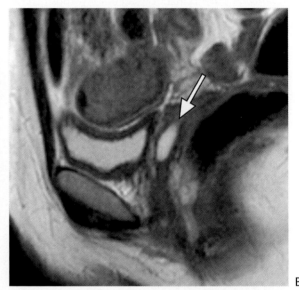

FIGURE 19.10. Gartner duct cyst (*arrows*) involves right upper vagina on axial **(A)** and sagittal **(B)** T2WI.

Canal of Nuck Cyst

The round ligament of the uterus inserts at the anterior aspect of the labia majora, surrounded by a peritoneal outpouching called the canal of Nuck, analogous to the processus vaginalis. If patent, inguinal hernia may result. Alternately, partial closure of this peritoneal recess may result in cyst formation (Fig. 19.11). These are much more anterior and less common than the other female perineal cysts.

Miscellaneous Others

Other cystic or partially cystic lesions of the vulva and perineum include posttraumatic hematomas (Fig. 19.12) or clitoral inclusion cysts, perianal and perineal fistulas and abscesses (Fig. 19.13), and rare lymphatic or lymphovascular malformations. In most cases, these lesions will be more complex and contain other tissue

elements or vascularity, in contrast to the simple, well-circumscribed appearance of most perineal cysts.

FUNCTIONAL DISORDERS OF THE PELVIC FLOOR

Functional problems of the pelvic floor, including urinary and defecatory dysfunction and pelvic organ prolapse, are very common and associated with significant quality of life impact for affected women. Pregnancy and vaginal delivery cause pelvic floor injuries in many women. Muscular and fascial defects and laxity may be associated with immediate clinical symptoms, or subclinical injuries may remain latent until postmenopausal muscular atrophy and/or weight gain unmask them in later years. An introduction to this complex anatomy and physiology is provided, and interested readers are referred to one of several detailed reviews.

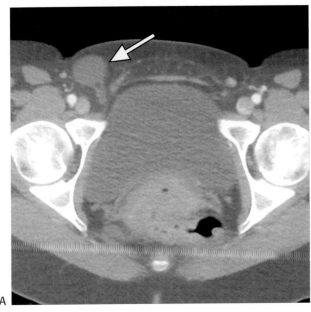
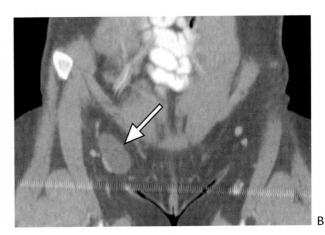

FIGURE 19.11. Axial **(A)** and coronal **(B)** CECT images show a canal of Nuck cyst (*arrows*) as a teardrop-shaped fluid density structure at the inguinal ring, directed toward the labia.

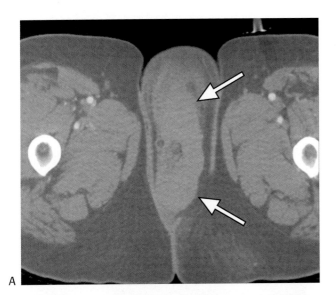

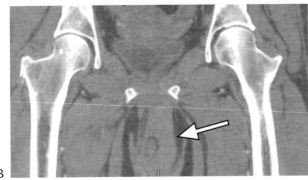

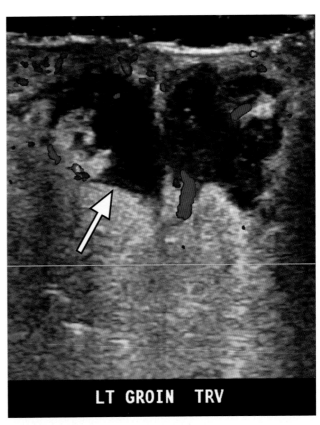

FIGURE 19.12. Left vulvar hematoma (*arrows*) on **(A)** axial and **(B)** coronal CECT images after Bartholin cyst excision. Foley catheter is displaced to the right.

FIGURE 19.13. Vulvar abscess manifests as irregularly marginated fluid collection (*arrow*) on translabial ultrasound.

Imaging Techniques

Functional imaging of the pelvic floor can be performed under fluoroscopy, ultrasound, or MRI guidance. There are many variations on patient preparation for each, with the broad goals of visualizing important structures and mimicking the physiologic processes of evacuation. In conventional fluoroscopic defecography (also called proctography), barium paste of one or more consistencies is instilled into the rectum and usually the vagina. In many centers, the patients also drink thin barium 1 to 2 hours prior to the study to opacify the small bowel, and in some centers, the bladder is also opacified with dilute iodinated contrast via a catheter. Patients are positioned in an upright seated position and are asked to sequentially relax and contract the pelvic floor and then to evacuate the barium into the fluoroscopic commode. This series of maneuvers is also described as rest–squeeze–push or relax–Kegel–strain. This is an inexpensive and time-honored method, which is thought to best approximate the physiologic processes of defecation, enabling ready assessment of opacified structures, but uses some ionizing radiation and lacks direct evaluation of muscular support and organ prolapse.

Ultrasound does not require any prep or enema and is performed with supine transperineal and transvaginal imaging during relaxation, squeezing, and coughing. This emerging technique is only performed in select centers and may be limited by the absence of a true evacuation component. However, the low cost, absence of radiation exposure, and wide availability make ultrasound appealing as a screening approach in pelvic floor dysfunction.

Rectal and vaginal gels are widely used in preparation for functional pelvic floor MRI. Patients are positioned supine (knees flexed if possible), unless an open magnet with upright position is available. A series of sagittal midline T2-weighted single-shot FSE (SSFSE) cine sequences with the patient relaxing, squeezing, and evacuating gel into absorbent pads provide the dynamic evaluation of pelvic floor function, while small field of view high-resolution T1WI and T2WI in multiple planes provide structural information about muscular support. MRI offers the advantage of direct evaluation of pelvic organs, muscles, and prolapse, with limitations including cost, patient difficulties with compliance, and nonphysiologic supine position in a closed magnet in most centers.

With all methods, patient education and support are essential to reduce patient embarrassment and ensure maximal push effort. If patients do not forcefully squeeze or push, evaluation is very limited and important diagnoses may be missed.

Compartment Concept

The pelvic floor has been artificially divided into anterior (bladder and urethra), middle (vagina and uterus), and posterior (anus and rectum) compartments corresponding to the urologists, gynecologists, and general surgeons who treat disorders in each compartment, respectively. However, the muscular support is shared by all of these structures, and many patients have elements of multicompartment dysfunction.

Dyssynergia

The normal anorectal angle at rest is between 90 and 110 degrees. When defecation is initiated, the angle becomes more obtuse and the canal straightens. In some patients, there is instead paradoxical contraction of the puborectalis sling and failure of pelvic floor relaxation, causing obstruction to defecation, also known as anismus or dyssynergia (Fig. 19.14). This can be successfully treated with biofeedback in some patients.

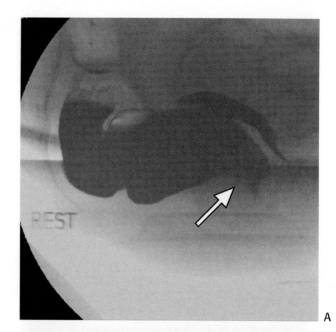

A

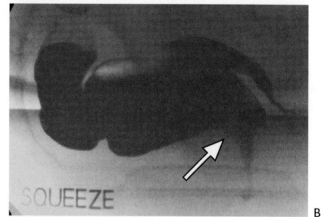

B

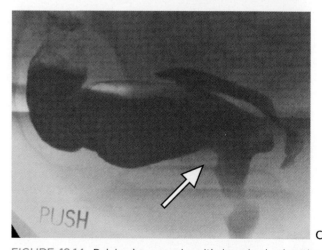

C

FIGURE 19.14. Pelvic dyssynergia with impaired relaxation of puborectalis sling impeding defecation. Defecography images at **(A)** rest, **(B)** squeeze, and **(C)** push phases of exam show little change in anorectal angle (*arrows*), which should become more acute with squeeze and more obtuse with push. The puborectalis indentation on the contrast column becomes more pronounced with push (*arrow*, **C**), indicating paradoxical contraction.

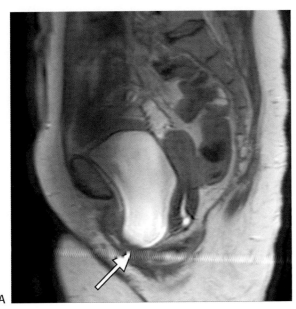

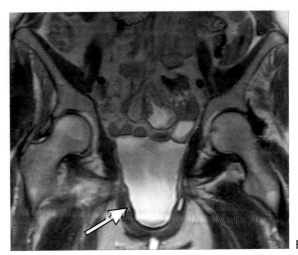

FIGURE 19.15. Cystocele with inferior herniation of urinary bladder (*arrows*) below the pubic symphysis with strain on **(A)** sagittal and **(B)** coronal T2WI. Note descent of the entire pelvic floor.

Cystocele and Urethral Hypermobility

Cystocele is the abnormal herniation of the bladder along the anterior vaginal wall. This is evident as an extrinsic compression on the opacified vaginal vault at fluoroscopy or is directly observed at MRI when the bladder descends below the pubococcygeal line (Fig. 19.15). Cystoceles are caused by weakening or defects of the endopelvic fascia, usually in multiparous women. The normal urethral orientation is near vertical but may rotate toward horizontal at rest or with straining in women with loss of urethral support after vaginal delivery or hysterectomy, leading to stress urinary incontinence.

Rectocele

The typical rectocele is anterior bulging of the rectum, causing abnormal convexity of the rectovaginal septum and posterior vaginal wall. An anterior bulge of <2 cm from the anal canal axis

is considered physiologic. Larger rectoceles are often associated with incomplete evacuation (Fig. 19.16). Laxity or defects in the levator ani complex, best diagnosed with MRI, are sometimes associated with lateral protrusion of the rectum into the ischiorectal space.

Enterocele and Sigmoidocele

Enterocele and sigmoidocele are descent of the small bowel or the redundant sigmoid, respectively, into the deep pelvis, with compression of the anterior/superior rectal wall and obstructed defecation in severe cases (Fig. 19.17). The enterocele or sigmoidocele may descend deeply into the rectovaginal space and even prolapse through the anus (Fig. 19.18) or vaginal introitus. These conditions are most commonly seen in women who have lost continuity of the endopelvic fascia after hysterectomy or multiple pregnancies, and surgical repair involves suspension of peritoneal contents to prevent herniation.

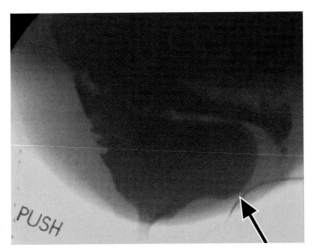

FIGURE 19.16. Rectocele on conventional defecography with large anterior bulge (*arrow*) during push. Note that the vagina is also opacified by barium and that the vagina and rectovaginal septum are nearly horizontal due to distortion by the rectocele.

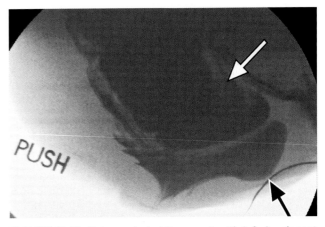

FIGURE 19.17. Enterocele (*white arrow*) with inferior decent of opacified small bowel into rectovaginal space during push, compressing rectum (*black arrow*), which also exhibits a rectocele.

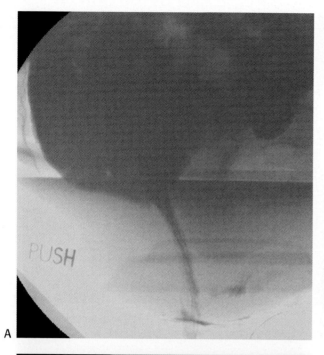

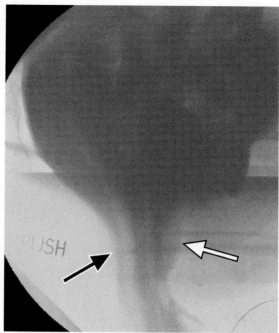

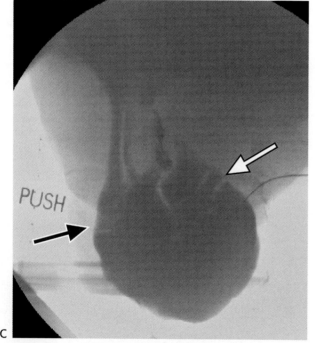

FIGURE 19.18. Peritoneocele containing small- and large bowel prolapses through anus with increasing push effort **(A–C)**. The rectum is seen posteriorly (*black arrows*) with sigmoid and small bowel anteriorly (*white arrows*).

Pelvic Floor Descent and Prolapse

When the entire muscular pelvic floor bulges inferiorly with straining or defecation, it is termed perineal descent (Fig. 19.15). In patients with normal pelvic floor function, the anorectal angle is located <2 cm below the pubococcygeal line at maximal strain, with severe descent being >6 cm below the pubococcygeal line. By contrast, when pelvic organs actually protrude through the pelvic floor hiatus, it is termed prolapse. The vagina, cervix, and/or uterus may prolapse in the middle compartment (Fig. 19.19), more directly appreciated by MR than by conventional defecography. In the posterior compartment, the rectum may telescope or intussuscept (internal prolapse) or actually invert through the anus (external

prolapse) (Fig. 19.20). Reduction of prolapse may be spontaneous or require manual assistance by the patient or physician. Depending on its extent and severity, pelvic organ prolapse has the potential to cause a substantial negative impact on quality of life, and appropriate imaging can provide valuable information for surgical planning.

PELVIC FLOOR NEOPLASMS

Urethra

Urethral cancer encompasses several histologies, including squamous cell carcinoma at the urethral meatus, urothelial cancer involving the upper and midurethra, adenocarcinoma arising

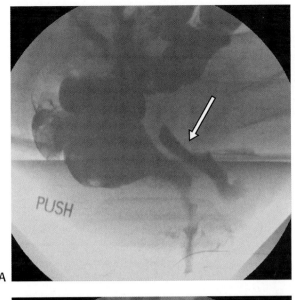

A

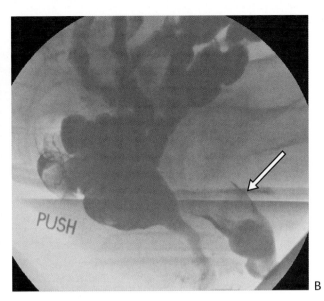

B

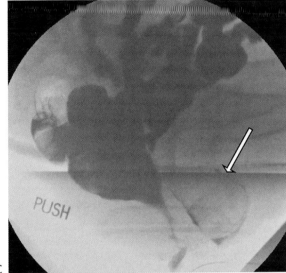

C

FIGURE 19.19. Uterine prolapse, with increasing protrusion of cervix (*arrows*, **A–C**) into vagina and through vaginal introitus with push effort.

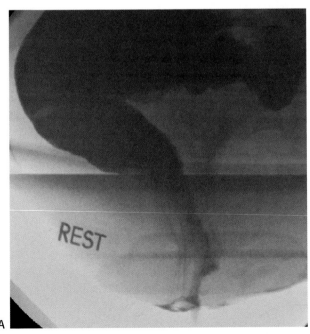

A

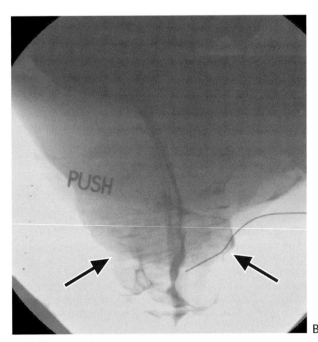

B

FIGURE 19.20. Normal rectum at rest **(A)** with external rectal prolapse **(B)** (*arrows*) with push. The folds of the inverted distal rectum are highlighted by barium.

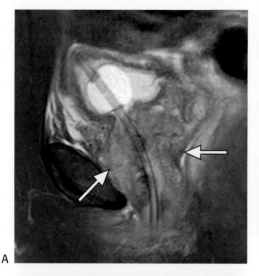

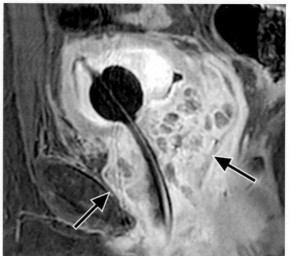

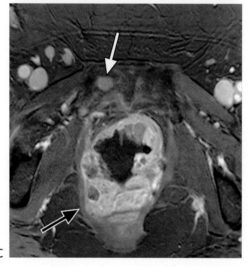

FIGURE 19.21. Clear cell adenocarcinoma of urethra, originally arising in a urethral diverticulum, with **(A)** heterogeneous intermediate signal mass (*arrows*) on sagittal T2WI, **(B)** mottled enhancement (*arrows*) and loss of adjacent fat planes on sagittal T1WI postcontrast, and **(C)** central necrosis on axial T1WI postcontrast. The final image also shows a pubic bone metastasis (*white arrow*) and bowing of the right puborectalis sling with likely invasion (*black arrow*).

from periurethral glands or diverticula (Fig. 19.21), and metastatic (Fig. 19.22) or direct involvement by other neoplasms. The appearance varies with tissue type, generally including solid masses with varying degrees of enhancement, central necrosis, and local invasiveness. Urethral leiomyomas are rare and difficult to distinguish from other masses by imaging. The role of the radiologist in such cases is precise anatomic delineation to enable surgical planning, usually requiring 3T MRI with small field of view T2WI and T1WI postcontrast, and systemic staging with CT or PET/CT when appropriate.

Vagina

Vaginal leiomyomas are much less common than uterine leiomyomas and exhibit similar imaging characteristics. Primary vaginal cancer is also uncommon, usually squamous in histology and frequently associated with human papilloma virus (HPV) infection. Vaginal cancer is evident on T2WI as an intermediate signal plaque or polyp (Fig. 19.23), sometimes with ulceration, with associated enhancement on T1WI postcontrast, and high signal on diffusion-weighted imaging (DWI). If superficial or limited to the upper vagina, vaginal cancer can sometimes be surgically resected. If infiltrative, it is often treated with primary chemoradiotherapy, which can be image guided (Fig. 19.24). Nodal metastatic sites depend on location, with inguinal node involvement from lesions near the introitus and obturator and iliac involvement from upper and mid-vaginal cancers.

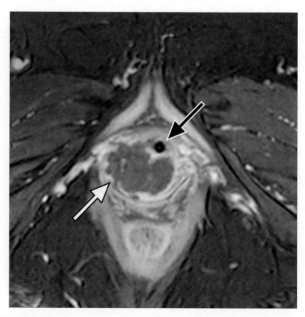

FIGURE 19.22. Urethral metastasis from cervical cancer with hypoenhancing mass (*white arrow*) eccentrically encasing ureter, with Foley catheter in lumen (*black arrow*) on axial T1WI postcontrast.

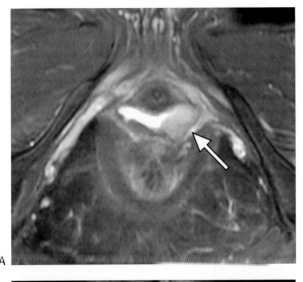

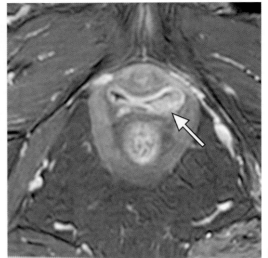

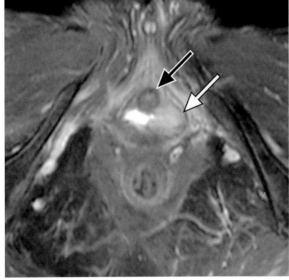

FIGURE 19.23. Primary squamous cancer of vagina with **(A)** intermediate signal mass (*arrow*) on axial T2WI and **(B)** thick, irregular enhancement (*arrow*) compared to normal mucosa on axial T1WI postcontrast. **C:** Axial T2WI more inferiorly shows superficial involvement of the urethra (*black arrow*) by tumor (*white arrow*).

Vaginal metastases or local tumor recurrence are more common than primary vaginal cancer and may appear years after hysterectomy for endometrial or cervical carcinoma (Fig. 19.25). Attention to the vaginal cuff is an important part of imaging surveillance in such patients. Vaginal lymphoma is rare, often submucosal, and should be diagnosed by biopsy.

Vulva

Most vulvar cancer is primary squamous cell carcinoma. Although vulvar cancer is less common than other gynecologic malignancies, 6,000 new cases are projected in the United States in 2016. Vulvar cancer in younger women is associated with HPV 16 and 18, tends to be multifocal and recurrent, and can be highly morbid due to the need for multiple surgeries. Vulvar cancer in older women is associated with chronic inflammation such as lichen planus. Vulvar cancer is a clinical diagnosis and a surgical disease whenever possible, so the utility of imaging is to evaluate for local extent and inguinal node involvement. FIGO staging is most widely used for vulvar cancer, summarized in Table 19.2. As with other perineal lesions, preoperative MR imaging should include small field of view, high-resolution T2WI, T1WI pre- and postcontrast, and DWI. As in other sites, vulvar squamous carcinoma has intermediate signal on T2WI with spiculated or microlobulated margins,

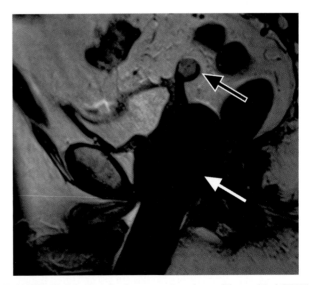

FIGURE 19.24. Brachytherapy planning with sagittal T2WI showing low-signal vaginal brachytherapy cylinder in the lumen (*white arrow*) and nodular endometrial cancer recurrence (*black arrow*) at the apex of the vaginal cuff.

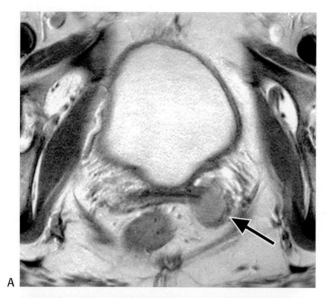

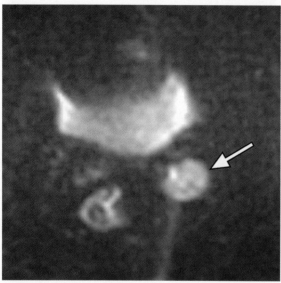

FIGURE 19.25. Cervical cancer recurrence at left vaginal cuff (*arrows*) with **(A)** intermediate signal mass on axial T2WI and **(B)** marked hyperintensity on axial DWI.

TABLE 19.2		
FIGO and TNM (AJCC) Staging of Vulvar Cancer		
FIGO Staging	TNM Staging	Description
I		Tumor confined to vulva
IA	T1a N0 M0	Lesions ≤2 cm in size and stromal invasion ≤1 mm, no nodes
IB	T1b N0 M0	Lesions >2 cm in size or stromal invasion >1 mm, no nodes
II	T2 N0 M0	Tumor any size, involves adjacent perineal structures (lower urethra or vagina, anus), no nodes
III		Tumor any size, ± local invasion, positive inguinofemoral nodes
IIIA	T1-2 N1a or b M0	1–2 nodal metastasis <5 mm or 1 node ≥5 mm
IIIB	T1-2 N2a or b M0	≥3 nodes <5 mm or ≥2 nodes ≥5 mm
IIIC	T1-2 N2c M0	Positive nodes with extracapsular spread
IV		Tumor involves regional or distant structures
IVA	T3 N0-2 M0 or T1-2 N3 M0	(T3) Transmural involvement of upper urethra or vagina, bladder, rectum, or adherence to pelvic bone OR (N3) fixed, ulcerated inguinofemoral nodes
IVB	T3 N0-3 M1	Distant metastasis including pelvic lymph nodes

variable enhancement and central necrosis, and high signal on DWI. Involvement of adjacent organs (clitoris, urethra, bladder, anus, rectum), muscles, bones, vasculature, and nodes should be detailed (Fig. 19.26) in preparation for surgical resection. Alternately, CT or PET/CT can be used for inguinal node evaluation. Lymph nodes involved by squamous carcinomas are often necrotic and may appear cystic (Fig. 19.27). Inguinal and femoral node involvement is a dire prognostic sign, indicating stage III disease and expected 5-year survival of about 50%. Thus, it is very important for radiologists to evaluate and specifically comment on the size and morphology of these lymph nodes. Pelvic nodes are considered distant metastases as they are further up the chain of drainage and indicate stage IV disease.

Vulvar melanoma, sweat gland tumors, Bartholin gland adenocarcinoma, and metastatic disease (Fig. 19.28) are other diagnostic considerations best diagnosed by tissue biopsy.

Rare Tumors

Perineal mesothelial tumors include fibromas, rare sarcomas, and the unusual but highly characteristic aggressive angiomyxoma (Fig. 19.29). Neurogenic tumors (Fig. 19.30) are also rare but underscore the importance of a multiparametric approach to distinguish solid masses from apparent "cysts" at imaging.

CONCLUSION

The female perineum is an anatomically and functionally complex space where a variety of benign and malignant pathologies may arise. Both fluoroscopic and MR defecography can provide important information about pelvic floor function and organ prolapse. Ultrasound and MRI have primary diagnostic roles in the soft tissues of the perineum, contributing to the diagnosis of benign pathologies and staging and surveillance of perineal malignancies. Ongoing refinements in the spatial and contrast resolution of these modalities allow radiologists to visualize and assess perineal structures that were not previously detectable by imaging, offering new opportunities for contributions to patient care.

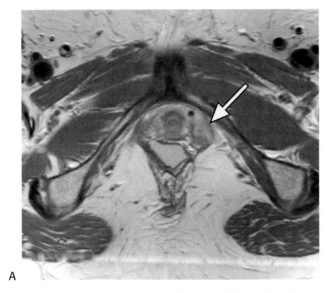

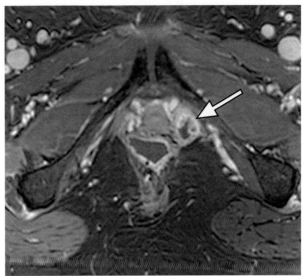

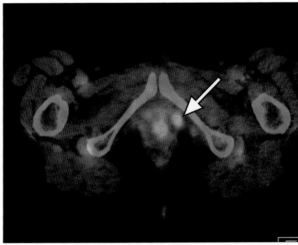

FIGURE 19.26. Squamous cell carcinoma of vulva with **(A)** intermediate signal mass (*arrow*) on axial T2WI, approaching but not involving the urethra or left clitoral crus, **(B)** peripherally enhancing mass (*arrow*) on axial T1WI postcontrast, and **(C)** corresponding focal ¹⁸FDG hyperavidity (*arrow*) on fused PET/CT. PET/CT is particularly helpful in this context because positive inguinal or femoral lymph nodes or distant disease may substantially impact surgical plan.

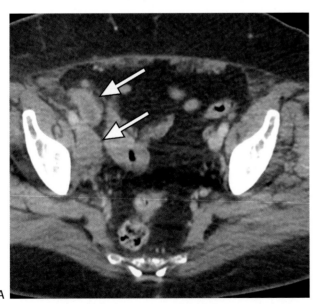

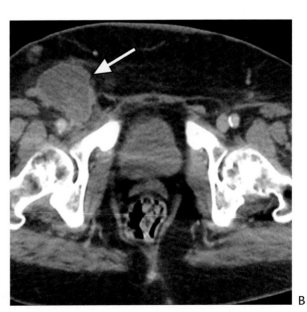

FIGURE 19.27. Lymph node metastases (*arrows*) from right-sided vulvar squamous cell carcinoma in the **(A)** obturator and external iliac and **(B)** inguinal node groups on CECT. Note that the largest lymph nodes become centrally necrotic and cystic in appearance.

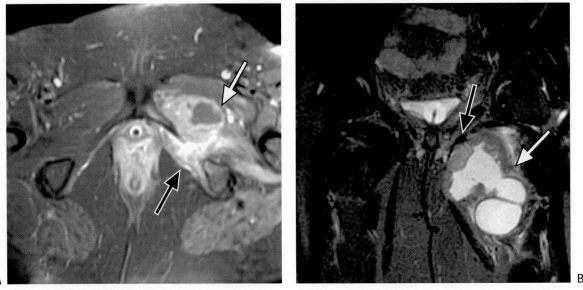

FIGURE 19.28. Endometrial cancer metastasis presenting as a vulvar mass. Axial T1 postcontrast **(A)** and coronal T2WI **(B)** illustrate an expansile mass (*white arrows*) with central necrosis involving obturator fossa and extending into upper thigh, with involvement of ischiocavernosus muscle (*black arrows*).

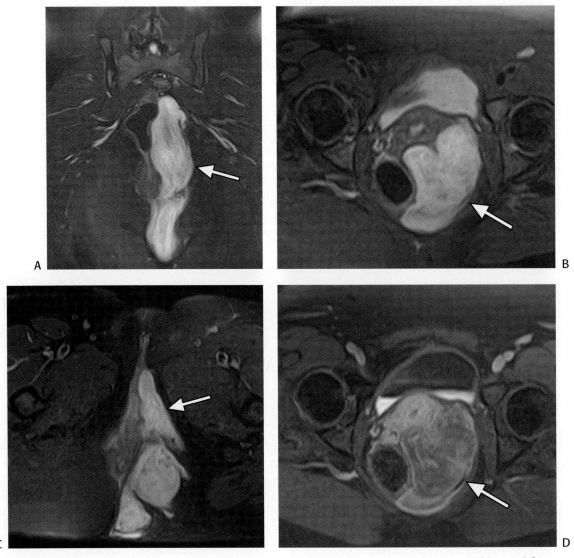

FIGURE 19.29. Aggressive angiomyxoma of vulva (*arrows*) involving mesorectal space, ischiorectal fossa, and labia, evident as a very high-signal mass on **(A)** coronal and **(B, C)** axial T2WI with fat saturation and **(D)** exhibiting definite enhancement on T1WI postcontrast. This is a histologically benign tumor with an infiltrative growth pattern and propensity for local recurrence.

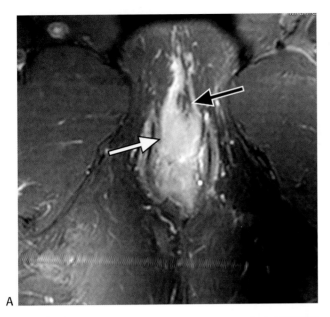

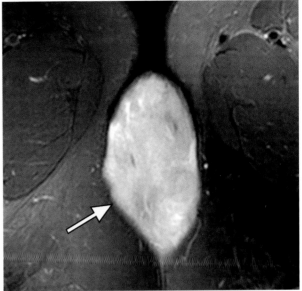

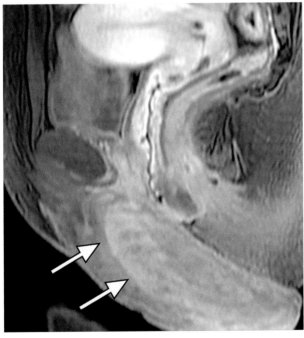

FIGURE 19.30. Perineal schwannoma with **(A, B)** very high signal (*white arrows*) and intimate association with clitoral body (*black arrow*) on axial T2WI and **(C)** diffuse enhancement of the mass (*arrows*) on T1WI postcontrast.

SUGGESTED READINGS

Agarwal MD, Resnick EL, Mhuircheartaigh JN, et al. MRI of the female rerineum: clitoris, labia, and introitus. *Magn Reson Imaging Clin N Am.* 2017, in press.

Bitti GT, Argiolas GM, Ballicu N, et al. Pelvic floor failure: MR imaging evaluation of anatomic and functional abnormalities. *Radiographics.* 2014;34:429–448.

Brandon CJ, Lewicky-Gaupp C, Larson KA, et al. Anatomy of the perineal membrane as seen in magnetic resonance images of nulliparous women. *Am J Obstet Gynecol.* 2009;200(5):583.e1–583.e6.

Dahiya K, Jain S, Duhan N, et al. Aggressive angiomyxoma of vulva and vagina: a series of three cases and review of literature. *Arch Gynecol Obstet.* 2011;283(5):1145–1148.

Heller DS. Benign tumors and tumor-like lesions of the vulva. *Clin Obstet Gynecol.* 2015;58(3):526–535.

Hosseinzadeh K, Heller MT, Houshmand G. Imaging of the female perineum in adults. *Radiographics.* 2012;32:E129–E168.

Khatri G, Diaz de Leon A, Lockhart M. MR imaging of the pelvic floor. *Magn Reson Imaging Clin N Am.* 2017, in press.

Lakhman Y, Nougaret S, Micco M, et al. Role of MR imaging and FDG PET/CT in selection and follow-up of patients treated with pelvic exenteration for gynecologic malignancies. *Radiographics.* 2015;35(4):1295–1313.

Langer JE, Oliver ER, Lev-Toaff AS, et al. Imaging of the female pelvis through the life cycle. *Radiographics.* 2012;32:1575–1597.

Lee SI, Oliva E, Hahn PF, et al. Malignant tumors of the female pelvic floor: imaging features that determine therapy: pictorial review. *AJR Am J Roentgenol.* 2011;196:S15–S23.

Micco M, Sala E, Lakhman Y, et al. Imaging features of uncommon gynecologic cancers. *AJR Am J Roentgenol.* 2015;205(6):1346–1359.

NCCN Guidelines: Vulvar Cancer. National Comprehensive Cancer Network Clinical Practice Guidelines in Oncology. Version I. 2017. nccn.org

Ravier E, Lopex JG, Augros M, et al. Case report and review of the literature: a perineal schwannoma. *Prog Urol.* 2011;21:360–363.

Shetty AS, Menias CO. MR imaging of vulvar and vaginal cancer. *Magn Reson Imaging Clin N Am.* 2017, in press.

20

Urinary Tract Trauma

Urinary tract injuries, which represent up to 10% of traumatic abdominal injuries, can be categorized as blunt, penetrating, or iatrogenic. In many patients, especially those who have suffered from blunt trauma, the severity of a urinary tract injury is difficult to judge from physical examination. For this reason, imaging studies are frequently obtained in patients in whom urinary tract injuries are possible.

RENAL INJURIES

Clinical Features: Blunt Trauma

Blunt trauma accounts for about 80% of all renal injuries. Approximately three-fourths of reported renal injuries occur in men younger than 50 years of age, and when they occur, they tend to be more severe in children than adults. Motor vehicle crashes account for at least one-half of reported blunt trauma injuries to the kidneys, with falls, altercations, industrial accidents, and sports injuries accounting for most of the remainder.

Most blunt trauma renal injuries occur in patients suffering multisystem trauma, with the only exception being sports-related injuries, where even severe renal injuries can be isolated. The liver and spleen are the other abdominal organs most commonly associated with renal injury, followed by the pancreas, colon, and small bowel.

While hematuria is commonly encountered after blunt abdominal injury, most adults and children with traumatic renal injuries after blunt trauma do not require surgical treatment. It has been argued that normotensive patients with microscopic hematuria do not need imaging, since even if any renal injuries are present, no treatment will be necessary. In comparison, imaging of the kidneys should always be performed in hypotensive patients with microscopic hematuria or in normotensive patients with gross hematuria.

Some of these patients may have active bleeding detected on imaging studies, in which case angiography is usually obtained, followed by embolization, if a bleeding artery can be identified.

Clinical Features: Penetrating Trauma

Penetrating renal injuries fall into two major categories: (1) those related to stabbings and (2) those related to gunshot wounds. Many stab wounds to the kidneys are not associated with other injuries. In contrast, more than 80% of gunshot wounds of the kidney are associated with other abdominal injuries, usually of the bowel, pancreas, diaphragm, liver, or spleen. In comparison to blunt trauma, any hematuria after a penetrating injury is a sign of renal damage, and further evaluation is needed.

In the past, most patients with penetrating injuries in whom a renal injury was suspected (due to either the mechanism of injury or the presence of hematuria) underwent surgical exploration. The mere demonstration that the kidney was in the path of a penetrating injury, even in the absence of hematuria, was an indication for surgical exploration; however, it has been shown that limited posterior stab wounds that do not penetrate the renal fossa can be managed conservatively. It has also been recently suggested that patients who have had gunshot wounds, who have no clinical evidence of peritonitis and no hypotension, and who can be evaluated reliably with serial physical examinations can be managed conservatively. Surgery may not be needed in many of these patients.

Anatomy and Mechanism of Injury

The kidneys are protected from injury by the rib cage, the vertebral column, and the psoas muscles. The fascial coverings of the kidneys and the retroperitoneal fat provide additional protection.

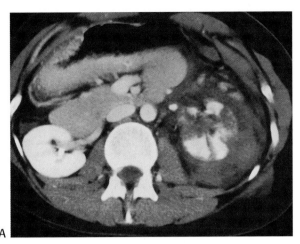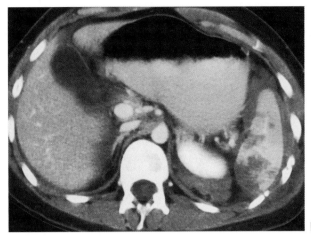

FIGURE 20.1. Renal and splenic injuries. A contrast-enhanced nephrographic-phase axial CT image through the mid left kidney shows multiple renal lacerations **(A)** with a large perinephric hematoma and **(B)** multiple splenic lacerations.

When this protection fails and there is blunt injury to the lower ribs or vertebrae, there is a higher incidence of renal injury. Splenic injury frequently accompanies injury to the left kidney (Fig. 20.1), whereas liver injury often accompanies injury to the right kidney (Fig. 20.2).

Blunt injuries of the kidneys occur as a result of a direct blow to the flank or from deceleration. With a direct blow, the kidney is crushed, causing intrarenal, subcapsular, or perinephric hematomas or any combination of these. Bleeding within the renal parenchyma results in an intrarenal hematoma. Bleeding that occurs between the renal parenchyma and the renal capsule results in a subcapsular hematoma. If the capsule is also torn, hemorrhage spills into the perinephric space but is confined by Gerota fascia, resulting in a perinephric hematoma. Bleeding into the perinephric space is frequently self-limited because Gerota fascia provides a tamponade effect. Only rarely does hemorrhage extend beyond Gerota fascia into other spaces of the retroperitoneum.

Some blunt injuries produce one or more lacerations of the renal parenchyma. Lacerations may be superficial or deep. When a laceration extends entirely through the kidney, separating it into

two or more fragments, the kidney is said to be fractured. With an acute deceleration injury, acute tension on the renal pedicle may produce a laceration of the renal vein or artery, resulting in an intimal tear in the vessel that may cause complete thrombosis of the renal artery, renal pedicle avulsion, or, rarely, avulsion of the ureteropelvic junction (UPJ).

Penetrating trauma, when it affects the kidney, usually results in direct injury of the renal parenchyma, vascular pedicle, or collecting system. Iatrogenic renal injuries may occur from renal biopsy, from percutaneous nephrostomy placement, or during surgery (Fig. 20.3). Iatrogenic injuries may result in bleeding (subcapsular or perinephric hematoma), pseudoaneurysm, arteriovenous fistula, or urinoma formation.

Diagnostic Approach to Imaging Renal Trauma

After blunt trauma, patients who are normotensive and who have no or only microscopic hematuria are exceedingly unlikely to have a significant urinary tract injury. For this reason, imaging is not

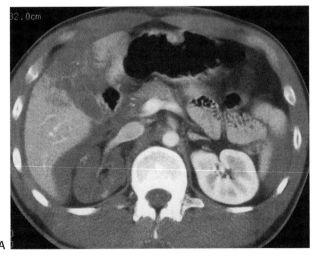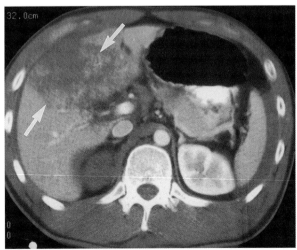

FIGURE 20.2. Renal and hepatic injuries. **A:** A contrast-enhanced corticomedullary-phase axial CT image demonstrates absent enhancement of the right kidney as a result of renal infarction. Adjacent intraperitoneal fluid represents a hemoperitoneum. There is also heterogeneous diminished perfusion of the liver adjacent to the gallbladder and **(B)** a large liver laceration (*arrows*).

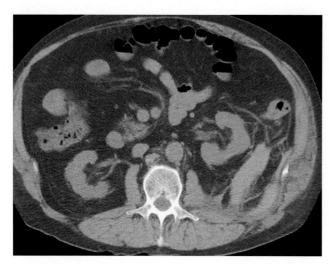

FIGURE 20.3. Perinephric hematoma. An unenhanced axial CT image obtained in a patient after a renal biopsy demonstrates poorly defined high-attenuation material adjacent to the posterior and posterolateral aspects of the left kidney, representing a large perinephric hematoma.

needed, if solely performed to evaluate the urinary tract in these patients. In comparison, renal imaging should always be performed in patients with gross hematuria (whether they are normotensive or hypotensive) as well as in patients with microscopic hematuria who are also hypotensive.

Indications for imaging after penetrating renal trauma are different from those suffering blunt trauma. It is recommended that imaging be performed in any patient with any degree of hematuria after penetrating trauma. In addition, imaging should be performed even in the absence of hematuria, when the mechanism of injury raises concern for urinary tract trauma.

As a rule, evaluation of the lower urinary tract in a patient who has had blunt trauma to the pelvis (with or without abdominal trauma) should precede evaluation of the upper urinary tract. In male patients, retrograde urethrography should precede cystography, to evaluate the patient for a urethral injury. Conventional cystography can then be performed to evaluate the bladder. When computed tomography (CT) is performed to assess all of the abdominal organs, CT cystography can be performed at the same time as standard abdominopelvic CT and substituted for conventional cystography.

Radiologic Examination

Ultrasound

Ultrasound (US) is used as the initial imaging examination for evaluating patients with blunt abdominal trauma in some centers in the United States. US is portable and inexpensive, avoids ionizing radiation, and does not interfere with ongoing resuscitation. However, this examination is limited in patients with a large body habitus and when there is a large amount of bowel gas. Additionally, the quality of the US exam is operator dependent.

US is usually performed in emergency departments to determine if there is fluid or blood in the peritoneal cavity. On US, free intraperitoneal fluid may appear as a hypoechoic or anechoic region, most easily seen in the hepatorenal fossa, around the tip of the spleen or in the pelvis. If a screening US examination is positive, the patient must then have a CT examination for further evaluation.

A substantial limitation of US is the fact that a negative US does not exclude the presence of an abdominal visceral organ

injury. This is because acute hematomas, including those in the renal subcapsular or perinephric regions, may be echogenic rather than hypoechoic and may be difficult to detect. It may not be easy to distinguish hyperechoic perinephric hematomas from echogenic perinephric fat. For this reason, CT is often performed even after a patient has a "normal" US examination in the emergency department.

US may occasionally be useful to follow renal injuries that have been identified earlier by CT, especially in cases where it is desirable to limit radiation exposure to the patient (as in children and pregnant women); however, its utility is limited even as a follow-up study, as US is not able to evaluate the kidneys, renal collecting systems, and ureters with the same detail as CT.

Computed Tomography

Abdominal and pelvic CT remains the most commonly performed and most useful examination for imaging patients after blunt trauma. CT is also usually performed as a first-line study in patients who have suffered penetrating injury. Standard multirow detector CT (MDCT) images should be obtained after the intravenous administration of contrast material, usually as a dynamic bolus of 100 to 125 mL of iodinated nonionic contrast media at a concentration of 300 to 370 mg of iodine/mL. Imaging is typically obtained beginning 65 to 70 seconds after contrast media administration, during the portal venous phase of enhancement (when the kidneys are in the corticomedullary phase and when there are differences between renal cortical and medullary enhancement). This phase is utilized, because, although not ideal for the kidneys, it is optimal for evaluating all of the other abdominal organs. Arterial phase imaging may be obtained when a vascular injury is suspected in advance of imaging. Delayed or excretory-phase images obtained after contrast material has been excreted into the renal collecting systems should be performed whenever fluid is identified adjacent to the kidney, in order to exclude a urine leak, even when the renal parenchyma appears to be intact, as, on rare occasions, the renal collecting system or ureter can be disrupted in the absence of a renal parenchymal injury (Fig. 20.4).

Magnetic Resonance Imaging

The role of magnetic resonance imaging (MRI) in trauma patients is limited, particularly in the acute setting. MRI is often more logistically difficult to perform, as MR scanners are often located at a distance from the emergency department, while CT scanners are often located in emergency departments. Also, patients cannot be monitored in an MR scanner as easily as they can be during a CT examination.

In patients in whom there is a strong relative contraindication to contrast material administration (such as a history of a severe allergy to iodinated contrast media), MRI may be preferred over CT, however. MRI would be used preferentially in these patients to assess the vascular integrity of the kidney and the integrity of the renal collecting system. Occasionally, follow-up MR imaging of acute injuries documented on CT may also be performed.

Angiography

The use of angiography for diagnostic evaluation of renovascular injuries is no longer felt to be necessary; however, angiography is often obtained emergently in patients in whom CT has detected active arterial bleeding. Embolization can then be performed if an injured artery is identified (Fig. 20.5).

Classification of Traumatic Renal Injuries

Renal injuries can be classified into five grades according to the American Association of Surgeons in Trauma (AAST) system

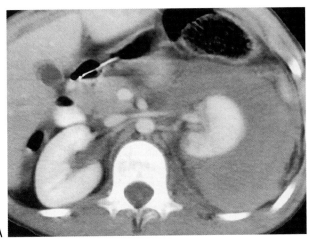
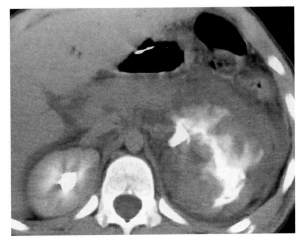

FIGURE 20.4 Perinephric hematoma and urine leak. **A:** Contrast-enhanced nephrographic-phase axial CT image shows a large amount of fluid surrounding the left kidney. The renal parenchyma appears to be intact. **B:** An excretory-phase image shows extravasation of excreted contrast material from the left renal collecting system into the perinephric space from a laceration that extends into the collecting system.

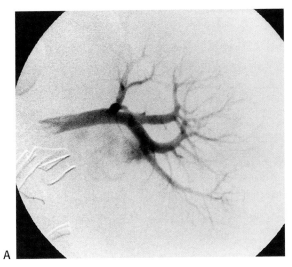
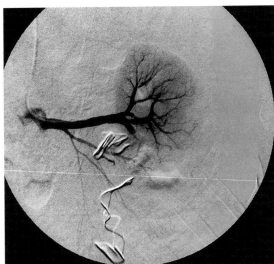

FIGURE 20.5. Traumatic renal hemorrhage. **A:** Conventional arteriogram obtained after selective injection of the left renal artery shows frank bleeding from a laceration of a lower segmental artery. **B:** After embolization with Gelfoam (Upjohn, Kalamazoo, Michigan), the bleeding was controlled.

(Table 20.1) or merely divided into three categories, as minor (including AAST grade I and II injuries), intermediate (including grade III and IV injuries), and major (grade V injuries). The AAST classification is generally used when renal injuries are detected on CT.

About 80% of AAST renal injuries are classified as grade I injuries. These include parenchymal contusions and small subcapsular hematomas. The remaining 20% of renal injuries are divided evenly among the remaining four grades of injuries (about 5% each).

TABLE 20.1	
Renal Injury Scale of the American Association of Surgeons in Trauma	
Grade	Injury Description
1	• Nonenlarging subcapsular hematoma with no laceration
	• Contusion with no laceration
2	• Nonexpanding perirenal hematoma confined to the retroperitoneum
	• Superficial laceration (<1 cm depth) in the renal cortex, which does not involve the renal collecting system
3	• Laceration > 1 cm depth in the renal cortex that do not involve the collecting system (with no urinary extravasation seen on delayed enhanced imaging)
4	• Expanding subcapsular hematoma
	• Laceration extending into the renal pelvis
	• Extravasation of urine from the renal collecting system
	• Injury to main renal artery or vein, with contained hemorrhage
	• Segmental infarctions without lacerations
5	• Shattered kidney
	• Intimal dissection with complete renal artery thrombosis
	• Avulsion of renal pedicle with renal devascularization

Problems with AAST classification system include the fact that it does not take into account CT identification of active bleeding, which can be due to disruption of a renal artery or renal artery branch, a pseudoaneurysm, or an arteriovenous fistula. Visualized active bleeding is generally considered to be an indication for emergent angiography with embolization, if the source of bleeding can be identified during angiography. Additionally, isolated UPJ disruption is not included in this system, an injury, which usually requires prompt treatment. Due to these limitations, a complete description of renal injuries on imaging studies requires that information additional to the AAST classification be provided. Specifically, comments should be made about any active bleeding or evidence of an isolated renal collecting system or ureteral injury.

Minor Renal Injuries

Minor injuries (AAST grade I and II injuries) may be treated expectantly and rarely require surgical intervention. The vast majority of minor renal injuries, most of which do not involve a break in the renal capsule, consist of small- to moderate-sized intrarenal hematomas or renal contusions. Other injuries in this group include small subcapsular or perinephric hematomas, small cortical lacerations, and subsegmental renal infarcts. While most of these injuries result from blunt trauma, they can also be seen after penetrating trauma and can occasionally be iatrogenic (such as after extracorporeal shock wave lithotripsy).

On US, intrarenal hematomas are seen as poorly marginated areas of either decreased or increased echogenicity within the cortex (Figs. 20.6 and 20.7). On CT, intrarenal hematomas are seen as rounded or ovoid, poorly marginated areas of decreased attenuation within the renal parenchyma (Fig. 20.8). In some cases, renal lacerations may be visualized extending into the hematoma itself (Fig. 20.9).

On US, subcapsular and perinephric hematomas may be seen as collections of varying echogenicity that abut the kidneys (Fig. 20.10). On CT, subcapsular hematomas appear as rounded or elliptical areas of decreased attenuation located between the renal cortex and the renal capsule. Such hematomas indent or flatten the renal margins, as they exert a compressive force against the renal parenchyma (Fig. 20.11). Perinephric hematomas are located between the renal capsule and Gerota fascia. They do not indent or

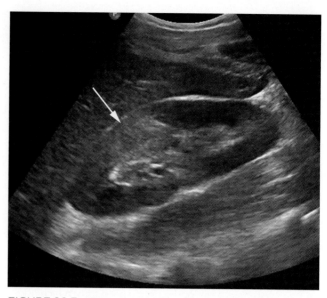

FIGURE 20.7. Ultrasound of a renal contusion and intrarenal hematoma. Longitudinal ultrasound image of the right kidney shows increased renal parenchymal echogenicity in the area of a renal contusion, due to the presence of an intrarenal hematoma (*arrow*).

flatten the renal contour (Fig. 20.12). They may be associated with an intrarenal hematoma or with a concomitant subcapsular hematoma (Fig. 20.13). Perinephric hematomas may be quite large and may extend inferiorly into the true pelvis following the cone of renal fascia. They can also displace the kidney anteriorly. Conversely, on occasion, perinephric hematomas may be quite localized and simulate a subcapsular collection. This is because the blood can be accumulated between the bridging septa that are located in the perinephric space.

The CT attenuation of hematomas depends upon their age, with acute hematomas having a higher attenuation value than unenhanced renal parenchyma (Fig. 20.14). With time, hematomas will develop areas of decreased attenuation due to liquefaction of the clot. A subacute or chronic hematoma may also develop a thin enhancing rim (Fig. 20.15).

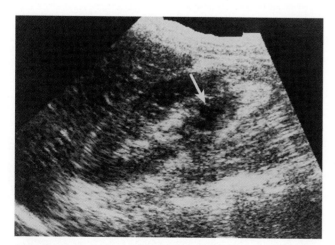

FIGURE 20.6. Ultrasound of a renal contusion and intrarenal hematoma. Longitudinal ultrasound image of the right kidney shows decreased renal parenchymal echogenicity in an area of renal contusion, due to the presence of an intrarenal hematoma (*arrow*). There is anterior displacement of the lower pole of the right kidney.

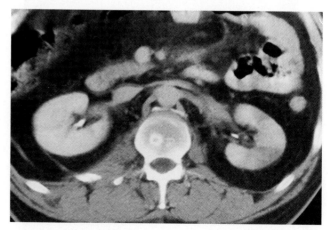

FIGURE 20.8. CT of a renal contusion and intrarenal hematoma. A contrast-enhanced nephrographic-phase axial CT image shows two subtle low-attenuation areas in the left kidney, representing renal contusions.

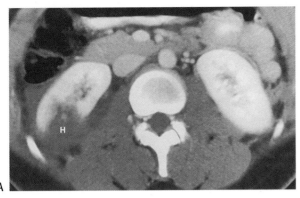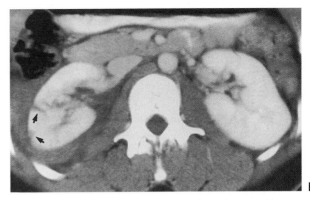

FIGURE 20.9. CT of an intrarenal hematoma and renal lacerations. **A:** A contrast-enhanced nephrographic-phase axial CT image shows a large hematoma in the right kidney (H). **B:** A more caudal image shows two small adjacent linear renal lacerations (*arrows*), as well as a small right perinephric hematoma.

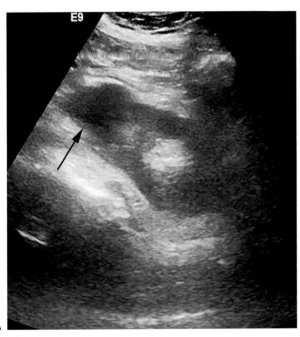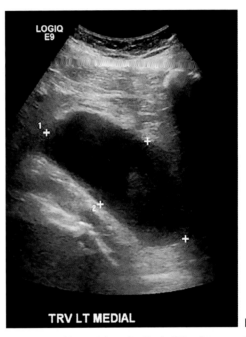

FIGURE 20.10. Ultrasound of a subcapsular hematoma. Transverse **(A)** and longitudinal **(B)** ultrasound images in a patient who sustained blunt trauma show a heterogeneous subcapsular hematoma along the medial aspect of the left kidney (*arrow*).

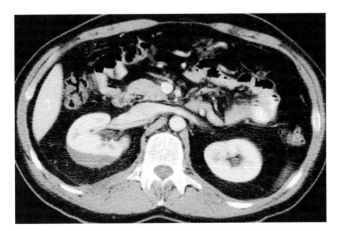

FIGURE 20.11. CT of a subcapsular hematoma. A contrast-enhanced corticomedullary-phase axial CT image demonstrates a small subcapsular hematoma adjacent to the posterior aspect of the right kidney. The contour of the kidney is deformed due to pressure from the hematoma, a characteristic feature.

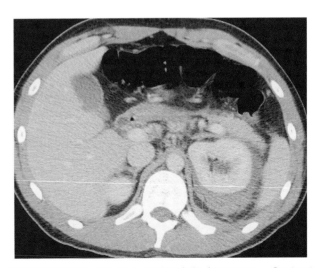

FIGURE 20.12. CT of a perinephric hematoma. Contrast-enhanced nephrographic-phase axial CT image demonstrates a hematoma in the left perinephric space. Note that the hematoma does not compress or deform the renal parenchyma.

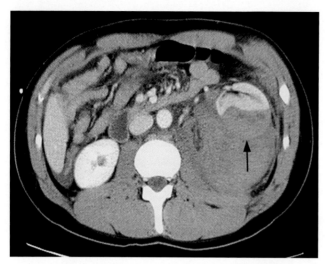

FIGURE 20.13. CT of combined subcapsular and perinephric hematoma. A contrast-enhanced corticomedullary-phase axial CT image demonstrates a large hematoma adjacent to the left kidney. A subcapsular component (*arrow*) deforms the renal contour. A large perinephric component is located more posteriorly.

Intermediate Injuries

Approximately 10% of traumatic renal injuries are intermediate in severity (AAST grade III and IV injuries). These intermediate injuries, which are well seen on CT, are usually managed conservatively. On occasion, surgical intervention may be required, particularly if clinical deterioration develops. Injuries in this category include major renal lacerations that extend beyond the renal capsule. Extensive perirenal hematomas are usually present in these cases. Many of these deep lacerations also extend to involve the renal collecting systems, with resultant extravasation of contrast medium into the retroperitoneum seen on CT images (or even conventional radiographs) obtained after renal excretion of previously administered intravascular contrast material. Vascular

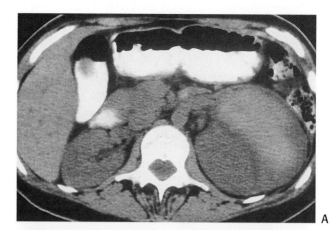

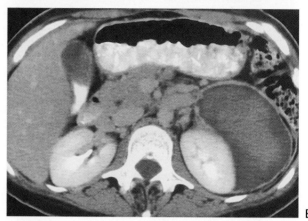

FIGURE 20.15. CT of a large subacute subcapsular hematoma. **A:** An unenhanced axial CT image shows high-attenuation and low-attenuation components of blood in a large fluid collection adjacent to the left kidney. **B:** On a subsequently obtained contrast-enhanced excretory-phase axial image, a relatively thick rind is seen surrounding the hematoma, indicating that the hematoma is organizing and consistent with its being subacute rather than acute.

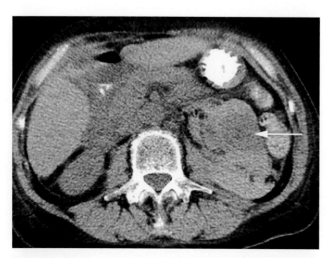

FIGURE 20.14. Noncontrast CT of an acute perinephric hematoma. An unenhanced axial CT image shows a complex fluid collection surrounding the left kidney. The collection has higher attenuation than does the unenhanced kidney (*arrow*).

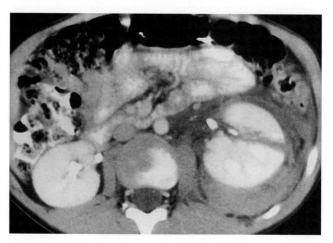

FIGURE 20.16. CT of a large renal laceration. A contrast-enhanced excretory-phase axial CT image shows a large linear laceration in the left kidney with an associated left perinephric hematoma.

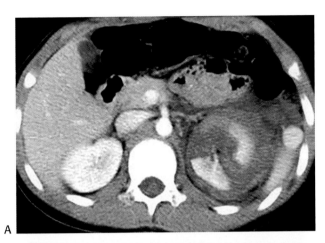

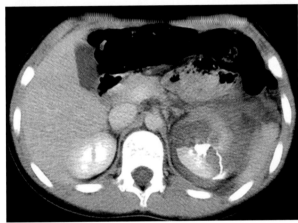

FIGURE 20.17. CT of a renal fracture with renal collecting system injury. **A:** A contrast-enhanced corticomedullary-phase axial CT image shows two completely separate enhancing fragments of the left kidney. There is a large amount of associated perinephric fluid. **B:** A delayed enhanced image obtained after excretion of contrast material into the renal collecting systems demonstrates excreted contrast material extravasating into the posterior component of the perinephric fluid.

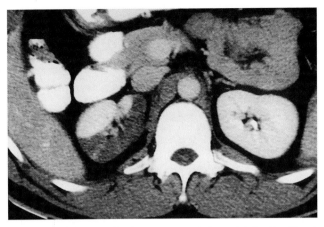

FIGURE 20.18. CT of a large segmental renal infarct without a cortical rim sign. A contrast-enhanced excretory-phase axial CT image shows a large nonenhancing area in the upper pole of the right kidney, which resulted from traumatic occlusion of the posterior segmental branch of the right renal artery. Note that there is no cortical rim sign surrounding the infarct at this time.

a traumatic infarction has occurred. It may take several hours for a cortical rim to appear.

Major Injuries

Major injuries (ASST grade V Injuries), which account for approximately 5% of all renal injuries, may pose a threat to the viability of the kidney or result in life-threatening hemorrhage. In such situations, immediate transcatheter embolization is often performed if any active bleeding is identified. Major renal injuries include multiple renal lacerations, resulting in a shattered kidney, or injury of the renal pedicle, including thrombosis or laceration of one or more renal arteries or avulsion or laceration of one or more of the renal veins. With multiple lacerations, large

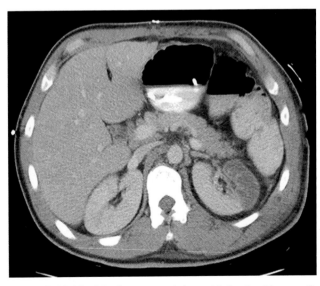

FIGURE 20.19. CT of a segmental renal infarct with a cortical rim sign. A contrast-enhanced nephrographic-phase axial CT image demonstrates nonperfusion of a wedge-shaped area in the lateral aspect of the left kidney. There is a thin cortical rim of enhancement around the periphery of the infarct, due to preserved flow through the capsular branch of the left renal artery.

injuries involving the segmental renal vessels are also included in this category.

On CT, the diagnosis of a major laceration can be made when a hematoma-filled cleft extends through the renal capsule and into the renal parenchyma (Fig. 20.16). If the laceration extends into the renal collecting system, opacified urine will extravasate into the perinephric space on delayed images (Fig. 20.17). If the lacerated segment has become devitalized, this portion of the kidney will not enhance after contrast material administration. Because this segment is surrounded by hematoma and does not enhance, it may be difficult to appreciate as a separate fragment.

Occlusion of a segmental renal vessel is the most common vascular injury of the kidney after blunt renal trauma. Such occlusion results in segmental renal infarction. On CT, infarcts appear as sharply demarcated wedge-shaped areas of diminished or absent contrast enhancement that extend to the renal cortex (Fig. 20.18). If the capsular blood supply remains intact, perfusion of the outer layer of cells results in characteristic enhancement of the cortical rim (Fig. 20.19). This cortical rim sign along the periphery of renal infarcts may not be apparent immediately after

perinephric hematomas are commonly seen, and the tamponade effect of the renal fascia may be lost if the fascia is also torn. Multiple devitalized segments of renal parenchyma may be present (Fig. 20.20). Arterial injuries will be discussed in more detail in an ensuing section on vascular injuries.

Renal Collecting System Injuries

By definition, patients with traumatic renal injuries that result in extravasation of urine from the renal collecting systems have AAST grade IV or V injuries. These leaks are almost always detected on delayed enhanced (excretory-phase) series obtained at the time of the initial trauma CT. In one study by Fischer et al., only one of 26 patients had a subsequently diagnosed leak that was missed on excretory-phase images from the initial CT. The reason for this delayed diagnosis was uncertain; however, it is possible that in some patients, a hematoma may initially tamponade a defect in the renal collecting system. Fortunately, more than 90% of intrarenal collecting system leaks will resolve spontaneously (Fig. 20.21).

Vascular Injuries

A variety of traumatic vascular injuries can be encountered, including active arterial bleeding, renal artery dissections and avulsions, pseudoaneurysms, and arteriovenous fistulae. Renal venous

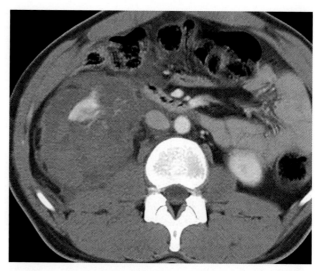

FIGURE 20.20. CT of a major renal injury. Only a single small vascularized segment of a shattered right kidney can be seen within a large right perinephric hematoma on this contrast-enhanced corticomedullary-phase axial CT image.

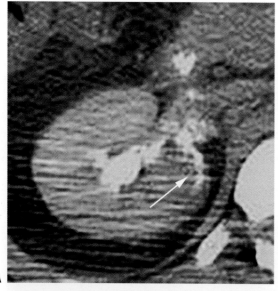

A

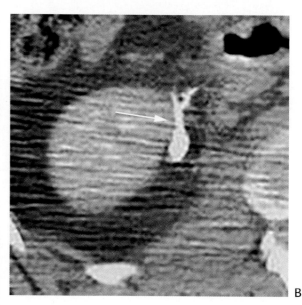

B

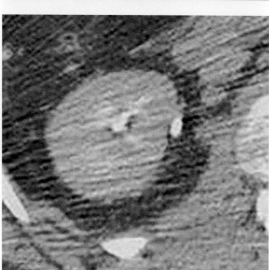

C

FIGURE 20.21. Resolution of a renal collecting system injury. **A, B:** A coned-down contrast-enhanced excretory-phase axial CT image of the midportion **(A)** and lower pole **(B)** of the right kidney shows contrast material leaking from the right renal collecting system into the renal sinus (*arrows*). **C:** One day later, the leak has already resolved.

injuries also occur, but these are difficult to diagnose on imaging studies, since they merely result in the development of hematomas. For these reason, they will not be addressed in any detail.

After blunt trauma, the most common severe main renal artery injuries are traumatic dissections of the renal artery or frank tears of the renal artery (occurring as a result of contrecoup tearing of the intima of the renal artery in patients suffering acute deceleration) or, less commonly, true renal pedicle avulsions. In traumatic dissections, the resulting intimal flap causes thrombosis of the renal artery, which is usually complete. In the majority of patients with these injuries, there is no significant associated perinephric or subcapsular hematoma (unless the injury has been caused by a penetrating wound or is associated with injuries to other organs). The net result of these injuries, if untreated, is usually global renal infarction with irreversible loss of renal function and parenchymal atrophy. There are isolated reports of spontaneous recovery of some renal function. In such cases, it is presumed that collateral renal circulation is able to preserve a small amount of functioning parenchyma.

Unfortunately, surgical repair of renal artery thrombosis or renal artery avulsion is seldom successful. Warm ischemia times for human kidneys (the maximum time allowed for reperfusion to be successful) have been reported to be as short as 1 to 6 hours by some investigators, whereas others report successful revascularization after much longer periods of time (12 to 20 hours). However, even when revascularization is attempted within this window, successful return of renal function usually does not occur. The majority of renal pedicle injuries occur in patients suffering multisystem trauma. Since associated injuries to other organs are often life threatening, it is not uncommon for several hours of warm ischemia to have occurred before consideration of renal-sparing surgery is even possible. In such circumstances, and in view of the absence of a significant incidence of late complications associated with even global renal infarction, many experts now feel that attempts at revascularization should be limited to the uncommon patient with bilateral renovascular injuries.

Pseudoaneurysms and traumatic arteriovenous fistulae almost always result from penetrating or iatrogenic renal injury. The majority of these injuries occur after percutaneous renal biopsy, are not hemodynamically significant, and close spontaneously. Clinically, pseudoaneurysms are often asymptomatic. In comparison, patients with arteriovenous fistulae, if the arteriovenous fistulae are large, may present with hypertension, left heart failure, and/or an audible bruit on physical examination.

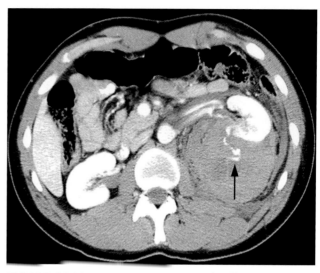

FIGURE 20.22. CT of active arterial bleeding into a perinephric hematoma. A contrast-enhanced corticomedullary-phase axial CT image shows a linear collection of contrast-enhanced blood extravasating into a large left perinephric hematoma (arrow). This patient subsequently underwent angioembolization of the bleeding vessel.

All renal arterial injuries can be diagnosed easily with CT. Diagnostic angiography is not needed for diagnosis; however, it is routinely performed prior to attempted embolization of bleeding vessels, pseudoaneurysms, or arteriovenous fistulae.

On CT, active arterial bleeding can be seen on arterial- or portal venous–phase images, as a brisk, often linear, area of enhancement within a subcapsular or perinephric fluid collection. This represents extraluminal extension of contrast-enhanced blood (Fig. 20.22). The degree of enhancement of the area of active bleeding is identical to that of the abdominal aorta. If delayed images are obtained, the amount of extravascular enhancement usually increases and becomes more amorphous as the blood diffuses into the adjacent hematoma.

On CT, thrombosis or avulsion of the main renal artery usually results in complete absence of contrast enhancement when imaging is performed shortly after injury (Figs. 20.23 and 20.24).

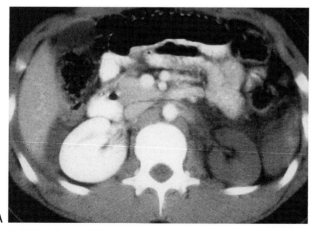
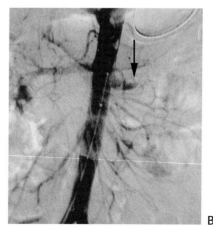

FIGURE 20.23. CT of traumatic renal artery thrombosis. **A:** A contrast-enhanced corticomedullary-phase axial CT image demonstrates complete lack of perfusion of the left kidney. **B:** An abdominal aortogram performed following the CT shows that there has been complete occlusion of a single left renal artery. Note that the "cutoff" involves the proximal portion of the renal artery (arrow).

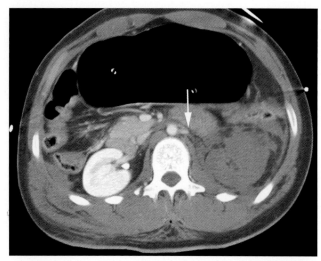

FIGURE 20.24. CT of traumatic renal artery thrombosis. A contrast-enhanced corticomedullary-phase axial CT image demonstrates uniform absence of perfusion of the left kidney. There is a small left perinephric hematoma. Note that the renal artery is occluded just a few centimeters distal to its origin (*arrow*).

Occlusion of a main renal artery usually occurs in the proximal one-third of the vessel (Figs. 20.23 and 20.24). In kidneys supplied by more than one renal artery, supply through the unaffected vessels may prevent total renal infarction from occurring (Fig. 20.25). In the majority of patients with renal pedicle injuries, there is no perinephric or subcapsular hematoma, unless this injury has been

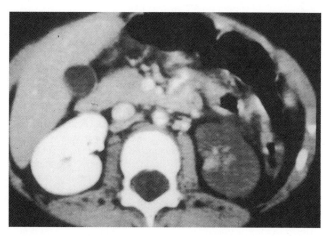

FIGURE 20.26. CT of traumatic renal artery thrombosis, with central perfusion due to periureteric collaterals. Contrast-enhanced corticomedullary-phase axial CT image obtained in a patient sustaining blunt trauma, shows near complete absence of perfusion of the left kidney. There is a small area of enhancement centrally, due to collateral flow from periureteric vessels.

caused by a penetrating wound or is associated with an injury of another organ.

In some cases, especially when the diagnosis of a renal pedicle injury is delayed, a rim of enhancement in the outer renal cortex may be present (cortical rim sign), because of circulation from capsular and collateral vessels (Fig. 20.19), or some renal parenchyma may be perfused in the renal sinus, because of circulation from periureteral collateral vessels (Fig. 20.26).

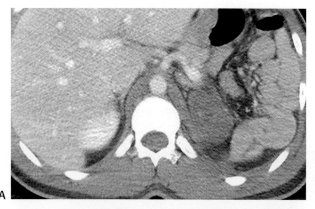

A

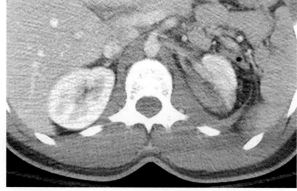

B

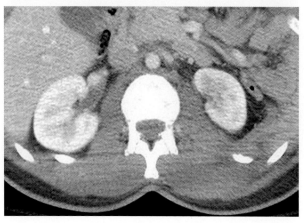

C

FIGURE 20.25. CT of traumatic occlusion of one of two left renal arteries. Contrast-enhanced corticomedullary-phase axial CT images through the upper pole **(A)**, midportion **(B)**, and lower pole **(C)** of the left kidney in a patient who sustained blunt trauma show the upper pole to be nonperfused, only the posterior aspect of the midkidney to be nonperfused, and the lower pole to be well perfused. This discrepant enhancement is due to traumatic thrombosis to an upper pole artery in a patient with two left renal arteries.

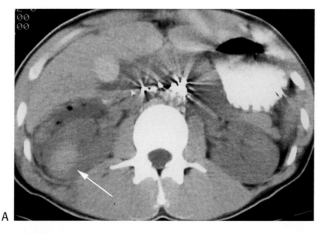

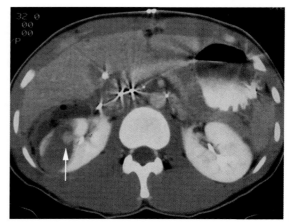

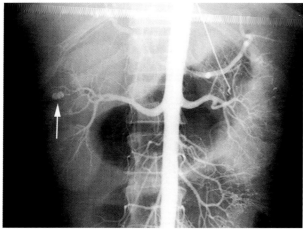

FIGURE 20.27. CT of a traumatic renal artery pseudoaneurysm after penetrating trauma. **A:** An unenhanced axial CT image in a patient who had undergone penetrating trauma shows high-attenuation material within the right kidney, consistent with an intrarenal hematoma (*arrow*). There is fluid and extraluminal gas along the anterior aspect of the right kidney. **B:** After contrast material administration, an excretory-phase axial CT image shows a large pseudoaneurysm within the intrarenal hematoma (*arrow*). Note that the pseudoaneurysm enhances to the same extent as the abdominal aorta. **C:** An aortogram shows the pseudoaneurysm arising from a right renal artery branch (*arrow*).

Pseudoaneurysms can be easily diagnosed on US, CT, or MRI. A focal rounded area is detected in the kidney, which on US demonstrates blood flow and on CT or MRI enhances with contrast material administration to the same extent as the adjacent abdominal aorta (Fig. 20.27).

Arteriovenous fistulae can also be easily detected on US, CT, or MRI. These result in the formation of prominent vessels, with dilated veins that demonstrate early and brisk enhancement.

There is early filling of the renal vein and the interior vena cava. In some instances, the adjacent nephrogram may be decreased (due to preferential flow of blood into veins rather than kidney parenchyma).

Renal venous injuries are much more difficult to diagnose than arterial injuries. They can be suspected in patients with expanding subcapsular or perinephric hematomas in whom no arterial source of bleeding can be identified (Fig. 20.28).

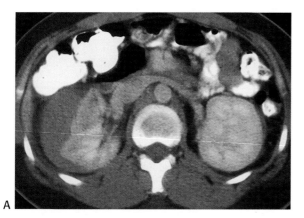

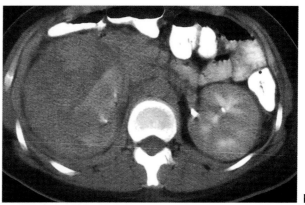

FIGURE 20.28. CT after a traumatic renal vein laceration. **A:** Contrast-enhanced corticomedullary-phase axial CT image shows a moderate-sized hematoma with compression of the lateral margin of the kidney. **B:** Three days later, after a further drop in the patient's hemoglobin, a repeat study performed without IV contrast material administration showed a marked increase in the size of the collection. At surgery, a laceration of the right renal vein was found.

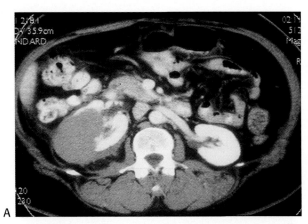

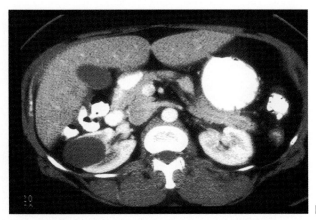

FIGURE 20.29. CT of a traumatic rupture of a right renal cyst. **A:** A contrast-enhanced corticomedullary-phase axial CT image shows a large hematoma in the mid right kidney, extending into the perinephric space. There is a large renal cortical defect. **B:** A contrast-enhanced corticomedullary-phase axial CT image obtained 2.5 years earlier shows that there was a large simple cyst in this area previously.

Traumatic Injuries to Abnormal Kidneys

In patients with a preexisting renal abnormality, even relatively minor trauma may cause disproportionate symptoms that bring the patient to medical attention. Such underlying conditions include renal calculi, renal tumors, renal cysts, and some congenital conditions, including UPJ obstructions, pelvic kidneys, and horseshoe kidneys.

Traumatic injuries to abnormal kidneys are often easily detected on CT (Fig. 20.29). Special care should be given to CT evaluation of patients with congenitally abnormal kidneys, particularly horseshoe kidneys, because, during blunt trauma, the isthmic portion (composed of either functioning renal parenchyma or a fibrous band, which crosses the midline) of a horseshoe kidney can be compressed directly against the spine without the protection of overlying anterior ribs (Figs. 20.30 and 20.31).

Imaging after Renal Trauma

There are a number of occasionally encountered early and late complications of renal trauma. Early complications include bleeding, infection, fistula, and urine leak with urinoma formation.

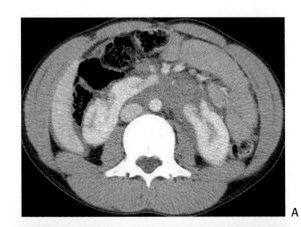

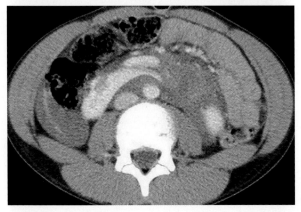

FIGURE 20.31. CT of a traumatic injury to a horseshoe kidney. **A:** A contrast-enhanced corticomedullary-phase axial CT image shows a large hematoma within and surrounding the medial aspect of the left moiety of a horseshoe kidney. **B:** An axial image obtained several centimeters more caudally again demonstrates the large hematoma, as well as discontinuity and irregularity of the perfused portions of the kidney.

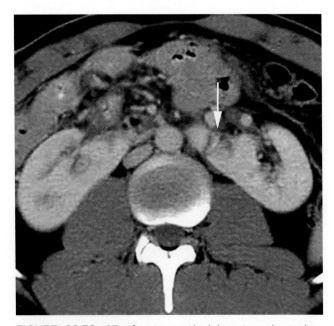

FIGURE 20.30. CT of a traumatic injury to a horseshoe kidney. A contrast-enhanced nephrographic-phase axial CT image shows a small heterogeneous linear defect in the medial aspect of the left moiety of a horseshoe kidney (*arrow*), representing a small area of renal laceration and contusion.

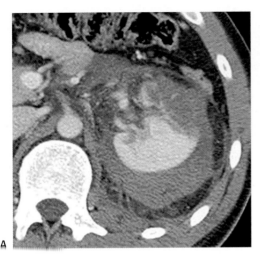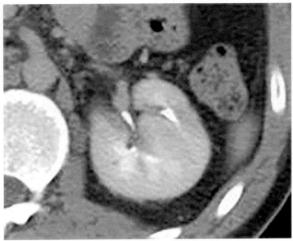

A   B

FIGURE 20.32. Resolution of a major traumatic renal injury. **A:** A contrast-enhanced corticomedullary-phase axial CT image of the left kidney shows a large area of disruption anteriorly, with perinephric hematoma. Excreted contrast material extravasated into the hematoma on delayed images (not shown), confirming the presence of renal collecting system leak. **B:** A contrast-enhanced excretory-phase axial CT image obtained 9 months later demonstrates complete healing of the injury. There is now only minimal irregularity of the renal contour and there is no perinephric fluid.

Late complications include persistent or new bleeding, urinary tract obstruction, fistula formation, and, rarely, hypertension (<5% of patients). Despite these complications, routine CT follow-up of patients after renal trauma, whether or not the patient has required treatment, is rarely necessary, providing the patients are asymptomatic and the initial renal injuries are not the most severe (< AAST grade V injuries). This is because the vast majority of patients who have complications after renal trauma are symptomatic (e.g., having pain, fever, leukocytosis, and/or hypertension), which indicates a need for imaging. It is not necessary to identify occasionally encountered asymptomatic posttraumatic renal abnormalities, such as renal parenchymal scarring, segmental infarctions, and persistent subcapsular or perinephric fluid (Fig. 20.32).

URETEROPELVIC JUNCTION INJURIES

Isolated tears or avulsions of the UPJ are rare. When they occur, the vascular supply of the renal pedicle remains intact, but the UPJ is sheared from its attachment to the renal pelvis, resulting in a urinoma. Injuries of the UPJ may be partial or complete. Distinction between these two types of injury is critical, as partial injuries may be treated with a stent, whereas complete disruptions require open surgery.

On imaging studies, patients with UPJ disruptions will always have abnormal fluid along the medial aspect of the perinephric space. This fluid may be present in the absence of any imaging evidence of a renal parenchymal injury (Fig. 20.33A). When such fluid is visualized on unenhanced or early enhanced CT images, delayed excretory-phase images should always be obtained, at which point excreted contrast material will be seen to accumulate within this fluid (Fig. 20.33B). With partial UPJ injuries, some contrast medium will be demonstrated in the ureter below the site of injury on excretory-phase contrast-enhanced imaging studies (Fig. 20.34). With complete disruptions, no continuity of the ureter is present and there will be no opacification of the ureter distal to the UPJ (Fig. 20.35), unless there is reflux of excreted contrast material from the bladder.

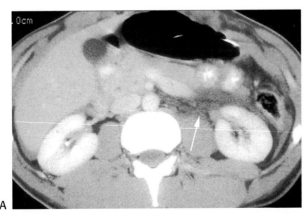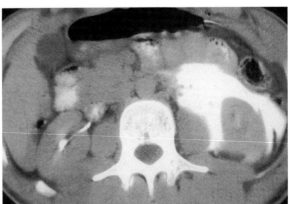

A   B

FIGURE 20.33. CT of a complete traumatic ureteropelvic junction disruption. **A:** A contrast-enhanced early excretory-phase image shows a small amount of fluid adjacent to the anteromedial aspect of the left kidney (*arrow*). The renal parenchyma is intact. **B:** A markedly delayed axial CT image shows that excreted contrast material has extravasated into the perinephric space.

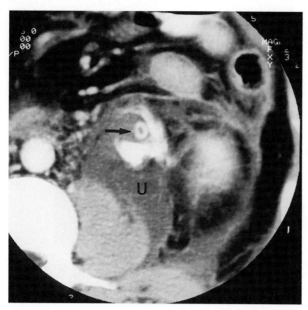

FIGURE 20.34. CT of a partial traumatic ureteropelvic junction disruption. A contrast-enhanced corticomedullary-phase axial CT image shows extravasation of contrast/urine adjacent to the left psoas muscle with formation of a urinoma (U). There is contrast material in the ureter (*arrow*), which surrounds a small filling defect, representing a blood clot. The ureteral opacification indicates that the UPJ disruption is only partial.

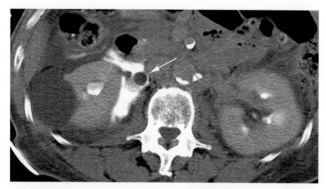

FIGURE 20.35. CT of a complete traumatic ureteropelvic junction disruption. Contrast-enhanced delayed excretory-phase axial CT image shows extensive extravasated contrast material along the medial aspect of the right kidney. There is no opacification of the right ureter (*arrow*), which is outlined by the contrast material, suggesting that the UPJ disruption is complete.

URETERAL INJURIES

Ureteral injuries are rare, accounting for <1% of all urinary tract injuries. Most ureteral injuries are iatrogenic, with many of these occurring during surgery and others during urologic procedures. They are also encountered after penetrating trauma. Ureteral injuries include partial or complete lacerations and ureteral contusions, the latter being injuries of the ureter that produce ureteral wall damage, but no frank laceration. As with UPJ disruptions, ureteral disruptions can be partial or complete.

Surgical injuries to the ureter have been seen after a variety of abdominal and pelvic procedures, with the greatest frequency of injuries reported after gynecologic operations, most commonly

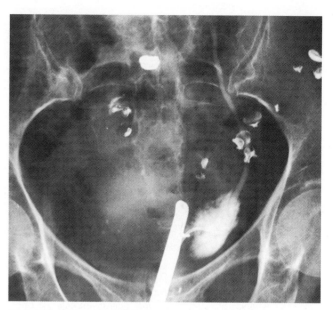

FIGURE 20.36. Ureteral injury demonstrated with retrograde pyelography. An anteroposterior abdominal radiograph obtained after cystoscopic cannulation of the distal left ureter in a patient who previously had a traumatic ureteral stone basketing procedure shows an amorphous collection of contrast material surrounding the distal left ureter.

hysterectomy. Injury of the ureters may also complicate abdominal–perineal resections, sigmoid colon resections, enterolysis, resection of abdominal aortic aneurysms, and lumbar laminectomies. The mechanism of surgical injury is often inadvertent ligation of the ureter; however, injury may also develop when the blood supply of the distal ureters is compromised during pelvic lymph node dissection. When the blood supply to the ureter is damaged, ureteral necrosis can ensue, with acute or subacute urinoma formation and development of a ureteral stricture. Surgical transection of the ureter can also result in urinoma formation. Given the mechanism of most surgical ureteral injuries, it is not surprising that the majority involve the distal rather than the proximal or mid ureter.

About half of all surgical ureteral injuries are recognized at the time of surgery. This allows for the injuries to be repaired during the operation. Unilateral ureteral injuries not recognized at surgery are often difficult to diagnose afterward. It may take weeks to even months to make a diagnosis. When symptoms occur, they are relatively nonspecific, consisting of ipsilateral flank pain and/or fever. A considerable minority of patients with ureteral injuries (25% to 50%) do not have hematuria, so the absence of hematuria does not mean that there is no ureteral damage. When ureteral injuries are unrecognized for long periods of time, fistulae may develop, often to the vagina or skin. Ureterovaginal fistulae usually result from leakage of extravasated urine through an anastomotic staple line at the vaginal vault and may become clinically apparent due to leakage of urine through the vagina.

In comparison to partial or complete unilateral ureteral disruptions, complete bilateral disruptions are generally recognized in the immediate postoperative period because of anuria.

Ureteral injuries may be encountered after a number of urologic procedures, including ureteroscopy, ureteral stone basketing, retrograde pyelography, and ureterolithotomy. Of these, ureteroscopy is the highest risk procedure. In most cases, the injury results from ureteral perforation. Ureteral injuries can be identified when they occur during some fluoroscopic urologic procedures, such as retrograde pyelography, where leakage of contrast material into the adjacent tissue is easily identified (Fig. 20.36).

Ureteral injuries after penetrating trauma can occur following gunshot wounds or stabbings. Nearly all ureteral injuries from penetrating trauma are associated with injuries to other organs. Ureteral contusion is most commonly seen after gunshot wounds, resulting from a blast effect of a bullet or bullet fragment on the ureter. Contusions are rarely encountered after other types of trauma, including stabbing or surgery.

Since surgical ureteral injuries may not be clinically suspected, abdomen and pelvic CT examinations may be obtained in postoperative patients to search for the source of fevers or pain. These are usually performed during the portal venous phase of contrast enhancement or, if the patient has a contrast allergy or compromised renal function, without intravenous contrast material administration. In these instances, the ureteral injury cannot be detected directly. Affected patients may have developed pelvocaliectasis or periureteric fluid collections representing urinomas, although these collections may not be distinguishable from seromas or abscesses if excretory-phase contrast-enhanced images are not obtained (Fig. 20.37). If these collections are subsequently aspirated, their etiology can be determined due to their very high creatinine levels.

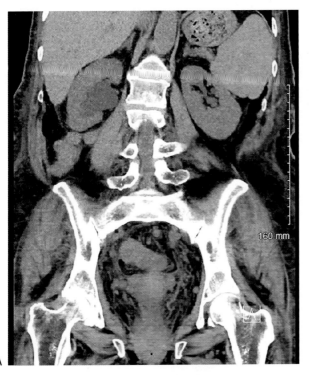
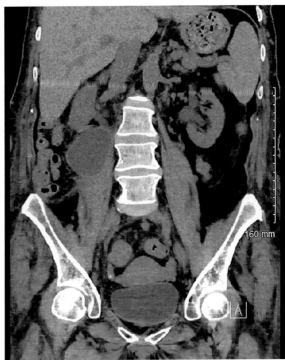
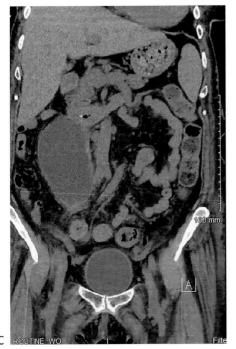

FIGURE 20.37. CT of a ureteral injury occurring during a right hemicolectomy. **A:** An unenhanced coronal reformatted CT image shows that the right renal calices and pelvis are dilated. **B:** A more anterior image shows a dilated right proximal ureter to be contiguous with a right-sided extraluminal fluid collection. **C:** The fluid collection, which was unexpected, representing a urinoma, is seen to be very large on an even more anteriorly obtained image.

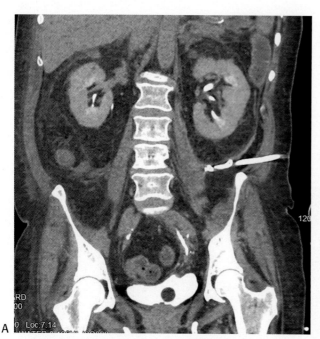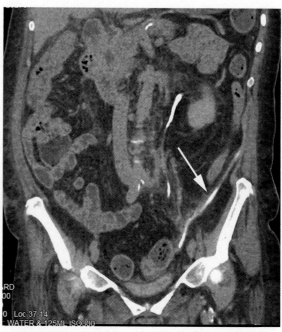

FIGURE 20.38. CT of ureteral injury occurring during an endoscopic procedure. **A:** A contrast-enhanced excretory-phase coronal reformatted CT image shows contrast material in both renal collecting systems. There is no renal collecting system dilatation. A percutaneous drainage catheter had been previously inserted into a left-sided extraperitoneal urinoma, which is now decompressed. **B:** A more anterior image demonstrates contrast material opacifying segments of a nondilated left ureter; however, some of the contrast material has extravasated into a linear tract in the extraperitoneal space (*arrow*), confirming the presence of a ureteral leak. No contrast material was identified in the distal ureter, suggesting that the ureteral disruption was complete. The patient subsequently underwent surgical repair of the distal left ureter.

On CT, a specific diagnosis of ureteral injury can be established only when excretory-phase contrast-enhanced images are obtained and when extravasation of excreted contrast medium outside the ureter can be detected. If the ureter is opacified distal to the site of injury, a partial injury is most likely. Rarely, however, such opacification could be the result of vesicoureteral reflux from an opacified bladder in a patient with a complete disruption (with the opacification of the bladder due to normal excretion of contrast material into the contralateral renal collecting system, ureter, and then bladder). If the ureter is not opacified distally, a complete injury must be considered (Fig. 20.38); however, the significance of a nonopacified ureteral segment distal to the site of injury is also not necessarily definitive. This finding could also merely be due to peristalsis of an intact more distal ureter in a patient with a partial ureteral disruption. It has been suggested that such nonopacification can be suspected to be due to peristalsis in a partially, rather than a completely disrupted ureter, if there is only a small amount of extravasated periureteral contrast material adjacent to the injured ureter.

On occasion, active extravasation from the ureter may not be seen after a ureteral disruption, even when excretory-phase images are obtained (presumably, because the leak is intermittent or has healed). In these instances, periureteral fluid is still often present. Another finding that can be seen in patients who have had ureteral injuries is ipsilateral pelvocaliectasis. This dilatation, which likely results from scarring at the injury site, can be seen chronically but can sometimes even develop within a few days of the injury.

Imaging studies can be used to identify complications of ureteral injuries, when the diagnosis is not made promptly after the injury occurs. This includes chronic urinomas and fistulae (Fig. 20.39).

Partial ureteral injuries often can be managed successfully with interventional uroradiologic procedures. Some patients can be treated with percutaneous nephrostomy drainage alone or with nephrostomy combined with ureteral stenting. In many instances, nephrostomy and stent placement is required for long periods of time (often between 1 and 2 months). In comparison, complete ureteral injuries usually require open surgery, with ureteroureterostomies performed for proximal or mid ureteral injuries and distal ureteral injuries often treated with ureteral resection and reimplantation into the bladder.

BLADDER INJURIES

While injury of the bladder may occur as a result of blunt, penetrating, or iatrogenic trauma, the vast majority of bladder injuries are due to blunt trauma in patients who are involved in motor vehicle crashes. The susceptibility of the bladder to injury is felt to vary with its degree of filling at the time of the trauma; a collapsed or nearly empty bladder is less vulnerable to injury than is a distended bladder.

Clinical Features

Clinical signs of bladder injury are nonspecific. Suprapubic tenderness is usually present, as is hematuria. The urge to void may be absent or normal. In some forms of bladder rupture, the organ may still act as a reservoir; thus, a normal urge to void may be present.

Radiologic Examination

Retrograde cystography has been the traditional examination for the diagnosis of bladder rupture. Although it is preferably performed in a fluoroscopy suite, it can be performed with portable fluoroscopy equipment or merely by obtaining overhead portable radiographs when the clinical situation demands it. An attempt to instill at least 300 mL of dilute (30%) contrast medium should be made in order to achieve adequate bladder distention (Fig. 20.40); however, some patients with pelvic hematomas will tolerate substantially less

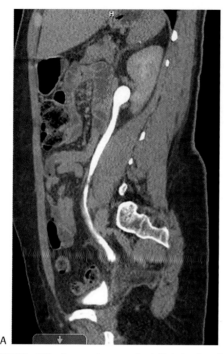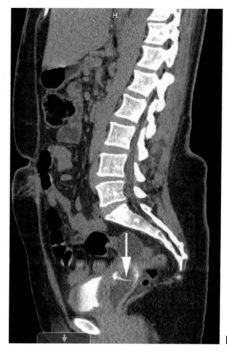

FIGURE 20.39. CT of a ureterovaginal fistula developing after ureteral injury during a hysterectomy. **A:** A contrast-enhanced excretory-phase sagittal CT image shows a dilated left ureter. **B:** A more medial image demonstrates opacification of a fistulous tract between the distal left ureter and the vagina (*arrow*). A small amount of contrast material also layers dependently in the vagina more posteriorly.

bladder distention before complaining of marked discomfort (due to compression of the filling bladder by a pelvic hematoma). Since the object is only to distend the bladder under pressure, smaller instilled volumes are sufficient under these circumstances. Contrast material instillation should, therefore, be titrated with the patient's symptoms. A patient who feels that his or her bladder is full after

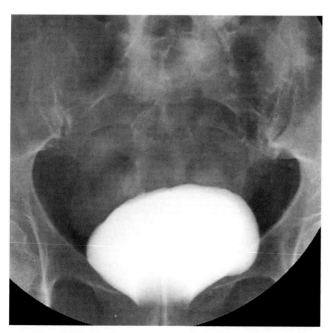

FIGURE 20.40. Normal conventional cystogram. An antero-posterior abdominal radiograph obtained after instillation of 350 mL of contrast material into the bladder via a Foley catheter fails to demonstrate any extravasation of contrast material. The patient did not have a bladder rupture.

instillation of <300 mL of contrast material should still have sufficient bladder distention to detect a bladder rupture.

Both scout and postdrainage radiographs are an essential component of the conventional trauma cystogram, the former to detect any preexisting radiopacities that might be confused for extravasated contrast material on subsequent radiographs and the latter to exclude the possibility that any extravasated contrast material was previously obscured by a full bladder. Some images should include the upper abdomen, as this coverage may be helpful in facilitating detection of intraperitoneal bladder rupture. When fluoroscopic equipment is not used, an initial radiograph after instillation of approximately 100 mL of contrast medium can be obtained to check for gross extravasation. If none is present, the remainder of the contrast medium can then be infused.

The accuracy of cystography for the diagnosis of bladder injury has been reported to be 85% to 100%. A false-negative cystogram is most likely to occur in patients who have suffered penetrating bladder injury, especially when caused by small caliber bullets. In such cases, it is assumed that the small bladder tear is sealed by a hematoma or by surrounding mesentery.

Since most trauma patients undergo a CT examination of the abdomen and pelvis, CT is now commonly used to evaluate the bladder for traumatic injury rather than cystography (Fig. 20.41); however, assessment of the bladder using CT performed with passive contrast filling only from excreted contrast media is not adequate to exclude bladder injury. Bladder ruptures can be missed if only this approach is utilized. Instead, as with conventional cystography, active filling of the bladder via a Foley catheter or a suprapubic tube is required. Such active bladder filling is referred to as a CT cystogram.

Performance of CT cystography should be considered in any patient who has sustained blunt trauma to the pelvis, when there is any amount of extraluminal pelvic fluid (either extraperitoneal or intraperitoneal). While bladder ruptures are more likely if pelvic fractures are present, they can also occur in the absence of pelvic bone injury. CT cystography should also be considered after penetrating trauma, if the mechanism of injury and/or clinical presentation is

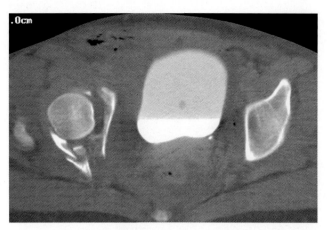

FIGURE 20.41. Normal CT cystogram. An axial CT image obtained after active instillation of 300 mL of dilute contrast material into the bladder via a Foley catheter fails to demonstrate any extravasation of contrast material. There is an extensive pelvic hematoma, subcutaneous gas, and a complex comminuted right acetabular fracture. The patient did not have a bladder rupture.

concerning for bladder injury. In comparison, a bladder rupture is exceedingly unlikely if no extraluminal fluid is identified in the pelvis on a CT examination that includes the abdomen and pelvis. Thus, conventional or CT cystography need not be performed in patients in whom no extraluminal pelvic fluid is present.

To perform CT cystography, the bladder is filled in a retrograde fashion with very dilute contrast media (3% to 5%) and contiguous images are acquired through the pelvis. An appropriate dilution of contrast media can be obtained by instilling 30 to 35 mL of 300 mg I/mL contrast material into a bag of 500 mL of normal saline. As with conventional cystography, instillation of at least 300 mL of dilute contrast material is preferred but should be titrated with the degree of patient discomfort. CT cystography performed in this fashion has an accuracy that is at least as high as that of conventional cystography.

Bladder Injury after Blunt Pelvic Trauma

The greatest risk factor for bladder injury in a blunt trauma patient is the presence of pelvic bone fracture. Still, only a minority of patients with pelvic fractures will have bladder injury, with the incidence estimated to be approximately 5% to 10%. Conversely, the vast majority (80% to 90%) of patients with bladder injuries will also have pelvic bone fractures.

The different types of bladder injuries include bladder contusions, interstitial bladder injuries, and bladder ruptures.

Bladder contusions occur when there is an incomplete tear of the bladder mucosa. This results in ecchymosis in a localized segment of the bladder wall. Bladder contusion is generally regarded as the most common form of traumatic bladder injury. Both fluoroscopic and CT cystography are normal in patients with bladder contusions. Thus, this diagnosis is one of exclusion and is considered likely in patients who have hematuria after pelvic trauma, but in whom no other cause of hematuria can be found. Cystoscopy is rarely performed for confirmation and no treatment is necessary.

Interstitial bladder injury occurs as a result of an incomplete tear of the serosal surface of the bladder. On fluoroscopic and CT cystography, an irregular mural defect in the bladder wall, representing the site of injury, can usually be identified; however, there is no extravasation of contrast medium from the bladder (Fig. 20.42). This injury is rare, with only a few confirmed cases having been reported. This injury heals spontaneously and no treatment is needed.

Bladder ruptures are the most important of the traumatic bladder injuries. They are divided into extraperitoneal, intraperitoneal,

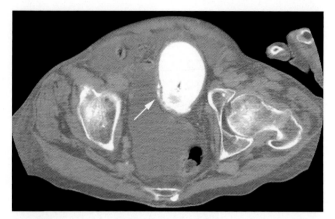

FIGURE 20.42. CT cystogram of an interstitial bladder injury. An axial CT image obtained through the pelvis during a CT cystogram demonstrates an irregular mural defect along the right lateral wall of the bladder (arrow); however, there is no leakage of instilled contrast material from the bladder lumen into either the intraperitoneal or extraperitoneal spaces.

and combined ruptures (with the latter having both extraperitoneal and intraperitoneal components).

Extraperitoneal Bladder Rupture

The most common type of bladder rupture, by far, is extraperitoneal bladder rupture. Extraperitoneal bladder ruptures are nearly always associated with one or more fractures of the pubic rami or diastasis of the symphysis pubis. Classically, the injury occurs when there is a laceration of the extraperitoneal portion of the bladder

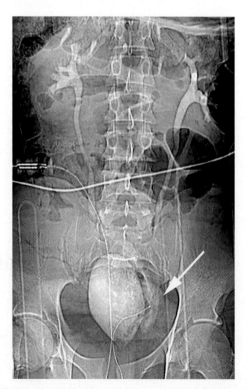

FIGURE 20.43. Abdominal radiograph of an extraperitoneal bladder rupture. A digital scout radiograph from a CT scan after injection of contrast material demonstrates an amorphous irregular collection of contrast material along the left lateral side of the bladder (arrow). The appearance is characteristic of an extraperitoneal bladder rupture.

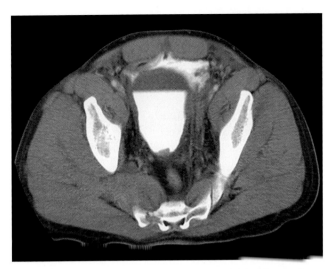

FIGURE 20.44. CT of an extraperitoneal bladder rupture. A contrast-enhanced excretory-phase axial CT image shows an amorphous collection of contrast material in the prevesical space, diagnostic of an extraperitoneal bladder rupture. Additional fluid, representing hematoma, is noted laterally in both the right and left hemipelvis.

wall by a bone spicule associated with the fracture. However, the site of extravasation can also be far removed from the site of pelvic fracture, suggesting that this injury can be caused by another mechanism. One such explanation is that bladder injury results when stress is applied to the hypogastric wings or to the puboprostatic ligaments, causing the bladder wall to tear. In still other cases, this may represent a contrecoup injury.

In extraperitoneal rupture, contrast media extravasation is limited to the pelvic extraperitoneal space. On both conventional and CT cystography, extraperitoneal contrast material generally has a "streaky" irregular appearance, as it invaginates into extraperitoneal fat (Figs. 20.43 and 20.44). Leakage of contrast material occurs characteristically along the lateral aspects of the bladder and/or into the extraperitoneal prevesical space (Fig. 20.45). As previously mentioned, if conventional cystography is to be performed, it is important to obtain postdrain radiographs, as some ruptures can be hidden by the distended bladder on radiographs obtained with the bladder distended (Fig. 20.46). On CT, the

extraperitoneal contrast material has been described as having "a molar tooth" configuration as it opacifies the extraperitoneal space adjacent to the lateral and anterior aspects of the bladder (Fig. 20.47). Occasionally, a fat–fluid level can rarely be detected in the ruptured bladder lumen. This has been speculated to be due to leakage of extravesical fat into the bladder lumen via the defect in the bladder wall.

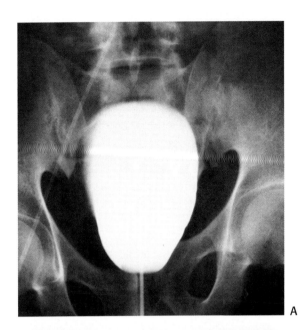

A

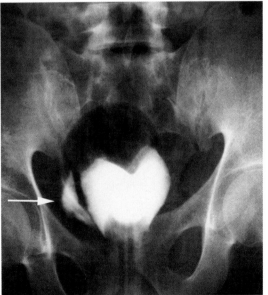

B

FIGURE 20.46. Conventional cystography of an extraperitoneal bladder rupture not seen on an anteroposterior image obtained after the bladder is filled. **A:** An abdominal radiograph obtained after active instillation of contrast material into the bladder shows the bladder to be well distended. No extraluminal contrast material is identified. **B:** A postdrain film obtained several minutes later demonstrates an irregular collection of contrast material along the right lateral aspect of the bladder (*arrow*), representing an extraperitoneal bladder rupture. This was previously obscured by contrast material in the distended bladder.

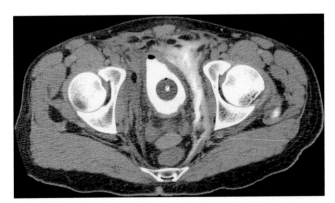

FIGURE 20.45. CT cystography of an extraperitoneal rupture. An axial image from a CT cystogram shows extraperitoneal contrast material extravasating into the extraperitoneal space in the left hemipelvis. A Foley catheter and small amount of gas are seen within the bladder.

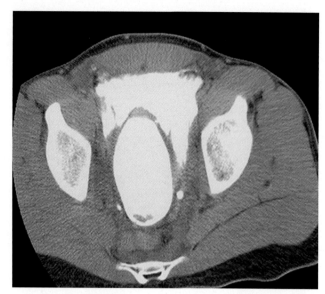

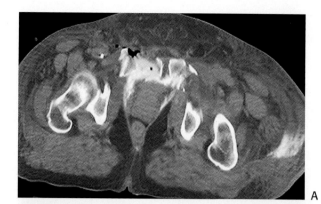

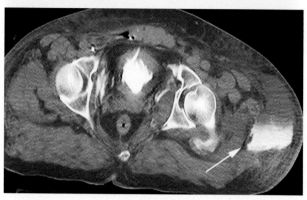

FIGURE 20.47. CT cystography of an extraperitoneal bladder rupture: the "molar tooth" sign. An axial image from a CT cystogram shows an amorphous extraperitoneal collection of contrast material anterior and lateral to the bladder. The configuration of the extravesical contrast material has been suggested to resemble a molar tooth.

In rare instances, extravasation can extend beyond the perivesical space and into the perineum, scrotum, penis, thigh, or pelvic soft tissues (Figs. 20.48 and 20.49), presumably as a result of traumatic disruption of the fascial boundaries of the pelvis, as well as of the bladder. Extravasation into the perineum can be present with a bladder injury alone, as a result of a urethral injury (see below) or as a result of a combination of both bladder and urethral injury.

FIGURE 20.49. CT cystography of an extraperitoneal bladder rupture with extension into overlying soft tissues. **A:** An axial CT image from a CT cystogram demonstrates an irregular collection of extravesical contrast material surrounding a disrupted symphysis pubis, consistent with an extraperitoneal bladder rupture. **B:** A more cephalad image shows that some contrast material has tracked into the soft tissues of the lateral portion of the pelvis (*arrow*).

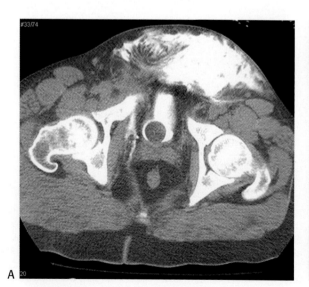

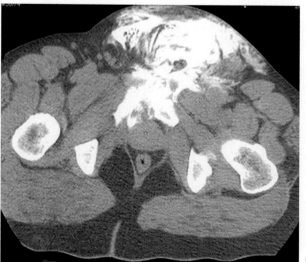

FIGURE 20.48. CT cystography of an extraperitoneal bladder rupture with extension into overlying soft tissues. **(A, B)** Axial CT images from a CT cystogram, in a patient with a large extraperitoneal bladder rupture, show a large amount of extraluminal contrast material having leaked outside of the bladder into the anterior pelvic wall.

Extraperitoneal bladder ruptures can usually be treated conservatively, with several weeks of indwelling Foley catheter drainage. Most of these ruptures will resolve within this time period. Surgery is generally reserved for patients with very large bladder disruptions or for patients who require operative repair of other abdominal or pelvic organ injuries.

Intraperitoneal Bladder Rupture

Intraperitoneal bladder ruptures account for approximately 15% to 25% of bladder injuries. They occur when there is a sudden increase in intravesical pressure as a result of a blow to the lower abdomen in patients who have a distended bladder. The weakest portion of the bladder wall, the dome, then ruptures. This is the only bladder surface that is in direct contact with the peritoneal surface. Intraperitoneal ruptures commonly occur due to sudden abdominal or pelvic compression by seat belts or steering wheels. In comparison to extraperitoneal bladder ruptures, many patients with intraperitoneal bladder ruptures do not have pelvic bone fractures.

On conventional or CT cystography, contrast material instilled into the bladder in patients with intraperitoneal bladder ruptures will opacify the peritoneal cavity, eventually outlining loops of bowel and extending into the paracolic gutters (Figs. 20.50 to 20.52). In comparison to the irregular appearance of extraperitoneal contrast material, intraperitoneal contrast material has a characteristic smooth configuration (Fig. 20.53). Sometimes, the liver

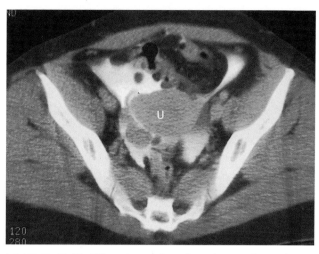

FIGURE 20.51. CT cystography of an intraperitoneal rupture. An axial image from a CT cystogram shows contrast material extravasated into the peritoneal cavity and outlining the uterus (U) and pelvic loops of bowel, clearly demonstrating its intraperitoneal location.

and the spleen will also be outlined by the extravasated contrast material (Fig. 20.54).

While moderate or large amounts of intraperitoneal fluid can be present, intraperitoneal bladder ruptures can result in only a small amount of fluid present in the cul-de-sac. Thus, this diagnosis can be overlooked if conventional or CT cystography is not performed (Fig. 20.55).

Intraperitoneal ruptures are treated surgically. This is because when urine extravasates into the peritoneal space, it is resorbed

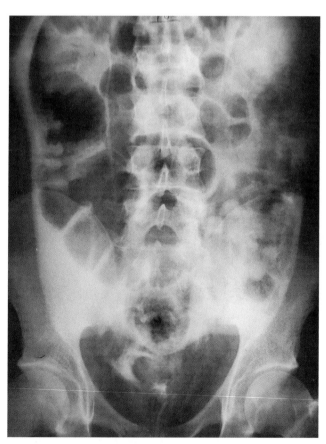

FIGURE 20.50. Conventional cystography of an intraperitoneal bladder rupture. An anteroposterior radiograph from a conventional cystogram shows that contrast media has leaked from the bladder into the peritoneal cavity. Extensive intraperitoneal contrast media is seen outlining multiple loops of bowel. The excreted contrast material in the renal collecting systems and ureters is from an earlier CT.

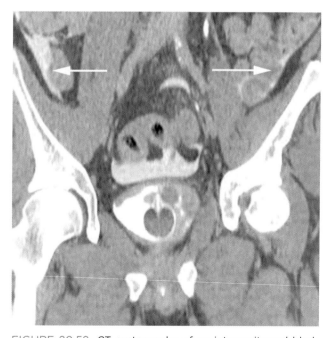

FIGURE 20.52. CT cystography of an intraperitoneal bladder rupture. A coronal reformatted image from a CT cystogram demonstrates that some of the contrast material instilled into the bladder has extravasated into the peritoneal cavity above the dome of the bladder and into both paracolic gutters (arrows).

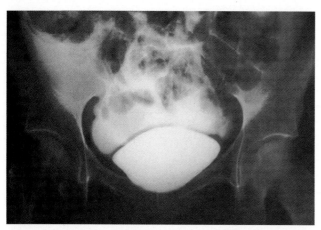

FIGURE 20.53. Conventional cystography of an intraperitoneal bladder rupture. An anteroposterior radiograph obtained during a conventional cystogram shows a large amount of contrast material opacifying the peritoneal cavity, outlining loops of bowel in the pelvis. The intraperitoneal contrast material has a smooth configuration.

through the peritoneum and electrolyte disturbances can result. Patients with intraperitoneal bladder ruptures can also develop chemical and/or infectious peritonitis.

Combined Bladder Rupture

Combined bladder rupture is a term used for the simultaneous presence of intraperitoneal and extraperitoneal bladder rupture.

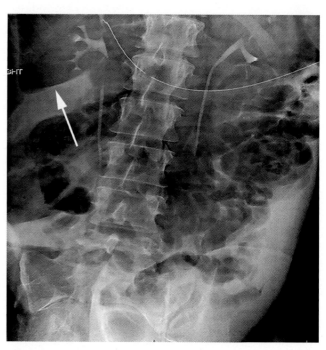

FIGURE 20.54. Conventional cystography of an intraperitoneal bladder rupture. An anteroposterior radiograph from a conventional cystogram shows that a large amount of contrast material has extravasated into the peritoneal cavity and outlines the edge of the liver (*arrow*).

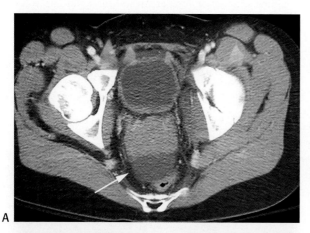

A

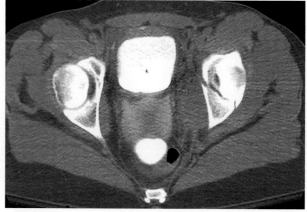

B

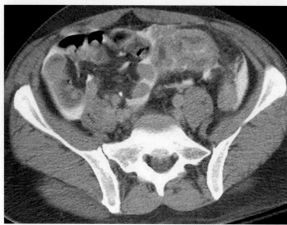

C

FIGURE 20.55. CT cystography of an intraperitoneal bladder rupture. **A:** A contrast-enhanced corticomedullary-phase axial CT image shows a small amount of fluid in the cul-de-sac (*arrow*). There is a fracture at the dome of the left acetabulum with an adjacent left pelvic sidewall hematoma. A CT cystogram **(B)** was subsequently performed, which confirms extravasation of contrast material into the cul-de-sac and **(C)** outlining loops of bowel.

This is the least common type of bladder rupture, accounting for only 5% to 10% of bladder ruptures. On conventional cystography, both types of extravasation may be demonstrated; however, in some cases, only one component is apparent. This can be problematic, as failure to detect an intraperitoneal component of a combined rupture can lead to inappropriate conservative management. On CT cystography, both components of the rupture are more easily detected; however, sometimes, it can be difficult to differentiate small intraperitoneal from extraperitoneal components.

Bladder Injury after Penetrating Trauma

Penetrating injury of the bladder may occur as a result of a bullet wound or as a result of impalement of the bladder by various objects. Penetrating bladder injury may result in intraperitoneal, extraperitoneal, or combined bladder ruptures.

Patients who have had penetrating trauma and in whom a bladder injury is suspected can be imaged with conventional or CT cystography. As is the case with renal injuries, the high association of injury to other visceral organs mandates surgical exploration in the majority of cases of penetrating bladder injury. In particular, vascular injuries are commonly associated with bladder injuries following gunshot wounds. In comparison, with knife wounds of the bladder, there is a high incidence of associated bowel injury.

Iatrogenic Bladder Injury

The bladder is the urinary tract organ most likely to be injured at surgery (usually during gynecologic procedures, but also after other operations). Obstetric bladder injury may result from laceration of the bladder during cesarean birth, injury secondary to trauma from obstetric forceps, or pressure necrosis of the bladder wall during labor. Transurethral urologic procedures, especially transurethral biopsy of bladder tumors, or, occasionally, complications of bladder repair or prostatectomy may also result in bladder injuries or leaks (Figs. 20.56 to 20.58). Injury of

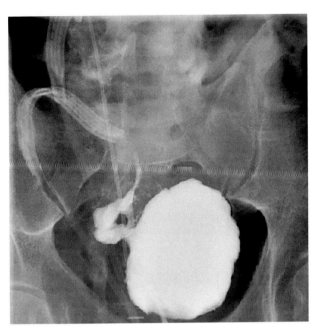

FIGURE 20.57. Conventional cystogram of a bladder leak following partial cystectomy. An anteroposterior radiograph obtained during a cystogram in a patient who has had a partial cystectomy for removal of a benign bladder mass demonstrates a linear tract of extraluminal contrast material along the right lateral aspect of the bladder, indicating a bladder leak. There are two right-sided surgical drains and a ureteral stent is in place.

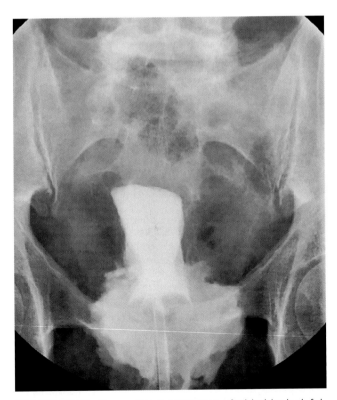

FIGURE 20.56. Conventional cystogram of a bladder leak following prostatectomy. An anteroposterior radiograph obtained following instillation of 250 mL of contrast material into the bladder shows a large amorphous collection of extraluminal contrast material contiguous with the bladder base, indicating a leak at the anastomosis between the bladder neck and the urethra. Most leaks after prostatectomy occur at this location.

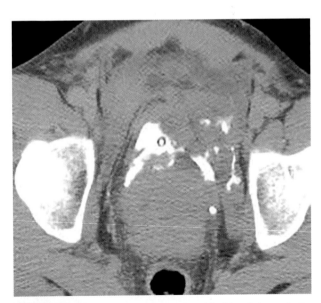

FIGURE 20.58. CT cystogram of a bladder injury during prostatectomy. An axial image from a CT cystogram shows a Foley catheter in the bladder in this patient who is status post recent prostatectomy. Some of the instilled contrast material is leaking into the extraperitoneal space.

the bladder may also occur in as the result of migration of surgically placed devices. Instruments that may damage the bladder include intrauterine contraceptive devices, Foley catheters, orthopedic hardware, surgical drains, and ventriculoperitoneal shunt catheters.

When bladder injuries are unrecognized, fistulae may develop to adjacent organs. This is more common to the vagina after hysterectomy, with the urine eventually tracking into and through the vaginal vault anastomosis. Vesicouterine fistulae rarely occur as a delayed complication of cesarean section.

Spontaneous Bladder Injury

Spontaneous bladder rupture refers to the extremely rare occurrence of a bladder rupture in the absence of any known antecedent trauma. In most cases, an underlying pathologic condition of the bladder is responsible. Such conditions include bladder tumors, inflammation, adjacent lesions that infiltrate the bladder, and bladder outlet obstruction.

The term idiopathic bladder rupture is used to refer to the occurrence of bladder rupture when there is no known trauma or known underlying or adjacent bladder pathology. Most of these cases occur in patients with alcoholism, and it is postulated that the bladder injury results from trauma that the patient is unable to recall.

URETHRAL INJURIES

Male Urethral Injuries

Blunt Urethral Injury

Urethral injuries following blunt trauma in men occur either in association with a pelvic fracture or as a result of a straddle injury. From 3% to 25% of blunt trauma patients with pelvic bone fractures have urethral injuries, with these injuries almost always involving the posterior urethra. Posterior urethral injuries are more commonly associated with unstable fractures of the pelvic ring. There is a correlation between the degree of severity of the urethral injury and the severity of the pelvic ring disruption. Conversely, severe pelvic fractures may sometimes result in no or relatively minor urethral injury, and, in some instances, severe urethral injury may occur with relatively minor pelvic fractures. In fact, posterior urethral rupture has rarely been reported without a pelvic fracture. In general, however, patients with urethral injury and pelvic fractures commonly also have other organ injuries, and have relatively high mortality rates, of 9% to 33%.

Urethral injury with pelvic fracture is associated with significant local morbidity including bulbomembranous urethral stricture, impotence, and urinary incontinence.

While the single most suggestive clinical sign of urethral injury is blood at the external urethral meatus, this finding may be absent. On rectal examination, there may be a high-riding prostate gland; but in young male patients, it is often difficult to distinguish the prostate from a pelvic hematoma. Blind urethral catheterization should be avoided in patients with suspected urethral injury, due to the risk of converting a less severe into a more severe injury. Thus, retrograde urethrography should be performed prior to attempted Foley catheter insertion in these patients.

Many trauma patients arrive in the radiology department with a Foley catheter already in place. The catheter may be correctly or malpositioned. On occasion, emergency department physicians or trauma surgeons may have concern about a urethral injury, even when a properly positioned Foley catheter has been inserted and may request a urethrogram. In these instances, the indwelling Foley should never be removed, since if a urethral injury is present, it is already being appropriately treated (with the catheter). Furthermore, if a urethral injury is present and a Foley catheter is removed for a retrograde urethrogram, one cannot be certain that a catheter will be subsequently reinserted safely after the procedure has been completed. In these cases, a pericatheter urethrogram can be attempted (see below).

Mechanism of Injury

The urogenital diaphragm (UGD) is attached to the medial surface of the inferior pubic rami. The prostate gland is attached to the pubis by the puboprostatic ligaments. As a result, pubic ramus fractures with separation or displacement of the symphysis pubis may result in disruption of the UGD and puboprostatic ligaments, causing proximal/cephalad displacement of the prostate gland.

The classically described urethral injury after blunt trauma is complete separation/disruption of the urethra at the junction of the prostatic and membranous urethra, produced by shearing at the time of injury. Less severe trauma may result in a partial urethral injury, producing a laceration in the urethra at this site, but not complete disruption. Although a membranous urethral tear is still described in the literature as the classic injury, retrograde urethrography has shown that urethral injuries most commonly extend into the proximal bulbous urethra, below, rather than at, the UGD, due to discontinuity of the UGD. Although the apex of the prostate intermingles with fibers of the external sphincter at the UGD, it is not firmly fixed. When injury occurs, the prostate can readily separate from the anterior urethra. The prostate moves superiorly, taking with it the prostatic urethra and portions of the membranous urethra.

A straddle injury usually occurs when a male patient falls astride a hard object such as the crossbar of a bicycle, a steel or wooden beam, or the edge of a manhole cover. Kicks to the perineum may also injure the bulbous urethra. The urethra and corpus spongiosum are compressed between the hard object and the inferior aspect of the pubis. This may result in urethral contusion with an intact urethra or partial or complete rupture of the bulbous urethra. Due to their anterior location, straddle injuries are not usually associated with pelvic fractures.

Radiologic Examination

In patients with suspected urethral injury, retrograde urethrography should be performed, as it remains the best study for determining the presence and nature of a urethral injury. A radiograph should be exposed during the active injection of 10 to 20 mL of contrast media, via a Foley catheter, with the tip inserted just beyond the urethral meatus, in the fossa navicularis. The Foley balloon is inflated gently so that the catheter will remain in place. Enough contrast material should then be hand injected slowly to ensure filling of the deep bulbar and prostatic portions of the urethra. It is desirable to ensure that at least some contrast material enters the bladder during urethrography, to exclude the possibility of a type II injury (which results in contrast extravasation above the UGD; see description of urethral injury types below).

Pericatheter urethrograms are performed by placing a small catheter (such as a pediatric nasogastric tube or a small-gauge Foley catheter without the balloon being inflated) alongside the indwelling Foley catheter, exerting pressure on the meatus (using a gloved hand or the patient's hand, if the patient is alert and able to cooperate). Contrast material is then slowly injected. These studies are often performed successfully; however, sometimes, sufficient pressure cannot be applied to allow for opacification of the urethra alongside the indwelling Foley catheter.

TABLE **20.2**		
Blunt Male Urethral Injury Imaging Classification System		

I—Posterior urethra intact, but stretched
II—Pure posterior injury with tear of membranous
  urethra above the UGD—partial or complete
III—Combined anteroposterior urethral injury with
  disruption of the UGD—partial or complete
IV—Bladder neck injury with extension into the
  urethra
IV(a)—Injury of the base of the bladder without
  extension into the urethra, but with periurethral
  extravasation, such that the appearance mimics a
  type IV urethral injury
V—Pure anterior urethral injury, including straddle
  injury—partial or complete

Classification of Male Urethral Injuries

An imaging classification of blunt posterior and anterior male ure-thral injuries, initially proposed by McCallum and Colapinto and modified by Sandler, has been widely used by radiologists for many years. This classification system categorizes urethral injuries into five types, which are discussed in detail in the paragraphs that fol-low and also summarized in Table 20.2:

Type I male urethral injuries result from rupture of the pubo-prostatic ligaments in the absence of any urethral disruption. A hematoma develops in the prostatic fossa, resulting in elevation of the bladder base, with resultant stretching of the intact posterior urethra (Figs. 20.59 and 20.60). True type I injuries are uncom-mon. Mere extrinsic compression of the posterior urethra by a periurethral hematoma without dislocation of the bladder should not be considered a type I injury.

With type II male urethral injuries, there is rupture of the pubo-prostatic ligaments AND disruption of the urethra above the UGD (Fig. 20.61). The UGD remains intact. This prevents extraurethral contrast material introduced during a retrograde urethrogram

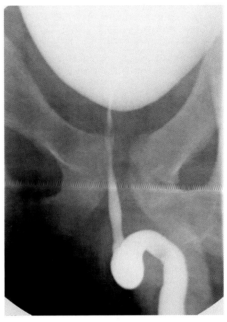

FIGURE 20.60. Retrograde urethrogram of a type I urethral injury. An anteroposterior spot radiograph obtained during a retrograde urethrogram shows the base of the bladder to be elevated, being displaced cephalad to the superior pubic rami. The prostatic urethra is elongated and the bladder base is slightly elevated, secondary to rupture of the puboprostatic ligaments.

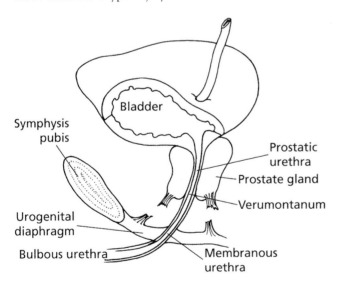

Type I

FIGURE 20.59. Diagram of a type I urethral injury. A draw-ing in the sagittal plane through the pelvis shows the mecha-nism of a type I urethral injury. The puboprostatic ligaments are ruptured, resulting in elevation of the prostate, including the prostatic urethra; however, the urethra remains intact.

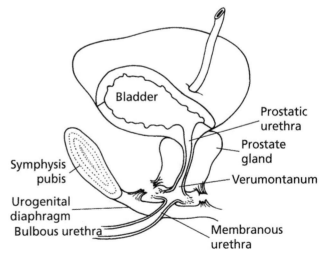

Type II

FIGURE 20.61. Diagram of a type II urethral injury. A draw-ing in the sagittal plane shows the mechanism of a type II urethral injury. The puboprostatic ligaments are ruptured and there is also disruption of the urethra above the level of the UGD. On retrograde urethrography, this would result in accumulation of extraurethral contrast material in the pelvis above, but not below, the UGD.

from extending below the pelvis (and into the perineum and scrotum). Instead, contrast material extravasates from the urethra into the extraperitoneal space in the pelvis. This injury is also relatively uncommon. Type II injuries can be complete, in which case contrast material instilled during a retrograde urethrogram does not opacify the bladder (Fig. 20.62), or partial, in which case the entire urethra is opacified and some contrast material can enter the bladder (Fig. 20.63). On occasion, a partial injury may appear to be complete, because contrast media instilled during a retrograde pyelogram fails to enter the bladder due to spasm or blood clot blocking an only partially disrupted urethra.

Type III male urethral injuries are the most common urethral injuries. With type III injuries, the puboprostatic ligaments are again disrupted; however, there is urethral rupture with extension of the urethral injury from the posterior urethra, through the UGD and into the proximal bulbous urethra (Fig. 20.64). Thus, these injuries are not true posterior urethral injuries. They are more accurately classified as combined anteroposterior urethral injuries. On retrograde urethrography, type III injuries result in contrast material extravasation below the UGD into the perineum and/or scrotum, with or without simultaneous extravasation into the extraperitoneal space in the pelvis. Because the degree of disruption of the UGD varies depending on the severity of the injury, the amount of contrast material extravasation into the perineum also varies. As long as some extravasation extends into the perineum and/or scrotum (which indicates that at least some disruption of the UGD is present), the injury should be classified as type III. As with type II injuries, type III injuries may be partial or complete (Figs. 20.65 and 20.66).

Type IV male urethral injuries are injuries of the urethra and adjacent bladder base (Fig. 20.67). This is in contrast to type IVa injuries where only the bladder base is disrupted. Thus, type IVa injuries are actually extraperitoneal bladder ruptures. Type IV and IVa injuries are considered together, because an imaging distinction between them is generally not possible. During retrograde urethrography, both result in the accumulation of extraurethral contrast material adjacent to the posterior urethra at the bladder base (Figs. 20.68 and 20.69).

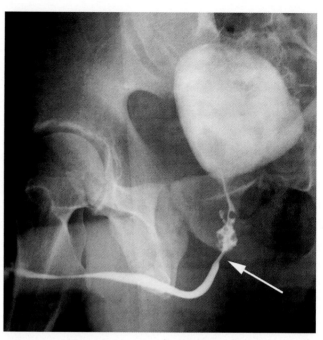

FIGURE 20.63. Retrograde urethrogram of a partial type II urethral injury. A pelvic radiograph obtained during a retrograde urethrogram with the patient in a right posterior oblique position demonstrates a small accumulation of extraurethral contrast material. The disruption is only partial, since some of the contrast material traverses the entire urethra and enters the bladder. This can be characterized as a type II injury, because all of the extraurethral contrast material is located above the UGD (with the UGD demarcated by the *arrow*).

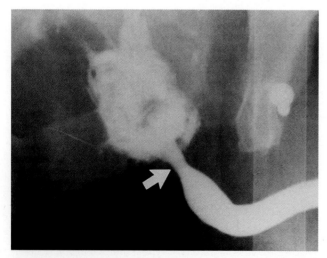

FIGURE 20.62. Retrograde urethrogram of a complete type II urethral injury. A left posterior oblique radiograph obtained during a retrograde urethrogram shows complete disruption of the urethra above the level of the UGD (*arrow*). There is no accumulation of contrast material in the scrotum. There is also no opacification of the bladder.

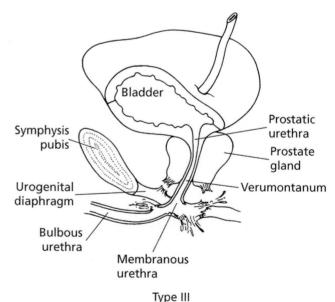

Type III

FIGURE 20.64. Diagram of a type III urethral injury. A drawing in the sagittal plane shows the mechanism of a type III urethral injury. The puboprostatic ligaments are ruptured. There is disruption of the urethra extending to and involving the UGD. On retrograde urethrography, this would result in accumulation of extraluminal contrast material in the scrotum, below the level of the UGD with or without extraluminal contrast material in the pelvis.

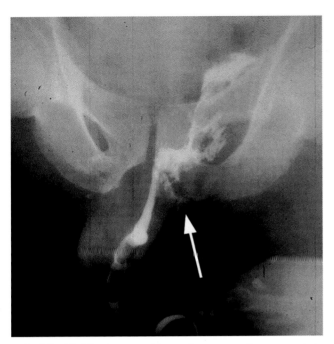

FIGURE 20.65. Retrograde urethrogram of a complete type III urethral injury. An anteroposterior pelvic radiograph obtained during a retrograde urethrogram shows a moderate amount of contrast material leaking from the urethra, both above and below (*arrow*) the UGD. The appearance is diagnostic of a type III urethral injury. There is no opacification of the prostatic urethra or bladder, suggesting that the urethral disruption is complete.

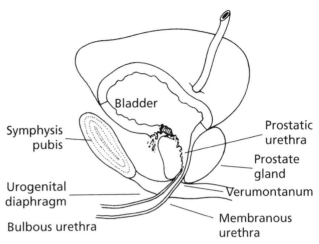

FIGURE 20.67. Diagram of a type IV urethral injury. A drawing in the sagittal plane shows the mechanism of a type IV urethral injury. There is partial or complete disruption of both the urethra and the bladder neck. On retrograde urethrography, this would result in accumulation of extraluminal contrast material adjacent to the bladder neck and the prostatic urethra.

Type V male urethral injuries are injuries to the anterior urethra, usually the bulbous urethra (Fig. 20.70). Most type V injuries are straddle injuries. With type V injuries, when retrograde urethrography is performed, there is extravasation of contrast material only outside of the anterior urethra (Fig. 20.71).

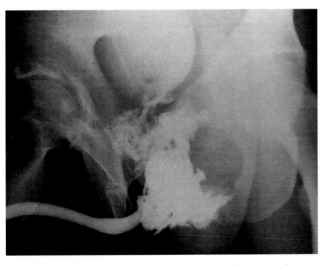

FIGURE 20.66. Retrograde urethrogram of a partial type III urethral injury. A pelvic radiograph obtained during a retrograde urethrogram with the patient in a right posterior oblique position demonstrates extensive extraurethral contrast material both above and below the UGD, characteristic of a type III injury. Some of the contrast material traverses the entire urethra and enters the bladder, indicating that this is a partial disruption.

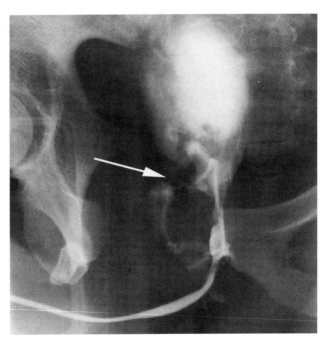

FIGURE 20.68. Retrograde urethrogram of a type IV urethral injury. An anteroposterior pelvic radiograph obtained during a retrograde urethrogram demonstrates contrast leakage from both the bladder neck and the prostatic urethra (*arrow*). There is also a wide diastasis of the symphysis pubis. The appearance is indistinguishable from a type IVa injury.

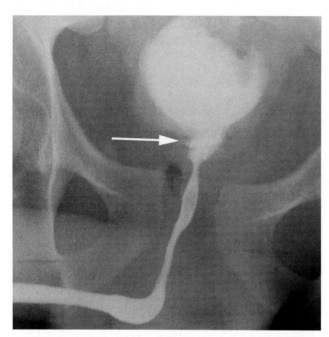

FIGURE 20.69. Retrograde urethrogram of a type IVa urethral injury. An anteroposterior radiograph from a retrograde urethrogram shows contrast material extravasation around the bladder neck and the prostatic urethra (*arrow*). There is also diastasis of the symphysis pubis. This patient was subsequently found to have only a bladder neck injury. The prostatic urethra was intact. The radiographic appearance is indistinguishable from a type IV injury.

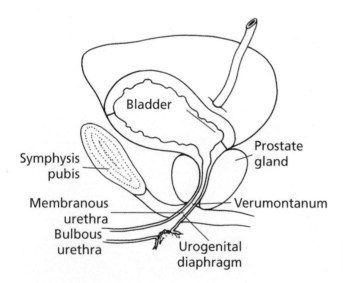

Type V

FIGURE 20.70. Diagram of a type V urethral injury. A drawing in the sagittal plane shows the mechanism of a type V urethral injury. There is disruption of the anterior, usually the bulbous, urethra. On retrograde urethrography, this would result in accumulation of extraluminal contrast material adjacent to the bulbocavernous urethra. As with other urethral injuries, type V injuries can be partial or complete.

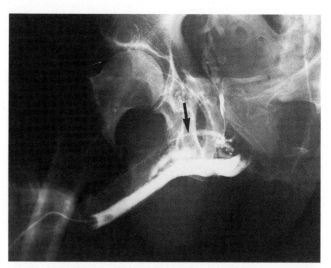

FIGURE 20.71. Retrograde urethrogram of a type V urethral injury. A right posterior oblique pelvic radiograph obtained during a retrograde urethrogram in a patient after a straddle injury demonstrates contrast leakage from the bulbar urethra. Some of the contrast material has also extravasated into the venous system, and the dorsal vein of the penis is opacified (*arrow*).

If Buck fascia is lacerated, contrast medium can extravasate into the scrotum (Fig. 20.72). Contrast media may also rarely extend into the anterior abdominal wall beneath Scarpa fascia, particularly if a large volume of contrast material has been injected for the urethrogram. As with type II and III urethral injuries, type V injuries may be partial or complete, with partial injuries being more common.

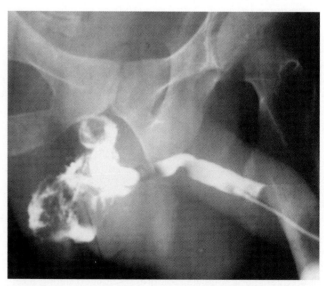

FIGURE 20.72. Retrograde urethrogram of a type V urethral injury. A left posterior oblique radiograph obtained during a retrograde urethrogram in a patient with a straddle injury demonstrates a complete urethral disruption. Contrast medium extravasates into the scrotum because of simultaneous rupture of Buck fascia.

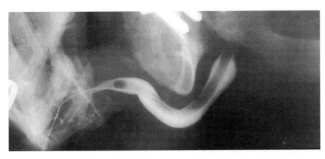

FIGURE 20.73. Normal pericatheter urethrogram. A right posterior oblique pelvic radiograph obtained during a pericatheter urethrogram fails to demonstrate any extravasation of contrast material outside of the urethra. The long tubular filling defect in the urethra represents the indwelling Foley catheter.

Pericatheter Urethrography

Occasionally, a patient in whom a Foley catheter has already been inserted (by emergency medical technicians or in the emergency department) may have a mechanism of trauma suggesting that a urethral injury is present. In these cases, the indwelling catheter should not be removed to assess the urethra's integrity. If an injury is present, it is already being treated appropriately by the inserted catheter. If the catheter is removed, it is possible that a partial disruption could be converted to a complete disruption during attempted catheter reinsertion. For this reason, pericatheter urethrograms should be performed. When successfully performed, these studies are often successful in excluding (Fig. 20.73) or confirming (Fig. 20.74) the presence of a urethral injury.

Clinical Management

Type I urethral injuries generally require no surgical intervention. The initial urethrogram showing an intact urethra is used to help

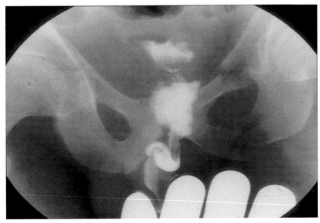

FIGURE 20.74. Pericatheter urethrogram of a type III urethral injury. An anteroposterior pelvic spot radiograph obtained during a pericatheter urethrogram shows that some of the instilled contrast material has extravasated outside of the urethra. The extraurethral contrast material extends into the perineum both above and below the UGD, confirming a type III urethral injury. The filling defect is the indwelling Foley catheter. There are fractures of the superior and inferior pubic rami.

to guide the subsequent careful insertion of a small, well-lubricated catheter into the bladder. The bladder can then be filled through this catheter and a cystogram performed to exclude bladder injury. If no extravasation occurs from the bladder, the catheter can be removed and the patient allowed to void at will. Repeat retrograde and voiding urethrogram in 3 months, if performed, should demonstrate resorption of the pelvic hematoma and return of the bladder and prostate to a normal position.

The prognosis for patients suffering complete type II and type III urethral injuries is much worse. These urethral disruption injuries, often with associated pelvic fractures, must be treated surgically. Open primary repair of a complete urethral injury has been performed in the past. This involves surgical intervention soon after the injury and has fallen out of favor, unless there are simultaneous bladder neck or rectal injuries.

The conventional treatment of complete urethral disruption is delayed repair. This approach involves the insertion of a suprapubic catheter for drainage at the time of the injury. Because there is no initial attempt at repair, a urethral stricture will subsequently develop in all patients. The suprapubic catheter is usually left in place for approximately 3 months, after which time the urethra will be repaired by a one- or two-stage urethroplasty. This delayed method of repair has been favored, because immediate surgery is so difficult. At the time of the injury, there is often associated soft tissue injury and a large hematoma, and the urethral fragments may be distracted. After 3 months, many of the acute soft tissue abnormalities will have resolved. Delayed repair is associated with lower incidences of incontinence and impotence compared with immediate primary repair (up to 12% and 2%, respectively for delayed, rather than 25% and 40% for patients for immediate surgery).

If a delayed repair of a complete type II or type III urethral disruption is to be performed, a retrograde urethrogram may be obtained immediately before the urethroplasty. For this study, the bladder is filled through the suprapubic cystostomy tube and a retrograde urethrogram is performed at the same time. The patient is then asked to attempt to void. Such an examination can outline the full length of the strictured urethral segment, provided that the patient is able to open the bladder neck when attempting to void (Fig. 20.75). Rarely, the bladder neck does not open because the bladder capacity is small, and the bladder neck has not opened for 3 months because of the suprapubic drainage. In this instance, the suprapubic catheter can be clamped for 6 to 8 hours to increase the bladder capacity before attempting a second voiding study.

Partial type II and type III urethral ruptures have lower long-term morbidity than do complete ruptures, thus further demonstrating the importance of accurate radiologic diagnosis by retrograde urethrography at the time of the trauma. Patients with partial type II and type III urethral injuries can be treated with an indwelling catheter.

Type IV injuries need careful clinical assessment, because of the potential for injury of the internal urethral sphincter (at the bladder neck). Because the internal urethral sphincter is the primary continence sphincter, such injuries, if unrecognized, may lead to incontinence and/or bladder neck stricture.

Type V injuries usually result in a focal stricture in the proximal third of the bulbous urethra. With minor straddle injuries, if the retrograde urethrogram shows an intact urethra, the patient can be allowed to void normally, with no treatment needed. If the urethra is compressed or distorted by hematoma, but intact, and there is no extravasation, a small, well-lubricated catheter may be carefully inserted into the bladder and left for a few days.

In more severe straddle injuries, retrograde urethrography generally shows a complete or partial rupture. A complete rupture should be treated acutely by suprapubic tube placement and will

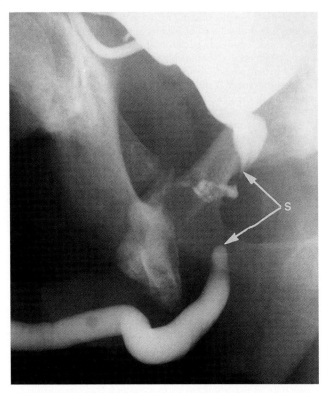

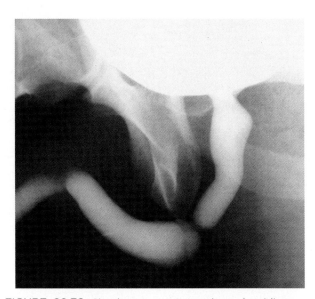

FIGURE 20.76. Simultaneous retrograde and voiding cystourethrogram after type V urethral injury. A dynamic retrograde and voiding cystourethrogram (performed through a suprapubic tube) was obtained 3 months after partial urethral rupture from straddle injury. The short length of the resultant high-grade well-defined fibrotic stricture is easily determined.

FIGURE 20.75. Simultaneous retrograde and voiding cystourethrogram 3 months after a type III urethral injury. A right posterior oblique radiograph is obtained after simultaneous instillation of contrast material through a suprapubic tube and a retrograde urethral catheter with the patient asked to attempt to void. The bladder neck is open, and the proximal prostatic urethra is filled. A small amount of extravasation has occurred, indicating persistent urethral disruption. The concomitant injections allow for the resultant urethral stricture length to be estimated. Hard fibrous scarring has developed along the occluded portion of the urethra (S).

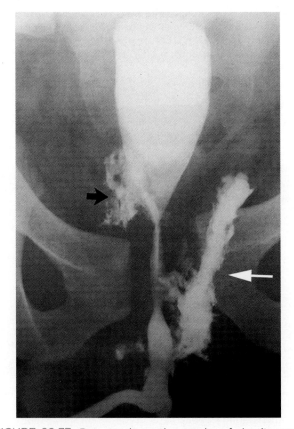

always result in a stricture. If a partial rupture is present, attempted catheterization may complete the rupture. So suprapubic cystostomy tube insertion is also recommended by many for treatment of partial type V injuries. Although small partial ruptures may heal without stricture, many will result in short, focal strictures (Fig. 20.76), some of which may be amenable to endoscopic management. Scarring does not extend to the membranous urethra. Complete and some partial ruptures (when severe) in the bulbous urethra will require urethroplasty.

Simultaneous Bladder and Urethral Injuries

Up to 20% of male patients with urethral injuries due to blunt trauma also have bladder injuries. Occasionally, the bladder injury may be shown on the retrograde urethrogram (Fig. 20.77); however, this is often not the case. Thus, conventional fluoroscopic or CT cystography should be performed after retrograde urethrography, either via a carefully inserted Foley catheter in a patient without a complete urethral disruption or via a suprapubic tube. In those instances in which an open primary repair is attempted for partial or complete type II or type III injuries in the absence of cystography,

FIGURE 20.77. Retrograde urethrography of simultaneous urethral and bladder ruptures. An anteroposterior radiograph from a retrograde urethrogram demonstrates a partial type III urethral injury (*white arrow*) as well as an extraperitoneal bladder rupture (*black arrow*). Note is also made of a diastasis of the symphysis pubis.

the bladder must be carefully inspected at the time of surgery to exclude a simultaneous bladder tear.

Penetrating Urethral Injuries

Penetrating injuries usually result from gunshot or knife wounds. They most commonly affect the anterior rather than the posterior urethra. They generally require immediate surgical exploration and antibiotic therapy to contain superimposed infection. Gunshot wounds may deform (Fig. 20.78) or even destroy portions of the urethra. Patch or pedicle grafting may be necessary, performed surgically as a one-stage urethroplasty or as the first stage of a two-stage procedure. Knife wounds may result in focal lacerations or focal disruptions of the anterior urethra. Such injuries can generally be treated by anastomosis of the injured segment of bulbous urethra. On rare occasions, the urethra may be injured as a result of foreign body insertion (Fig. 20.79).

Iatrogenic Urethral Injuries

Iatrogenic urethral injuries can occur during instrumentation, most commonly Foley catheter insertion, but also during cystoscopy. Injuries during attempted Foley catheter insertion may become apparent because the involved health care worker experiences difficulty when advancing the Foley. Urethral disruption sometimes occurs as a result of Foley catheter balloon inflation in the urethra.

Problems in Foley catheter insertion are more common when the health care worker is inexperienced. Since Foley catheters are often placed by nurses and junior house officers, it is essential that these health care providers receive sufficient training so

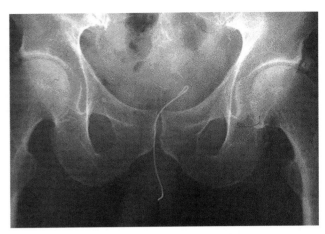

FIGURE 20.79. Pelvic radiograph of a foreign body urethral injury. An anteroposterior radiograph of the pelvis shows a long thin metallic structure in the region of the urethra, one end of which appears to extend into the bladder. This represents the metallic wire in a pipe cleaner self-inserted in an unsuccessful attempt to treat urinary difficulty.

that the procedure can be performed correctly. Effective training has been demonstrated to reduce the frequency of urethral injuries.

When an iatrogenic urethral injury occurs, the affected patient almost always complains of penile or perineal pain. Hematuria is usually present. Fortunately, most such injuries are only contusions and resolve without untoward sequelae; however, occasional patients will develop long-term complications, usually urethral stricture disease. Imaging studies (most often retrograde urethrography or CT) will demonstrate the incorrect positioning of the catheter (Fig. 20.80).

Female Urethral Injuries

Traumatic rupture of the female urethra is rare. It is usually the result of instrumentation, vaginal operation, or obstetric complications. Approximately 1% of urethral injuries in women are caused by pelvic fractures. Most reported cases have occurred in girls or young women. The rarity of this lesion is likely due to the short length of the urethra and to its mobility, because the female urethra is only loosely fixed by the UGD. In patients with pelvic fractures, rupture of the female urethra should be suspected when deep vaginal lacerations are also present or when there is inability to void or to pass a Foley catheter. The urethra may be avulsed at or within 2 cm of the bladder neck. As with male injuries, female urethral ruptures may be partial or complete.

Diagnosis of urethral injury in women is generally established endoscopically. In rare instances, voiding cystourethrography can be performed (with the bladder opacified via a suprapubic tube). Retrograde urethrography is rarely, if ever, performed in women. In the past, these studies had been performed for nontraumatic indications with special double-balloon catheters. Double-balloon female retrograde urethrography was technically difficult to perform and often very uncomfortable for the patient. This procedure has largely been abandoned.

Partial disruptions and contusions of the female urethra can be treated by stenting the urethra with a catheter. If there is a complete disruption, primary repair is recommended. Complete avulsion at the bladder neck requires a suprapubic surgical approach with anastomosis of the separated urethral ends. More distal complete

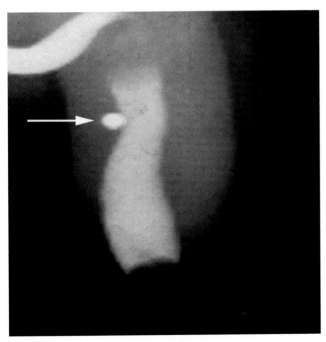

FIGURE 20.78. Retrograde urethrography in a patient who is status post gunshot wound. A spot radiograph obtained during a retrograde urethrogram in a patient who was accidentally shot with a BB gun demonstrates the metallic BB immediately adjacent to and deforming the anterior urethra (arrow). There is no extravasation of contrast material outside the urethra, demonstrating an intact urethra.

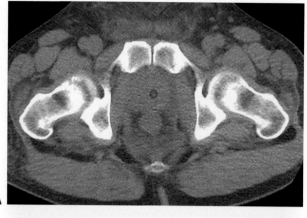

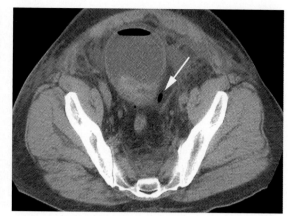

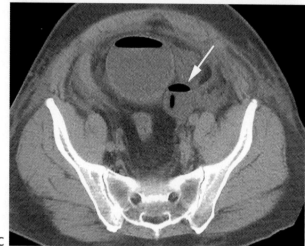

FIGURE 20.80. CT of a malpositioned Foley catheter. **A:** An unenhanced axial CT image shows a portion of the shaft of a Foley catheter in the prostatic urethra. **B:** A more cephalic image demonstrates a portion of the air-filled catheter posterolateral to the bladder rather than within the bladder lumen (*arrow*). **C:** An even more cephalic image shows that the inflated balloon of the Foley catheter (*arrow*) lies outside the bladder lumen.

urethral rupture is often approached transvaginally, with an end-to-end urethral anastomosis performed over a catheter used to stent the urethra. Delayed urethral repair is not advised, as patients with delayed surgery have a higher incidence of strictures and fistulae.

PENILE INJURIES

Rupture of the corpus cavernosum is an uncommon injury that generally occurs during strenuous sexual activity when the erect penis is forcibly bent. This injury is often referred to as a penile fracture. With penile fractures, the patient experiences intense pain and the penis becomes deformed and ecchymotic. During erection, the urethra is stretched and more vulnerable to injury, so the urethra can also be affected when the corpora cavernosum is disrupted.

Concomitant Urethral Rupture and Penile Fracture

Urethral injury, which occurs in 10% to 30% of patients with penile fracture, should be suspected in patients with penile fractures when gross hematuria is present, when blood is seen at the urethral meatus, or when the patient is unable to void. Retrograde urethrography is effective in excluding or diagnosing urethral injury in patients with penile fractures (Fig. 20.81). Urethral injuries can also be identified during flexible cystoscopy.

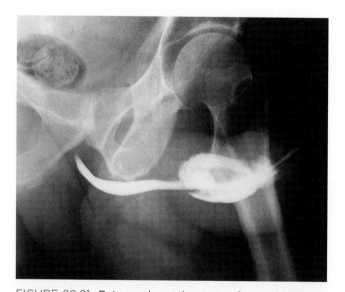

FIGURE 20.81. Retrograde urethrogram of a urethral injury in a patient with a penile fracture. A left posterior oblique radiograph obtained during a retrograde urethrogram demonstrates extensive extravasation of contrast material from the penile urethra, which was located adjacent to the site of an associated injury of the corpus cavernosum.

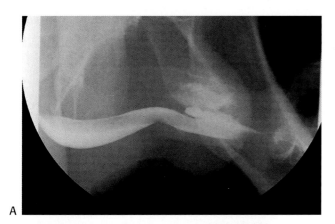

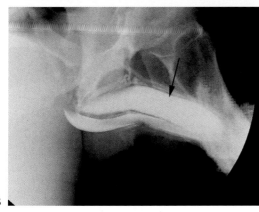

FIGURE 20.82. Retrograde urethrogram of a traumatic urethrocavernous fistula following penile fracture. **A:** An oblique radiograph obtained during a pericatheter urethrogram shows a small amount of contrast material extravasating from the urethra into the more cephalically located corpora cavernosa. **B:** An image obtained after additional contrast material was injected showing increased opacification of the corpora cavernosa (*arrow*). Additional tubular structures are opacified penile veins.

Cavernosography has also been used for preoperative evaluation of patients with known or suspected penile fractures. Since patients with fractures of the erect penis have tears in the tunica albuginea, cavernosography may demonstrate the exact site and the extent of the tear. This may be useful, as the site of a tunica albuginea tear may not be obvious at operation. Urethrocavernous fistulae may also occur in patients with a fractured penis. These fistulae can be demonstrated on urethrography and cavernosography (Fig. 20.82).

Prompt surgical repair of a corporal tear is generally recommended, as this reduces the likelihood that the posttraumatic complications of impotence and penile curvature will be encountered. Blood clot evacuation can be performed at the time of surgery.

SUGGESTED READINGS

General

Eisenstat RS, Whitford AC, Lane MJ, et al. The flat cava sign revisited what is its significance in patients without trauma. *AJR Am J Roentgenol.* 2002;17:21–25.

Hewitt JJ, Free KS, Sheafor DH, et al. The spectrum of abdominal venous CT findings in blunt trauma. *AJR Am J Roentgenol.* 2001;176:955–958.

Holly BP, Steenburg SC. Multidetector CT of blunt traumatic venous injuries in the chest, abdomen, and pelvis. *Radiographics.* 2011;31:1415–1424.

Lubner M, Menias C, Rucker C, et al. Blood in the belly CT findings of hemoperitoneum. *Radiographics.* 2007;27:109–125.

Nunes LW, Simmons S, Kinback R, et al. Diagnostic performance of trauma US in identifying abdominal or pelvic free fluid and serious abdominal or pelvic injury. *Acad Radiol.* 2001;8:128–136.

Sirlin CB, Brown MA, Andrade-Barreto OA, et al. Blunt abdominal trauma clinical value of negative screening US scans. *Radiology.* 2004;230:661–668.

Stuhlfaut JW, Soto JA, Lucey BC, et al. Blunt abdominal trauma performance of CT without oral contrast material. *Radiology.* 2004;233:689–694.

Yao DC, Jeffrey RB, Mirvis SE, et al. Using contrasted-enhanced helical CT to visualize arterial extravasation after blunt abdominal trauma incidence and organ distribution. *AJR Am J Roentgenol.* 2002;178:17–20.

Renal Injuries

Amerstorfer EE, Haberlik A, Riccabona M. Imaging assessment of renal injuries in children and adolescents: CT or ultrasound? *J Pediatr Surg.* 2015;50:448–455.

Breen KJ, Sweeney P, Nicholson PJ, et al. Adult blunt renal trauma: routine follow-up imaging is excessive. *Urology.* 2014;84:62–67.

Dahlstrom K, Dunoski B, Zerin JM. Blunt renal trauma in children with pre-existing renal abnormalities. *Pediatr Radiol.* 2015;45:118–123.

Fischer W, Wanaselja A, Steenburg SD. Incidence of urinary leak and diagnostic yield of excretory phase CT in the setting of renal trauma. *AJR Am J Roentgenol.* 2015;204:1168–1173.

Gross JA, Lehnert BE, Linnau KF, et al. Imaging of urinary system trauma. *Radiol Clin North Am.* 2015;53:773–788.

Harris AC, Zwirewich CV, Lyburn ID, et al. CT findings in blunt renal trauma. *Radiographics.* 2001;21:S201–S214.

Hass CA, Dinchman KH, Nasrallah PF, et al. Traumatic renal artery occlusion: a 15-year review. *J Trauma.* 1998;45(3):557–561.

Heller MT, Schnor N. MDCT of renal trauma: correlation to AAST organ injury scale. *Clin Imaging.* 2014;38:410–417.

Kawashima A, Sandler CM, Corl FM, et al. Imaging of renal trauma: a comprehensive review. *Radiographics.* 2001;21:557–574.

McPhee M, Arumainayagam N, Clark M, et al. Renal injury management in an urban trauma centre and implications for urologic training. *Ann R Coll Surg Engl.* 2015;97:194–197.

Miller KS, McAninch JW. Radiologic assessment of renal trauma: our 15-year experience. *J Urol.* 1995;154:352–355.

Navsaria PH, Nicol AJ, Edu S, et al. Selective nonoperative management in 1106 patients with abdominal gunshot wounds: conclusions on safety, efficacy, and the role of selective CT imaging in a prospective single-center study. *Ann Surg.* 2015;261:760–764.

Park SJ, Kim JK, Kim KW, et al. MDCT findings of renal trauma. *AJR Am J Roentgenol.* 2006;187:541–547.

Patel DP, Redshaw JD, Breyer BN, et al. High-grade renal injuries are often isolated in sports-related trauma. *Injury.* 2015;46:1245–1249.

Rhyner P, Federle MP, Jeffrey RB. CT of trauma to the abnormal kidney. *AJR Am J Roentgenol.* 1984;142:747.

Sandler CM, Toombs BD. Computed tomographic evaluation of blunt renal injuries. *Radiology.* 1981;141:461–466.

Serafetinides E, Kitrey ND, Djakovic N, et al. Review of current management of upper urinary tract injuries by the EAU trauma guidelines panel. *Eur Radiol.* 2015;67:930–936.

Ureteropelvic Junction and Ureteral Injuries

Boone TB, Gilling PJ, Husmann DA. Ureteropelvic junction disruption following blunt abdominal trauma. *J Urol.* 1993;150(1):33–36.

Gross JA, Lehnert BE, Linnau KF, et al. Imaging of urinary system trauma. *Radiol Clin North Am.* 2015;53:773–788.

Patel BN, Gayer G. Imaging of iatrogenic complications of the urinary tract: kidneys, ureters, and bladder. *Radiol Clin North Am.* 2014;52:1101–1116.

Bladder Injuries

Avey G, Blackmore CC, Wessells H, et al. Radiographic and clinical predictors of bladder rupture in blunt trauma patients with pelvic fracture. *Acad Radiol.* 2006;13:573–579.

Chan DPN, Abujudeh HH, Cushing GL, et al. CT cystography with multiplanar reformation for suspected bladder rupture experience in 234 cases. *AJR Am J Roentgenol.* 2006;187:1296–1302.

Martinez-Moya M, Dominguez-Perez AD. Letter: fat-fluid intravesical level: a new sign of bladder rupture. *AJR Am J Roentgenol.* 2011;197:W373–W374.

Morgan DE, Nallamala LK, Kenney PJ, et al. CT cystography: radiographic and clinical predictors of bladder rupture. *AJR Am J Roentgenol.* 2000;174:89–95.

Pao DM, Ellis JH, Cohan RH, et al. Utility of routine trauma CT in the detection of bladder rupture. *Acad Radiol.* 2000;7:317–324.

Patel BN, Gayer G. Imaging of iatrogenic complications of the urinary tract: kidneys, ureters, and bladder. *Radiol Clin North Am.* 2014;52:1101–1116.

Sandler CM, Hall JT, Rodriguez MB, et al. Bladder injury in blunt pelvic trauma. *Radiology.* 1986;158:633–638.

Sandler CM, Phillips JM, Harris JD, et al. Radiology of the bladder and urethra in blunt pelvic trauma. *Radiol Clin North Am.* 1981;19(1):195–211.

Urethral Injuries

Gomez RG, Mundy T, Dubey D, et al. SIU/ICUD consultation on urethral strictures: pelvic fracture urethral injuries. *Urology.* 2014;83(suppl 3a):S48–S58.

Goldman SM, Sandler CM, Corriere JN Jr, et al. Blunt urethral trauma: a unified, anatomical–mechanical classification. *J Urol.* 1997;157:85–89.

Ingram MD, Watson SG, Skippage PL, et al. Urethral injuries after pelvic trauma: evaluation with urethrography. *Radiographics.* 2008;28:1631–1643.

Johnsen NV, Dmochowski RR, Mock S, et al. Primary endoscopic realignment of urethral disruption injuries—a double-edged sword. *J Urol.* 2015;194:1022–1026.

Kashefi C, Messer K, Barden R, et al. Incidence and prevention of iatrogenic urethral injuries. *J Urol.* 2008;179:2254–2258.

Kommu SS, Illahi I, Mumtaz F. Patterns of urethral injury and immediate management. *Curr Opin Urol.* 2007;17:383–389.

Latini JM, McAninch JW, Brandes SB, et al. SIU/ICUD consultation on urethral strictures: epidemiology, etiology, anatomy, and nomenclature of urethral stenosis, strictures, and pelvic fracture urethral disruption injuries. *Urology.* 2014;83(suppl 3a):S1–S7.

Lumen N, Kuehhas FE, Djakovic N, et al. Review of the current management of lower urinary tract injuries by the EAU trauma guidelines panel. *Eur Urol.* 2015;67:925–929.

Sandler CM, Goldman SM, Kawashima A. Lower urinary trauma. *World J Urol.* 1998;16:69–75.

Penile Injuries

Pariser JJ, Pearce SM, Patel SG, et al. National patterns of urethral evaluation and risk factors for urethral injury in patients with penile fracture. *Urology.* 2015;86:181–186.

Wani I. Management of penile fracture. *Oman Med J.* 2008;23:162–165.

Index

Note: Page numbers followed by *f* and *t* indicate figures and tables, respectively.